VOLUME I

THIRD EDITION

CLINICAL UROGRAPHY

An Atlas and Textbook of Roentgenologic Diagnosis

JOHN L. EMMETT, M.D., M.S. (Urology)
Emeritus Consultant, Section of Urology, Mayo Clinic;
Emeritus Professor of Urology, Mayo Graduate School of
Medicine (University of Minnesota); Rochester, Minnesota.

DAVID M. WITTEN, M.D., M.S. (Radiology)
Formerly Consultant, Section of Diagnostic Roentgenology,
Mayo Clinic; Assistant Professor of Radiology, Mayo Graduate
School of Medicine (University of Minnesota); Rochester, Minnesota.

W. B. SAUNDERS COMPANY
Philadelphia • London • Toronto • 1971

W. B. Saunders Company: West Washington Square
                          Philadelphia, Pa.

                          12 Dyott Street
                          London, WC1A   1DB

                          1835 Yonge Street
                          Toronto 7, Ontario

Vol. I   SBN 0-7216-3377-3

CLINICAL UROGRAPHY

Print No.   9   8   7   6   5   4   3   2   1

CONTRIBUTORS

HAROLD W. CALHOON, M.D.
Tulsa, Oklahoma; formerly Resident in Urology, Mayo Graduate School of Medicine (University of Minnesota), Rochester, Minnesota.

J. CRAIG CLARK, M.D.
Methodist Hospital, Philadelphia, Pennsylvania.

JAMES H. DeWEERD, M.D., M.S. (Urology), F.A.C.S.
Department of Urology, Mayo Clinic; Professor of Urology, Mayo Graduate School of Medicine (University of Minnesota), Rochester, Minnesota.

LAWRENCE G. FEHRENBAKER, M.D.
Resident in Urology, Mayo Graduate School of Medicine (University of Minnesota), Rochester, Minnesota.

ELWIN E. FRALEY, M.D.
Professor of Surgery and Chairman, Division of Urology, University of Minnesota School of Medicine, Minneapolis, Minnesota.

WILLIAM L. FURLOW, M.D., M.S. (Urology)
Department of Urology, Mayo Clinic, Rochester, Minnesota.

LAURENCE F. GREENE, M.D., PH.D. (Urology)
Department of Urology, Mayo Clinic; Professor of Urology, Mayo Graduate School of Medicine (University of Minnesota), Rochester, Minnesota.

KAMAL A. HANASH, M.D.
Resident in Urology, Mayo Graduate School of Medicine (University of Minnesota), Rochester, Minnesota.

GLEN W. HARTMAN, M.D.
Department of Diagnostic Radiology, Mayo Clinic; Instructor in Urology, Mayo Graduate School of Medicine (University of Minnesota), Rochester, Minnesota.

JAMES C. HUNT, M.D., F.A.C.P.
Chairman, Division of Nephrology, Mayo Clinic; Associate Professor of Clinical Medicine, Mayo Graduate School of Medicine (University of Minnesota), Rochester, Minnesota.

PANAYOTIS P. KELALIS, M.D., M.S. (Urology), F.A.C.S.
Department of Urology, Mayo Clinic; Assistant Professor of Urology, Mayo Graduate School of Medicine (University of Minnesota), Rochester, Minnesota.

OWINGS W. KINCAID, M.D., M.S. (Radiology)
Department of Diagnostic Radiology, Mayo Clinic; Associate Professor of Radiology, Mayo Graduate School of Medicine (University of Minnesota), Rochester, Minnesota.

FRANK J. LEARY, M.D., M.S.
Department of Urology, Mayo Clinic; Instructor in Urology, Mayo Graduate School of Medicine (University of Minnesota), Rochester, Minnesota.

STANLEY R. LEVINE, M.D., F.A.C.S.
Attending Urologist, Highland Park Hospital, Highland Park, Illinois; Lake Forest Hospital, Lake Forest, Illinois; Consultant in Urology, Spinal Cord Injury Center, Hines Veterans Administration Hospital, Hines, Illinois; formerly Resident in Urology, Mayo Graduate School of Medicine (University of Minnesota), Rochester, Minnesota.

REZA S. MALEK, M.B., B.S. (Lond.)
Resident in Urology, Mayo Graduate School

of Medicine (University of Minnesota), Rochester, Minnesota; formerly Senior House Officer, St. Thomas' Hospital, London University, London, England.

VICTOR F. MARSHALL, M.D., F.A.C.S.
Professor of Surgery (Urology), Cornell University Medical College; Attending Surgeon in Charge (Urology), James Buchanan Brady Foundation of the New York Hospital; Associate Attending Surgeon, The Memorial Center for Cancer, New York, New York.

W. EUGENE MILLER, M.D., M.S. (Radiology)
Department of Diagnostic Radiology, Mayo Clinic; Instructor in Radiology, Mayo Graduate School of Medicine (University of Minnesota), Rochester, Minnesota.

GEORGE H. MYERS, JR., M.D.
Staff Urologist and Senior Investigator, Surgery Branch—National Cancer Institute, National Institutes of Health, Bethesda, Maryland; formerly Resident and Associate Consultant, Mayo Graduate School of Medicine (University of Minnesota), Rochester, Minnesota.

DENIS C. O'SULLIVAN, M.B., B.Ch., F.R.C.S., F.R.C.S.I., F.A.C.S.
Urologist, Bon Secour Hospital and St. Finbarr's Hospital, Cork, Ireland; formerly Resident in Urology, Mayo Graduate School of Medicine (University of Minnesota), Rochester, Minnesota.

CHARLES C. RIFE, M.D.
Department of Urology, Mayo Clinic, Rochester, Minnesota.

CHARLES E. SHOPFNER, M.D.
Professor of Radiology, University of Missouri School of Medicine; Director, Department of Radiology, Children's Mercy Hospital, Kansas City, Missouri.

LYNWOOD H. SMITH, M.D., F.A.C.P.
Division of Nephrology, Mayo Clinic; Instructor in Medicine, Mayo Graduate School of Medicine (University of Minnesota), Rochester, Minnesota.

RANDALL G. SPRAGUE, M.D., PH.D. (Medicine), F.A.C.P.
Division of Endocrinology, Mayo Clinic; Professor of Medicine, Mayo Graduate School of Medicine (University of Minnesota), Rochester, Minnesota.

KENNETH E. STANLEY, M.D., M.S. (Urology), F.A.C.S.
Staff Urologist, Wichita Clinic, St. Francis Hospital and Wesley Hospital, Wichita, Kansas; formerly Resident in Urology, Mayo Graduate School of Medicine (University of Minnesota), Rochester, Minnesota.

BARRY L. STERN, M.D.
Resident in Urology, Mayo Graduate School of Medicine (University of Minnesota), Rochester, Minnesota.

CAMERON G. STRONG, M.D., M.S., F.A.C.P.
Division of Nephrology, Mayo Clinic; Instructor in Medicine, Mayo Graduate School of Medicine (University of Minnesota), Rochester, Minnesota.

JOSE M. TALAVERA, M.D.
Resident in Urology, Mayo Graduate School of Medicine (University of Minnesota), Rochester, Minnesota.

W. NEWLON TAUXE, M.D., M.S. (Pathology)
Department of Clinical Pathology, Mayo Clinic; Associate Professor of Clinical Pathology, Mayo Graduate School of Medicine (University of Minnesota), Rochester, Minnesota.

HARRY W. ten CATE, M.D.
Consultant in Urology, Academisch Ziekenhuis Wilhelmina Gasthuis, Clinical Professor of Urology, University of Amsterdam, Amsterdam, Netherlands; formerly Resident in Urology, Mayo Graduate School of Medicine (University of Minnesota), Rochester, Minnesota.

DAVID C. UTZ, M.D., M.S. (Urology), F.A.C.S.
Department of Urology, Mayo Clinic; Associate Professor of Urology, Mayo Graduate School of Medicine (University of Minnesota), Rochester, Minnesota.

PREFACE
TO THE THIRD EDITION

The question may be asked why a third edition of *Clinical Urography* is necessary so soon (7 years) after publication of the second edition. Such a question seems reasonable inasmuch as the subject matter consists primarily of roentgenographic demonstrations of anatomic deformities and (to a lesser extent) of physiologic aberrations which result from disease and trauma. On first thought it might appear that such data are more or less constant and change little from year to year in contrast to the material found in medical and surgical texts, especially those which deal extensively with therapy, where constant change is the rule.

There are several reasons for undertaking this revision. First, the authors wish to constantly improve the quality of the book by deleting some illustrations and substituting, as well as adding, better ones. The number of illustrations has been increased by 30%; approximately 30% are new. Also important in this regard was the decision by the publishers to change to "offset" printing. This has required that all illustrations be rephotographed from original gloss prints or x-ray films. The dramatic improvement in the quality of the illustrations, however, more than compensates for the enormous effort and expense involved.

Second, in the past 7 years dramatic advances have been made in urographic methods and techniques which now permit unusual accuracy in diagnosis. Probably the greatest single advance in urography has been the demonstration that larger amounts and greater concentrations of contrast medium may be safely used. This factor plus the use of tomography (when necessary) in routine excretory urography has greatly increased the diagnostic yield of this modality. The excellent urograms now obtainable have almost completely eliminated the need for retrograde pyelography. This subject is discussed in Chapter 1.

Since the second edition was published (1964) there has been a tremendous increase in the use of angiography in many fields of diagnosis, including urology. The ability to demonstrate the vascular tree of the kidney plus the ability also to opacify the renal parenchyma (nephrogram) has opened new fields of diagnosis which previously were not considered possible. Because of the importance of this new modality, a full chapter concerning its use and application has been written by Dr. Owings W. Kincaid (Chapter 2). Also a liberal

v

number of angiograms have been added throughout the other chapters of the book.

A relative newcomer to the field is the procedure of lymphangiography (Lymphography, Chapter 19). Although this subject was briefly considered in the second edition, it has now assumed sufficient importance that we have devoted a full chapter to it. This chapter has been written by Dr. W. Eugene Miller who performs almost all of these examinations at the Mayo Clinic. Although the final place of this diagnostic procedure has not yet been determined, we think it deserves description here.

Renovascular hypertension, which is often amenable to surgical correction, continues to receive front-page attention. Since the last edition considerable diagnostic and therapeutic progress has been made concerning it. At the Mayo Clinic this problem is now the responsibility of a new diagnostic Division of Nephrology headed by Dr. James C. Hunt. A completely new chapter (Chapter 13) on this subject has been written by Dr. Cameron G. Strong and Dr. James C. Hunt, which will bring the reader up-to-date on this fast-changing subject.

Trauma to the urinary tract and fistulas and sinuses have been brought together into a new chapter (Chapter 15) by Dr. Panayotis P. Kelalis. The subject of urinary diversion also has been enlarged into a new chapter (Chapter 16) by Dr. James H. DeWeerd. Urologic problems related to gynecology have been grouped together in a new chapter (Chapter 18).

Several chapters have been extensively rewritten and updated. In Chapter 5, the currently debated problem of ureteral reflux versus obstruction of the vesical neck as the cause of persistent urinary infection in children has been considered in some detail. The role of reflux as a cause of pyelonephritis, renal atrophy, and hydronephrosis of adults has been explored in greater depth than in the second edition. Chapter 7 (Nontuberculous Infections of the Genitourinary Tract) likewise has been revised by Dr. Glen W. Hartman, with special emphasis on the importance of urography in the diagnosis of pyelonephritis. A major revision of the material on renal cystic disease (Chapter 9), with special attention to the important subject of congenital cystic disease, will make this chapter of much greater value to the urologist and the pediatrician than was the analogous chapter in the last edition.

Chapter 10 (Tumors of the Genitourinary Tract) has been enlarged and made more complete. Differential diagnosis between tumor and cyst by means of various new diagnostic modalities has been considered at some length. Newer concepts are described, such as that concerning the "functioning" nature of neuroblastoma, which now permits great accuracy in differentiation of this lesion from Wilms' tumor.

Chapter 12 (Anomalies of the Urinary Tract) has been completely rewritten and expanded. Sections on the subjects of intersexuality and ectopic anus (imperforate anus; anal atresia) in this chapter have been written by Dr. Charles E. Shopfner, who has advanced fresh new concepts concerning etiology, embryology, and diagnosis of these anomalous states.

In Chapter 17 (Miscellaneous Subjects) several new subjects such as Renal Transplantation, Chyluria, and Amyloid Disease have been added. More complete treatments than in the prior edition, of the subjects of Renal Papillary Necrosis and Bilateral Cortical Necrosis also have been added.

As is the case in all definitive works of this type, the authors are indebted to many colleagues for help in the preparation. Those who have written parts for this edition are acknowledged in the list of contributors. As was true of the second edition, several of the contributors are currently residents in training in the Department of Urology who have written on subjects of particular interest to them or on which they previously had done investigative work for other studies.

Appreciation is due several members of the Mayo Clinic staff for critically reviewing various portions of the manuscript. As they are experts in their individual fields, their suggestions and help have been invaluable in maintaining an optimal degree of accuracy in selected subjects, as follows: Dr. Edgar G. Harrison, Jr., and Dr. George M. Farrow of the Department of Surgical Pathology for advice on many pathologic problems in numerous chapters; Dr. Robert B. Wilson, Department of Obstetrics and Gynecology, for reviewing the material on placentography; Dr. W. Henry Hollinshead, Department of Anatomy, for reviewing Chapter 11 (Embryology of the Genitourinary Tract) and for advice on Chapter 12 (Anomalies of the Urinary Tract); Dr. Donald A. Scholz, Division of Endocrinology, and the late Dr. F. Raymond Keating, Jr., for reviewing the subjects of hyperparathyroid disease and nephrocalcinosis; Dr. Sheldon G. Sheps, Division of Cardiovascular Diseases, for reviewing the material on tumors of the adrenal medulla.

Most of the films for *Clinical Urography* have been selected from the files of the Mayo Clinic. A substantial number, however, have been generously and freely supplied by urologists and roentgenologists both in this country and abroad. Our sincere thanks and gratitude go to these men who are too numerous to mention here. However, acknowledgment of the source has been made in the legend under each such illustration.

It is with great pleasure that I announce the association of Dr. David M. Witten as a coauthor of this book. Dr. Witten is a consultant in the Department of Diagnostic Radiology of the Mayo Clinic with special responsibility for urologic radiology. The recent shift of responsibility for urologic radiology from the Department of Urology to the Department of Diagnostic Radiology has already resulted in substantial improvement in quality of our radiologic examinations. It is anticipated that Dr. Witten's association will help assure the continued improvement and excellence of quality in future editions of this book. Also it is hoped that the combined disciplines of both a clinical urologist and roentgenologist will assure proper balance and perspective which will prove most acceptable and helpful to the maximal number of physicians and students.

Much of the "heavy" work in the preparation of this book has fallen on the Section of Photography of the Mayo Clinic. Members of that section have been most willing and cooperative in remaking photographs, varying techniques to suit special situations, and providing, in innumerable other ways, individual and "custom" treatment for an enormous quantity of work.

It is with gratitude that I mention the tremendous help afforded us by the Section of Publications of the Mayo Clinic, without which this book would have been nearly impossible to produce. Special thanks go to Dr. Carl M. Gambill and Dr. Robert D. Knapp, Jr., who edited the manuscript, to Mrs. Betty Calkins, who did the final checking of the manuscript, and to Mrs. Nancy Nelson, who handled the proof.

JOHN L. EMMETT, M.D.

CONTENTS

VOLUME II

VOLUME III

Chapter 13

RENOVASCULAR AND RENAL HYPERTENSION: CLINICAL
FEATURES, DIAGNOSIS, AND MANAGEMENT.......................... 1605
By Cameron G. Strong and James C. Hunt

Chapter 14

MISCELLANEOUS VASCULAR LESIONS AFFECTING THE
URINARY TRACT.. 1637
By Frank J. Leary and David C. Utz

Chapter 18

GYNECOLOGIC PROBLEMS RELATED TO THE
URINARY TRACT... 1949

Chapter 19

LYMPHOGRAPHY 2017
By W. Eugene Miller

Chapter 20

UROLOGIC APPLICATIONS OF RADIOACTIVE MATERIAL 2041
  By W. Newlon Tauxe

CHAPTER 1

Methods in Urographic Diagnosis

THE CONTROVERSIAL HISTORY OF EXCRETORY UROGRAPHY*

by

Victor F. Marshall

Priorities are prone to be controversial. If the subject concerns a great and lasting achievement, the argument not only may be prolonged but it also is likely to be soon confused by nonessentials. Personalities often play a role and the separation of facts from wishes can be extremely difficult. There is no doubt that the introduction of practical excretory urography was a great and lasting achievement. It is a fact that excretory urography was grossly impractical and rarely performed even experimentally before 1929, but this method of examination

---

*Dr. Marshall conducted a very thorough, meticulous, and time-consuming investigation into the events which led to the discovery and development of excretory urography. As a result of his findings, Dr. Moses Swick was presented with the 1965 Valentine Award of the New York Academy of Medicine, which is given yearly to a living scientist who has made outstanding contributions to urology. This dissertation clarifies a subject which for years has been riddled with confusion and controversy. (J.L.E.)

was common and practical by 1931. As will be noted, the priorities were promptly obscured.

In 1906, Voelcker and Lichtenberg demonstrated the practicality of pyelography by the retrograde method, and the status of the individual upper urinary tract was largely removed from the arena of clever guessing. However, instrumentation was required—not invariably successful—and the contrast media tended to be irritating and even toxic if absorbed. No doubt, many persons dreamed of a nontoxic injectable or orally administrable compound which would outline reliably the open parts of the urinary system. Urologists today are so accustomed to highly efficient excretory urography that they may forget the earlier time when it was not available. Of course, that direct descendant of excretory urography, angiography, was not available then either.

Osborne, Sutherland, Scholl, and Rowntree at the Mayo Clinic tried intravenous sodium iodide about 1923. They obtained dim visualization, but severe reactions occurred routinely. Later, Roseno (1929a; 1929b) combined sodium iodide with urea which improved the visualization somewhat, but the compound, Pyelognost, was quite toxic. There were others (Hryntschak; Lenarduzzi and Pecco; Ziegler and Köhler) who experimented with the idea, but nothing safe or efficient was developed.

About 1928, Drs. Binz and Räth, biochemists at the chemical institute of the agricultural college in Berlin, were synthesizing pyridone compounds with components of arsenic and iodine. Their objective was a bactericidal agent against coccal infections, a sort of "magic bullet" in the tradition of Ehrlich and his Salvarsan. After some hopeful developments in controlling infections, their compounds were being tested clinically by Professor Leopold Lichtwitz, an internist, at the Städtisches Krankenhaus in Hamburg-Altona. Dr. Emanuel Libman of the Mt. Sinai Hospital in New York had just awarded a fellowship for foreign travel to one of his promising medical interns, Dr. Moses Swick. While studying pathology in Berlin, Swick heard of these new drugs and sensed that they might opacify the urinary tract. It was generally realized that much of these injected compounds was excreted in the urine, but Swick saw the prospect of radiographic visualization of the kidneys. Soon he was at work on this possibility under Lichtwitz in Altona.

All did not concatenate at once! The compounds were toxic; some were insoluble. But excretion was shown to be mainly in the urine, and some faint shadows of the bladder could be noted in animals. The goal of the biochemists' productions thus became excretory urography, and the antibacterial aspect faded away. Using Swick's suggestions as well as their own reoriented ideas, these biochemists made many variants with a resulting reduction in toxicity and an increase in solubility, which improved application. The bladder could be visualized regularly, but the pyelograms were usually absent or, at most, faint.

Trials on patients had been under way, but they had given variable and equivocal results until an attempt was made on a patient who had an obstructing ureteral stone; the pyeloureterogram on the obstructed side was quite clear (Swick, 1968)! Obviously more urologic patients were needed for study. Accordingly, an arrangement was made for Swick to transfer to St. Hedwigskrankenhaus in Berlin, a 200-bed urologic hospital under the direction of the famous Professor Alexander von Lichtenberg.

Shortly thereafter this German baron departed for urologic meetings in the United States where he was enthusiastically received. At about this time, Binz and Räth sent to Swick a soluble, relatively nontoxic, compound which was excreted in a high concentration in the urine. A principal compound of earlier studies, **Selectan neutral**, had been modified by substituting a sodium acetate radical for a methyl group to produce the famous **Uroselectan** (Joseph; Swick, 1966) (Fig. 1–1). After several consecutive successes on patients, Swick cabled the momentous news to his benefactor, Dr. Libman, in July 1929 and requested that von Lichtenberg be informed. In the United States, the latter apparently spoke with enthusiasm of this development; at least, a considerable American experience had accrued within 1 year thereafter (von Lichtenberg). Work continued, von Lichtenberg returned, and a presentation at the 1929 meeting in Munich of the German urologic society was planned.

Here the controversy began, and the facts started to be obfuscated. Evidently von Lichtenberg felt that he should be the principal author, since the final work was done in his institution. Regardless of the merits of this attitude, the situation was understandable from von Lichtenberg's viewpoint. He was an internationally famous urologist directing the world's largest urologic hospital, and directing it from the top of the geheimrat

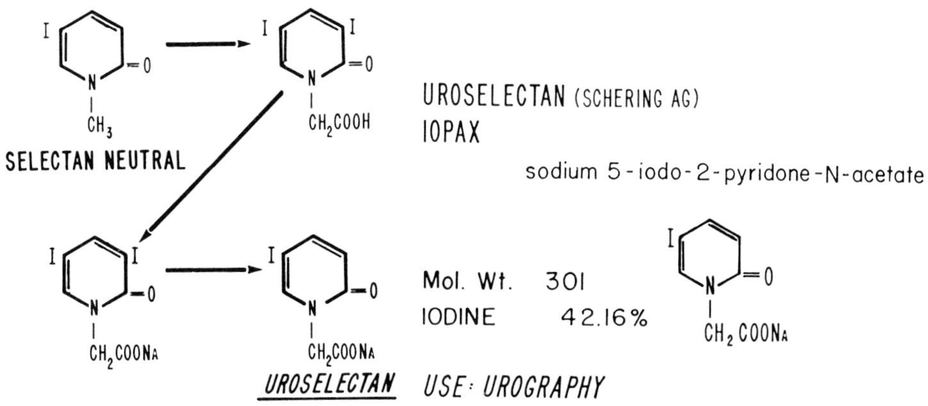

UROSELECTAN (SCHERING AG)
IOPAX

sodium 5-iodo-2-pyridone-N-acetate

Mol. Wt. 301
IODINE 42.16%

UROSELECTAN *USE: UROGRAPHY*

Figure 1–1. Structural formulas of Selectan neutral and Uroselectan. (From Swick, M., 1966.)

system. Evidently Swick was to be relegated to a minor role in the presentation. His name might well have entered oblivion had not his earlier mentor, Professor Lichtwitz, arranged a conference with von Lichtenberg, von Salle (editor of *Klinische Wochenschrift*), Renner (chief associate of Lichtwitz), and Swick. There are unfortunately no minutes of this conference, but the outcome is clearly recorded. The first presentation at this historical meeting was by Swick alone (1929). It concerned the developmental work on animals and human beings, mostly at Altona. The second presentation was on clinical applications and was offered by von Lichtenberg and Swick. Binz and Räth were credited as the actual makers of the compounds. It is almost inconceivable that an unknown, isolated, young internist from a foreign country (the United States of America) could have hoodwinked the important sophisticated personages at that conference into permitting such a sequence of presentations and authorship, if he had not done what these papers indicated. It would have been morally wrong for them to have permitted Swick to create what they would have known to be a fraud, and very simple for these powerful doctors to have stopped him. (Indeed, it would have brought credit and glory to them, not only in preventing the perpe-

tration of a fraud but also in enhancing their personal images.)

Despite these beginning circumstances, Swick was soon ushered into the background. Professor von Lichtenberg occupied a very prestigious position among American urologists. For the convention of The American Urological Association in New York, in June, 1930, a symposium on intravenous pyelography had been organized by Dr. Joseph Francis McCarthy, the president. Swick who was back in New York was not invited to attend. He was not then a member of The American Urological Association. Thus, von Lichtenberg alone gave the American premier on "The Principles of Intravenous Urography." He referred to Swick just once: "Lichtwitz's assistant, Swick, from this standpoint, continued the work in my clinic under my direction." In addition to the insinuation that von Lichtenberg's direction was vital, the statement does demonstrate that he realized that the fundamental preliminary work had been done in Lichtwitz's clinic. This distinction was already clearly indicated in the authorship of the two papers before the German urologic society, which have been referred to. Lichtwitz never made claim to a major role but he did back Swick. (Repeated rumors that Lichtwitz and von Lichtenberg became increasingly unfriendly do not seem farfetched!) In the remaining six papers (Binz; Braasch; Bugbee and Murphy; Herbst; Lowsley; Sweetser) and nine recorded discussions on the subject at that convention, only Binz mentioned Swick: "In March, 1929, I discussed matters with Prof. Lichtwitz and Dr. Swick." and "Prof. von Lichtenberg...appointed Dr. Swick to clinically try out the preparations that I would give him." The evidence is that both statements are essentially correct (actually Swick never had a formal appointment), and the first indicates Swick's involvement, and suggestions, before he went back to Berlin. There seems to be no argument that Binz and Räth actually prepared the compounds. Exactly how important Swick's individual suggestions were is unprovable; but his role, in reorienting the biochemists' goals and in carrying the development through animal and human experimentation to practical fruition, shines through the dust of this scramble for priorities. Von Lichtenberg's role was an important, albeit secondary one: He provided Swick with the facilities to expand his continuing studies.

In spite of being emotionally upset by these events, Swick did not immediately give up his studies on returning to the United States. He became associated with Dr. Victor Wallingford, a chemist at the Mallinkrodt Chemical Works, and together they developed Hippuran for which they received the Billings Gold Medal of the American Medical Association in 1933 (Swick, 1933b). Thus, Swick was a major developer, again with a chemist's aid, for the Hippuran series as well as the Uroselectan series of radiopaque materials (1933a). The descendants of these are being used widely and increasingly more than 35 years later. At the present time, 1970, the common commercial names of the descendants of Uroselectan are Neo-iopax and Diodrast. The current descendants of the Hippuran series are Urokon, Hypaque, Renografin, and Conray. The fact is readily notable

from these incomplete lists that these compounds are now used in a variety of procedures, not only in the field of urology but especially in angiography. In 1965, Dr. Swick received the Valentine Award of the New York Academy of Medicine, which is given each year to the living scientist considered by the selection committee to have made outstanding contributions to urology.

THE PLAIN FILM (OTHER TERMS: KUB AND SCOUT FILM)

Necessity for Plain Film Before Urogram

The first principle of accurate diagnosis is to make a plain roentgenogram, commonly referred to as a *plain film* of the urinary tract, before any opaque medium is injected. It is surprising how often diagnosis is inaccurate because a preliminary plain film of the area of the kidneys, ureter, and bladder was not made. The necessity of this procedure will become more apparent as the problem of urologic diagnosis unfolds in the subsequent pages of this book. Two examples here, however, will serve to impress this point on the student's mind. The first example is that of "silent" urinary calculi. By this term is meant urinary calculi that do not produce symptoms. Only too often one sees a physician unsuccessfully treat for several weeks what he considers a common, uncomplicated infection of the urinary tract, before obtaining a plain film and discovering the real cause to be calculi in some part of the urinary tract. The second example is that of a physician who attempts to interpret a retrograde pyelogram or excretory urogram in a case in which no preliminary plain film has been made. Areas of increased density in the region of the calyces or where the ureter is

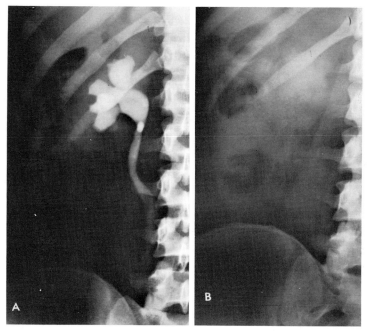

Figure 1–2. A, *Retrograde pyelogram*. **Increased density of medium** below ureteropelvic juncture, where ureter bends back on itself, might be erroneously interpreted as calculus if no preliminary plain film had been made. **B,** *Plain film*. Shows no calculus to be present.

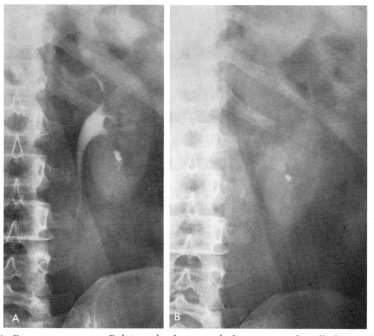

Figure 1–3. A, *Excretory urogram*. Pelvis and calyces might be erroneously called normal, if preliminary plain film were not available. **B,** *Plain film*. Shows **stone forming cast of lower calyx of left kidney.**

kinked or doubled back on itself may be interpreted erroneously as calculi (Fig. 1–2*A* and *B*). Conversely, when calculi are present they may be missed entirely by being obscured by the opaque medium (Fig. 1–3*A* and *B*).

It is important that the plain film be made *before* the urogram, rather than as an afterthought. The reason for this is apparent; even though the plain film is made several hours or days after the urogram, it is possible for medium to be retained in the kidney or ureter if stasis is present. Obviously this may seriously confuse interpretation. *Never attempt to interpret any urogram if a preliminary plain film is not available.*

Technique of Making a Plain Film

Careful roentgenographic technique in the making of a plain film is important if satisfactory roentgenograms are to be obtained. The *preparation of the patient* for this roentgenogram is not standardized. Some roentgenologists prefer no catharsis of any kind. They feel that catharsis irritates the intestinal tract and tends to produce more gas than when no preparation is used. Those who adhere to this method give a laxative only to those patients whose plain film is unsatisfactory without preparation. However, the majority of roentgenologists prefer to purge the patient before roentgenograms are made. The most common type of preparation is to advise the patient to eat no evening meal. About 6 p.m. he is given 1 to 2 fluidounces (about 30 to 60 ml) of castor oil, and he reports for the roentgenologic examination the following morning before breakfast is eaten. In some clinics multiple enemas are advised on the morning of the examination in addition to the castor oil the evening before examination. Many roentgenologists are opposed to this procedure because they feel that air is introduced into the bowel with the enemas. The object of prepara-

tion is, of course, to eliminate fecal material and intestinal gas, which produce troublesome shadows that obscure the urinary tract. It is our opinion that the advantages of preparation far outweigh the disadvantages and that for plain films of the highest diagnostic quality preparation with a laxative is required in most cases.

A detailed *description of the actual roentgen technique* is hardly necessary here, since it has been included in many textbooks on roentgenography and it is described in detail by many manufacturers of x-ray equipment. Furthermore, improvements in x-ray equipment are so rapid that any detailed description here would be obsolete as soon as written. However, a few fundamental points may be helpful. All roentgenograms should be made with a Bucky diaphragm. Films should be placed in cassettes that are equipped with intensifying screens of good quality. These cassettes must be kept very clean so that confusing artifacts do not appear in the developed roentgenogram. The roentgenograms are taken with the patient in the supine position, and the abdomen is compressed with an inflated rubber bag. The bag is compressed tightly by means of a band controlled by a roller and ratchet that are part of the equipment of most combination cystoscopic and x-ray tables. The patient is instructed to hold his breath at the end of expiration, and it is advisable to tell him to pinch his nose in order to ensure complete cessation of breathing. He must also be instructed not to move in any way while the exposure is being made, since the slightest amount of motion may completely ruin the roentgenogram for interpretation.

It is always well to use two 14 by 17-inch (about 36 by 43 cm) films so that the entire urinary tract is visualized. The *lower film* should be placed so that the symphysis pubis is situated 2½ inches (about 6.4 cm) above the lower border of the cassette. In exposing the film the x-ray tube should be rotated so that the central beam of rays is directed toward the patient's feet at an angle of 10° with a vertical line perpendicular to the body. This will permit the roentgen rays to pass beneath the symphysis pubis. The position of the *upper film* depends on the stature of the patient. If the patient is short-waisted, the symphysis pubis should be just on the cassette; if the patient is medium-waisted, the symphysis should be about 1 inch (about 2.5 cm) below the lower border of the cassette; if the patient is long-waisted, the symphysis should be approximately 3 inches (about 7.5 cm) below the lower border of the cassette. In exposing the film the x-ray tube should be rotated so that the central beam of rays is directed toward the patient's head at an angle of 10° with a vertical line perpendicular to the body. This permits the roentgen rays to pass beneath the costal margin. It is important that the roentgen beams be directed as described for both the upper and lower films so that the upper and lower portions of the urinary tract will not be obscured by the ribs or the pubic rami. One of the most common errors seen in the making of roentgenograms of the urinary tract is failure to place the lower film low enough. When this occurs, prostatic calculi, vesical calculi, and stones in the intramural portion of the ureter may be missed entirely.

THE UROGRAM

TERMINOLOGY

Strictly speaking, the term *urogram* indicates the roentgenographic delineation of the entire urinary tract with opaque contrast medium. The term does not state whether the medium was introduced by the retrograde or the excretory method. Some writers on urology have somewhat confused the terminology by employing the word *urogram* to mean roentgenograms made by the excretory method as contrasted to the word *pyelogram,* which they use to indicate a roentgenogram made by the retrograde injection of opaque medium. It is obvious that such terminology is inaccurate. We prefer to use the term *urogram* to denote the roentgenogram that visualizes the urinary tract by means of opaque contrast medium, regardless of the method of its administration. If the descending or excretory method is used, we speak of it as *excretory urography.* If the retrograde method is employed, it is called *retrograde pyelography.*

The term *pyelogram* is rather loosely used. When one speaks of a pyelogram he usually means a roentgenogram that outlines with opaque contrast medium the calyces, renal pelvis, and ureter. The term *pyelogram* in itself means only the delineation of the pelvis. Nevertheless, the term has become so widely used that it probably will always be accepted in the literature to mean a film which includes the calyces, pelvis, and ureter. It must of necessity be modified by the adjective *retrograde* or *excretory* to denote the method by which it was made.

As stated previously, if one uses the term *urogram,* it should include the visualization by means of opaque contrast medium of the entire urinary tract; namely, the renal parenchyma, the calyces, pelves, ureters, bladder, and urethra. For the purpose of clarity, however, we shall arbitrarily employ the term *urogram* in this book to mean only the visualization of the upper part of the urinary tract, which includes the renal parenchyma, the calyces, pelves, and ureters. Because the roentgenologic visualization of the bladder usually requires a special technique and films, we shall speak of such roentgenograms as *cystograms* and of the roentgenologic visualization of the urethra with opaque contrast medium as a *urethrogram.*

Retrograde Pyelography

TECHNIQUE OF URETERAL CATHETERIZATION

The technique involved in making a retrograde urogram should claim our attention first. The patient is prepared in the same manner as for the making of a plain film of the urinary tract. The retrograde method requires that catheters must be introduced through the ureters into the renal pelves by means of cystoscopic manipulation. Two main types of *ureteral catheters* are used: *opaque* and *nonopaque*. Most urologists prefer the opaque or "x-ray" catheter, since it outlines the course of the ureter and will localize shadows over the ureteral area without the necessity of completely filling the ureter with opaque medium. It has one disadvantage, however; when one is endeavoring to localize minute shadows located in the course of the ureter, the width of even a 5-F catheter may completely obscure the shadow and defeat the purpose of the investigation (Fig. 1-4A and B). Ureteral catheters are made with both blunt and pointed or olive tips. The blunt-tipped catheter is less likely to traumatize and irritate the ureter. The point-tipped catheter is easier to introduce into small ureteral orifices and is more readily passed beyond points of ureteral obstruction. When local anesthesia is being employed for cystoscopy, the cystoscopist should not employ too large a ureteral catheter for the routine type of investigation. A 5-F catheter is the most frequently used size, as it is easily accommodated by the average ureter and yet is large enough to permit fairly rapid collection of specimens of urine from the renal pelvis. If difficulty is experienced in passing a 5-F

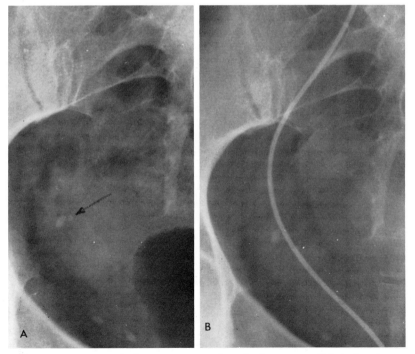

Figure 1-4. A, *Plain film.* Two shadows opposite right ischial spine; medial shadow is **stone** and lateral shadow **phlebolith.** B, *Plain film with lead catheter in right ureter.* Shadow of stone is completely obscured by catheter and would be missed if no preliminary film were available.

catheter, a 4-F catheter will often pass easily. Some urologists prefer the routine use of 4-F catheters, which they believe cause less discomfort to the patient.

Extreme care should be exercised in catheterizing the ureters if satisfactory films are to be obtained. If a ureter is traumatized by rough manipulation, it becomes spastic and the ureterogram will suggest narrowing or stricture. The most common cause for failure in ureteral catheterization is the attempt to introduce the catheter into the ureteral orifice too rapidly. The orifice should be approached slowly and carefully, avoiding poking its periphery, which results in ureteral spasm and may completely defeat any attempt to introduce the catheter. After the catheter has been introduced into the ureteral orifice, it should be slowly and carefully passed up the ureter.

The distance the ureteral catheter should be passed varies in different patients. The tip of the catheter should be introduced well into the renal pelvis. If the catheter is introduced too far, it enters a calyx (Fig. 1–5) and if the cystoscopist uses too much force, it may penetrate the renal cortex. Such penetration also may be apparent rather than real. If medium is injected into the cortex, the patient may experience a severe febrile reaction. This is especially true if such a medium as sodium iodide is used. This matter will be discussed more fully later. When the catheter is fairly soft and pliable, if introduced too far, it may coil back on itself in the pelvis or ureter, so that on withdrawal it may form a knot (Fig. 1–6). When this occurs it may be difficult to remove the catheter, as the knot holds up at the intramural portion of the ureter on withdrawal. It is the usual custom to introduce the catheter slowly and carefully until a slight obstruction is encountered. If a normal length of catheter has been introduced, this usually indicates that the tip of the catheter is in the renal pelvis. Catheters

which are too rigid and stiff should not be employed. On the other hand, catheters that are flaccid from too much boiling are very difficult to use.

Some urologists prefer to leave the cystoscope in place while the medium is being injected into the catheters to make the urogram. The reason for this procedure is that if, when the urogram is developed, it is found that the catheter is not in the proper place, its position can be changed without the reintroduction of the cystoscope.

Since the development of image-intensification fluoroscopy with television monitoring, fluoroscopic control of both the placement of ureteral catheters and the injection of contrast medium for retrograde pyelography has become practical. With this technique the ureteral catheters can be placed in any position needed and the volume of medium injected can be controlled to demonstrate to best advantage any lesion encountered. This results in films of higher diagnostic quality than are obtained with the average retrograde pyelogram done without fluoroscopy, and lessens the chance of improper placement of the catheter.

Use of "Acorn-" or Bulb-Tipped Catheters

It is difficult to visualize the entire ureter in the manner just described. An attempt to fill the ureter by continuing the injection of contrast medium as the catheter is withdrawn is sometimes effective, but more often it fails. The best technique is to employ an "acorn-" or bulb-tipped ureteral catheter of about the same caliber as the ureteral orifice. It is introduced just inside the ureteral orifice and kept in this position under cystoscopic vision while contrast medium is injected. It fits tightly enough within the intramural ureter so that the medium runs up the ureter rather than leaking back down around the catheter. Injection

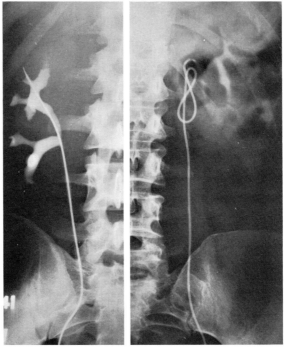

Fig. 1–5   Fig. 1–6

Figure 1–5. *Right retrograde pyelogram.* Catheter has been introduced too far, so that tip of catheter is well up in fornix of lateral branch of upper calyx, and gives impression of apparent penetration of cortex.

Figure 1–6. *Plain film, with lead catheter in left ureter.* Catheter has been introduced too far and has coiled itself into knot in region of renal pelvis.

is done slowly and carefully, and at the first twinge of flank pain, injection is terminated and a film exposed. This type of pyeloureterogram is the best that can be obtained; the drawbacks are (1) the cystoscope must be left in place during injection and (2) specimens of urine cannot be obtained from the kidney.

TYPE OF CONTRAST MEDIUM AVAILABLE

Before the introduction of the organic iodides, preparations of a 12% solution of sodium iodide or bromide were used routinely. This makes an excellent contrast medium as far as roentgenologic visualization is concerned, but it may be irritating to the mucosal lining of the urinary tract, and occasionally very severe reactions result. This is especially true if the injected medium is retained, as is the case, for instance, in a hydronephrotic kidney (Fig. 1–7). In such a kidney a retrograde pyelogram made with sodium iodide or bromide frequently has precipitated a severe febrile reaction in the patient, associated with multiple fulminating cortical abscesses requiring immediate nephrectomy to save the life of the patient.

Since the advent of excretory urography most urologists have come to employ the same organic iodide preparations for retrograde purposes that are employed intravenously or orally for excretory urography. Generally speaking, a 20% to 30% solution of any of those preparations now used for excretory urography will be of sufficient opacity to make an excellent retrograde urogram. Though the cost of such media is considerably higher than that of sodium iodide, it cannot be considered expensive when one considers the safety of the patient.

In more recent years the manufacturers

of the intravenous contrast media have become aware of this potential market and have placed suitable solutions on the market for retrograde pyelography (see section on "Urographic Contrast Media Available" later in this chapter for detailed discussion of the newer contrast media). For the purpose of reducing post-pyelographic reactions, some of the manufacturers have added an antibiotic (2.5% to 4.2% solution of neomycin sulfate). Opinions differ concerning the efficacy of this additive. Bloom and Richardson; Roth, Kaminsky, and Hess; and Samellas, Biel, and Draper have been favorably impressed with the antibiotic additive. On the other hand, Hoffman and de Carvalho's studies have suggested that it is ineffective. In their opinion postpyelographic reactions are caused by the injection of too much medium rather than by bacterial contamination. They advocated the injection of 2.5 to 3 ml of medium rather than 5 to 10 ml (or more) as is customary. The retrograde media currently on the market are as follows:

Pyelokon-R*=20% solution of sodium acetrizoate (Urokon).

Retropaque†=20% solution of methiodal sodium (Skiodan) with 4.2% neomycin sulfate.

Retrografin‡=30% solution of sodium and methylglucamine diatrizoate (Renografin) with 2.5% neomycin base.

METHOD OF INJECTING CONTRAST MEDIUM

There are two principal methods of introducing retrograde opaque solutions: by gravity and by syringe. The danger of overdistending the pelvis and calyces, with subsequent extravasation of opaque medium, is less on use of the gravity method than with the syringe method.

---

*Mallinckrodt Chemical Works is the manufacturer.
†Winthrop Laboratories is the manufacturer.
‡E. R. Squibb and Sons is the manufacturer.

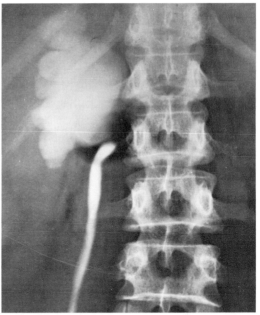

Figure 1–7. *Right retrograde pyelogram.* Hydronephrosis with obstruction at ureteropelvic juncture. Type of case in which retrograde medium might be retained and possibly might produce systemic reaction.

The buret containing the medium should be elevated not more than 18 inches (about 46 cm) above the level of the kidney. When the syringe method is used, the injection should be made slowly and carefully, with as little manual pressure as possible being used. In either case, injection should be terminated as soon as the patient complains of a sense of fullness or pain in the renal region. As a general rule, 5 to 10 ml of medium will make a satisfactory pyelogram. It is wise not to inject more than this amount, even though the patient does not complain of distress, until the first urogram has been taken and developed. If the urogram shows incomplete filling, a larger amount of medium may then be quite safely introduced.

In our experience the syringe method of injection requires less time than the gravity method and has proved entirely satisfactory. No matter which method is used, however, one must constantly be on the alert to avoid overdistention of the pelvis and calyces, with subsequent extravasation of opaque medium. Though this is not a serious complication if the newer types of organic iodide solutions (such as those employed in excretory urography) are used, nevertheless it can produce a reaction uncomfortable to the patient, characterized by pain, fever, and at times chills. Fortunately the reaction usually is transient and in most cases terminates within 24 to 48 hours, unless infection has been introduced by means of contaminated solutions.*

ROENTGENOGRAPHIC TECHNIQUE

The roentgenographic technique used in making a retrograde urogram is essentially the same as that described for the plain film, except that usually only one film is used instead of two, the x-ray tube being placed over the center of the film, with no rotation of the tube as used in taking plain films. After 4 or 5 ml of the contrast medium has been injected, the catheter is withdrawn about 2 inches (about 5 cm), and the injection is continued, to allow the ureter to fill. The urogram is taken with the patient lying on his back and in the horizontal position. At times it is important to determine the amount of excursion of the kidney. In such a case a second urogram should be made, with the position of the table changed so that the patient is as near the erect position as possible. The urograms are made at the moment the injection is stopped and before the medium has time to run back around the catheter into the bladder. More recently, as was pointed out above, fluoroscopic control of retrograde pyelography has made it possible to monitor filling of the ureter and renal pelvis and to obtain spot films of

the areas of interest when they are best demonstrated.

At times it is impossible, with the ordinary pyelogram made in the anteroposterior position, to include or exclude shadows which may lie in apposition to the pyelographic outline of the kidney or ureter. In such a case an *oblique* (angulated) pyelogram (Fig. 1-8A, B, and C) or *lateral* pyelogram (Fig. 1-9A, B, and C) may be invaluable. The necessary degree of rotation of the patient will vary in each case. The patient lies on the side being investigated, with the opposite side rotated away from the table to an angle of about 45°. He is supported there by sandbags placed under the shoulder and thigh. At times it may be necessary to make several oblique pyelograms with different degrees of rotation before the desired result is achieved. The completely lateral position is not routinely used because the vertebral column tends to obscure the pyelogram. At times, however, it may be distinctly useful, as, for instance, in determining anterior displacement of the kidney and ureter or in visualizing the profile of minor calyces in cases of malrotation. (See discussion of lateral pyelogram, Chapter 4.)

The Delayed Pyelogram

Of considerable help in selected cases is the *delayed pyelogram* (Fig. 1-10A and B). This type of pyelogram is used when one suspects the presence of stasis in the pelvis or ureter. To determine this a pyelogram is made as usual in the horizontal anteroposterior position. The catheter is immediately removed and the patient is allowed to sit or stand for 5 to 20 minutes. After this, another film is exposed. If any contrast medium remains in the pelvis or ureter, it usually denotes a delay in emptying time, although one must always remember the possibility of the stasis being due to spasm of the ureter or ureteropelvic junction produced by irritation from the catheter.

---

*See discussion of pyelorenal backflow, Chapter 4.

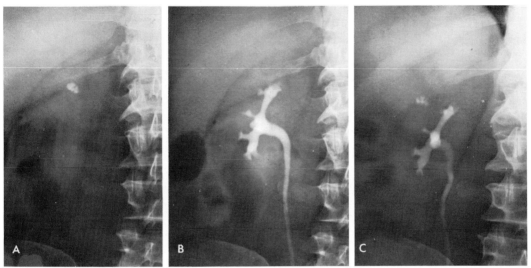

Figure 1–8.   A, *Plain film.* Calcific shadow over upper pole of right kidney. B, *Retrograde pyelogram, anteroposterior position.* Shadow obscured by upper calyx. C, *Retrograde pyelogram, oblique position.* Shadow is projected laterally and is definitely excluded from urinary tract.

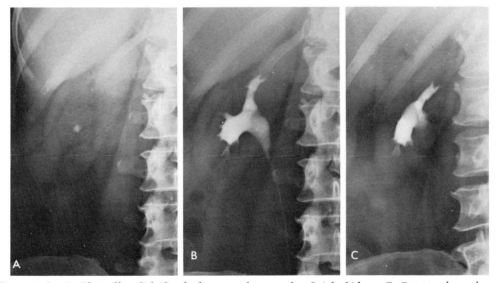

Figure 1–9.   A, *Plain film.* Calcific shadow over lower pole of right kidney. B, *Retrograde pyelogram, anteroposterior position.* Shadow obscured and apparently included in lower calyx. C, *Retrograde pyelogram, lateral position.* Shadow still obscured by lower calyx, indicating that shadow is produced by **stone in lower calyx.**

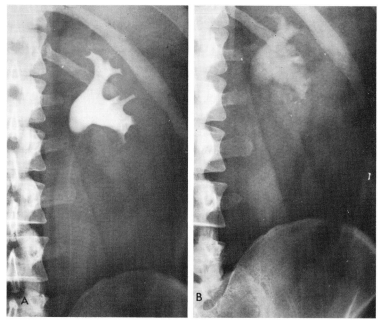

Figure 1–10. A, *Retrograde pyelogram*, left. **Pyelectasis graded 1+** (on basis of 1 to 4, in which 1 designates mildest and 4 most severe condition). Suggestion of obstruction at ureteropelvic juncture. **B,** *Thirty-minute delayed pyelogram.* Medium retained in pelvis and calyces, indicating **definite obstruction at ureteropelvic juncture.**

Excretory Urography

TECHNIQUE

A technically satisfactory excretory urogram demonstrates clearly and completely both the renal parenchyma and the urinary collecting system, including the calyces, renal pelvis, ureters, and urinary bladder. Failure to demonstrate one or more of the parts of the urinary tract is a leading cause of diagnostic error and one which can, to a large degree, be eliminated if care and attention to detail are exercised in making the examination.

Preparation

There is considerable difference of opinion regarding the need for **preparation of patients for excretory urography.** Some hold that preparation, especially catharsis, is unnecessary and in fact undesirable. The weight of opinion, however, favors the view that adequate preparation including both dehydration of the patient and cleansing of the bowel to help eliminate feces and gas is an essential requirement if excretory urograms of the highest quality are to be made.

Withholding of food and drink for 6 to 12 hours before examination causes the kidneys to produce a relatively concentrated urine. The opacity of the excreted contrast medium consequently is increased and better visualization of anatomy is obtained. Catharsis with 1 to 2 ounces of castor oil or its equivalent in one of the proprietary laxative preparations eliminates fecal material from the colon in most cases and helps to reduce the amount of gas in the bowel in some. It has been our experience at the Mayo Clinic that mild cathartics do not remove fecal material from the colon in the case of most sedentary, elderly, or hospitalized patients and only the stronger cathartics such as castor oil are effective. Enemas, especially the tap-water or soapsuds type, have likewise been ineffective in our experience and in some cases tend to increase rather than decrease the amount of bowel gas. Some proprietary enema preparations, especially Lavema,[*] are quite effective in cleansing the bowel and are used by some radiologists for preparation of both children and adults.

The need for both dehydration and catharsis is reduced somewhat when large doses (50 ml or more) of one of the modern urographic contrast media are used and when conventional filming technique is supplemented by tomography. Even in these cases, however, the overall quality of the examination is improved by preparation and unless there are specific contraindications we believe preparation should be a part of the examination.

Ureteral Compression

Since the introduction of excretory urography, many different procedures have been adopted to produce partial urinary stasis and prevent the excreted contrast medium from leaving the renal pelvis too rapidly. The simplest is to position the table with the patient's head tilted down at an angle of from 10° to 15° in a **moderated Trendelenburg position.** For many patients, this position places the calyces lower than the ureteropelvic junction. Since the contrast medium is hypertonic as compared to the urine it tends to settle in the dependent upper and posterior calyces and to produce more complete filling.

A more effective method for retention of medium in the renal pelvis and calyces is partial occlusion of the ureters by means of **external ureteral compression** (Cimmino). A variety of devices have been used for this purpose, including small wooden blocks, rolls of gauze, single solid or air-filled rubber balls, and others. The most effective and comfortable have been devices consisting of two

small inflatable rubber balloons which are held in place by a sponge-rubber or a plastic-foam block and a flexible cloth band which passes around the patient (Daughtridge) (Figs. 1–11 and 1–12). The balloons are placed over the ureters where they cross the promontory of the sacrum and are fixed snugly in place by the supporting plastic foam block and band. Inflation of the balloons must be adequate to occlude or partially occlude the ureters at this point but should not be great enough to produce pain. An example of the effectiveness of this procedure is demonstrated in Figure 1–13.

A compression device of this type can be used on both children and adults. It should not be used on patients who have had recent surgical operations on the abdomen because of the discomfort it will produce, and it should not be used on patients who have had recent operations on the kidneys or ureters as extravasation of medium and urine may result. Compression should only be used with caution or not at all on patients with known aneurysm of the abdominal aorta, depending on its size and location.

Ureteral compression produces few complications if carefully applied. An occasional patient will develop syncope apparently as the result of vagal stimulation or of inferior vena caval obstruction with decreased return of blood to the heart. This is quickly corrected by release of the compression. In rare cases extravasation of contrast medium from a calyx occurs (Fig. 1–14) and produces transient flank pain. This stops as soon as compression is relieved and no significant sequelae result.

Interval Between Injection of Contrast Medium and Exposure of Films

Immediately before injection of the contrast medium the **patient should be instructed to void.** If this is not done, the diffusion of contrast medium in a bladder

---

[*]Winthrop Laboratories, New York, N.Y.

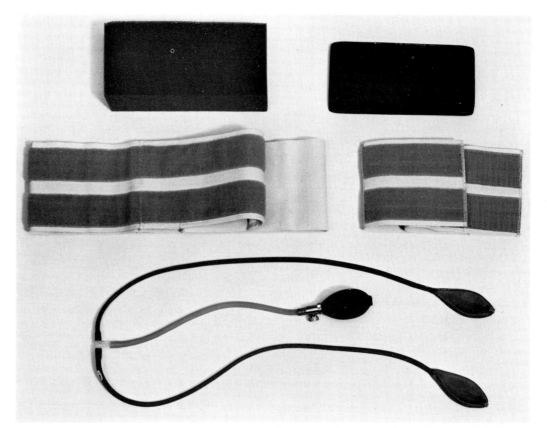

Figure 1–11. Components of compression device (from top left): plastic foam block, plexiglass plate, canvas belt with Velcro strips, additional lengths of belt, and balloons with tubing and inflation bulb. (From Daughtridge, T. G.)

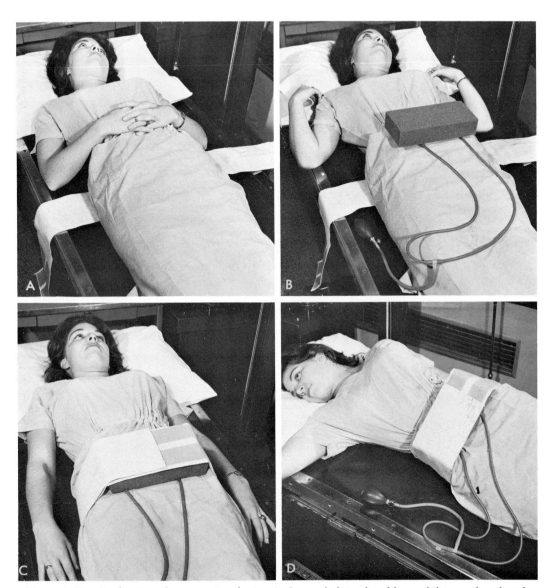

Figure 1-12.   Application of compression device. **A,** Canvas belt is placed beneath hips so that plexiglass plate will lie over lower part of abdomen. **B,** Balloons are placed on either side of midline and plastic foam block is in place. **C,** Belt is securely in place, and patient is positioned for anteroposterior roentgenogram. **D,** Patient is positioned for oblique projections with compression device unchanged. (From Daughtridge, T. G.)

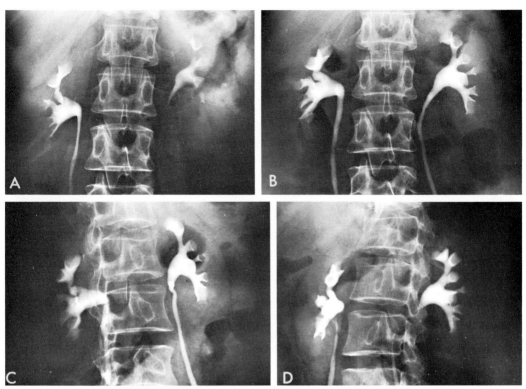

Figure 1–13. Value of external ureteral compression in excretory urography. Normal *excretory urograms.* A, Without compression, lower calyceal groups on left are incompletely filled. B, With compression, all calyceal groups are well opacified. C and D, *Oblique roentgenograms with compression,* showing value of visualizing pelvis and calyces completely filled in more than one projection. (From Daughtridge, T. G.)

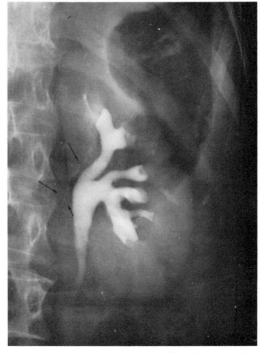

Figure 1–14. *Excretory urogram, 10-minute compression film.* Extravasation of medium from calyx with pyelolymphatic backflow (*arrows*), resulting from ureteral compression. Normal kidney. This is rarely of clinical significance.

filled with urine may produce a cystogram of sufficient size and density to obscure the lower parts of the ureters.

The patient is then placed on a table equipped with a Bucky diaphragm, and the x-ray machine is put in place. An upper and a lower film (plain film) are first exposed, processed, and inspected by the physician in order that any technical faults in the positioning or exposure can be corrected and additional plain films (oblique, lateral, and so on) can be made if needed before the contrast medium is injected. (The development of rapid automatic film processing machines in recent years has greatly facilitated the careful control of every step in the excretory urogram.)

Filming Technique

There are no specific rules governing either the timing of roentgenographic exposures or positioning of the patient for excretory urography and as a result there is wide variation from institution to institution depending on the preferences of the examining physician. However, since much of the contrast medium is excreted within 15 to 20 minutes after injection, the films must be made during this period. In most instances, multiple films are required.

It is our custom at the Mayo Clinic to use two slightly different basic filming sequences for adults and a third for children.

For Adults. *Suspected Urinary Tract Disease.* The adult patient with suspected urinary tract disease is positioned on the x-ray table for preliminary plain films in the anteroposterior projection (see previous discussion of plain film). These are processed and inspected and additional plain films are made if indicated. Contrast medium is injected and ureteral compression is applied. Films, centered to demonstrate the kidneys, are exposed 5 and 10 minutes after injection with the compression on. After the 10-minute film, the compression device is released, and the third film is exposed immediately. The final film, centered to demonstrate the bladder, is exposed approximately 20 minutes after injection. This filming sequence provides generally adequate visualization of the kidneys, ureters, and bladder: (1) The renal parenchyma is well demonstrated on the 5- and 10-minute films. (2) The pelvis and calyces are ordinarily filled by 10 minutes, and their appearance both with and without compression can be studied. (3) After release of compression, the ureters and bladder are shown to best advantage (Fig. 1–15A through D).

Hypertension. For adults studied because of arterial hypertension (see Chapter 13), compression is not applied initially and carefully timed films are made 2 and 3 minutes after injection to demonstrate the kidneys during the earliest stages of opacification of the collecting system. By this technique any difference in the times of appearance of medium in the two kidneys can be detected. (Many prefer "minute sequence" films made 30 seconds and 1, 2, 3, 4, and 5 minutes after injection. We have found the 2- and 3-minute films to be of greatest value for screening purposes and reserve the more extensive filming sequence for selected cases.) Ureteral compression is applied after the 3-minute film, and a 10-minute film, with compression, is exposed. Compression is removed when the renal calyces and pelvis are seen to be adequately filled, and a 20-minute film is exposed to show the bladder.

Tomography and Reinjection. With rapid automatic processing of films (90 seconds), the progress of each examination can be followed carefully. If necessary, at any point in the examination, additional special films (oblique, prone, lateral, upright, tomograms, and so on) can be made to clarify anatomic details. **Tomography** with three or four films made at different levels through the kidneys and exposed 10 to 15 minutes after injection is a tremendously valuable adjunct to conventional filming technique (Figs. 1–16*A* and *B* and 1–17*A* and *B*). This procedure is used as needed in our outpatient practice and routinely in our hospital practice, where adequate bowel preparation is difficult. In cases where urinary tract anatomy is not adequately demonstrated by the conventional techniques, **delayed films** are made after **45 minutes or longer**; or the patient is immediately **reinjected with a large dose of concentrated medium** (usually 50 ml or more of Hypaque-M 90% or its equivalent), and both tomograms and conventional roentgenograms are made with the patient in various positions. With these methods, urinary tract anatomy can be demonstrated adequately in almost every case, *and the need for retrograde pyelography is reduced sharply or largely eliminated* (Figs. 1–18*A* and *B* and 1–19*A* and *B*).

For Children. For children under the age of 5 or 6 years, compression is dispensed with and the gonadal areas are shielded with a radiopaque lead rubber mask to keep radiation exposure to a minimum. For the same reason, the number of films made also is reduced: Other than the preliminary plain film, a film of the kidney region made from 3 to 5 minutes after injection and a second film at 7 and 12 minutes to include both the kidneys and the bladder are sometimes adequate. More often, however, the urinary tract is obscured by bowel shadows and additional films are necessary. When this is the case it is helpful to give a **carbonated beverage (soda pop) to distend the stomach with gas** and displace bowel from over the kidneys. A straight anteroposterior film shows the left kidney in most cases but a right oblique is usually needed to project the gas-filled stomach over the right kidney (Fig. 1–20*A* through *D*). Occasionally, both obliques are required. Additional films can be made as needed when obstruction is present or renal function is poor.

UROGRAPHIC CONTRAST MEDIA AVAILABLE
(Table 1–1 and Fig. 1–21)

From the inception of excretory urography (1931 to 1932) until about 1951, the two most universally used preparations were sodium iodomethamate (Neo-Iopax) and iodopyracet (Diodrast). Sodium iodohippurate (Hippuran) proved to be definitely inferior for intravenous injection, and its oral use proved impracticable. For this reason it was used primarily for retrograde pyelography.

About 1950 a definite advance resulted from the development of the triiodobenzoic acid derivatives, which provided compounds containing three atoms of iodine to the molecule instead of the conventional two in the older media. The first of these compounds to be given extensive clinical trial was sodium acetrizoate (Urokon). Following this, other compounds employing the basic triiodinated benzoic acid nucleus were developed: sodium diatrizoate (Hypaque) in 1954, methylglucamine diatrizoate (Renografin, Cardiografin), and mixtures of sodium and methylglucamine diatrizoates (Renovist, Hypaque-M) in 1953 and 1954, and shortly thereafter sodium dipotrizoate (Miokon). In 1962, the iothalamate group of media including both sodium (Conray-400, Angio-Conray) and methylglucamine salts (Conray) became available. More recently another triiodobenzoic acid compound, metrizoate (Isopaque), has been subjected to extensive clinical trial in Europe and is currently under investigation in the United States.

In the relatively short time that has elapsed since the introduction of these new contrast media, a rather voluminous literature has accumulated concerning their comparative merits, especially on the quality of urograms and the incidence and severity of side reactions. Three such studies are summarized as examples in Table 1–2. Sodium acetri-

(Text continued on page 29.)

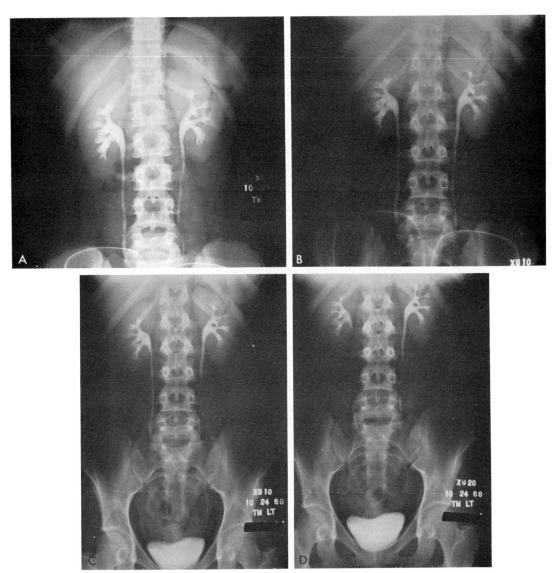

Figure 1–15. Excretory urographic technique. Typical *excretory urograms*. **A,** *Five-minute film,* centered to show kidneys. Ureteral compression is on. **B,** *Ten-minute film* with ureteral compression. Note that calyces, pelvis, and upper parts of ureters are well filled. **C,** *Ten-minute film* without ureteral compression. Renal pelvis, calyces, and upper parts of ureters remain filled but are not distended. Lower parts of both ureters are demonstrated. **D,** *Twenty-minute film.* Film is centered with its lower edge 1 to 2 inches below symphysis pubis in order that entire bladder region is included.

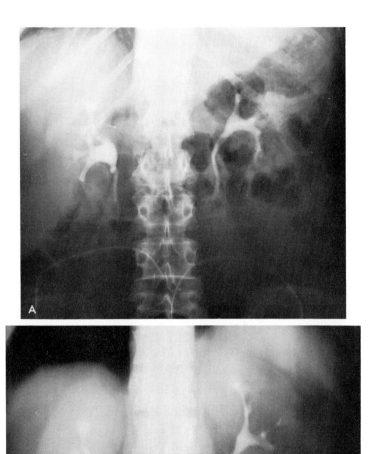

Figure 1–16.   Value of tomography. **A,** *Excretory urogram, 10-minute film.* Renal outlines and some calyces are badly obscured by overlying gas. **B,** *Tomography, 15-minute film.* Renal outlines and calyces are clearly demonstrated.

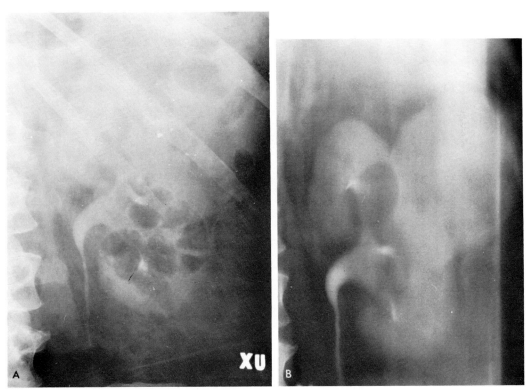

Figure 1–17. Value of tomography. **A,** *Excretory urogram.* Renal outline partially obscured and calyces not well filled—interpreted as grossly normal. **B,** *Tomogram* reveals large mass (**hypernephroma**) which was not suspected from conventional urographic films.

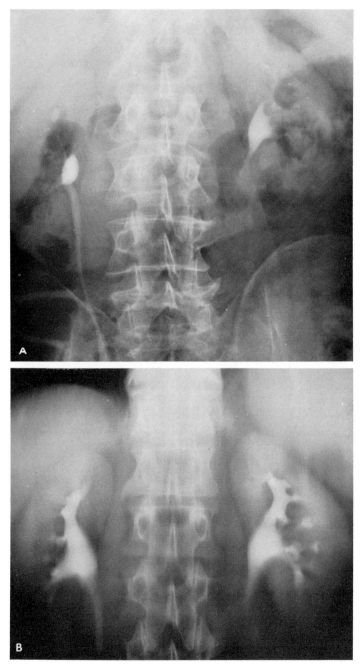

Figure 1–18. Value of reinjection and tomography. **A**, *Excretory urogram, 10-minute film.* Collecting system is poorly filled, and renal parenchyma is partially obscured. Examination is unsatisfactory. **B**, *Tomography after reinjection* (50 ml Hypaque-M 90%). Renal parenchyma, pelvis, and calyces of both kidneys are well demonstrated, and retrograde pyelography is unnecessary. (**Normal findings.**)

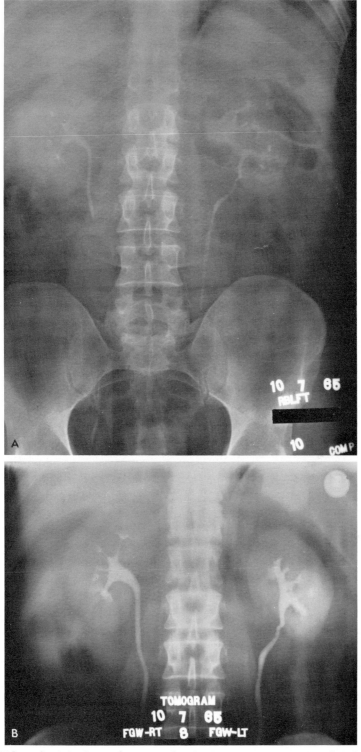

Figure 1–19. Value of reinjection and tomography. **A,** *Excretory urogram.* Renal outlines are partially obscured and collecting system is poorly opacified. **B,** *Reinjection and tomography.* Renal parenchyma and collecting system are well demonstrated, thus avoiding retrograde pyelography.

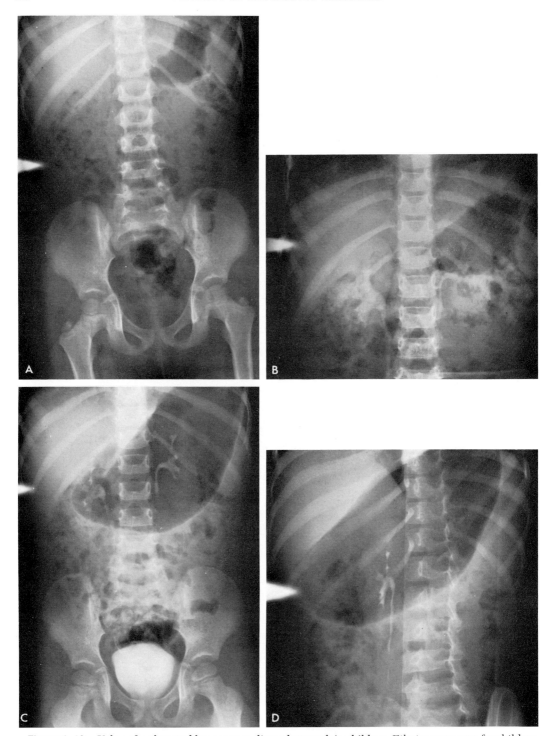

Figure 1–20.   Value of carbonated beverage to distend stomach in children. Filming sequence for children. *Excretory urograms.* **A,** *Plain film.* **B,** *Five-minute film,* showing localized exposure of renal areas. Gonads are shielded with lead rubber mask. Kidneys are badly obscured by bowel shadows. **C,** *Ten-minute film,* showing kidneys, ureters, and bladder. Stomach is distended with gas from drinking carbonated beverage. **D,** *Right oblique film,* projecting gas-filled stomach over right kidney to eliminate obscuring bowel shadows.

Table 1–1. Urographic Contrast Media

TRADE NAME*	GENERIC NAME	CHEMICAL NAME	IODINE CONTENT	CONCENTRATION OF DRUG IN COMMERCIALLY AVAILABLE SOLUTION, % (WT/VOL)	MANUFACTURER'S SUGGESTED DOSE, ML	
					Adults	Children†
Conray	Meglumine iothalamate	5-Acetamido-2,4,6-triiodo-N-methyl-isophthalamic acid, methylglucamine salt	282 mg/ml	60	25 to 30	Less than 6 mo—5 6 to 12 mo—8 1 to 2 yr—10 2 to 5 yr—12 5 to 8 yr—15 8 to 12 yr—18 12 to 14 yr—20 to 30
Conray-400	Sodium iothalamate	5-Acetamido-2,4,6-triiodo-N-methyl-isophthalamic acid, sodium salt	400 mg/ml	66.8	25	
Hypaque	Sodium diatrizoate	Sodium 3,5-diacetamido-2,4,6-triiodobenzoate	300 mg/ml	50	30	
Renografin 60	Sodium (8%) and methylglucamine (52%) diatrizoate	Sodium and methylglucamine 3,5-diacetamido-2,4,6-triiodobenzoate	293 mg/ml	60	25	
Renografin 76	Sodium (10%) and methylglucamine (66%) diatrizoate	Sodium and methylglucamine 3,5-diacetamido-2,4,6-triiodobenzoate	370 mg/ml	76	20	
Renovist	Sodium (35%) and methylglucamine (36%) diatrizoate	Sodium and methylglucamine 3,5-diacetamido-2,4,6-triiodobenzoate	372 mg/ml	69.3	25	

*Names of the manufacturers of these products follow: Conray and Conray-400—Mallinckrodt Chemical Works; Hypaque—Winthrop Laboratories; Renografin 60, Renografin 76, and Renovist—E. R. Squibb and Sons.
†Recommended doses for children are the same or (Renografin 76) approximately the same for all agents.

EARLY UROGRAPHIC MEDIA

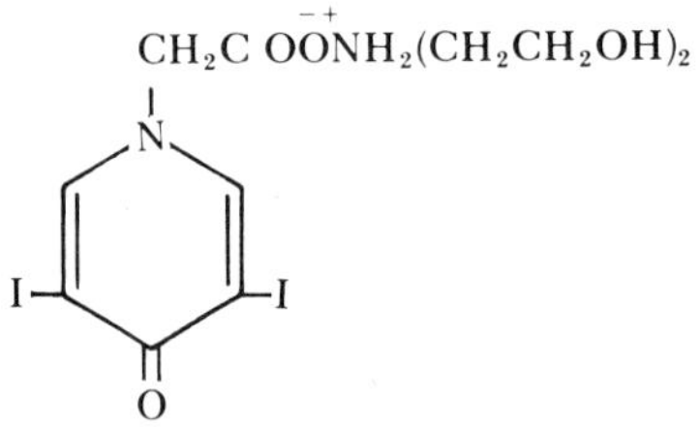

$CH_2C\overset{-}{O}O\overset{+}{N}H_2(CH_2CH_2OH)_2$

Iodopyracet group —
diethanolamine salt of 3,5-diiodo-
4-pyridone-N-acetic acid
Diodrast (Winthrop)

ICH_2SO_3Na

Iodomethamine group —
sodium iodomethane sulfonate
Skiodan (Winthrop)

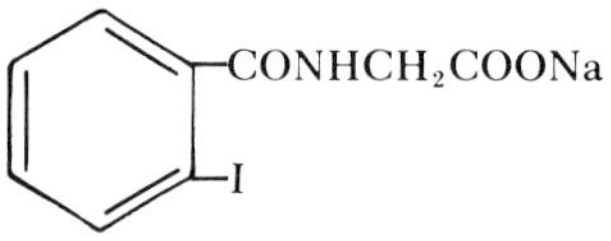

CONHCH$_2$COONa

Iodohippurate group —
sodium *o*-iodohippurate
Hippuran (Mallinckrodt)

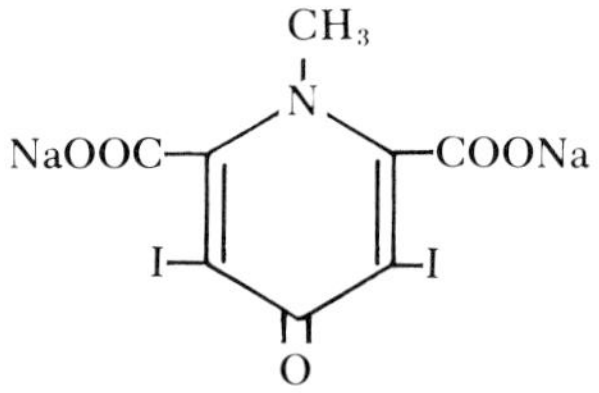

NaOOC—COONa

Iodomethamate group —
disodium salt of N-methyl-3,5-
diiodochelidamic acid
Neo-Iopax (Schering)

MORE RECENT UROGRAPHIC MEDIA

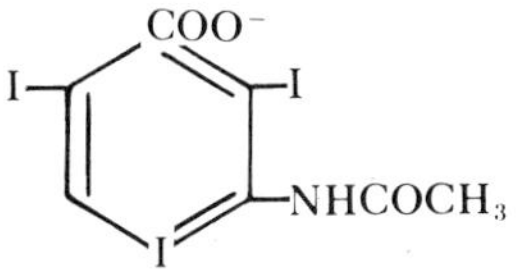

COO⁻

NHCOCH$_3$

Acetrizoate group —
3-acetamido-2,4,6-
triiodobenzoic acid
Urokon (Mallinckrodt)

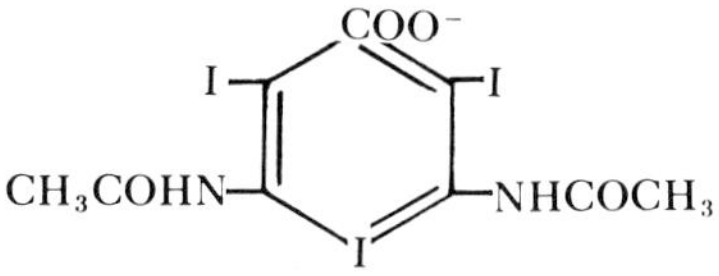

COO⁻

CH$_3$COHN—NHCOCH$_3$

Diatrizoate group —
3,5-bisacetamido-2,4,6-
triiodobenzoic acid
Hypaque (Winthrop)
Renografin (Squibb)
Renovist (Squibb)

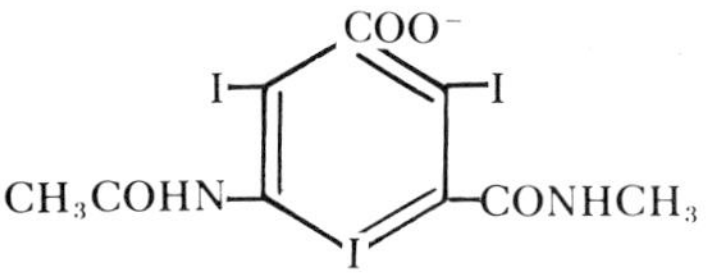

COO⁻

CH$_3$COHN—CONHCH$_3$

Iothalamate group —
5-acetamido-2,4,6-
triiodo-N-methylisophthalamic acid
Conray (Mallinckrodt)

Figure 1–21.   Structural formulas of various urographic media.

zoate (Urokon) was definitely superior to the older media both in quality of urograms and lower incidence of side reactions (Culp, Van Epps, and Edwards; Utz and Thompson), but this substance was found to be considerably more toxic than the diatrizoate (Eyler, Drew, and Bohne) and iothalamate (Strain and Rogoff) compounds and is no longer available for intravenous urography.

Most authors now consider all of the diatrizoate and iothalamate compounds to be excellent contrast media. The sodium salts, being smaller molecules, contain relatively more iodine per molecule and are therefore slightly more radiopaque than are their methylglucamine counterparts at equal concentrations. The sodium salts are also less viscous, a desirable property when large doses of highly concentrated solutions must be delivered rapidly through small caliber needles or catheters. However, the methylglucamine salts are thought by most investigators to be less toxic than the sodium salts (Fischer and Cornell), and they are also somewhat more soluble in water. Concerning the comparative merit of these for clinical use, however, opinions differ—one author reporting superior results with one and another favoring a different product. At the present writing the problem seems to have resolved itself into individual preference as the result of personal experience.

METHODS OF ADMINISTRATION OF CONTRAST MEDIUM

Intravenous injection, when feasible, is the method of choice. **In the case of adults** it is usually easy to find a suitable vein in the antecubital fossa or on the back of the hand. **In the case of infants,** however, suitable veins may be difficult to locate. The most satisfactory *site of injection* in such cases is the external jugular vein. To do a venipuncture in this area it is necessary to immobilize the in-

fant by wrapping his arms and body in a large towel or sheet. The head is tilted to the opposite side, and as he cries or strains, the vein stands out in relief, making venipuncture an easy procedure. The so-called scalp vein needles which are commercially available in sterilized disposable form are widely used in pediatric practice for this purpose and are much easier to use on children than are conventional needles. **Subcutaneous or intramuscular administration** has been used in the past when intravenous administration failed. This procedure usually produces urograms of poor quality and is not an adequate substitute for intravenous administration of contrast medium. Fortunately, with the development of the "scalp vein" needles, it is rarely, if ever, necessary to use the subcutaneous or intramuscular route for administration of these substances.

In the event that venipuncture of an infant is impossible and subcutaneous injection necessary, Cerny, Kendall, and Nesbit recommend dilution of 30 ml of 50% sodium diatrizoate to a volume of 100 ml with 5% dextrose in water. Half (50 ml) of this mixture is injected subcutaneously over each scapula through a 21-gauge needle. X-ray exposures are then made at 15, 30, 45, and 60 minutes.

Dose for Adults

In the case of adults, the commonest dose for injection is that recommended by the manufacturer (Table 1-1). These doses range from 20 to 30 ml for media which vary in strength from 50% to 76%. As far as can be determined, however, the doses are not based on any specific physiologic, pharmacologic, clinical, or roentgenographic data which would indicate that these are maximal or even optimal doses; rather, they seem to represent the smallest doses which will produce an "acceptable" excretory urogram of the average patient. As experience with the modern contrast media (diatrizo-

Table 1–2. Comparison of Quality of Urograms and Incidence of Reactions With Various Contrast Media

CASES	MEDIUM	QUANTITY INJECTED, ML	QUALITY OF FILMS, % OF CASES			INCIDENCE OF REACTIONS, %		DEATHS
			Good*	Fair*	Total Diagnostic	Total	Serious	
			Study of 1,400 cases by Utz and Thompson					
200	Neo-Iopax, 75%	20	43	42	85	86†	0.5	0
200	Urokon, 50%	25	52	36	88	36	0.5	0
200	Urokon, 50%, with Benadryl	25	49	40	89	34	0.5	0
200	Renografin, 76%	20	78	17	95	8	0	0
200	Renografin, 60%	25	82	14	96	8	0	0
200	Hypaque, 50%	25	73	20	93	12	0	0
200	Miokon, 50%	25	65	28	98	14	0	0
			Study of 2,122 cases by Culp, Van Epps, and Edwards					
774	Urokon, 70%	—	70.8	24.6	95.4	9.3	10‡	1
644	Diodrast, 35%	—	71.8	19.3	91.1	6.05	5‡	0
179	Neo-Iopax, 50%	—	59	21	80	16.2	2‡	0
155	Miokon, 50%	—	89	6.8	95.8	49.0§	4‡	0
235	Renografin, 76%	—	82.4	13.4	95.8	6.4	1‡	0
135	Hypaque, 50%	—	84.6	8.1	92.7	16.29	2‡	0
			Study of 2,234 cases by Macht, Williams, and Lawrence					
683	Hypaque, 50%	20	78	13	91	7.2	0	0
921	Renografin, 60%	20	83	12	95	4.1	0	0
630	Conray-400	20	88	8	96	5.4	0	0

*Good = prompt concentrated excretion of medium; urinary stream outlined sufficiently well to eliminate need for retrograde studies. Fair = density not comparable to retrograde pyelogram, yet sufficient outline of calyces and pelvis so that a diagnostic statement could be made.
†Chiefly pain in arm.
‡Urticaria, difficult breathing, or cardiovascular collapse.
§Principally flushing and bitter taste in mouth.

ates and iothalamates) has accumulated, it has become evident that the doses recommended by the manufacturers tend to be too small to produce urograms of the highest quality in many cases. Friedenberg and Carlin have advocated doses of 50% sodium diatrizoate or 60% methylglucamine diatrizoate ranging from 30 to 100 ml, depending on body surface area. They found the frequency of excellent to good urograms is increased from about 65% in examinations made with standard volumes to about 95% in those made with larger doses. Hemley, Gallagher, and Cusmano; MacEwan; Gronner, Arkoff, and Burhenne (among others) have recommended doses roughly double those recommended by the manufacturers, as both useful and safe for routine use. Powell and associates evaluated doses of 20, 40, and 80 ml, and of 0.5 ml/lb of body weight and 1 ml/lb of body weight, along with other factors, and concluded that the more contrast agent used the greater the percentage of excellent results. They found no significant increase in side effects with large doses. Schencker; Wendth; Hartley; Feldman, Goade, Bouras, and Bargoot; and others have recommended drip-infusion techniques with doses of contrast medium ranging from 1 ml/lb of body weight of 50% sodium diatrizoate or its equivalent to 300 ml or more of 30% methylglucamine diatrizoate. The advocates of these high-dose techniques report no significant increase in incidence or severity of reactions as compared to that obtained with standard low-dose urography and have demonstrated that the larger doses of medium will substantially improve demonstration of the urinary tract, increase diagnostic accuracy, and sharply reduce the need for retrograde pyelography. Our own experience with the routine use of large doses of urographic contrast medium (50 ml of either sodium and meglumine diatrizoate 69% or meglumine iothalamate 60%) has convinced us of the safety and utility of this method for increasing the diagnostic yield from this examination.

Dose for Children

As for adults, the commonest dose for injection in children is the dose recommended by the manufacturer (Table 1-1). But, like the recommended dose for adults, the dose for children can be increased in proportion to body weight with a substantial improvement in quality of urograms and without any increase in incidence or severity of reactions to the medium (Voltz and associates). Some recommend doses approximately double those recommended by the manufacturer (MacEwan, Dunbar, and Nogrady), and Standen, Nogrady, Dunbar, and Goldbloom have reported using doses of 5 ml/kg of Renografin 60 up to a maximum of 25 ml for infants up to 1 year of age with no serious reactions.

It is our practice at the Mayo Clinic to use the following dose schedule for routine examinations of infants and children. The dose schedule is based on the use of sodium and meglumine diatrizoate (Renovist) 69%:

Newborn	10 ml
6 months to 2 years	10 to 15 ml
2 to 5 years	15 to 20 ml
5 to 12 years	20 to 25 ml
More than 12 years	30 ml

Rate of Injection

For the most part, manufacturers suggest injection times varying from 1 to 3 minutes or more to minimize side effects, especially flushing, nausea, and vomiting. More rapid injections are well tolerated, however, and experience with rapid injection of large volumes of concentrated medium for nephrotomography, angiocardiography, and arteriography as well as rapid injection (less than 30 seconds) for urography has demonstrated no apparent increase in severe or life-threatening reactions attributable to rapid intravenous injection of the diatrizoates or iothalamates.

REACTIONS TO CONTRAST MEDIA

Reactions have always been a problem with intravenous injection of contrast media. Mild reactions (a better term is "side effects") are relatively common and include such manifestations as pain in the arm, flushing, metallic taste in the mouth, nausea, vomiting, faintness, tingling, numbness, and cough. The more serious reactions are distinctly uncommon but constitute a hazard to the patient and may be life-threatening. Such conditions as urticaria, edema, and asthma may be considered in this category or there may be severe acute shock-like episodes with hypotension, convulsions, cyanosis, shock, cardiac arrest, and death.

In the largest single study of this problem, Ochsner, Little, Buchtel, Giesen, and Morel observed untoward reactions of some type in 8.53% of 10,000 patients. In a subsequent study of the same group of patients, Coleman, Ochsner, and Watson observed that of the 10,000 patients studied only 1.68% had reactions considered to be "allergic" (shock [0.08%], asthma [0.02%], nasal and conjunctival symptoms [0.25%], or dermal reactions [1.33%]). No deaths occurred. The remaining reactions were considered to be nonallergic (nausea, vomiting, local pain, faintness, and other miscellaneous mild side effects).

The ultimate and most feared reaction, of course, is death. Pendergrass and associates in 1955 collected reports of 156 deaths from excretory urography since 1930. They estimated that during the 10-year period, 1942 to 1952, 6,370,000 excretory urograms had been made in the United States, with 42 known deaths, an incidence of 6.6 deaths per million. From a similar study, 1942 through 1956, they

estimated the mortality rate from 1942 through 1956 at 8.6 per million. Approximately 90% of fatal reactions occurred during or immediately after injection.

There is, without question, an association between a history of allergy and the occurrence of reactions to urographic contrast media. The nature of this association and its significance are not entirely clear, however. (Coleman, Ochsner, and Watson observed that in their series of 10,000 cases more than twice as many "allergic" reactions occurred among patients with no history of allergy as occurred among patients with a history of allergy.) Thus, it has been the opinion of some that a history of allergic disease and even a history of previous mild reaction (that is, flushing, urticaria, nausea, and pain) to iodinated contrast agents is not a contraindication to repeat examination (Finby, Evans, and Steinberg, 1958). Further data on this point are contained in a recently completed study at the Mayo Clinic (Witten and Hirsch) (Table 1-3). In this study, a substantial increase in incidence of reactions was found among patients who gave a history of allergy. Despite the fact that reactions were more common, no major reactions were recorded in such patients in this series, including those who gave a history of previous reaction (primarily urticaria but including nasal congestion, asthma, and other milder reactions) to urographic contrast medium. Deaths of patients with a history of allergy have been reported, however, and we have observed two such cases in the past 11 years: one patient had a history of asthmatic bronchitis and the second had a history of hives from eating shrimp and swordfish.

We are of the opinion that a history of allergy does not preclude excretory urography, and even a history of previous reaction (urticaria, for example) to urographic contrast medium is not in itself an absolute contraindication to repeat examination. In such cases, how-

Table 1-3.   **Relationship Between History of Allergy and Reaction to Urographic Contrast Agents***

ALLERGIC HISTORY	PATIENTS EXAMINED	PATIENTS HAVING REACTIONS	
		No.	*%*
None	7,445	89	1.2
Asthma	140	9	6.4
Hay fever	316	13	4.1
Urticaria of unknown cause	69	5	7.2
Food allergy†	276	14	5.1
Reaction to urographic contrast medium‡	121	24	19.8
Iodine sensitivity	39	5	12.8
Other§	1,854	37	2.0

*Mild side effects—such as flushing, nausea and vomiting, and pain in arm—not included.
†Includes allergy to seafoods.
‡Primarily urticaria—no patient was reexamined who had had a previous major reaction (such as shock) to a contrast medium.
§Primarily cutaneous reactions to penicillin or sulfa or "reactions" (usually intolerance) to other drugs.

ever, prudence would dictate careful evaluation of the need for the examination and it should not be done in the absence of a clear-cut indication and then only when no other diagnostic method will suffice.

Cause of Reactions

The cause of reactions has evoked much study and conjecture, but the mechanism is still far from clear (Bergman and Ellner; Knoefel; Landsteiner; Landsteiner, Levine, and Van Der Scheer; Mann; Sandström). The most common assumption has been that the serious reactions represent a definite allergic manifestation; yet, as pointed out by Sandström and by Lasser, experimental proof of a true anaphylactic reaction mediated by an antigen-antibody mechanism is lacking. Hildreth and co-workers at the University of Pennsylvania considered this subject exhaustively and stated that the three most plausible causes of reactions are "toxicity, pharmacological idiosyncrasy and allergy." They pointed out that the vast majority of drug reactions are caused by a few relatively potent allergens of which the iodides are prime offenders. To explain the mechanism of reaction, they made use of the Landsteiner haptene theory (1930; 1936) which postulates that the iodide combines with protein to form haptenes. They finally concluded that "while proof of the mechanism of reactions occurring during intravenous urography is lacking, the available evidence strongly suggests allergy as the chief cause."

In contrast to this view, Lasser pointed out in a recent review of this subject that there is a substantial body of evidence against the concept that the radiopaque media function as haptenes and produce antibodies by combining with body proteins. He cited the fact that not a single instance of a demonstrated antibody against contrast media can be found in the literature and pointed to this as well as his own unsuccessful efforts in attempting to produce antibodies against sodium acetrizoate (Urokon) as strong evidence that reactions to injectable contrast media are probably not antibody-antigen in nature. He also indicated that iodine itself is tightly bound in urographic contrast media and suggested that the role of hypersensitivity to iodides per se in reactions to contrast media is probably small. It is his concept that these adverse effects are primarily chemotoxic reactions which are most closely related to the poorly understood effects of hypertonicity of contrast media and contrast-protein interactions. At the biochemical level, he thinks contrast-protein interactions may produce alterations in the diffusibility of certain endogenous substances (for example, histamine), alterations in the fluid and electrolyte composition of tissues, and inhibition or activation of a number of enzyme systems. At the cellular level, he thinks these biochemical effects may be manifested by effects on red blood cells (crenation and sludge formation),* on white blood cells (activation or inhibition of contained enzymes or both), on blood vessel walls (altered permeability and relaxation of smooth muscle components), on nerves (production of motor activity or motor defects), and on clot formation (production of coagulation defects).

Histamine Theory of Allergy and Anaphylactic Shock. If the cause of serious reactions from contrast media is on an allergic basis, then theoretically the antihistamine drugs should offer some help for both prophylaxis and treatment. In 1945 Loew and Kaiser demonstrated that anaphylaxis in the guinea pig is due in large part to bronchospasm resulting from the action of histamine which is liberated from the lung. These authors, with Moore, also demonstrated that

---

*The rapid injection of large doses of concentrated urographic medium has been demonstrated to cause aggregation or agglutination of the erythrocytes into clumps too large to pass through capillaries. This phenomenon which is known as *sludging* has been observed in a wide variety of conditions in which hypertonic solutions including the more concentrated urographic media have been injected. It is thought that sludged erythrocytes can block pulmonary capillaries, causing a marked increase in pulmonary vascular resistance, acute cor pulmonale, and death. Bernstein and Evans, in 1960, found that by administration of dextran of low molecular weight the suspension stability of the blood could be maintained and sludging prevented. This concept aroused considerable interest among physicians doing arteriography, angiography, and nephrotomography; but, to date, neither the efficacy nor practicability of premedication with dextran of low molecular weight prior to these examinations has been demonstrated.

diphenhydramine hydrochloride (Benadryl) inhibits the action of histamine on the bronchi and ileum of the guinea pig. Experiments by Wells, Morris, and Dragstedt suggested that the inhibition was due in part at least to "competition of Benadryl with histamine for its site of action." They recognized, however, that this did not fully explain the modification of anaphylaxis and postulated the possibility that Benadryl also "prevents the release of histamine." An experiment was set up in which dogs were subjected to severe anaphylactic shock. Some of the dogs were protected with preliminary injection of Benadryl, while the others were used as controls. None of the 22 animals protected with Benadryl died, but 9 of 26 dogs not protected died. These authors pointed out that in the protected dogs, Benadryl reduced but did not obliterate the vasodepressor effects of histamine. They were unable to state, therefore, that histamine was the sole factor in vasodepression and anaphylactic shock. In the years that have elapsed since these experiments, the evidence accumulated still points to histamine release as the major factor in allergic anaphylactic shock. On the basis of these experimental data considerable clinical and experimental efforts have been made to control reactions from contrast media with antihistamine drugs. This work will be described shortly.

Tests for Sensitivity to Contrast Media

Although tests to determine sensitivity to contrast media have fallen into disrepute, for the sake of completeness they will be described herein.

Oral Test. In 1940 Dolan described an oral test which consists of placing 1 to 2 ml of contrast medium under the tongue. After 10 minutes, if there has been no reaction, the patient is instructed to swallow it. If there is no reaction within 30 seconds, one proceeds with the intravenous administration of the medium. Numbness of the lips, a feeling of thickness of the tongue, and swelling of the tongue are signs of sensitivity.

Ocular Test. For this test, first described by Archer and Harris in 1942, a drop of contrast medium is put on the conjunctiva of one eye (the other being used as a control). The eyes are closed, then opened and examined after 1½ and after 3½ minutes. The degree of injection of the blood vessels of the sclera and conjunctiva is the criterion of the test.

Cutaneous (Intradermal) Test. This test was described in 1942 (Naterman and Robins; Robins). Five tenths of a milliliter of the contrast medium is injected intradermally into the skin of the forearm beside a control injection of normal saline. The areas are examined after 10 to 15 minutes. A wheal or erythema or both indicate a positive reaction as follows: slightly positive, wheal 8 to 9 mm in diameter with no erythema or a wheal less than 8 mm in diameter plus erythema more than 10 mm in diameter; moderately positive, wheal 10 to 15 mm in diameter; and strongly positive, wheal more than 15 mm in diameter.

Intravenous Test. The most commonly used test consists of the intravenous injection of 0.5 to 1 ml of contrast medium and waiting at least 1 minute. (Wait 5 to 10 minutes if there is a strong history of allergy or sensitivity to iodine.) If no untoward reaction occurs, the entire dose is injected.

Evaluation of Pretesting. It is now quite generally conceded that sensitivity tests are grossly unreliable (Alyea and Haines; Finby, Evans, and Steinberg, 1958; 1960). Pendergrass and his co-workers in their 1955 survey pointed out that results of sensitivity tests before injection of the medium had been negative on three fourths of 31 patients who died. Some urologists and roentgenologists have abandoned preliminary tests, but a substantial number still pretest prin-

cipally with the intravenous test for medicolegal reasons (Nesbit, 1958; 1959). In some instances, however, reactions to the test dose are observed; and they may be severe, even resulting in death. An impending reaction is often indicated by itching, sneezing, vomiting, or faintness. If a reaction to the test dose does occur, all agree that the necessity for continuing the examination must be carefully reevaluated. In most instances it is prudent to discontinue the examination at this point and substitute cystoscopy and retrograde pyelography but if excretory urography is deemed essential the examination should proceed with all possible caution. Appropriate emergency drugs and equipment should be at the patient's side, and in many cases antiallergic drugs should be administered before further injection of the contrast agent is undertaken.

Prevention of Reactions With Antihistaminic Drugs

Since 1948, articles have appeared in the literature concerning the prophylactic use of antihistaminic drugs to prevent reactions from intravenous injection of contrast media. The first studies employed the *oral administration* of antihistamines an hour or two before injection of the contrast medium (Getzoff, 1948; 1951). Subsequently, *intravenous injection* of antihistamines, 3 to 5 minutes before injection of the contrast medium, was advocated. Finally, mixing of the antihistamine (Olsson) with the contrast medium came into use. The antihistaminic drugs which have been most commonly used (judging by reports in the literature) are diphenhydramine hydrochloride (Benadryl), chlorprophen-iramine maleate (Chlor-Trimeton), and tripelennamine hydrochloride (Pyribenzamine). Also reported in occasional studies are thenyldiamine hydrochloride (Thenfadil), brompheniramine maleate (Dimetane), and promethazine hydrochloride (Phenergan). Benadryl has been administered intravenously in 50-mg doses prior to injection of the contrast medium, but in the majority of reported studies a dose of 10 to 50 mg has been mixed with the contrast medium. By far the most commonly employed dose has been 20 mg. Chlor-Trimeton has been used in almost the same manner. Pyribenzamine has been favored as an oral medicament in doses of 50 to 100 mg given 1 hour or more prior to injection of the contrast medium.

The reported results of antihistaminic protection have been anything but uniform, being variously reported as effective,[*] slightly effective (Bersack and Whitaker; Gilg), and without effect.[†] Most of the reports are favorable, but a substantial number are definitely unfavorable. Few of the studies, however, are based on a large enough series of cases with suitable controls to be statistically significant. Curiously, some authors report that antihistaminic prophylaxis reduces the incidence and severity of the minor reactions (Gilg), but not the serious ones; others report that only the serious (allergic type) reactions are affected (Nesbit, 1958; 1959).

The foregoing brief summary indicates that there is as yet no general agreement as to the usefulness of the antihistamines. At the Mayo Clinic we do not use them routinely but occasionally do use them for patients who present with a strong allergic history. If antihistamines are to be used on ambulatory patients, however, their soporific properties should not be forgotten. Patients should not be allowed to leave the physician's office unescorted and should avoid driving until the effects of the drug have worn off.

---

[*](Doyle; Getzoff, 1948; 1951; Hart, Sachs, and Grabstald; Moore and Sanders; Nesbit, 1958; 1959; Olsson; Sanger; Simon, Berman, and Rosenblum; Wechsler, 1956; 1957)

[†](Crepea, Allanson, and DeLambre; Finby, Evans, and Steinberg, 1958; Hamm, Waterhouse, and Weinberg; Hildreth and associates; Pendergrass and associates, 1955, 1958; Utz and Thompson)

Treatment of Reactions

For the minor reactions such as pain in the arm, feeling of warmth, flushing, metallic taste in the mouth, nausea and vomiting, tingling, numbness, and cough, treatment is not usually necessary, as the reactions are transient.

Serious reactions, however, usually occur suddenly and must be treated promptly to avoid a fatal outcome (Barnhard and Barnhard). Equipment must be at hand for immediate use, and the personnel must be well trained in the technique of its use. Patients must be watched closely during the procedure so that reactions may be recognized at once. The difference of a few seconds or minutes in recognition and treatment may be the deciding factor between life and death. A physician must be in attendance at all times, and in hospital practice, arrangements should be made with the department of anesthesiology so that an anesthesiologist may be summoned instantly to help.

Fortunately, most "allergic" reactions are not serious. They manifest themselves with edema of the skin and mucous membranes, producing the symptoms and signs of conjunctivitis, rhinitis, urticaria, and edema of the face, tongue, and glottis with asthmatic symptoms. The immediate intramuscular or intravenous injection of 10 mg of Chlor-Trimeton or in more severe cases subcutaneous or intramuscular administration of 0.5 ml of 1:1000 epinephrine will eliminate the symptoms. When epinephrine is used, the dose may need to be repeated in 10 to 15 minutes. The blood pressure should be watched closely for hypotension and impending shock.

If the reaction proceeds to more serious proportions, vasomotor collapse is heralded with signs and symptoms of dyspnea, cyanosis, and shock. Convulsions may occur and usually indicate anoxia. One hundred per cent oxygen should be administered immediately through a face mask. An adequate airway must be maintained and if necessary an endotracheal tube should be introduced. Artificial respiration then may be carried out as necessary. If shock is profound, absorption of the subcutaneously or intra-muscularly injected epinephrine may be poor, in which case 0.25 ml should be given slowly intravenously. Benadryl, 25 to 50 mg, or Hydrocortisone, 100 mg, or both should be administered intravenously at once (Wright). Asthma and pulmonary edema may be combated with 0.5 gm of aminophylline given intravenously over a period of 5 to 20 minutes.

The hypotension is treated with the Trendelenburg position plus administration of vasopressor drugs such as a 1.0% solution of metaraminol (Aramine), 0.2 to 1 ml subcutaneously or intramuscularly or 1.5 to 10 ml in 500 ml of normal saline or 5% dextrose in water intravenously. If there is no response, levarterenol bitartrate (Levophed), 4 to 8 ml, in 500 ml of 5% glucose should be given intravenously, the rate of administration being governed by the blood pressure.

Convulsions or laryngospasm or both may be controlled with the intravenous injection of 2 to 3 ml of a 2.5% solution of thiopental sodium. Laryngeal edema if not controlled by epinephrine may require an emergency tracheotomy.

RADIATION DOSE FROM EXCRETORY UROGRAPHY

Estimation of the dose of radiation delivered to the patient during a roentgenographic procedure such as excretory urography is difficult. Measurements vary with the size of the patient, size of the field, filtration of the beam, and other physical factors, and when measured the dose is difficult to assess in terms of clinical and genetic significance. In all cases, however, it is prudent to keep the dose as small as possible yet at the same time as large as necessary to produce an examination which will provide the infor-mation needed to diagnose and treat the patient. The dose can be kept to a minimum if the following are true: (1) The x-ray apparatus is in good working order. (2) It is used only by or under the direction of an experienced, well-trained technologist. (3) The x-ray beam is adequately filtered to reduce undesirable "soft" radiation. (4) The x-ray beam is carefully collimated so that the field size does not exceed the film size in the plane of the film. (5) The field size is kept as small as is consistent with adequate examination. (6) The gonads of children and, when practical, of adults in the child-bearing age group are adequately shielded.

As examples of the wide range of doses of radiation reported from excretory urography the following can be cited: Izenstark and Lafferty reported an average skin exposure *per projection* of 1,465 mR (milliroentgens) for males and 1,047 mR for females, with an average total dose to the gonads *per examination*, of 751 mR for males and 577 mR for females. Spalding and Cowing reported skin doses ranging from 2,375 mR for thin patients to 2,750 mR for heavy patients from an average excretory urogram with five films. They also recorded doses of 475 mR to 550 mR with single films for the KUB. Penfil and Brown in a study of the radiation doses to the United States population reported an average testicular dose of 2,091 mrad (millirads) for males and an average ovarian dose of 407 mrad for females from a five-film intravenous or retrograde pyelogram. They also showed that collimation of the beam size to film size in the plane of the film would reduce gonadal doses by two thirds.

Of special practical significance to urologists doing urography in their private offices is the work of Pasternack and Heller who observed wide variations in doses between private offices and hospital departments. Average gonadal doses from excretory urography in private offices were 431 mrad for males less than

15 years old and 239 mrad for older males. For females less than 15, the average gonadal dose was 703 mrad and for older females 696 mrad. In hospitals and clinics, where greater care was apparently exercised in controlling the size of the x-ray field, the corresponding doses were 7 and 17 for males and 443 and 685 mrad for females.

INCREASED RISK OF EXCRETORY UROGRAPHY IN MULTIPLE MYELOMA

Acute oliguric renal failure has been reported as an uncommon but potentially fatal complication of excretory urography in cases of multiple myeloma. The incidence of this complication is unknown; but it appears to be quite low, since only small numbers of cases have been reported and retrospective studies of myeloma patients from Veterans Administration Hospitals by Morgan and Hammack and by Vix failed to demonstrate a single case among a total of 163 patients who had excretory urography. In our own experience at the Mayo Clinic, we have observed two patients with acute renal failure in a series of 201 patients with multiple myeloma who had this examination during a 10-year period (Myers and Witten).

It is postulated that acute oliguric renal failure results from sudden bilateral intratubular obstruction secondary to precipitation of Bence Jones protein and that there is a direct cause-and-effect relationship between the excretory urogram and the onset of acute renal failure (Leucutia).* It has been suggested that intratubular protein precipitation results either from a direct precipitating effect of urographic medium on urinary proteins

or from a lowered glomerular filtration rate due to dehydration. In vitro studies of the direct precipitating effect of contrast media (Lasser, Lang, and Zawadzki) have shown that protein precipitates sometimes will form when urine is mixed with the older urographic media such as iodopyracet (Diodrast) and sodium acetrizoate (Urokon) but that they will not form in urine mixed with methylglucamine (meglumine) diatrizoate (Renografin) or sodium diatrizoate (Hypaque). Since acute renal failure has been observed after urography with both meglumine and sodium diatrizoate, it appears that the contrast material itself may play only a secondary role or possibly no direct role at all in the genesis of the renal failure. This has led a number of authors to suggest that dehydration from water restriction or vomiting may be the chief cause of acute renal failure in these cases (Morgan and Hammack; Rees and Waugh). Because of the reported cases of acute renal failure with death, Leucutia considered myeloma an absolute contraindication to excretory urography, but the experiences of Morgan and Hammack led them to conclude that their study demonstrated no increased risk of excretory urography for patients with myeloma as compared to the risk for those with other diseases. Vix went even further and stated, "The indications and precautions for intravenous pyelography in multiple myeloma need be no different to those in other diseases with renal impairment." It is our own opinion, however, that a small but definite increased risk of excretory urography for patients with multiple myeloma does exist but that it does not appear to constitute enough of a risk to warrant classifying multiple myeloma as an absolute contraindication to excretory urography. However, excretory urography should be undertaken cautiously and only for well-defined indications in these cases; and, since dehydration may be a problem, as Morgan and Hammack have pointed out, it seems prudent to avoid

---

*The evidence supporting the tubular obstructive theory is not clear-cut, however, since the amount of tubular cast formation as seen at autopsy often does not correlate well with the severity of the renal functional impairment.

both dehydration and the administration of laxatives which will increase dehydration in preparing a patient for excretory urography.

Are Excretory and Retrograde Urography Competitive or Complementary Procedures?

There is still a difference of opinion as to the relative value of excretory and retrograde urography in urologic diagnosis. In some clinical centers excretory urography is used almost routinely in the diagnosis of urologic cases, whereas in others retrograde pyelography still holds the most important place. It will be possible here to describe only the advantages and disadvantages of excretory urography. Each physician must draw his own conclusions as to its worth. At the Mayo Clinic we make very liberal use of excretory urography; hence our statements may be somewhat more enthusiastic than other urologists might think justifiable. Its chief value, of course, lies in the diagnosis of lesions in the upper part of the urinary tract; namely, the kidneys and ureters. Nevertheless, at times it may be of value in diagnosis of lesions of the bladder.

INDICATIONS FOR EXCRETORY UROGRAPHY

The chief advantage of excretory urography is that it permits visualization of the upper part of the urinary tract, including both the renal parenchyma and the collecting system, without cystoscopic examination. Though cystoscopy is by no means a formidable procedure, still it is at best uncomfortable for the patient and should not be done without a definite reason. Important also is the fact that excretory urography accurately depicts the situation as it is; whereas a retrograde pyelogram tends to disturb the urinary tract and yield abnormal physiologic and anatomic findings that may be the result of trauma from ureteral catheterization rather than disease.

By means of excretory urography the kidneys may be visualized without danger of the typical reactions occasionally seen following retrograde pyelography, which consist of pain, colic, fever, and, rarely, an acute cortical infection of a kidney. Such reactions, though seen only occasionally in normal or almost normal kidneys, are encountered more frequently when retrograde medium is injected into a hydronephrotic kidney or in one in which a stone is present that may obstruct the normal drainage of the kidney. In renal tuberculosis the danger always exists of disseminating the infection by means of a retrograde pyelogram. In all of these cases, therefore, an excretory urogram would be the procedure of choice and, even though visualization was not sufficiently good and a subsequent retrograde pyelogram was found necessary, the physician would be aware of the situation before cystoscopy was started and would carry out the procedure in such a manner as to obviate, as far as possible, severe reactions.

There are certain urologic conditions in which catheterization of the ureters is either impossible or possible only with excessive trauma. These are such conditions as marked enlargement of the prostate gland, large tumors of the bladder which involve the regions of the ureteral orifices, extensive tuberculosis of the bladder in which the ureters cannot be identified, and impassable obstructions in the ureter caused by stone, stricture, or anatomic deformity. After transplantation of the ureters to the bowel, excretory urography is the only means of determining the condition of the kidneys.

Use for Infants and Children

Excretory urography is particularly well suited to use in the diagnosis of urologic conditions in children. Although there is no age at which cystoscopic examination is impossible, still it is a rather technical procedure in infants and young children and requires some sort of general anesthetic. Because the most common pathologic change in the urinary tract encountered in childhood is stasis of urine and because excretory urography visualizes the urinary tract best in the presence of stasis, it is in children that excretory urography achieves one of its greatest fields of usefulness. Diagnosis, however, is somewhat hampered by gas in the intestine, as it is almost impossible to secure good preparation of the bowel in children.

Use in Traumatic Lesions of the Urinary Tract

Another field in which excretory urography is almost indispensable is in the recognition of injury of the urinary tract, either from accidents or from surgical procedures. (This subject is fully discussed in Chapter 15, page 1696.)

Use for Patients With Fever

The presence of fever usually offers no contraindication to excretory urography. We have made excretory urograms, when necessary, in the presence of high fever and never have seen any unfavorable reaction because of it.

Demonstration of Anomalies

Before the days of excretory urography, anomalies of the upper part of the urinary tract were frequently missed in urologic investigation, chiefly because they were not suspected. For instance, a duplication of the renal pelvis in which the upper pelvis was hydronephrotic and produced symptoms, might easily have gone unrecognized if the lower pelvis and calyces were of fairly normal size and contour as outlined by a retrograde pyelogram. This was especially true if

there was incomplete duplication of the ureter, the two ureters joining before reaching the bladder so that only one ureteral orifice was present on either side. In such a situation there was nothing in the cystoscopic appearance of the bladder to suggest duplication. Since the advent of excretory urography the incidence of anomalies of the urinary tract has been found to be considerably higher than heretofore had been known. Duplication, ectopia, and fused kidneys are now recognized early in the diagnostic procedure, and repeated cystoscopic examinations in such cases have become quite uncommon (Fig. 1–22).

Excretory Urography as Routine Examination Preliminary to Cystoscopy

Excretory urography is being used more and more as a routine preliminary examination before cystoscopy. A plain film plus an excretory urogram supplies infinitely more information than the plain film alone and is almost as easily and economically obtained. If a urologic problem is of sufficient magnitude to warrant cystoscopy, it is usually desirable or mandatory to know the condition of the upper part of the urinary tract. At the Mayo Clinic we now employ excretory urography in the majority of patients undergoing cystoscopy. This practice greatly expedites cystoscopy, ensures greater accuracy, and requires fewer retrograde pyelograms with their attendant discomfort and febrile reactions. Knowledge of the function of each kidney prior to cystoscopic examination is of inestimable value to the urologist.

The value and convenience of preliminary excretory urography are exemplified well by the case of a patient being investigated for gross hematuria. Here a preliminary excretory urogram is almost imperative. If it is not made and the source of hematuria is not found to be in the bladder, it may be necessary to

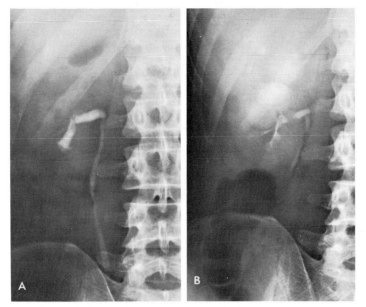

Figure 1–22. **A,** *Retrograde pyelogram.* Only pelvis and lower calyx are outlined. No medium enters middle and upper calyces. **Stones** are included in pelvis. **B,** *Excretory urogram.* Visualizes marked dilatation of upper and middle calyces, which have been obstructed by stones in pelvis. In this case excretory urography gives more information than retrograde pyelography.

make bilateral pyelograms or repeat the cystoscopy later to make a retrograde pyelogram. In such a case, even though the excretory urogram is poor, usually one kidney is sufficiently visualized to exclude it as a source of the hematuria so that only one retrograde pyelogram is necessary. Again, if an excretory urogram has been taken prior to cystoscopy, one will not make the mistake that is occasionally made of inadvertently injecting retrograde medium into a hydronephrotic kidney or above a point of obstruction.

DISADVANTAGES OF EXCRETORY UROGRAPHY

The disadvantages of excretory urography are chiefly those related to potential reaction to the contrast agent and to incomplete visualization of the urinary collecting system. The problem of reactions to contrast agents has been discussed, but it should be emphasized that indiscriminate use of this potentially hazardous examination should be avoided and that it should be ordered only when clearly indicated. Incomplete filling of the pelvis and calyces is occasionally a problem even with the use of large doses of contrast medium and ureteral compression, but it is not nearly so much of a problem as previously. When the renal pelvis, calyces, or ureter is incompletely demonstrated it is often necessary to supplement the examination by means of retrograde pyelography.

One of the greatest dangers in excretory urography is the tendency of the physician to guess at a diagnosis when interpreting a poor excretory urogram which does not satisfactorily visualize the urinary tract. It is extremely important to avoid such a habit, or the excretory urogram will fall into disrepute. When a retrograde urogram is necessary for accurate diagnosis, it should be made without hesitation.

CONTRAINDICATIONS AND DISADVANTAGES OF RETROGRADE UROGRAPHY

The chief disadvantages arise because of the procedure involved in administration of the medium. The necessity of a cystoscopic examination and catheterization of the ureters involves a procedure which is uncomfortable or painful to the patient and may be followed by temporary discomfort or a distinct reaction. The introduction of a catheter into a ureter is a traumatic procedure, no matter how carefully done, and may in itself initiate a spasm in the calyces, pelvis, or ureter which will give rise to a renal colic after removal of the catheter. The introduction of any medium into the renal pelvis may be irritating. In the days when sodium iodide was used as a retrograde medium, postpyelographic reactions were common and many patients required hospitalization for 24 to 48 hours afterward. Since urologists have begun using the organic iodides of the modern contrast media, the incidence of postpyelographic reactions has been sharply reduced. This subject has been more fully discussed previously under the subject of technique in making retrograde pyelograms. It is inadvisable to make retrograde pyelograms in the presence of urinary stasis or renal insufficiency. It is inadvisable to inject contrast medium above a point of obstruction such as a ureteral calculus (see Chapter 6). In such cases severe reactions may be encountered, varying from acute infection of the renal cortex accompanied by chills and fever to total anuria.

The question of the advisability of making *bilateral retrograde pyelograms* at one sitting has been discussed for years. There are those in the profession who do not hesitate to perform such a procedure in almost any type of case. The consensus, however, is that this should be done only when it seems absolutely necessary and only when the kidneys are expected to be in reasonably good condition. Since modern contrast media have been used in retrograde urography, the contraindications to making bilateral pyelograms at one sitting have become somewhat less. It is good insurance to leave the ureteral catheters in place for a period of at least 30 minutes after bilateral pyelograms have been made, in order to guarantee the complete evacuation of the contrast medium from the renal pelves and to minimize postpyelographic reactions.

Drip-Infusion Urography

Intravenous infusion of a large volume of dilute urographic contrast material to produce dense opacification of the renal parenchyma and complete filling of the urinary collecting apparatus is known as drip-infusion urography. This technique was first conceived of by Dr. H. H. Forsythe Winchell and was first used by him and by Dr. J. A. Arata both of whom were at that time radiologists at the US Army Hospital, Nurnberg, Germany (Arata). In 1964, Dr. Bernard Schencker published an account of the technique and subsequently it came into widespread use, both as a primary method of urography and as a supplement to conventional urography in difficult cases.

TECHNIQUE

According to Schencker (1964; 1966), the drip-infusion pyelogram achieves its excellence by virtue of hydration, diuresis, and complete filling of the urinary tract. In his original description, Schencker recommended a dose of 1 ml/lb of body weight of 50% sodium diatrizoate (Hypaque) mixed with 1 ml/lb of 5% dextrose in water. A minimal adult dose of 300 ml of this solution was suggested. Subsequently he has recommended a dose of 250 ml for most patients. This solution is administered by rapid drip (unrestricted) through an 18-gauge needle. The time of infusion is not critical, but usually it is 6 to 10 minutes. Films are made at the end of infusion, when opacification of the renal parenchyma is optimal. Subsequent films, made after 5 to 30 minutes, demonstrate the filled and distended collecting system, with maximal filling after 20 to 30 minutes. The patient is not dehydrated before the examination, since hydration favors diuresis. Tomography, with films made at various levels through the kidney, during the period of greatest parenchymal opacification has been widely used to supplement the routine films obtained with this technique (Pratt and White; Schencker, 1964; Wendth).

While this technique can be used for routine urography, most find that it is more practical to reserve it for use in selected difficult or problem cases. We have found it to be of greatest value if used in conjunction with tomography, in order that both the renal parenchyma and the renal collecting system can be fully demonstrated without interference from other abdominal soft-tissue and bowel shadows. Schencker pointed out that infusion urography is used most frequently after inadequate standard excretory urography, when a repeat double dose or retrograde study would otherwise be considered (Figs. 1-23, 1-24, and 1-25). The technique also has proved valuable in demonstrating the ureters when retrograde pyelography would otherwise be necessary, in studying patients with severely depressed renal function (Figs. 1-26 and 1-27), and in detecting adrenal tumors (see discussion of adrenal tumors, Chapter 10).

A number of authors—including Schencker, Marcure, and Moody; Neal, Howell, and Lester; and Genereux—have advocated use of this technique as a substitute for conventional nephrotomography done by the bolus technique (see discussion of nephrotomography below) for differential diagnosis of renal cyst and renal tumor. In our experience, the fact that the renal vasculature is not demonstrated by this technique substantially increases the chance that tumor will be misdiagnosed as cyst. The chance for error is greatest in the case of tumors (usually renal carcinomas of the dark cell type) which are well circumscribed and relatively small and from which the urographic medium is rapidly "washed out," leaving a mass which appears avascular on the nephrogram (Fig. 1-28). In these cases conventional "bolus type" nephrotomography or renal arteriography will clearly demonstrate the true character of the lesion whereas the infusion technique will not.

Excretory Urography as a Test of Renal Function

The excretion of urographic contrast agents is a physiologic process which depends, in the broadest terms, on the functional status of the kidney. This fact has led to a strong tendency among physicians to equate early appearance of medium and dense opacification of the renal pelvis with good renal function. As urographic techniques have improved and as more accurate measures of renal function have become available to the clinician, it has become clear that ordinary urography is not a reliable test for either the presence or the severity of renal functional impairment (Hoffman and Grayhack; MacEwan, Dunbar, and Nogrady; Schwartz, Hurwit, and Ettinger). A gross reduction in renal function resulting from obstruction, renal vascular insufficiency, or severe parenchymal disease is of course accompanied by delayed appearance of medium and poor opacification of the renal collecting system in most cases and is evident as a gross abnormality on the films. Even in these severe cases, however, only a qualitative and not a quantitative estimate of renal function is possible. In the presence of less advanced disease, the ordinary excretory urogram often fails to demonstrate either a delay in appearance or poor concentration of medium and the presence of mild or moderately severe functional impairment may not be sus-

(*Text continued on page 50.*)

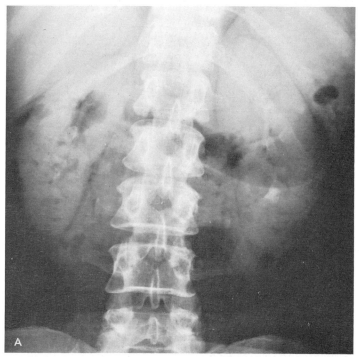
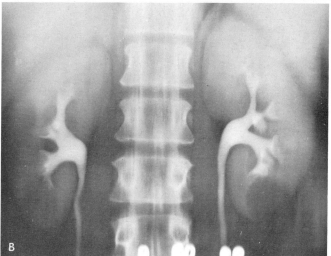

Figure 1–23. Value of drip-infusion urogram with tomogram. **A,** *Excretory urogram.* Poor visualization of renal pelvis and calyces. **B,** *Drip-infusion urogram with tomogram.* Excellent visualization of renal parenchyma and collecting system. Previously unsuspected mass (**simple cyst**) is present in lower pole of left kidney.

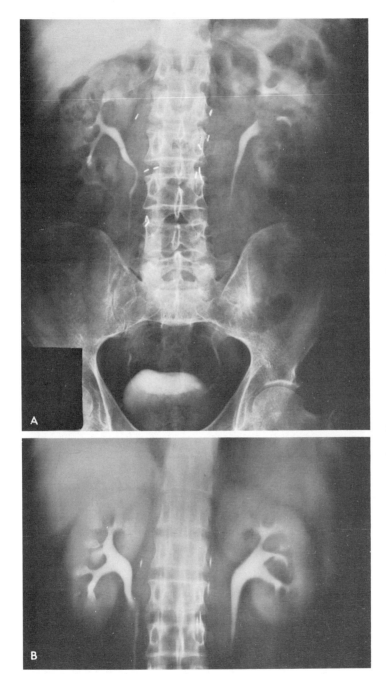

Figure 1–24.   Value of drip-infusion urogram with tomogram. **A,** *Excretory urogram.* Incomplete filling of pelvis and calyces of left kidney. Renal outlines are obscured. **B,** *Drip-infusion urogram with tomography.* Kidneys are well shown. **Small mass** distorts middle calyx on left.

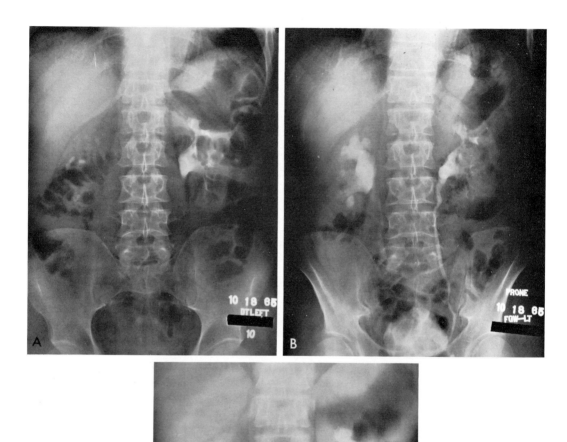

Figure 1–25. Value of drip-infusion urogram with tomogram. A, *Excretory urogram.* Renal outlines are obscured and collecting system is poorly visualized. B, *Drip-infusion urogram.* Renal collecting system is filled more completely, but anatomic detail is still not completely demonstrated. C, *Drip infusion with tomography.* Renal parenchyma and collecting system are well demonstrated. **Pyelonephritis with renal atrophy and pyelocalcycectasis** is present on right and previously unsuspected **nonopaque calculus** is present in renal pelvis.

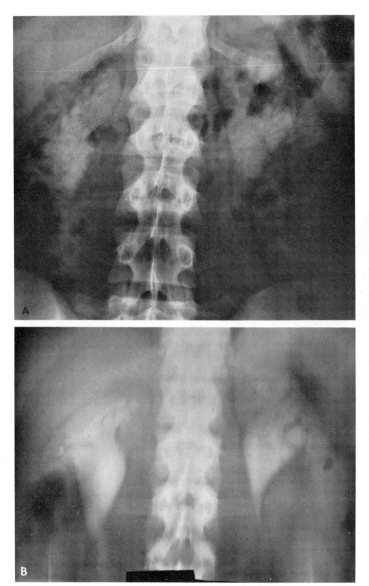

Figure 1–26. Value of drip-infusion urogram with renal insufficiency. *Drip-infusion urogram.* **Renal insufficiency.** (Serum creatinine 4.9 mg/100 ml; blood urea 105.) **A,** *Plain film.* Renal outlines and collecting system are poorly visualized and diagnosis is not possible. **B,** *Tomogram after drip infusion.* Kidneys are well demonstrated. Parenchyma is atrophic and calyces are blunted as result of **pyelonephritis.**

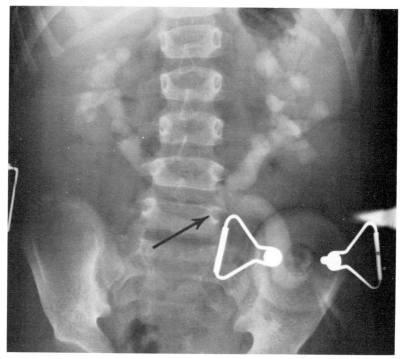

Figure 1–27. *Drip-infusion urogram* of child with **urinary diversion.** (Serum creatinine 2.15 mg/100 ml; blood urea 98.) Both **ureteroureterostomy** (*arrow*) and **cutaneous ureterostomy** are present and are well demonstrated by this technique.

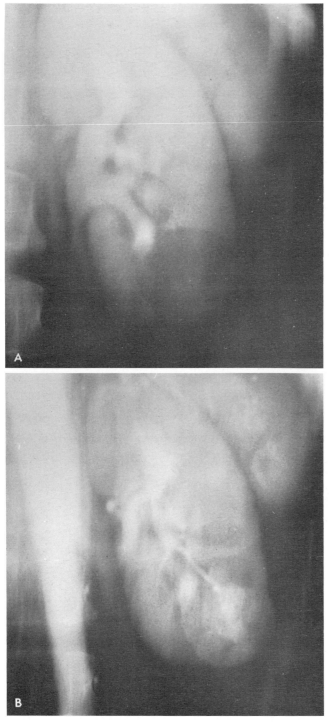

Figure 1–28. Example of possible error from drip-infusion type nephrotomogram. Hypernephroma simulating cyst. *Nephrotomograms.* **A**, *Nephrographic phase*, corresponding to nephrogram obtained by drip infusion. Mass simulates simple cyst. It appears avascular and is sharply circumscribed. **B**, *Arterial phase.* Solid, vascular character of mass is obvious, but would not have been suspected without arterial-phase films.

pected. With the larger doses of contrast medium (diatrizoates and iothalamates) that are now commonly used in excretory urography even severely depressed renal function may be masked because of dense opacification of the kidney (Cattell and associates; Fulton, Witten, and Wagoner; Sherwood and associates). (See Figs. 1-26 and 1-27.) The problem is further complicated by artifacts and technically inadequate examinations which seem to show differences in concentration and rate of excretion when in fact none are present. Among these, variations in shape, size, and position of the collecting system of the two kidneys, peristaltic emptying of one side before the other, overlying gas and fecal material, and examination of patients in a hydrated or partially hydrated state are leading causes of erroneous diagnoses of depressed function in one or both kidneys.

Part of the emphasis on excretory urography as a test of renal function (Edling and associates; Wigh, Anthony, and Grant) results from the need for reliable screening tests to help identify patients who have renal artery stenosis causative of hypertension. Two modifications of excretory urographic technique have been developed (minute-sequence urography and the urea-washout test). Both are qualitative tests and are useful primarily for identification of patients with unilateral disease.

MINUTE-SEQUENCE UROGRAPHY (RAPID-SEQUENCE PYELOGRAM)

Minute-sequence urography has been shown by Maxwell, Gonick, Wiita, and Kaufman as well as others to be a useful and practical adjunct to other clinical and laboratory data for evaluation of patients under study for suspected unilateral renal artery stenosis of functional significance. *The test is based on the fact that the rate of accumulation of contrast me-*

dium in the calyces and pelvis is reduced in renal ischemia severe enough to cause hypertension as a result of a reduction in the glomerular filtration rate. The minute-sequence urogram makes it possible to compare this parameter of function in the two kidneys, and if a unilateral delay is seen (in the absence of obstruction or renal parenchymal disease) it is strong evidence for functionally significant renal artery stenosis (Fig. 1-29) (Witten and associates). Unfortunately, this simple test has not proved to be sufficiently sensitive to detect functionally significant unilateral renal artery stenosis in one third or more of the cases and it is of no value in bilateral disease. The technique is merely an extension of conventional urography, the differences being that the dose of contrast medium is injected rapidly (20 seconds or less) and carefully timed films are made at 1, 2, 3, 4, and 5 minutes after injection. No ureteral compression is used. Some advocate a film at 30 seconds in an attempt to show a decreased nephrogram on the diseased side, but we have never been impressed with the value of this film. *In the large proportion of cases, the 2- or the 3-minute film shows the delay in appearance of medium to best advantage.*

UREA-WASHOUT TEST

The pyelogram-urea-washout test was proposed by Amplatz in 1962 as a simplified radiologic version of the split renal function test. It is based on the following oversimplified physiologic considerations (Schreiber and associates; Staab and associates): A hemodynamically significant renal artery stenosis results in a diminished pulse pressure downstream to the area of constriction, producing a decreased blood flow to the renal parenchyma. Partially as a result of this abnormality, the diseased kidney reabsorbs water and sodium at a more rapid rate than the opposite uninvolved kid-

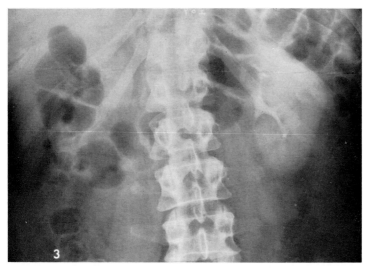

Figure 1–29. *Excretory urogram.* **Positive minute sequence study for hypertension.** Three minutes after injection contrast medium is seen in pelvis and calyces on left but not on right. This delay in appearance suggests **possible renal artery stenosis** on right. (From Witten, D. M., Hunt, J. C., Sheps, S. G., Greene, L. F., and Utz, D. C.)

ney. Since the presently available urographic contrast agents (diatrizoates and iothalamates) are filtered by the glomeruli and not reabsorbed by the tubules (at least to any significant degree), reabsorption of water on the diseased side results in hyperconcentration of contrast medium in this kidney. The intravenous infusion of urea produces a sharp diuresis which enhances the hyperconcentration effect so that **the side with arterial stenosis retains the contrast material and remains visible while the contrast material in the normal side becomes diluted and is "washed out."** The same effect can be obtained by diuresis with a nonreabsorbable osmotic diuretic such as mannitol (Witten and associates) (Fig. 1–30).

The technique as described by Staab, Amplatz, Stejskal, and Loken is as follows:

The routine intravenous pyelogram preparation and scout film are obtained. No compression is used. Fifty c.c. of 75 per cent sodium diatrizoate [Hypaque] are then injected rapidly and intravenously into a Y-tubing, which at one end has 500 c.c. of 8 per cent [urea in] saline. The routine fast intravenous pyelogram films are taken at 30 seconds, 1, 2, 3, 5, and 10 minutes.

The three-minute film is developed and inspected. If equal concentration in both collecting systems has resulted, then the **ureasaline mixture** is allowed to run wide open. The 5 and 10-minute films serve as a baseline. Usually the 500 c.c. take from 8 to 10 minutes to infuse. During this infusion five films are obtained, exposed every three minutes.

This test has been considered to be a valuable adjunct by Staab and his associates and by Schreiber and his associates, but Levitt, Amplatz, and Loken have recently pointed out that ureawashout tests and split renal function tests do not necessarily give identical results and that, in their hands, neither is particularly reliable in predicting surgical response. They found the urea-washout test was correct more often than was the split renal function test, but even so it was correct in only 11 of 17 cases (65%). Thus it appears that these special urographic tests of renal function (minute-sequence urography and ureawashout test) may be useful adjuncts to diagnosis when they are positive but that they cannot be relied upon as the sole

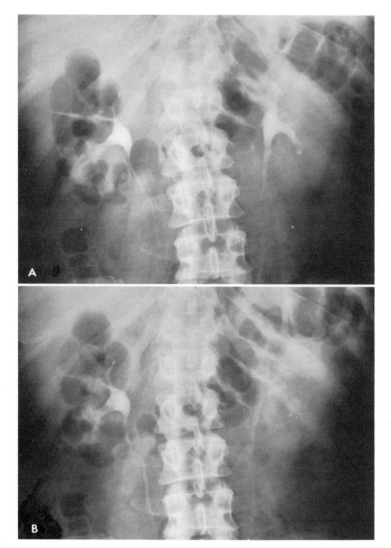

Figure 1–30. *Excretory urograms.* **Positive "mannitol washout" study for hypertension of possible reno-vascular origin. A,** Appearance just before start of infusion of osmotic diuretic (mannitol). Renal pelvis and calyces of both kidneys are well opacified. **B,** Appearance 10 minutes after start of infusion of diuretic. Contrast medium is retained on right where renal artery stenosis is present but has "washed out" from normal left kidney. (From Witten, D. M., Hunt, J. C., Sheps, S. G., Greene, L. F., and Utz, D. C.)

indicators of either the presence or absence of curable renovascular hypertension.

TOMOGRAPHY; NEPHROGRAPHY; NEPHROTOMOGRAPHY

Tomography

Tomography is a roentgenographic technique by which the roentgenologist is able to focus on any plane of the body parallel to the platform of the x-ray table on which the patient is lying. By adjustment of the roentgenographic apparatus the desired level comes into focus, and an exposure made at this level will show sharply defined structures at that particular plane in the body, whereas structures in other planes will be blurred and not well visualized.

The principle of tomography was first worked out in the United States by Kieffer in 1928, and he made a working model of the apparatus in 1929. He stated that, unknown to him at the time, three Frenchmen, Bage and Portes and Chausse, had developed and obtained French patents for a similar apparatus in 1922. Kieffer published his work in 1938. In the same year Moore described his results with tomography and gave Kieffer credit for its development. In Kieffer's 1938 paper he mentioned contributions of several other workers, namely, Vallebona in 1930, Bartelink in 1933, Ziedses des Plantes in 1932 and 1934, and Grossmann, and Chaoul in 1935. Andrews, in 1936, gave a historical discussion of this subject.

Kieffer described the principle of tomography as follows:

...the tube and film move during exposure in such a way that the roentgenographic shadow of a selected plane in a body remains stationary on the moving film while the shadows of all other planes have a relative displacement on the film, and are therefore blurred to varying amounts, depending mainly on the distance of such planes from the one selected.

Tomography first gained favor in the localization of lesions of the lungs (Fig. 1–31*A* and *B*). It now is especially helpful in investigation of the retroperitoneal region because it eliminates overlying shadows of gas and fecal material in the bowel and permits an unobstructed view of the plane in question. Exposures at different planes will show a soft tissue mass in several subsequent "cuts," and from these its position, relation to known landmarks in the body, and size may be determined.

Tomograms are usually made with the patient in the supine position on the x-ray table. With the patient lying supine, the kidney is usually in focus in planes between 5 and 12 cm above the level of the table. Tomography thus will locate an abdominal or retroperitoneal mass precisely. It will indicate not only whether it originates from the kidney (Burns) but also whether its main extension is on the ventral, dorsal, medial, or lateral aspect of the kidney. A suprarenal mass may be identified likewise.

Tomography can be easily combined with other techniques of examination (Hinman, Steinbach, and Forsham). Excretory urograms may gain remarkably in contrast when combined with tomography. The nephrographic phase in excretory urograms combined with this method will show a particularly clear outline of the kidney against a darkened background (Andersen; Pendergrass). For this purpose it has been combined with renal arteriography and retroperitoneal gas insufflation (see Fig. 1–46). It should be noted that both kidneys do not always lie at the same level, so that one kidney may be in focus while the other is not. The tomographic outlining of poorly defined shadows in the thorax may be of importance in the diagnosis of metastatic pulmonary disease secondary to renal, testicular, prostatic, vesical, and other neoplasms of urologic interest.

Nephrography (the Nephrogram)

In 1932 Wesson and Fulmer first described opacification of the renal parenchyma by means of excretory urography performed during an attack of renal colic. In 1935 Wilcox described the same phenomenon. In 1947 Weens and Florence described its occurrence in 10 of a series of 23 patients having renal colic. They tried to reproduce the phenomenon by artificially obstructing the ureters with balloon-tipped ureteral catheters. Opacification of the renal parenchyma during aortography was described in 1938 and 1939 by Steinberg and Robb. Opacification of the renal parenchyma was called a *nephrogram*. Wall and Rose in 1951 and Detar and Harris in 1954 made early observations.

In 1951 Weens and colleagues produced nephrograms by means of the rapid (1 to 2 seconds) intravenous injection of 50 ml of 70% solution of Diodrast through a large (12-gauge) needle. Their first film was exposed 6 seconds after the completion of injection. Several films were made at short intervals thereafter. They stated that their best films were usually obtained between 15 and 18 seconds after injection as compared with 15 to 30 minutes when using the technique of artificial ureteral obstruction combined with routine excretory urography.

PHYSIOLOGIC PRINCIPLES OF THE NEPHROGRAM

Weens and colleagues explained the nephrogram as "the presence of dye in the finer ramifications of the tubular system."

In 1959 Edling and Helander carried out some ingenious experiments on dogs in an effort to explain the mechanics of the nephrogram. They injected diprotrizoate (Miokon) into the renal artery on one side and thorium dioxide (which is not excreted by the kidney) into the renal artery on the other side. They noted that at 3½ seconds after injection the density of the parenchyma of both kidneys had increased; thereafter the density of the kidney receiving the thorium decreased whereas that of the other kidney increased for 27 seconds. After this time the density of the cortex diminished but that of the pyramids increased. At 45 seconds the apices of the pyramids were well shown. At 69 seconds the density of the entire renal parenchyma had returned to normal. They concluded that the nephrographic effect starts with the contrast filling of the intrarenal arteries but in the main is dependent on filtration and excretion of the medium by both the glomeruli and tubules. They added that tubular cells also concentrate the contrast medium after which it diffuses back into the veins. The 45-second stage of opacification is mainly from the contrast medium in the collecting tubules of the pyramids.

Intravenous Nephrotomography (the Nephrotomogram)

In 1954 Evans and colleagues combined tomography and nephrography and coined the word *nephrotomography*. At present many urologists (Post and Southwood) consider intravenous nephrotomography the primary method for use in the diagnosis of mass lesions of the renal parenchyma, especially for differentiation of cyst and tumor. It should be pointed out that a nephrotomogram also may be made an adjunct of an aortogram simply by exposing films during the "nephrographic phase" and employing the tomographic apparatus. Although the films exposed during the vascular phase of the aortogram would be considerably superior in outlining the renal vessels, still the procedure is too formidable to employ in routine diagnosis when a simpler technical procedure such as intravenous nephrotomography will provide adequate information for diagnosis. Figures 1-32 and 1-33 illustrate the excellent manner in which the renal parenchyma can be opacified by intravenous nephrotomography. It is also apparent from these illustrations that the renal vessels are not too well outlined. For this reason the method is not reliable enough for diagnosis of lesions and anomalies of the renal artery and its branches. Indications for nephrotomography are thus mainly limited to preoperative differentiation of renal masses and demonstration of damage to the renal parenchyma from infarcts, infection, and so forth (see Chapter 7). Evans has reported that simple cyst or tumor may be diagnosed by this method with 90% to 95% accuracy (Fig. 1-34). In our experience, diagnostic accuracy has been very high in cases where the renal anatomy is well visualized and the characteristics of the lesion are well demonstrated on the nephrotomogram. We find, however, that in approximately 20% of the cases this technique does not demonstrate the lesion with enough clarity for diagnosis. When this occurs, we recommend further study by renal arteriography, percutaneous needle puncture of the mass, or exploration for definitive diagnosis.

TECHNIQUE

With the patient lying supine on the x-ray table, preliminary renal tomograms are made, and the desired level of tomography is determined. A 12-gauge Robb-Steinberg needle or a 13-gauge angiographic needle is inserted into the antecubital vein of the left or right arm, and 5 ml of 20% dehydrocholic acid (Decholin) is injected intravenously to determine the arm-to-tongue circulation time. Usually the patient will experience the bitter taste on his tongue in 10 to 14 seconds after injection. For all practical purposes the arm-to-tongue circulation time is identical to the arm-to-kidney circulation time.

After the circulation time is measured, an initial (loading) dose of 30 ml of a 50% solution of sodium diatrizoate (Hypaque) is injected through the needle in the antecubital vein. This is given to increase the nephrographic density and also to provide an outline of the collecting system (thus providing an excretory urogram). About 5 minutes later, 50 to 80 ml of a 90% solution of Hypaque is injected as rapidly as possible by hand into the vein. The first film is exposed at the predetermined end of the circulation time. If properly timed this film should show the renal artery and its main branches as well as the kidneys, all of which are opacified in what is termed the *arterial phase.* Immediately thereafter, during the period of intense nephrographic blush known as the *nephrographic phase,* additional films spaced 1 cm apart are made through the entire thickness of both kidneys to demonstrate the renal parenchyma and any lesion present. The complete series of films should be exposed within 60 to 90 seconds. The number of "cuts" will vary in individual cases depending on the problem. Precise timing of serial exposures is essential for good results.

INTERPRETATION OF FILMS

In the dense opacification of the renal parenchyma a *solitary cyst* will stand out as a radiolucent dark rounded shadow almost completely avascular (Fig. 1-34; see also Chapter 9). Its margins are sharply defined and perhaps even somewhat accentuated by the surrounding opacified parenchyma. This is in contrast to renal tumors, whose density is usually greater than that of the normal parenchyma; ab-

---

*At the Mayo Clinic we are now using a tomographic multileaf cassette with seven films separated from each other by 1 cm. All seven are exposed at the same instant so that seven "cuts," 1 cm apart, are obtained of the arterial phase (Witten, Greene, and Emmett).

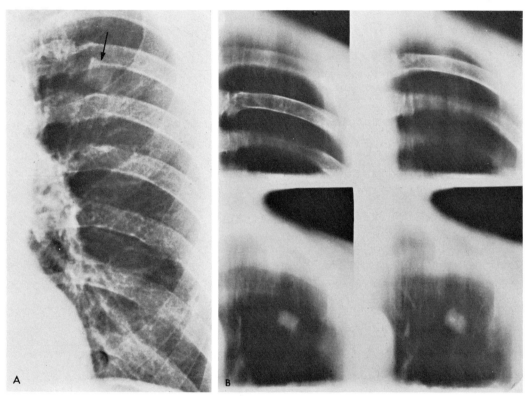

Figure 1–31. **A,** Thorax of 56-year-old man who proved to have **hypernephroma of left kidney.** Poorly defined shadow (*arrow*) in second intercostal space on left suggests possible metastatic lesion. **B,** *Tomogram* of left upper thoracic area. Shadow is well defined in two "cuts" as **definite metastatic nodule.** (Courtesy of Dr. H. W. ten Cate.)

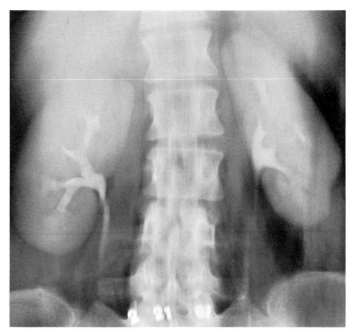

Figure 1–32. *Nephrotomogram, nephrographic phase.* Irregularity of lateral border of left kidney. Probably remains of **fetal lobulation.**

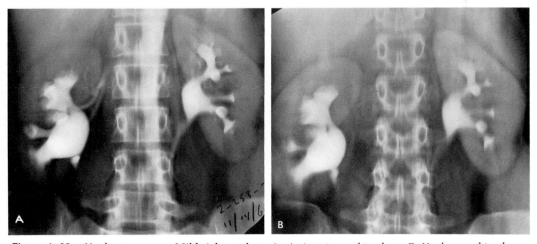

Figure 1–33. *Nephrotomogram.* **Mild right pyelectasis. A,** *Arteriographic phase.* **B,** *Nephrographic phase.*

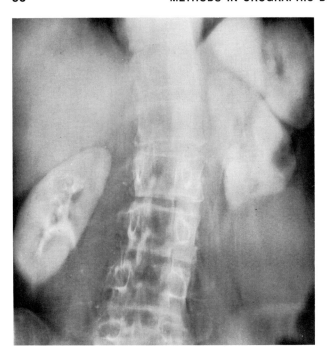

Figure 1–34. *Nephrotomogram.* Large simple cyst at lower pole of left kidney. Note excellent opacification of liver and spleen as well as kidneys. Cyst is radiolucent.

normal vascularization is also seen ("puddling," tumor staining, and so forth). Central necrosis in a tumor reduces vascularity and density. It is characterized by a blotchy and irregular appearance that is not easily confused with the translucency of a renal cyst. (See Chapters 9 and 10 for a more complete discussion.) At the present writing we have examined more than 4,000 patients by this technique with no mortality and only one serious reaction—acute laryngospasm precipitated by the injection of dehydrocholic acid (Decholin) for determination of the circulation time.

CYSTOGRAPHY AND CYSTOURETHROGRAPHY

The Cystogram

Roentgenographic visualization of the urinary bladder by means of contrast medium is called *cystography*. During excretory urography sufficient contrast medium often is excreted to produce an *excretory cystogram*. Although the quality of the excretory cystogram is usually not good enough to permit accurate diagnosis, it is surprising how much preliminary information can be gained from such films. Excretory cystourethrograms of fairly good quality can be made during the act of voiding as part of the excretory urographic study. Finally, a postvoiding film may permit a rough estimate of the amount of residual urine present. Excretory cystograms, owing to incomplete filling, however, are misinterpreted easily, and one should hesitate to express a definite opinion from such films only.

Endoscopic examination of the bladder and urethra is the most reliable method of confirming or excluding the presence of suspected disease of the lower part of the urinary tract. Since some diseases and pathologic conditions are extremely difficult to diagnose at the time of cystoscopy (Marion), retrograde urographic studies are indicated in such cases.

Retrograde cystograms are usually

more reliable than excretory cystograms. They can be made by filling the bladder with a radiopaque medium, air, or a combination of both through a urethral catheter. For *retrograde cystourethrograms* both bladder and urethra are filled to obtain an outline of both structures. A *micturition cystourethrogram* will result if, after filling of the bladder with contrast medium, the patient voids and a film is exposed during voiding.

Cystograms and cystourethrograms are particularly important in children. Most urologists perform these tests routinely in their pediatric practice since they have learned how often pathologic lesions and vesical and ureteral dysfunction may be detected by this means. For instance, recurrent attacks of urinary infection or other urologic signs and symptoms in children may be caused by such conditions as lower urinary tract obstruction (vesical neck hypertrophy, congenital urethral valves, and others) and vesicoureteral reflux, which may be missed during cystoscopy but easily recognized with a cystourethrogram. As a matter of fact, cystourethrography is the only method which will demonstrate these conditions.

TECHNIQUE OF CYSTOGRAPHY

The Simple Retrograde Cystogram

The simple retrograde cystogram is made as follows. The patient is encouraged to empty his bladder as completely as possible. He is then put on the x-ray table in the supine position. The glans penis and external meatus are cleaned as they usually are for catheterization. A 16- or 18-F straight or coudé catheter is inserted, and the bladder is evacuated. The residual urine is measured. A plain film of the area from the fifth lumbar vertebra to below the symphysis pubis is exposed.

From 150 to 200 ml of contrast medium* is instilled in the bladder through the catheter, and the catheter is removed. No attempt is made to overdistend the bladder, but it is filled, within the limits of comfort to the patient.

The safest way to introduce contrast medium into the bladder is by gravity. The supply of contrast medium* is held 20 to 30 inches (50 to 76 cm) above the bladder and is allowed to flow in through the catheter until the flow ceases. The first film provides an anteroposterior view. A second and a third exposure are made with the patient in the left and right semilateral or oblique positions. Films exposed in these positions will show a profile of the bladder from either side. They are of advantage in distinguishing diverticula and filling defects from vesical neoplasms in almost any location.

For the last film, made after the patient has emptied his bladder as completely as possible, an anteroposterior projection is used. If he is unable to void, the bladder is evacuated by catheter. This film will show the collapsed bladder (any remaining contrast medium) and any vesical diverticula observed in the first films. The amount of retention in diverticula can be estimated from it also. Filling defects caused by neoplasms may be delineated after the bladder has been emptied, so that comparison of the films showing the emptied bladder with those showing the filled bladder may demonstrate the degree of fixation of the vesical wall. If the main objective of retrograde cystography is to show vesicoureteral reflux, the first exposure in the anteroposterior projection should be made on a 14 by 17 inch (36 by 46 cm) film to include both ureters and kidneys.

---

*A 10% to 30% solution of any of the diiodinated or triiodinated compounds used for excretory urography is satisfactory. (See discussion of contrast media.)

Semilateral or Oblique Positions. For exposures with the patient in the right oblique or semilateral position, the patient, having the right hip on the table, is tilted with the top of the table to an angle of 45°. The right hip is flexed with the thigh on the abdomen to almost 90° while the left leg is extended (see Fig. 1–39). For the left oblique exposures the position is reversed.

The Air Cystogram

Air may be introduced into the bladder in an amount of 100 to 200 ml by catheter with a syringe. The air casts a radiolucent negative shadow that outlines the bladder almost as distinctly as the positive shadow obtained from contrast medium. Air cystograms are usually not as diagnostically satisfactory as cystograms made with contrast medium, since gas shadows from intestinal contents may be difficult to distinguish from areas of diminished density resulting from the air in the bladder. Vesical tumors sometimes cause a soft-tissue shadow of sufficient density to stand out in contrast to the negative air shadow. After injury, air cystography is sometimes employed. The demonstration of air under the diaphragm in such films is evidence of intraperitoneal rupture of the bladder if intestinal injury has been excluded.

Fatal air embolism has been described as a complication of air cystography.

The Polycystogram and Superimposition Cystography

Sometimes in cases of vesical neoplasm or of apparent involvement of the bladder by a pathologic process originating from neighboring organs, cystography can be of help in determining the degree of fixation of the bladder against adjacent structures. For this purpose either a polycystogram or a superimposition cystogram (Cobb and An-

derson) may be useful.* The technique of polycystography involves the making of three exposures on one film in the anteroposterior projection, each exposure being one third of the normal exposure time. The bladder is filled with 200 ml of contrast medium, and the first exposure is made with one third of the usual exposure time. About 120 ml of contrast medium is evacuated through the catheter, and a second exposure (again for one third of the normal exposure time) is made without changing the cassette. The last exposure (again for only one third of the usual exposure time) is made after another 50 ml of contrast medium has been evacuated by the catheter. In this way the film is exposed three times and shows the vesical outline three times with different degrees of filling (Figs. 1–35 and 1–36).

The technique of superimposition cystography as described by Cobb and Anderson involves, like the polycystogram, the making of multiple exposures on one film. A 16-F Foley catheter is passed into the bladder, the bladder is emptied, and the balloon is inflated. After a plain film has been taken, the cassette is changed and 30 ml of 50% sodium diatrizoate, or other suitable contrast material, is instilled into the bladder. At the end of maximal expiration a film exposure is made. Without changing the cassette additional exposures are made after instillation of 30, 40, and 50 ml of sterile saline. The bladder is then emptied, the Foley catheter is removed, and the single film is developed. (See also Figs. 10–313, 10–314, and 10–315.)

If the vesical wall in one region is fixed to surrounding tissues, the three outlines are not concentric but converge toward the area of fixation. In this way the polycystogram may be helpful in

---

*See also (1) "Double Contrast Cystograms" and (2) "Combined Perivesical Insufflation of Oxygen and CO_2 Cystograms" under discussion of Bladder Tumors, Chapter 10, pages 1257–1259.

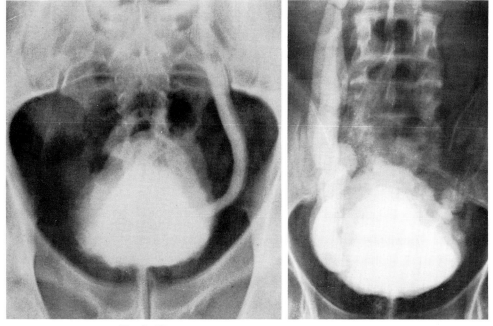

Fig. 1–35   **Fig. 1–36**

Figure 1–35. *Polycystogram* of man, 56 years of age, with **transitional cell epithelioma of bladder wall** on the right side. *Retrograde cystogram with three exposures on one film,* each for one third of usual exposure time with 200, 80, and 30 ml of contrast medium, respectively, in bladder. Note concentricity of outlines as evidence of noninfiltrating tumor. **Bilateral vesicoureteral reflux,** particularly on the left side. (Courtesy of Dr. H. W. ten Cate.)

Figure 1–36. *Polycystogram* of man, 75 years of age, with **prostatic hypertrophy and vesical tumor.** Tumor on right side of bladder wall is shown by concentric outlines. Bladder wall in area of tumor is not fixed. Note **right vesicoureteral reflux and small vesical diverticulum on left.** (Courtesy of Dr. H. W. ten Cate.)

planning a therapeutic program since marked fixation to neighboring structures could be considered a sign of inoperability of a vesical neoplasm.

Delayed Cystogram

Suspected vesicoureteral reflux is an important indication for retrograde cystography. Curiously enough, the first film exposed immediately after filling the bladder with opaque medium does not always demonstrate reflux. Stewart (1953; 1955) showed that reflux can be demonstrated in one or two films of a series of cystographic exposures whereas it may not be apparent in earlier or later films in the same series. He called attention to the value of delayed cystograms for dem-

onstration of vesicoureteral reflux particularly in children. Bunge (1953; 1954) and St. Martin, Campbell, and Pesquier confirmed his findings.

To make a delayed cystogram, the bladder is emptied by catheter and contrast medium is introduced by gravity. The dose is 30 to 120 ml for children and 120 to 240 ml for adults. Contrast medium may be left in the bladder for as long as 3 hours, if necessary, to demonstrate the reflux. One film is exposed immediately after instillation; other films are exposed at 15 to 30-minute intervals. The bladder should not be overdistended. Best results are obtained when the bladder is filled only to a degree compatible with comfort. Recognition of vesicoureteral reflux is of great importance both in children and adults. Delayed cystography is a necessity in the detection of reflux because excretory urography and cystoscopy may be misleading and the diagnosis may be missed without the evidence from the delayed cystogram.

The Triple-Voiding Cystogram

The technique of triple-voiding cystography was described first by Lattimer, Dean, and Furey for use in the diagnosis of residual urine and vesicoureteral reflux in children. Voiding in three installments often permits better emptying of a large atonic bladder than one simple micturition does. In order to verify the beneficial results of the triple-voiding technique films may be made after each voiding, the bladder initially having been filled with contrast medium. This series of films is called "the triple-voiding cystogram."

The patient's bladder is emptied by catheter then filled with contrast medium by gravity through the catheter according to the standard Columbia University cystographic technique (Dean, Lattimer, and McCoy), that is, the reservoir containing contrast medium is held exactly 24 inches (61 cm) above the symphysis pubis; a dilute solution of neomycin and contrast medium is allowed to drip in through the catheter at a rate of 120 drops/min until inflow ceases. One film is exposed immediately, and another, 30 minutes later. The patient is asked to void three times. After the first voiding, a film is exposed; the patient then walks around the room for 2 minutes, voids a second time, and another film is made. Again the patient walks around for 2 minutes, then voids the third time, and then the last film is made.

This technique provides data for an estimation of the amount of residual urine after each voiding. **It also may demonstrate vesicoureteral reflux, if present,** and supplies information concerning the degree of pyeloureterectasis present.

Sometimes ureters permit reflux but fail to empty promptly after voiding. Such trapping of refluxed urine is demonstrated on the triple-voiding cystogram. This technique is not applicable to children who are too young to cooperate.

Determination of Residual Urine by Means of Cystography

In most adult patients with lower urinary obstruction the ordinary postvoiding check by means of a urethral catheter gives accurate information concerning the amount of residual urine. Sometimes passage of a catheter is contraindicated or impossible owing to obstruction, as in some types of prostatic enlargement, urethral strictures, and urethral deformities. In such cases a postvoiding *excretory cystogram* is helpful in the detection of urinary retention. In other conditions a catheter can be introduced with ease, but it does not seem to drain all vesical contents owing to pathologic conditions of the bladder itself, for example, pronounced cystocele with a deep bas-fond or a vesical diverticulum that drains poorly because of position or narrowness of the stoma. In such cases shifting the position of the patient may give better results, but usually excretory cystography provides more accurate information. Occasionally, too, retrograde cystography is indicated to prove or disprove the presence of residual urine. The technique for the simple retrograde cystogram is followed. After the patient has emptied his bladder as completely as possible, another exposure is made to check roentgenographically the amount of contrast medium remaining in the bladder.

Delayed Cystography for Children. For infants and children cystographic demonstration of urinary retention has become an importnat diagnostic method. Small children are usually unable to void on command, and if they do, one is not at all certain whether they emptied the bladder as completely as possible. In order to know whether urinary retention is present or persistent, repeated catheterization would be needed with resultant frustration for both patient and doctor and the attendant risk of introducing infection. Delayed cystography is one of the methods used to check urinary retention in children.

Instillation of Mineral or Iodized Oil for Children. Howard and Buchtel in 1951 described a method for determining the residual urine in children by instillation of **mineral oil** into the bladder. If oil can be demonstrated in specimens of urine obtained 24 hours or more after instillation, urinary retention must be present. Young, Anderson, and King later substituted **iodized oil** (Lipiodol) for the mineral oil. This iodine-containing poppy-seed oil preparation floats in the bladder owing to its low specific gravity. It is adequately opaque and is well tolerated by children. Only 5 ml of a 10% solution of iodized oil is instilled into the bladder by catheter. A film is then exposed. For 24 hours the child is allowed to void at will and then another film is exposed. If oil, representing urinary retention, is noted, another film is exposed at 48 hours and further films are exposed, if indicated, at daily or even weekly intervals, with the child in the upright position. Vesicoureteral reflux can be demonstrated by the presence of the oily material in one or both kidneys.

The Cystourethrogram (Urethrocystogram)

Roentgenographic visualization of the male urethra can be effected in different ways: (1) by the retrograde urethrogram; (2) by the evacuation cystourethrogram; or (3) by a combination of these methods.

The Retrograde Urethrogram (Simple Urethrogram) and the Retrograde Cystourethrogram of Flocks

Retrograde urethrograms were first described in 1910 by Cunningham, who used a 10% solution of silver protein (Argyrol) as the contrast medium. This method has become an accepted diagnostic procedure for lesions of the anterior urethra. Injection of the contrast medium into the external meatus results in distention of the anterior urethra with good delineation of any irregularities, abscess cavities, diverticula, or obstructions that may be present. The resistance of the external urethral sphincter to the inflow of contrast medium usually provides adequate pressure to fill the anterior urethra. On the other hand, complete filling of the posterior (prostatic) urethra is not possible because the contrast medium runs freely and unimpeded through the vesical neck into the bladder. The simple retrograde urethrogram, therefore, is usually of little help in the diagnosis of lesions of the prostatic urethra and bladder neck.

Exposures in the semilateral position (Béclère and Henry), use of semisolid contrast materials (Flocks), and films exposed during the actual injection (Handek) have helped overcome this handicap to a certain extent. The method of Flocks for urethrocystography (a combination of air cystography and retrograde iodine-compound urethrography) also has done much to promote urethrographic diagnosis to the benefit of innumerable patients. This technique will be discussed in conjunction with other techniques later in this chapter.

The Evacuation Cystourethrogram (Micturition, Voiding, or Expression Cystourethrogram)

In order to delineate accurately the vesical neck and the prostatic urethra, the bladder is filled with opaque material just as it is in retrograde cystography, and films are exposed during active (micturition) or passive (expression) evacuation of the bladder. The opaque fluid, being propelled downward from the bladder into the urethra, will distend the prostatic urethra sufficiently to permit adequate visualization of that region (Hansen). As the external urethral sphincter opens and the bladder contents are forced out, a good picture of the anterior urethra is obtained as well. Voiding may be either "free" or "against resistance" (minimal compression of the meatus to provide greater distention and better filling). Micturition cystourethrograms are very satisfactory, since they provide a good anatomic study and also permit conclusions concerning vesical and urethral function.

The only limitation to a study of this nature is the patient's ability to cooperate and to void on command. Most adult patients are able and willing to do so if the purpose of the study is explained. Most older children also cooperate satisfactorily. The infant or young child may not be able or willing to void during such an examination. In such cases, with the infant under anesthesia, the bladder may be completely or almost completely emptied by suprapubic manual compression, the resulting films during this procedure being called *expression cystourethrograms*. Although such films may not be of perfect quality, most of them will permit accurate diagnosis of lower urinary tract disease (usually congenital obstruction).

CONTRAST MEDIA AVAILABLE FOR RETROGRADE CYSTOURETHROGRAPHY

In retrograde urethrography and retrograde cystourethrography almost all types of liquid, semisolid, watery, or oily opaque materials have been used. It is preferable to use a rather viscous material because such fluid on injection flows slower and distends the urethra better than nonviscous fluid. Oily substances, such as iodized oil (Lipiodol), although still in use, are distinctly inferior to water-soluble media because of poor wetting properties which result in poor adherence to the wet mucosal lining of the urethra. Furthermore, in simple

retrograde urethrograms the thin mucosa may easily break because of too forceful injection of medium, which causes too much distention (particularly in the presence of a stricture) or because of injury from the metal adaptor on the tip of the syringe that is used for introduction of medium into the urethra. Such small breaks in the mucosa may lead to urethrocavernous reflux; that is, the contrast material may enter the veins that lie immediately under the urethral mucosa (see Figs. 5-305, 5-307, 5-308, and 5-318). Fatal embolism has resulted from urethrocavernous reflux after use of oily contrast substances and suspensions of barium. We believe, therefore, that neither iodized oil nor barium preparations should be used in retrograde urethrography.

Semisolid Medium of Flocks

To increase the viscosity of liquid media, thickening materials such as tragacanth, sodium carboxymethylcellulose, or amylopectin may be added. The semisolid medium used by Flocks for urethrocystography is prepared as follows: A *water-soluble jelly* is made by thoroughly mixing 25 gm of powdered tragacanth, 40 ml of 95% alcohol, and 660 ml of distilled water. The mixture is allowed to remain in the refrigerator overnight. The next day it is autoclaved and stored for use over a period of several weeks.

The contrast medium is made up in the following proportions: 60 ml of Lipiodol (or an equal amount of full strength Neo-Iopax or Diodrast) is thoroughly mixed with 250 ml of the water-soluble jelly. Enough water is added to give the desired viscosity. This makes enough contrast medium for 12 to 14 urethrograms.

Semisolid Medium of Lowsley and Kirwin

Lowsley and Kirwin (1956) described a formula for jelly made with sodium hippurate (Hippuran) as follows:

Hippuran NNR	16.0 gm
Tragacanth USP (extra select scales)	1.5 gm
Glycerine USP	19.1 ml
Merthiolate 1:1000 sol.	10.0 ml
Distilled water q.s. ad.	100.0 ml

Add 50 ml of distilled water to the tragacanth to form a smooth paste. Add the glycerine and Merthiolate. Dissolve the Hippuran in the rest of the distilled water and add this solution to the paste with constant stirring. Strain through gauze if necessary.

Semisolid Medium of Morales and Romanus

Morales and Romanus exhaustively studied the advantages and disadvantages of a highly viscous material in urethrography in 1952. Their contrast medium (Umbradil-Viscous U) consists of iodopyracet (Umbradil or Diodrast) 35% with 3.25% sodium carboxymethylcellulose, lidocaine 0.25%, and distilled water added to make 100 ml. They stated that the addition of lidocaine (Xylocaine) helped the external urethral sphincter to relax sufficiently to permit adequate distention and visualization of the posterior urethra in retrograde urethrography. We have found a mixture of 50 ml of Renovist with ½ tube of sterile, water-soluble lubricating jelly (K-Y Sterile Lubricant) to be a satisfactory medium for adults and older children.

CONTRAST MEDIA AVAILABLE FOR EVACUATION CYSTOURETHROGRAPHY

The Triiodobenzoic Acid Compounds

Thickened media are not suitable for the voiding cystourethrogram, as patients often find it difficult to pass them freely. We have found a 30% solution of one of the triiodobenzoic acid compounds (Cystokon, Renografin, Renovist, or Hypaque), as suggested by Waterhouse, a most satisfactory medium, although it is irritating occasionally.

TECHNIQUE OF RETROGRADE CYSTOURETHROGRAPHY

Retrograde ("Simple") Urethrogram

In the Male. For retrograde urethrography a highly viscous contrast medium is injected into the anterior urethra with any type of syringe that carries an adaptor that will fit into the external meatus. Application of a local anesthetic agent to the urethra prior to the injection or use of a contrast medium to which such an agent has been added is advisable. Lidocaine (Xylocaine) added to the medium in a 0.25% solution is a rapid-acting anesthetic. The external meatus is pressed tightly against the metal adaptor of the syringe to prevent escape of medium around the adaptor. The penis is kept stretched to flatten mucosal folds and to straighten the penoscrotal angle. The contrast medium is injected slowly and gently, but with steady pressure on the piston of the syringe. During injection some resistance is encountered when the fluid reaches the closed external urethral sphincter. The sphincter usually will yield to steady gentle pressure, and injection of the remaining contrast medium is then easily accomplished. The film is exposed while the medium is still being injected when the surgeon thinks the contrast medium has passed through the external sphincter and prostatic urethra and is spilling over into the bladder. Sudden increase of pressure is contraindicated because this will stimulate the sphincter to close more tightly. The amount of medium varies individually, depending on the size and length of the urethra and the pathologic lesion present. Enough medium should be used, however, so that the entire urethra is adequately filled, with some flowing over into the bladder. Relaxation of the external sphincter can be facilitated by asking the patient to relax and feel as though he were voiding.

For a complete series, films are exposed (1) in the anteroposterior plane with the patient supine, (2) in the right oblique position, and (3) in the left oblique position. For all practical purposes, however, just one film in the right oblique position is usually sufficient (see Fig. 1-39).

With use of this technique for routine examinations, the hands of the surgeon are not properly protected from x-ray exposure. Injection of medium through a penile clamp (Brodny clamp) allows that protection, but the application of a clamp is not satisfactory for all patients. Use of a 16-F Foley catheter with a 5-ml bag may be tried in such instances. The catheter is introduced for about 1½ inches (3.8 cm), and the bag is gently distended with sterile water. Usually about 3 ml of water in the bag is sufficient to lock the catheter in position in the distal portion of the anterior urethra (fossa navicularis). The degree of distention of the bag can be readily palpated, and the patient will experience slight discomfort if overdistention occurs. By gentle traction on the catheter the penis can be kept extended throughout the exposures. It is advisable to first irrigate the catheter with water to evacuate any air that is present.

Retrograde urethrography is inadvisable immediately after urethral instrumentation or catheterization. Prior to the examination the bladder should be emptied by the catheter. Two or three days should elapse between any previous instrumentation and the making of retrograde urethrograms to allow healing of any small urethral injury from instruments or catheter. If retrograde injection of contrast material is performed while the urethral mucosa is injured from previous instrumentation, there is risk of urethrocavernous reflux (with possible embolism), urosepsis, or transient bacteremia (see Figs. 5-305, 5-307, 5-308, and 5-318). During the procedure injury to the urethra from the metal adaptor, from overdistention of the catheter bag, or

from too forceful injection of medium should be carefully avoided, for the urethral epithelium is less than 0.1 mm thick and may be injured easily.

Morales and Romanus suggested that the injection be performed under fluoroscopic control. The advantages of this procedure are obvious, but its disadvantage is an undue x-ray exposure of the genitalia of the patient, unless a device for image intensification can be applied. The same holds true for other techniques in this field, particularly when vesical and urethral functions are studied.

In the Female. Roentgenographic visualization of the female urethra is of less clinical importance than that of the male. Almost any lesion of the female urethra can be readily diagnosed by cystourethroscopy and vaginal palpation of the urethra, the only important exception being urethral diverticula or abscess cavities. The openings of such pockets may be so small that they are easily overlooked on urethroscopy even though the index of suspicion is high (Cook and Pool; Counseller). Also, vaginal palpation of the urethra is not always successful in expressing mucus or purulent material from the pocket.

Positive-Pressure Urethrograms. Retrograde positive-pressure urethrograms (Davis and Cian; Davis and Telinde; Lang and Davis) may be distinctly helpful in the female. For this purpose Davis and Cian developed a special type of catheter (Fig. 1-37). It carries a vesical balloon, which is inflated with 20 ml of air to tamponade the internal urethral orifice; a second, sliding balloon can be advanced along the stem of the catheter to occlude the external meatus. The intraurethral segment of the catheter has an opening through which the injected medium is delivered into the urethral lumen. With this instrument, better filling and delineation of the female urethra are effected than with simple retrograde injection or micturition (Fig. 1-38). See Chapter 18 for a more thorough evaluation of this subject.

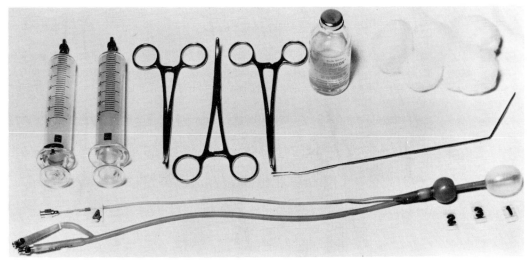

Figure 1–37. Sliding balloon type of catheter for making positive-pressure urethrograms in women. 1, Vesical balloon inflated with 20 ml of air to tamponade urethral orifice. 2, Sliding balloon, which is advanced to occlude external meatus. 3, Intra-urethral segment of catheter containing orifice for injection of contrast material. 4, Tubing for inflation of sliding balloon. Probe can be inserted through eye of catheter to facilitate its introduction into urethra. (From Lang, E. K., and Davis, H. J.)

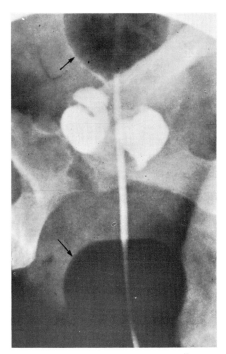

Figure 1–38. *Positive-pressure urethrogram* of female, using double-balloon catheter (*arrows* point to inflated balloons). **Two large urethral diverticula** arising as paired structures with fine sinus tracts communicating with urethra. Repeatedly overlooked at cystoscopy. (From Lang, E. K., and Davis, H. J.)

The Retrograde Cystourethrogram: Technique of Flocks

As has been mentioned previously, the method of Flocks for cystourethrography is of importance in the visualization of the posterior (prostatic) urethra in men, in addition to the anterior urethra. It consists essentially of a retrograde urethrogram combined with air cystography. The technique is as follows.

Four films are exposed at each examination: (1) a plain film exposed in the anteroposterior position and low enough to include the bladder, prostate gland, and urethra; (2) a retrograde cystogram (also made in the anteroposterior position) after introduction of a 5% solution of sodium iodide (or 7% solution of Hippuran) through a urethral catheter (150 ml of contrast medium usually is sufficient); (3) an air cystogram made in the right oblique position by evacuation of the contrast medium from the bladder through the urethral catheter followed by injection of air through the catheter into the bladder until the patient is aware of vesical distention; and (4) a film also exposed in the right oblique position after semisolid contrast medium has been injected.

This fourth exposure is made as follows: 30 ml of air is removed from the bladder with the syringe, and the catheter is withdrawn rapidly. The surgeon compresses the penis with the thumb and index finger to prevent the escape of more air. The semisolid contrast medium is injected into the urethra. In making the injection, a 30-ml Luer syringe equipped with a metal adaptor for urethral catheters is used. A piece of rubber tubing, 5 cm long, is attached to the metal adaptor and is introduced full length into the urethra. The metal adaptor is pressed tightly against the urethral meatus to prevent escape of medium around the tube. About 15 ml of opaque mixture is injected, at which time a sense of resistance is encountered as the medium reaches the tonic external sphincter. The sphincter gradually yields to steady flow pressure and allows the medium to pass into the prostatic urethra. An additional 10 to 15 ml is injected while a film is being exposed. It is imperative that the exposure be made while the medium is being injected so that the prostatic urethra will be well-filled.

TECHNIQUES OF EVACUATION (VOIDING OR EXPRESSION) CYSTOURETHROGRAPHY

Voiding Cystourethrogram

Ordinary Technique. The ordinary technique for micturition cystourethrograms in adults and children more than 4 years of age is as follows: The patient empties his bladder while standing. He is then placed on the x-ray table in the supine position. The glans penis and external meatus are cleaned as is done for catheterization. The urethra is anesthetized by injection of about 15 ml (or less, depending on age) of a sterile lubricating jelly containing a topical anesthetic agent. A soft sterile rubber catheter with a straight or coudé tip (for adults: 16-F; for children: according to size and age) is gently passed into the bladder. The contents are evacuated and measured for determination of residual urine. The opaque material is then introduced into the bladder through the catheter (see: technique for "The Simple Retrograde Cystogram," this chapter). For contrast medium in adults, a 25% to 35% solution of Diodrast or a 30% solution of Urokon, Hypaque, Miokon, Renografin, or Renovist may be used. (A less concentrated solution may be used in children to avoid irritation.) The opaque solution is gently injected or allowed to pass by gravity into the bladder. In adults 150 to 200 ml or more, depending on bladder capacity and comfort, is generally employed; for children smaller amounts are needed. The bladder should be filled without overdistention, the surgeon being guided by the patient's feeling of vesical distention, or by abdominal palpation. After the injection the catheter is removed.

The first cystogram is an anteroposterior view to show the bladder outline and possible vesicoureteral reflux. Then two exposures are made during the act of micturition, with the patient in the right oblique position (Fig. 1–39) and a fourth with the patient in the left oblique position if desired. If the patient is unable to void lying down, an upright position may be necessary. The fourth exposure, made after the patient has completely emptied his bladder, is to show any residual medium in the bladder or in urethral pockets or diverticula. Good cooperation from the patient is required for this test. When children have difficulty emptying their bladders on command, applying gauze moistened in ether to the skin over the suprapubic area or giving the child a whiff of ether in combination with manual pressure over the bladder may elicit spontaneous micturition.

Free Voiding Versus Voiding Against Resistance. Two types of voiding cystourethrograms have been described. One is free voiding; the other is voiding against resistance (Edling). The latter is used to obtain greater distention and better filling of the urethra. It is accomplished by partially occluding the urethral meatus by pinching the glans penis either with the fingers or with a penile clamp. It can be accomplished also by holding a syringe tightly against the meatus and having the patient void into the syringe against the resistance of the piston.

Technique of Waterhouse. Waterhouse has reduced the technique of the voiding cystourethrogram to its simplest elements by making only one x-ray exposure with the patient lying in the *right oblique position* (Fig. 1–39). His technique is as follows.

The patient is asked to void and is then placed on the examining table. A small soft catheter is passed and any residual urine is measured. A 30% solution of Renografin is introduced with a plunger syringe until the patient shows signs of a desire to void. (The bladder must be filled well or the patient will delay voiding.) The patient is then placed in the right oblique position with the left leg extended and the right flexed (Fig. 1–39) and is asked to void. One exposure is made when the patient is voiding well. Care should be taken to make the exposure when the patient is voiding well, as at the beginning or the end of micturition the sphincters may not be fully relaxed and artifacts may be produced. In children who are too young to cooperate, the bladder is filled to capacity, the child placed in position, and then given a bottle. Spontaneous voiding occurs shortly and the exposure is made.

The Expression Cystourethrogram: Technique of Williams

In the very young, evacuation of the bladder may be accomplished by manual expression over the suprapubic area. Wil-

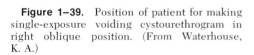

Figure 1–39. Position of patient for making single-exposure voiding cystourethrogram in right oblique position. (From Waterhouse, K. A.)

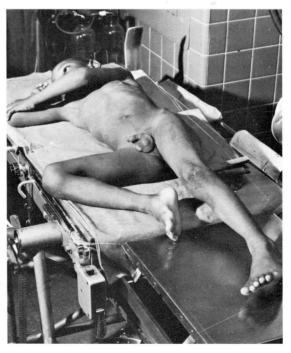

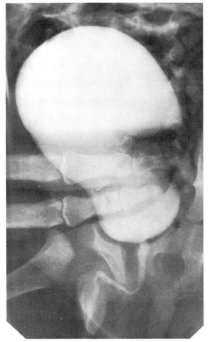

Figure 1–40. *Expression cystourethrogram.* Normal. Boy, 9 months of age, with unexplained uremia. (Courtesy of Dr. H. W. ten Cate.)

liams described this method in 1954, and it is as follows.

The procedure is carried out under general anesthesia. The bladder is first emptied by catheter. The bladder is filled with dye (Williams used a 10% to 15% solution of Diodrast) until it is distended and tight. The catheter is withdrawn, preliminary films are taken, and then firm manual pressure over the bladder propels urine down the urethra while further films are exposed. This expression is only possible in babies, and in older children when there is a nerve lesion of the bladder, but it is the babies about whom we most frequently require the information which the expression urethrogram can give us. In the expression cystourethrogram active relaxation of the internal sphincter is not obtained and the bladder neck therefore appears narrower than in the micturition films (Fig. 1–40).

Voiding Cystourethrography (Voiding Cinecystourethrography)

The technique of voiding cystourethrography combines the advantages of retrograde cystography, micturition cystography, and fluoroscopic (image-intensification) monitoring of both retrograde filling of the bladder and micturition. Most authors consider it a substantial improvement over older techniques for detection of vesicoureteral reflux and for studying the anatomic and physiologic aspects of voiding, especially as they pertain to the vesical neck and urethra. Davis, Lich, Howerton, and Joule have shown that a normal excretory urogram does not rule out urinary tract disease in infants and children and state that voiding cystourethrography is the best method of detecting obstructive changes in the bladder neck and urethra, diverticula of the bladder, urethral valves, and reflux. They express the commonly held view that "a voiding cystourethrogram should be part of the radiological work-up in all children with recurrent pyuria." Increasing experience with voiding cystourethrography in adults has shown that it is also of value in this group for detection of reflux and demonstration of urethral diverticula.

Voiding cystourethrography first came into widespread use about 1958 when image-intensification x-ray apparatus with attached cineroentgenographic equipment became generally available. Subsequently, it has gained steadily in popularity and is now a frequently used, routine examination in many centers and, to a large extent, has replaced older methods of cystography and urethrography, especially in children. The development of cineroentgenographic techniques resulted, to a large degree, from the work of Narath, Kjellberg and his associates, Benjamin and his associates, and Hinman and his associates. Numerous and detailed evaluations of this technique have been published by a number of investigators in recent years, including, as prominent examples, Davis and his associates, Garrett and Klatte, Tristan and his associates, and Shopfner.

Technique

Shopfner has pointed out that there are two schools of thought concerning the best method of performing cystourethrography, the cine and the spot-film method (Davis and associates; Rhamy, Garrett, and Carr; Shopfner; Thornbury and Immergut). His work demonstrates that the spot-film technique produces the most satisfactory overall results but that the essential feature of the examination is its performance with fluoroscopy and that the method of recording the examination on film is of secondary importance only. The basic technique is the same for both the cine and spot-film methods.

Voiding cystourethrography should ordinarily be performed after excretory urography. Some time (usually 1 day but a minimum of several hours) must have lapsed between these two examinations, since the presence of contrast material in the urinary tract after excretory urography may mask vesicoureteral reflux. No special preparation is necessary. In the radiographic room, the patient lies supine on the radiographic table and is prepared as for ordinary catheterization. In the case of small children or infants, immobilization by binding the arms and legs may be necessary and some (Tristan, Murphy, and Schoenberg) prefer to use a light anesthetic (we have never found this necessary or particularly desirable). Sterile catheterization is performed with a catheter of appropriate size (usually a size 8 or 10 F will do). The catheter is taped to the perineum to prevent its being expelled. A 15% to 30% solution of diatrizoate or iothalamate provides the most satisfactory medium available. The contrast medium is allowed to flow by gravity into the bladder until it is full enough for the patient to void. Often it is difficult to determine when the bladder is adequately filled, but strong complaints of discomfort, voiding around the catheter, and dorsiflexion of the toes usually indicate that the patient is ready to void. The amount of medium required varies widely but is usually less than 250 ml for children. For adults, however, and especially for women, micturition under the circumstances of this examination is difficult, and 500 to 750 ml or more is often required. When the bladder is full, small children and infants are allowed to void while lying in the oblique position on the table, but older children and adults void best in the upright position into a potty chair or other urine-collecting device.

Intermittent cine filming may be used to record the essential anatomic and pathologic features observed during filling and during micturition. The dose of radiation to the patient by this technique is relatively high, and film quality is often inferior. With the spot-film technique, anteroposterior and oblique (almost lateral) views of the filled bladder, four or more spot films of the urethra and bladder in the oblique view (taken in rapid succession) during voiding, and films of the bladder and renal region after voiding are usually adequate; but additional spot films may be needed to record abnormalities. Within the past 2 years we have adopted the practice of recording the entire fluoroscopic examination on video tape for temporary consultative and teaching purposes and of using 90-mm spot films made from the output phosphor of the image intensifier for permanent recording of the essentials of the examination. This permits a sharp reduction in radiation dose to the patient and facilitates both consultation and roentgenography.

PNEUMOGRAPHY (RETROPERITONEAL GAS [AIR] INSUFFLATION; PERIRENAL INSUFFLATION; PRESACRAL INSUFFLATION)

Injection of gas into the retroperitoneal space was introduced as a roentgenographic method by Carelli and Sordelli in 1921. Initially, Carelli injected carbon dioxide intraperitoneally to demonstrate echinococcal cysts, but he showed that the same gas introduced through the flank into the retroperitoneal area would outline the kidney and the adrenal gland (Fig. 1–41). The original technique was perfected by Cahill in 1935 and 1936 (Cahill 1935; 1944) and by Cope and Schatzki in 1939. Retroperitoneal insufflation of air through a flank gained favor in spite of the definite complications attendant on its use. Since the presacral route for gas insufflation was introduced by Rivas, this approach has gained more in popularity than that of the flank injection. The presacral technique is easier and carries less risk of complications than does that of the translumbar injection. *Still, it is not without danger. It should be performed, therefore, only for well-established indications.* Its most important complication is gas embolism.

GASEOUS MEDIA

Since Carelli first injected carbon dioxide retroperitoneally for roentgenographic contrast studies, other gases have been used for this purpose, including room air, filtered air, oxygen, helium, nitrogen, and nitrous oxide.

Air has the advantage of being cheap and readily available in liberal amounts. About 15 ml of air per kilogram of body weight is introduced. This is 800 to 1,500 ml for adults, and 100 to 200 ml for children. When a midline presacral injection is used, the air usually spreads easily to both sides. Thus bilateral presacral puncture is not necessary.

Many clinicians use *oxygen* on the presumption that it is dissolved and absorbed faster than air in blood and tissues, and that gas emboli are less likely. This difference may not be of enough significance to warrant use of oxygen, since gas embolism has been reported on several occasions during and after use of that gas (Harkins and Harmon; Ransom, Landes, and McLelland).

Carbon dioxide is so far the safest gas that can be used in pneumographic studies (Blackwood; Bland; Landes and Ransom; Pendergrass and Hodes). It is 20 times more soluble than oxygen in blood at body temperature. Intravenous injection of carbon dioxide in even large amounts does not produce any signs of clinical gas embolism. Its high solubility creates some problem in timing for satisfactory pictures. With the patient in the supine or lateral position, so much of the injected carbon dioxide will be absorbed in a short period that only a small amount has reached the perirenal spaces at the conclusion of the injection. To overcome this problem, Landes and Ransom injected the gas with the patient upright.

Translumbar Method (Flank Injection)

Most urologists now consider translumbar injection of gas for roentgenologic purposes an obsolete procedure because of the risk of gas embolism, but Robertson, Anderson, and Glenn in 1965 reported a simplified technique for bilateral perirenal carbon dioxide insufflation which, for them, has produced satisfactory and uncomplicated results (Figs. 1–42, 1–43, and 1–44). They describe their technique as follows:

The patient with suspected renal or adrenal tumor may be premedicated with narcotics or barbiturates and placed prone and semiupright on a routine urologic radiographic table. This position assures cephalad diffusion of the gas that is introduced. A preliminary plain film of the abdominal area delineates kidney position.

The entire lumbar area is prepared and draped as a sterile field and local skin anesthesia is effected bilaterally at the levels of the lower poles of the kidneys. Through the areas of local anesthesia, 20-gauge lumbar puncture needles with stylets are introduced in a slightly cephalad direction. Resistance of Gerota's fascia can usually be palpated and definite renal resistance is encountered, as with needle biopsy of the kidney. When renal resistance is felt, the needles are withdrawn approximately ½ cm. and the stylets are removed. Sterile Y-tubing of latex or plastic is then attached to the needles and connected to a 3-way stopcock. A tank of 95 per cent carbon dioxide is attached via a rubber inhalation bag to the stopcock and a 50 cc Luer-Lok syringe is used to withdraw carbon dioxide in 50 cc increments for injection.

With a clamp to alternately occlude first one arm of the Y-tubing and then the other, injection is made in each perirenal area until the patient observes flank fullness or discomfort. The average adult will experience such discomfort with approximately 300 cc gas in each perirenal area. However, injection of up to 1500 cc bilaterally has been accomplished without serious side-effects other than moderate shortness of breath, presumably occasioned by sub-diaphragmatic pressure of the insufflated gas.

Immediate radiographic exposures must be made, since carbon dioxide is rapidly diffused and absorbed. It has been our experience that virtually all of such insufflated carbon dioxide will be effectively resorbed within a half hour. If the initial films disclose an insufficient amount of gas for contrast, further injection is made of 100 to 200 cc bilaterally and further radiographic exposures are made.

This simple technique can be embellished by the addition of excretory urography or laminography.

Presacral Method (Presacral Insufflation)

The patient is placed on the examining or x-ray table in the knee-chest position. The area of the coccyx and adjacent buttocks is aseptically scrubbed and draped. The skin is infiltrated with a bleb of procaine at a point 1 cm below the tip of the coccyx. The gloved index finger of the left hand is placed in the rectum. A short 18-gauge needle is inserted with the right hand through the skin bleb and, with help of the palpating finger in the rectum, the needle is guided so that it slides along the sacrococcygeum and enters the area between rectum and coccyx. The tip of the needle is then advanced to a position 1 cm superior to the tip of the coccyx. If the needle enters the rectum inadvertently, no serious harm is done; it is withdrawn and readjusted into proper position. Careful aspiration is done to make sure that the needle has not entered a blood vessel. If blood is aspirated, it is best to postpone the pneumographic study for a few days because of the danger of a gas embolus. If no blood is aspirated, a short length of rubber tubing is attached to the needle. To the other end of the tubing a 50-ml piston syringe with a two-way stopcock is attached. Care should be taken not to change the position of the needle during these procedures. Once more the needle is aspirated to verify that no blood vessel has been punctured. As an additional precaution some 10 ml of sterile saline solution may be injected and aspirated. Room air, 50 ml at a time, is then injected slowly by hand pressure and with little force, until 800 to 1,200 ml has been introduced. The stopcock is closed prior to each refilling of the syringe to prevent air from escaping. Aspirations should be done repeatedly to ensure the proper position of the needle, and the needle should be held as stationary as possible throughout the whole procedure. The injection should be done gently; only little resistance is encountered. A pressure of not more than 20 to 30 cm of water is advocated; this may be determined by interposition of a manometric device, but simple hand pressure is safer. If more resistance is felt, the gas probably is infiltrating gluteal muscles. If no resistance is encountered, the gas is likely to be entering the rectum. Such failures do not harm the patient.

After the injection the head of the table is raised 15° to facilitate distribution of gas in the subdiaphragmatic retroperitoneal space. Good distribution of air occurs within 30 minutes in the majority of patients. Good films are obtained as long as 10 to 16 hours later. The exposed films show equal diffusion of gas on both sides in the retroperitoneal area, outlining the kidney, adrenal gland, and any mass originating from the pancreas or other retroperitoneal structures. If visualization of one side only is desired, the patient may be placed in a lateral position with that side up, prior to exposing the films. This change of position is not strictly necessary and the left-side-up position may be criticized on the grounds that it is the most unfavorable position in case of gas embolism. (See "Complications.")

Landes and Ransom's method for presacral injection of carbon dioxide consists of bilateral presacral puncture with a Tuohy needle when the patient is in the knee-chest position. A polyethylene tube is passed through the lateral hole in the needle into the presacral region on each side of the coccyx. The needles are removed, and the tubes remain in situ. The tubes are connected with a T tube. The patient now sits on the edge of the x-ray table with the plastic tubes taped in place. From 100 to 500 or 1,000 ml of 100% carbon dioxide is introduced to each side (at the rate of 100 ml/min) by alternately clamping one or the other of the limbs of the T tube. After, or even during, the procedure, films are exposed every 5 to 10 minutes. The upright position facilitates distribution of carbon dioxide in the retroperitoneal space. By having the polyethylene tubings in place, the exposed films can be viewed, and if unsatisfactory, more gas can be injected.

Complications

Usually the discomfort of pneumography is slight and temporary. Such symptoms as abdominal discomfort and the feeling of distention and some pain in the epigastric or retrosternal area or in the shoulders on deep inspiration may be present for a few to 48 hours after the injection. Subcutaneous emphysema may occur on the abdomen, genitalia, and neck; this may be annoying but is not serious, as it will be relieved on absorption of the gas. Moderate mediastinal emphysema causing significant thoracic pain should be considered a warning to stop further injection of gas. Occasionally free air will be seen under the diaphragm on the films.

Apart from gas embolism, complications of pneumography have been rare. Retroperitoneal infection with abscess has been described (Wilhelm, 1954) in a patient who had chills, high fever, and jaundice within 36 hours after presacral air insufflation.

GAS EMBOLISM

Gas embolism develops in an appreciable percentage of cases after translumbar injections but less after presacral injection (Glassman, Shapiro, and Robinson; Lefkovits). With the patient in the knee-chest or a Trendelenburg-lithotomy position the hemorrhoidal, middle, and lateral sacral veins are collapsed, as the pressure in them is very low or even negative. Thus, these vessels will not be punctured easily when the needle is inserted presacrally. If, however, laceration does occur and gas is introduced into a blood vessel while the patient is in this position, the gas will be sucked up by the open vessel, and a massive gas embolus will result. This may happen even if the vein has not been primarily injured by the needle but becomes lacerated from separation of tissue spaces by the increasing volume of injected gas. Ideally, therefore, gas should be introduced only when the patient is in a position in which the retrorectal venous plexuses lie well below the level of the right cardiac chambers. When so situated the vessels, when injured, will bleed instead of sucking up injected gas. Prophylaxis, therefore, would require a change of position after introduction of the needle, with the possibility of dislocation of the needle. Use of polyethylene tubing as suggested by Landes and Ransom is helpful in this respect. Some clinicians prefer to introduce the needle with the patient in the left decubitus, partial Trendelenburg position during the puncture and an anti-Trendelenburg position during injection of the gas, and finally, after removal of the needle, to change the patient to the supine position prior to exposing the films.

Gas embolism may be diagnosed by warning symptoms such as cyanosis, thoracic pain, nausea, irregular respiration, tachycardia, fall in blood pressure, perspiration, and other indications of shock. In the full blown case of gas embolism a typical "mill-wheel" murmur can be heard over the precordium. Constant observation of the patient is necessary to make an early diagnosis of gas embolism during the procedure. When any warning sign appears, the injection of gas is immediately discontinued and the patient is placed on his left side to relieve the air trap in the outflow tract of the right ventricle. The surgeon should be ready to perform thoracotomy and cardiac massage, evacuation of air by puncture, and electric stimulation of the heart muscle in the desperate case of cardiac arrest.

Although the incidence of gas embolism during pneumography is not accurately known, Landes and Ransom concluded from their nationwide survey that it may have occurred 122 times in some 12,000 pneumographies with 58 deaths, giving a mortality rate of about 0.5%.

Indications and Contraindications

Since pneumography is not completely without risk, it should be performed only on strict indications. The method may indeed provide information which is not easily obtainable by other, simpler techniques, but *nephrotomography and arteriography are rapidly replacing it and providing equally good visualization of the soft tissues in the retroperitoneal region* (see Figs. 1–32, 1–33, and 1–34). Suspicion of the presence of a suprarenal mass is one of its main indications. Pneumography may be helpful in the diagnosis of roentgenologically nonfunctioning kidneys, which may be absent, small, or ectopic. Retroperitoneal tumors of unknown origin present another indication. The problem of operability or inoperability of a renal tumor has been solved occasionally with the aid of pneumographic visualization providing information concerning extension of the tumor to surrounding tissues and organs (Fig. 1–45A and B). Often, however, pneumography only verifies a previously made diagnosis without adding much pertinent knowledge. It may, for more accurate details, be combined with excretory and retrograde urography, aortography, tomography, or nephrotomography.

Acute inflammatory lesions in the retroperitoneal and perirenal areas are contraindications of pneumography. The flank method is ill-advised in the presence of large renal tumors, as many veins in the region of the tumor may be dilated, and in cases of large malignant retroperitoneal tumor because of the danger of inadvertently puncturing it.

Visualization of the Normal and Abnormal Adrenal Gland

In the pneumographic diagnosis of adrenal masses the following points may be of interest (Harrison and Doubleday; Riches, Griffiths, and Thackray; Smith and associates; Steinbach, Hinman, and Forsham; Steinbach and associates; Walter and Goodwin). The normal right adrenal gland occasionally is identified on a plain film of the abdomen as a small

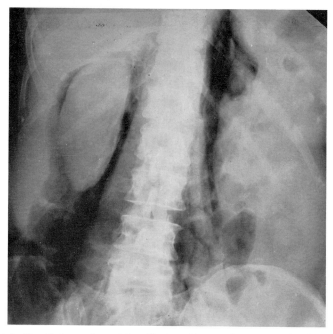

Figure 1–41. *Retroperitoneal insufflation of gas* outlines **normal right kidney.**

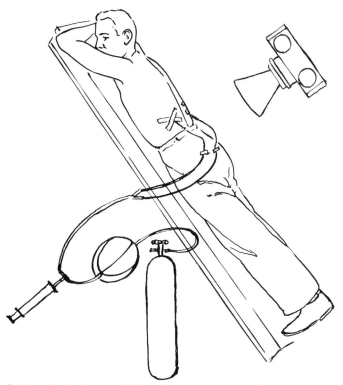

Figure 1–42. Technique of *simultaneous bilateral perirenal carbon dioxide insufflation.* Patient is prone and semi-upright on urologic radiographic table; 20-gauge spinal needles are introduced at level of lower poles of each kidney; and manual injection is made of 95% carbon dioxide in increments of 50 ml. (From Robertson, L. H., Jr., Anderson, E. E., and Glenn, J. F.)

triangular shadow above the upper pole of the right kidney. The left adrenal gland has a more semilunar shape and extends for a short length down the medial side of the upper pole of the left kidney. The kidney moves freely within Gerota's capsule, but the adrenal gland is attached to the upper portion of the capsule, which is, in turn, attached to the diaphragm. For this reason the adrenal maintains its normal position even in cases of marked renal ptosis. If the shadows of the kidney and adrenal are superimposed, they can be separated by taking films with the patient in the upright position (Steinbach and Smith).

Large adrenal masses displace the kidney downward; such renal displacement, however, is not diagnostic of an adrenal growth. Tumors of 2 inches (5 cm) in diameter or more are readily recognized on a scout film of good quality (Cope and Raker). Excretory and retrograde pyelograms are of little help in the diagnosis of adrenal enlargement. Presacral gas insufflation, preferably in combination with tomography, is helpful and may even permit preoperative differentiation between hyperplasia and tumor in Cushing's syndrome (Fig. 1–46A, B, and C). (See Chapter 10 for more complete discussion of adrenal tumors.)

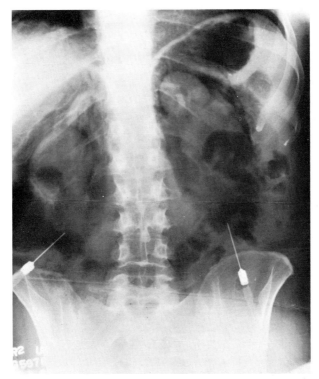

Figure 1–43. *Bilateral retroperitoneal carbon dioxide insufflation* demonstrates left adrenal adenoma. (From Robertson, L. H., Jr., Anderson, E. E., and Glenn, J. F.)

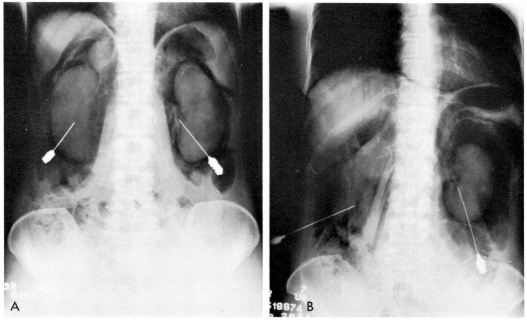

Figure 1–44. *Bilateral perirenal carbon dioxide insufflation.* **A,** Right adrenal adenoma. **B,** Right adrenal pheochromocytoma. (From Robertson, L. H., Jr., Anderson, E. E., and Glenn, J. F.)

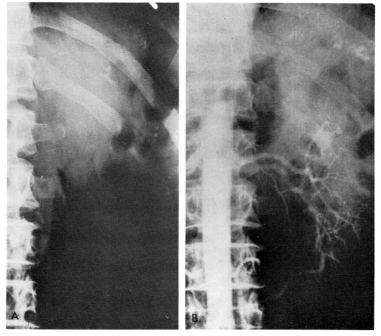

Figure 1–45. **A,** *Pneumogram after presacral insufflation of air* into man, 56 years of age. **Large hypernephroma on left.** Note that air does not penetrate around left kidney, showing large soft-tissue mass on that side. **B,** *Retrograde aortogram* in same case. At exploration tumor had invaded peritoneum and colon, had crossed midline to produce large mass around vena cava, and had produced multiple metastatic lesions. (Courtesy of Dr. H. W. ten Cate.)

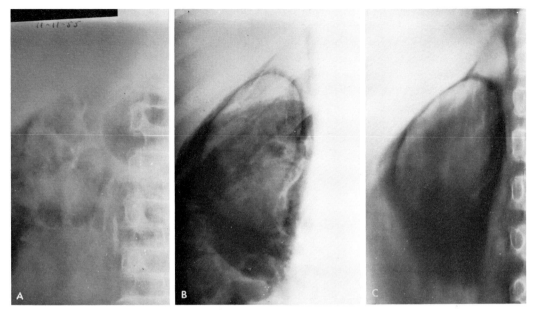

Figure 1–46. Comparison of various techniques in case of **functioning adrenal carcinoma. A,** *Plain film.* **B,** *Pneumogram.* **C,** *Pneumotomogram.* (From Hinman, F., Jr., Steinbach, H. L., and Forsham, P. H.)

SEMINAL VESICULOGRAPHY, EPIDIDYMOGRAPHY, AND UTRICULOGRAPHY

Seminal Vesiculography

Belfield in 1905 was one of the first genitourinary surgeons to call attention to chronic inflammatory diseases of the seminal vesicles. He recognized chronic vesiculitis as one of the causes of ill-defined pain in the perineal and sacrococcygeal regions and suggested injection of medicaments into the seminal ducts exposed through a small scrotal incision. In 1913 he described roentgenograms of seminal vesicles after injection of a 5% solution of colloidal silver (Collargol) into the vas deferens through a vasotomy opening (Belfield, 1913a; 1913b). Young and Waters followed with such studies the same year and in 1920 published the results of vesiculograms obtained after injection of contrast medium (thorium) into the ejaculatory ducts of the verumontanum during urethroscopy. Considerable work was done in this field by several investigators, among whom were McMahon, Peterson, Herbst and Merricks (1939; 1940; 1944), and Merricks. Wilhelm, in 1939, followed the technique of Belfield (1913b) with roentgenographic studies performed through the vasoseminal route. Excellent studies have been presented by the Brazilian urologist, Pereira, and in the United States by Abeshouse, Heller, and Salik and Golji.

INDICATIONS

Despite all the work done, seminal vesiculography has not achieved the wide attention among modern urologists that it probably deserves. Among the several factors responsible is the general feeling that chronic disease of the seminal vesicles as a cause of perineal distress has probably been exaggerated in the past and only rarely warrants elaborate surgical exploration of these organs. Other deterring factors to roentgenographic visualization of the seminal vesicles are the necessity for either bilateral surgical exposure of the vasa through scrotal incisions with needle puncture of the duct (which may result in infertility from injury or stricture) or difficult catheterization of the ejaculatory ducts with use of special urethroscopic equipment. It is also true that a number of patients complaining of ill-defined pains in the scrotum, testes, buttocks, perineum, and coccygeal region have psychosomatic disease, which calls for psychotherapy rather than urologic intervention. On the other hand, it is the task of the urologist to evaluate such symptoms and exclude organic disease as the underlying cause. Apart from the patients who may have complaints of chronic inflammatory disease of the epididymis, seminal vesicles, and prostate gland, there is the male with problems of infertility. In a number of sterile male patients roentgenographic examination of the seminal tract may be an important part of the overall examination.

Correct interpretation of vesiculograms requires considerable experience. For consultation of easily accessible contributions in the literature on this subject the reader is referred to the articles of Pereira and Golji. Most of the following descriptions are based on these papers.

TECHNIQUES

Seminal vesiculography can be performed through the vasoseminal route (vasopuncture or vasotomy) or through the transurethal approach (catheterization of ejaculatory ducts).

Vasoseminal Route

The patient is placed in the supine position on the x-ray table and the genital region is shaved, prepared, and draped as for bilateral partial vasectomy. Local anesthesia is employed, unless gen-

eral anesthesia is required for some particular reason. The vas is palpated in the scrotum about 4 cm distal to the external inguinal ring and separated from surrounding components of the funiculus. It is brought under the scrotal skin and held between thumb and index finger of the left hand. The vas is identified on palpation as a hard strand of tissue about the size of the lead in an ordinary pencil. The skin held between the urologist's thumb and index finger is infiltrated with 0.5% solution of procaine and incised for 2 cm in the direction of the vas. The vas is then lifted out of the wound with an Allis clamp and carefully separated from its fascial coverings to expose it for 2 cm. Gentle traction is exerted after encircling the vas with a short length of tape or suture material. A 20-gauge, short, bevelled hypodermic needle is now inserted into the lumen of the vas full length in the direction of the seminal vesicle. One may choose to do this without first making an incision into the vas (that is, a vasopuncture), being careful not to place the needle in an intramural position or to pierce the posterior wall of the vas. The alternative is to make a 2-mm longitudinal incision in the anterior wall of the vas and introduce a round blunt-tipped needle (that is, perform vasotomy). The vas need not be tied around the needle for fixation. The same procedure is carried out on the other side. With a 2-ml capacity syringe, 1.5 to 2 ml of a 70% solution of Urokon or other contrast medium is injected slowly and gently on each side. After the injections have been completed, one x-ray exposure is made in the anteroposterior projection with the roentgen tube centered over the symphysis pubis. Before closing the scrotal incision with a single, fine catgut suture, the film should be viewed. Closure of the opening in the vas is usually not necessary.

If seminal vesiculography is indicated as part of an examination for sterility in the male, the vasoseminal study is preferably carried out under general anesthesia and extended to provide opportunity for exploration of both testes, epididymides, and vasa. An epididymogram can be made by using the same incision, and testicular biopsy, if indicated, can be performed. The patency of the vasoseminal pathway can be studied by injection of 5 ml of methylene blue or indigo carmine into the vas just as has been described for contrast medium. The bladder is catheterized, and if the blue color is present in vesical urine, it provides evidence of patency of the seminal tract distal to the point of injection. If no blue is present, seminal vesiculography is indicated to show the location of the obstruction. This examination can be completed by bilateral epididymography.

Transurethral Route

Catheterization of the ejaculatory ducts through their openings on the verumontanum is possible with several types of urethroscopes. Of these, the McCarthy panendoscope with Foroblique telescope equipped with a special guide for catheterization of the ducts, designed by McCarthy and Wappler (Fig. 1–47), is the most widely used instrument. The tip of the catheter is bent downward and medially through the guide for easier introduction into the openings of the ejaculatory ducts. These are situated on the verumontanum, usually just distal and somewhat lateral to the utriculus (the utriculus being located on the top and near the center of the verumontanum) (McCarthy, Ritter, and Klemperer). Often these openings cannot be clearly seen, and their approximate position has to be known since the catheterization may have to be done more or less blindly. Sometimes anatomic variations are encountered, as described by McMahon; in other cases the openings are not visible owing to inflammatory changes of the verumontanum (colliculitis). The ejacula-

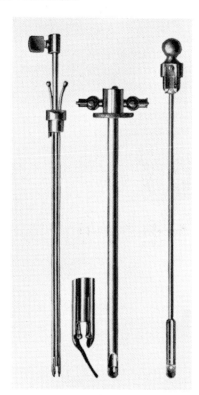

Figure 1–47. McCarthy ejaculatory duct instrument, consisting of special round sheath, 24 F, with obturator and catheterizing mechanism, and McCarthy Foroblique telescopes. (American Cystoscope Makers, Inc., New York.)

tory ducts are normally about 1 to 3 cm in length. They are delicate structures that are perforated easily by the probing catheter. For catheterizations, a 3- or 4-F ureteral catheter without wire stylet is used. The catheter is introduced for about 1 to 3 cm. On each side, 2 ml of 70% Urokon or another contrast medium is injected slowly. A film covering the area of the symphysis pubis and bladder is exposed in the anteroposterior direction, and the film is viewed before the catheters are withdrawn.

THE NORMAL VESICULOGRAM

The normal anatomic relationships of the ductus deferens, ampulla of the seminal vesicle, the seminal vesicle itself, ejaculatory duct, verumontanum, and prostate gland (Figs. 1–48 and 1–49) should be kept in mind (McCarthy, Ritter, and Klemperer) when interpreting seminal vesiculograms. When the vasoseminal routine is employed, the vas itself is depicted in the vesiculogram as a thin, sharply outlined channel with a tortuous course that can be seen from the site of injection to the ampulla, where it becomes wider, more irregular, and somewhat hazy. *The ampulla* is separately identified in normal cases because there is some free space between the distal portion of the vas and the seminal vesicle. *The vesicle* is delineated sharply as a convoluted wide channel consisting of a number of round or oval-shaped saccules regularly and closely joined. *The ejaculatory duct* is identified at its origin from the vesicle as a sharply outlined channel following a straight course downward toward the verumontanum. Both vesicles, ampullae, and ejaculatory ducts are in a symmetrical position in relation to the midline. The contrast medium flowing out into the prostatic urethra may either flow back into the bladder or come out through the external urethral meatus (Figs. 1–50 and 1–51).

THE ABNORMAL VESICULOGRAM

Golji described six groups of disorders of the seminal tract, which he classified as nonspecific infections, tuberculosis, obstructive lesions, malignant changes, traumatic lesions, and congenital anomalies.

In *nonspecific infections* some deviation of the distal end of the vas may be present due to perivesiculitis and fibrosis; the ampulla of the vas is hazy and ill-defined, drawn toward the seminal vesicle and sometimes incorporated in it or even in the opposite ampulla. The seminal vesicle is dilated and changed to a large irregular and ill-defined sac (catarrhal vesiculitis) or scarred with vague

contours; the free space between the seminal vesicle and the ampulla of the vas is partially or totally obliterated, and the ejaculatory ducts may be obstructed and not visualized or incorporated in each other (Figs. 1–52 through 1–61).

In *tuberculosis* of the distal genital tract destructive lesions characteristic of the disease, such as abscess cavities in the vas and vesicle or extensive calcifications in the vesicles and prostate gland, may be seen in addition to the changes characteristic of nonspecific chronic infection (Mygind). A "beaded" vas deferens is pathognomonic (Figs. 1–62, 1–63, and 1–64).

Obstructive lesions are usually due to chronic infections of specific or nonspecific nature. The obstruction can be caused by stricture or exudate and may be complete or incomplete. Complete obstruction due to chronic bilateral inflammation causes azoospermia and sterility. Such obstructions often are located in the tail of the epididymis, in the ampulla of the vas deferens, or in the ejaculatory ducts (Fig. 1–65). Vasography and epididymography may show the exact location of the obstruction.

Malignant changes of the distal seminal tract (vas, ampulla of vas, seminal vesicle, and ejaculatory duct) are usually due to infiltrative growths from the prostate gland. Occasionally a bladder cancer can extend into the seminal vesicles. The vesiculogram shows changes similar to those of chronic infection and are not characteristic of malignancy.

Traumatic lesions are rare but may occur in the course of prostatic surgery by tearing the ejaculatory ducts and verumontanum. Often such lesions will cause obstruction of the channels. In conservative open prostatic surgery the seminal vesicles are injured occasionally. Here again stricture and scarring are late results and produce bizarre vesiculograms.

Congenital anomalies are encountered only infrequently. Reduplication of the seminal tract or parts of it has been described. Agenesia or incomplete development is best diagnosed by surgical exploration if differentiation from obstruction is necessary. Vesiculography may be of help in demonstrating the seminal tract in cases of hypogonadism and pseudohermaphroditism.

(Text continued on page 88.)

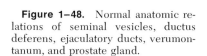

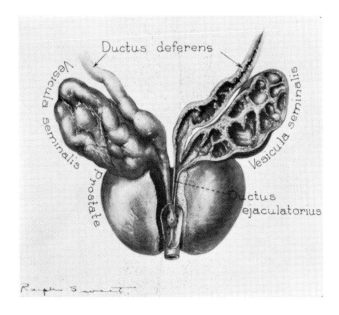

Figure 1–48. Normal anatomic relations of seminal vesicles, ductus deferens, ejaculatory ducts, verumontanum, and prostate gland.

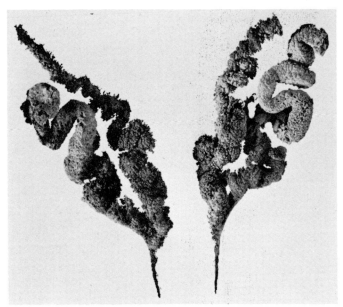

Figure 1–49. Plastic corrosion model of normal seminal vesicle. (From Nilsson, S. G.: The Human Seminal Vesicle [A Morphogenetic and Gross Anatomic Study With Special Regard to Changes Due to Age and to Prostatic Adenoma]. Acta chir. scandinav. Suppl. 296, 1962.)

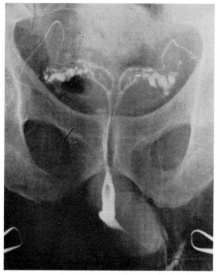

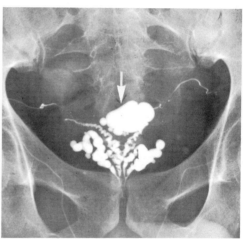

Fig. 1–50

Fig. 1–51

Figure 1–50. *Bilateral seminovesiculogram* made by injection through vasa. **Normal vesicles** in man, 74 years of age, with **marked prostatic hypertrophy.** Note **elongated prostatic urethra.** Owing to prostatic adenoma, the vesicles are displaced cephalad. Note also elongated ejaculatory ducts merge toward verumontanum, which is shown as a negative shadow. Owing to prostatic obstruction, most of the contrast medium flows out through the urethra. (Courtesy of Dr. H. W. ten Cate.)

Figure 1–51. *Bilateral seminal vesiculogram,* made by means of vasotomy (injecting contrast medium into each vas deferens through incision in scrotum). **Normal seminal vesicles and vasa deferentia.** Some medium has run into base of bladder (*arrow*). (See text.)

Fig. 1–52   Fig. 1–53

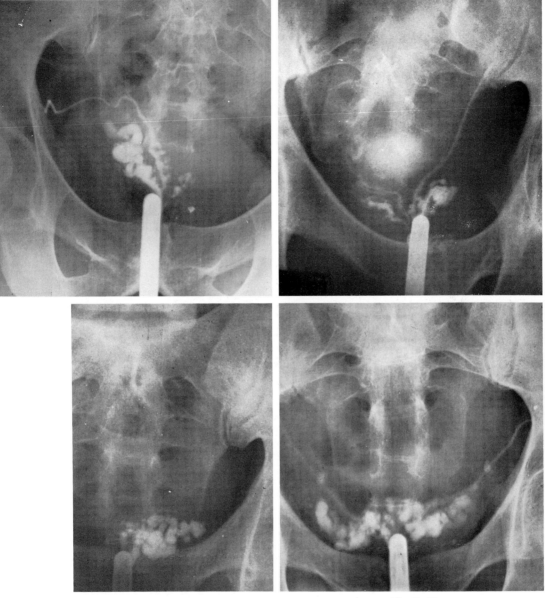

Fig. 1–54   Fig. 1–55

Figure 1–52. *Right seminal vesiculogram.* Advanced right seminal vesiculitis with distortion of ampulla and vas deferens. (Courtesy of Dr. J. W. Merricks.)

Figure 1–53. *Bilateral seminal vesiculogram.* Abscess of left seminal vesicle, with obliteration of upper (terminal) pole. Almost complete obliteration of right seminal vesicle, so that most of contrast medium has run into bladder. (Courtesy of Dr. J. W. Merricks.)

Figure 1–54. *Left seminal vesiculogram.* Abscess of lower (proximal) part of left seminal vesicle. (Courtesy of Dr. J. W. Merricks.)

Figure 1–55. *Bilateral seminal vesiculogram.* Bilateral seminal vesiculitis with dilatation and "fusion" of tubules, so that ampulla of vas on either side appears almost fused with vesicle. (Courtesy of Dr. J. W. Merricks.)

Fig. 1–56   Fig. 1–57

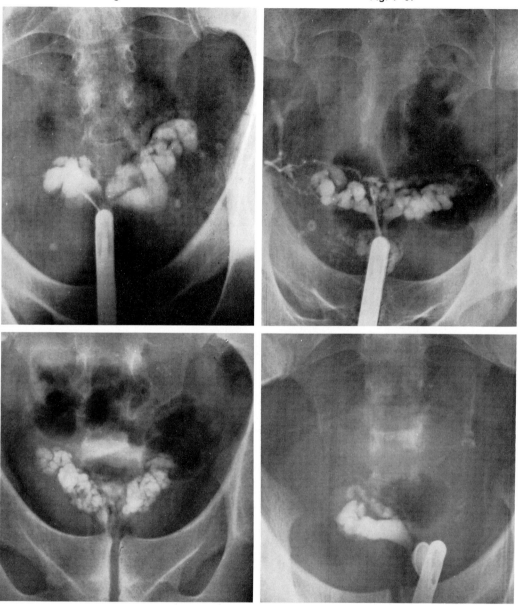

Fig. 1–58   Fig. 1–59

Figure 1–56. *Bilateral seminal vesiculogram.* Bilateral seminal vesiculitis, with advanced dilatation of tubules and partial obliteration of upper (terminal) portion of right vesicle. Dilatation was caused by obstruction of ejaculatory ducts. (This was relieved by dilating ducts.) (Courtesy of Dr. J. W. Merricks.)

Figure 1–57. *Bilateral seminal vesiculogram.* Bilateral seminal vesiculitis. Dilatation of tubules and "fusion" of tubules with ampulla of vas. Apparent lymphatic extravasation of contrast medium. Multiple prostatic calculi. (Courtesy of Dr. J. W. Merricks.)

Figure 1–58. *Bilateral seminal vesiculogram.* Bilateral seminal vesiculitis with dilatation and "fusion" of tubules. (Courtesy of Dr. J. W. Merricks.)

Figure 1–59. *Right seminal vesiculogram.* Right seminal vesiculitis. Dilatation and "fusion" of tubules with advanced changes in wall of vesicles as suggested by narrow, rigid appearance of wall of proximal part of vesicle. Note dilatation and irregularity of ampulla of vas. (Courtesy of Dr. J. W. Merricks.)

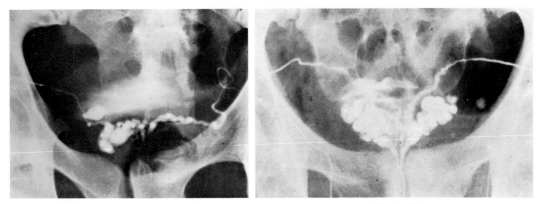

Fig. 1-60   Fig. 1-61

Figure 1-60. *Seminal vesiculogram.* **Chronic vesiculitis and perivesiculitis.** (From Golji, H.)
Figure 1-61. *Seminal vesiculogram.* **Catarrhal seminal vesiculitis.** (From Golji, H.)

Fig. 1-62

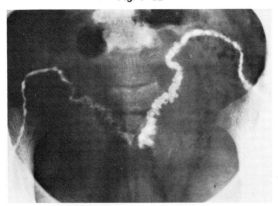

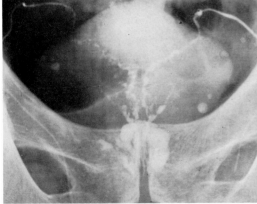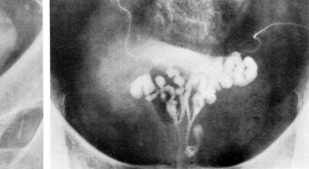

Fig. 1-63   Fig. 1-64

Figure 1-62. *Seminal vesiculogram.* **Genital tuberculosis.** Dilated vasa deferentia and ampullae with irregular beaded pattern. Stenosis of ejaculatory ducts. (From Mygind, H. B.)

Figure 1-63. *Seminal vesiculogram.* **Genital tuberculosis.** Beaded appearance of vasa deferentia and shrunken seminal vesicles. Large prostatic cavities partially filled with calcified material. (From Mygind, H. B.)

Figure 1-64. *Seminal vesiculogram.* **Genital tuberculosis.** Cavity in vicinity of left ejaculatory duct. Left seminal vesicle essentially normal. Right is incompletely filled. (From Mygind, H. B.)

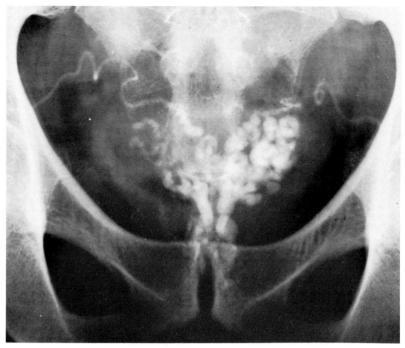

Figure 1–65. *Bilateral seminal vesiculogram.* **Obstruction of both ejaculatory ducts by prostatic calculi,** resulting in dilatation and "fusion" of tubules. Note marked dilatation of ejaculatory ducts. (Courtesy of Dr. J. W. Merricks.)

Epididymography

Roentgenographic studies of the epididymis were initiated by Boreau and associates in 1951 and evaluated by the same authors in 1952 and 1953. American experiences in this field have been described by Tucker, Yanagihara, and Pryde; Abeshouse, Heller, and Salik; and Golji. The indication for epididymography is mainly the study of sterility in the male. In cases of azoospermia, when testicular biopsies reveal active spermatogenesis, epididymography and vasoseminal vesiculography provide useful information on obstructions of the seminal tract. If obstruction appears to be present at the most proximal portion of the seminal tract, that is, at the globus minor (or even more proximally), reimplantation of the vas into a fertile area of the epididymis is the procedure of choice to reestablish normal fertility. Epididymography is not warranted for diagnosis of chronic or acute epididymitis since the usual physical and routine urologic examinations seem to provide sufficient information in such cases.

TECHNIQUE

The ductus deferens is isolated and brought into view in the same way as has been described for vasoseminal vesiculography. A short 20-gauge hypodermic needle (a finer needle, to 26-gauge, may be used also) is passed into the lumen of the vas and pointed in the direction of the epididymis; 1 ml of 70% Urokon or other contrast material in a 1-ml (tuberculin-type) capacity syringe is injected slowly and without force. The needle is then removed, and the same procedure is carried out on the opposite side. This operation can be performed under local anesthesia. If more elaborate exploration on both sides, eventually with bilateral vasoepididymostomy, is considered, general anesthesia is preferable. If local anesthesia is used, the patient may be turned to the prone position on the x-ray table after the wounds have been closed, and a small cardboard nonscreen film is used for exposures (Abeshouse, Heller, and Salik). In that case care should be taken to prevent contamination of the wounds.

THE NORMAL EPIDIDYMOGRAM

Beginning at the point of injection the normal vas is outlined as a thin line coursing downward and becoming convoluted toward the vasoepididymal junction. At this point (globus minor of the epididymis) the course of the convoluted tubule cannot be identified separately and the medium becomes feathery in appearance. The medium stops at the globus major, the body of the epididymis sometimes being forked (Fig. 1–66).

THE ABNORMAL EPIDIDYMOGRAM

Obstruction of the globus minor of the epididymis is shown in Figure 1–67. This is a bilateral epididymogram in one of Abeshouse, Heller, and Salik's patients, a man, 31 years of age, whose marriage has remained childless after 9 years. There was azoospermia but testicular biopsies revealed normal spermatogenesis. Figure 1–68 represents bilateral epididymograms in a 23-year-old man with *hypogonadism and female type of pubic hair,* who on exploration was found to have normal testes and epididymides, but in whom the left epididymogram shows a block in the region of the globus minor whereas only a faint shadow of medium is seen along the course of the right epididymis.

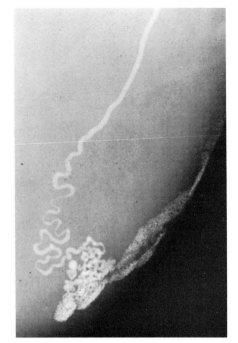

Figure 1–66. *Normal epididymogram.* (From Abeshouse, B. S., Heller, E., and Salik, J. O.)

Utriculography

Filling of the prostatic utricle with contrast medium during retrograde or micturition cystourethrography is seldom, if ever, successful. In 1957 Gullmo and Sundberg described a method for utriculography using the principle of positive pressure urethrography. The neck of the bladder is closed off from the bladder by a three-channel balloon-type urethral catheter, and the anterior urethra is closed by tying a soft rubber string around the shaft of the penis. Contrast medium is then delivered into the prostatic urethra through one of the channels of the catheter by an opening that has been cut approximately 1 cm below the balloon, that is, just opposite the colliculus seminalis. These authors succeeded in outlining the utriculus in 6 of their 22 patients. The procedure seemed to cause some discomfort. In two of the six patients the utriculus was shown to be pathologically enlarged. (See also discussion in Chapter 12, pages 1557–1558.)

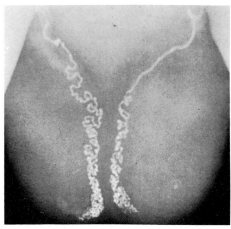
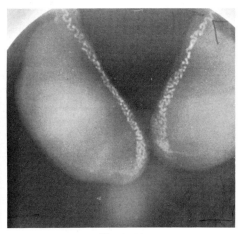

Fig. 1–67   **Fig. 1–68**

Figure 1–67. *Epididymogram.* Complete block in region of globus minor on both sides. (From Abeshouse, B. S., Heller, E., and Salik, J. O.)

Figure 1–68. *Bilateral epididymogram* of 23-year-old man with hypogonadism. Note obstruction of seminal duct at globus minor of left epididymis, whereas on right side only faint line of contrast is seen along body of epididymis. (Courtesy of Dr. H. W. ten Cate.)

INDICATIONS

Utriculography is rarely indicated since an enlarged utriculus can be recognized during urethroscopy and then, if necessary, can be catheterized with a ureteral catheter and subsequently filled with contrast medium for roentgenographic visualization. If utriculography with positive-pressure technique is to be performed, it is logical to try the double balloon type of catheter described by Davis and Cian for urethrography in the female (see also "Technique of Retrograde Cystourethrography in the Female" in this chapter, pages 66 and 67).

REFERENCES

History of Excretory Urography

Binz, A.: The Chemistry of Uroselectan. J. Urol. 25:297-301 (Mar.) 1931.

Braasch, W. F.: The Value of Uroselectan in Renal Lithiasis. J. Urol. 25:265-274 (Mar.) 1931.

Bugbee, H. G., and Murphy, A. J.: The Value and Limitations of Uroselectan as an Aid in Urological Diagnosis. J. Urol. 25:275-286 (Mar.) 1931.

Herbst, R. H.: Comparative Value of Uroselectan to Cystoscopic Pyelography. J. Urol. 25:287-291 (Mar.) 1931.

Hryntschak, T.: Discussion. Verhandl. deutsch. Gesellsch. Urol. 8:434, 1928.

Joseph, E.: Kriterium des normalen und abnormen Pyelo-Uretergramms: Intravenöse Pyelographien. Med. Welt. 4:197 (Feb. 8) 1930.

Lenarduzzi, G., and Pecco, R.: Iniezioni endovenose di ioduro di sodio. (Ricerche radiologiche sperimentali.) Arch. di. Radiol. 3:1055-1060 (Sept.-Oct.) 1927.

Lowsley, O. S.: Uroselectan in Urinary Tuberculosis. J. Urol. 25:293-295 (Mar.) 1931.

Osborne, E. D., Sutherland, C. G., Scholl, A. J., and Rowntree, L. G.: Roentgenography of Urinary Tract During Excretion of Sodium Iodid. J.A.M.A. 80:368-373 (Feb. 10) 1923.

Roseno, A.: Die intravenöse Pyelographie. II. Mitteilung. Klinische Ergebnisse. Klin. Wchnschr. 8:1165-1170 (June) 1929a.

Roseno, A.: Die intravenöse Pyelographie. Klin. Wchnschr. 8:1623 (Aug. 27) 1929b.

Sweetser, T.: Intravenous Urography in the Diagnosis of Renal Tuberculosis: Case Report. J. Urol. 25:311-312 (Mar.) 1931.

Swick, M.: Darstellung der Niere und Harnwege im Röntgenbild durch intravenöse Einbringung eines neuen Kontraststoffes, des Uroselectans. Klin. Wchnschr. 8:2087-2089 (Nov. 5) 1929.

Swick, M.: Excretion Urography by Means of the Intravenous and Oral Administration of Sodium Ortho-iodohippurate: With Some Physiological Considerations; Preliminary Report. Surg., Gynec. & Obst. 56:62-65 (Jan.) 1933a.

Swick, M.: Excretion Urography With Particular Reference to Newly Developed Compound: Sodium Ortho-iodohippurate. J.A.M.A. 101:1853-1855 (Dec. 9) 1933b.

Swick, M.: The Discovery of Intravenous

Urography: Historical and Developmental Aspects of the Urographic Media and Their Role in Other Diagnostic and Therapeutic Areas. Bull. New York Acad. Med. *42*:128-151 (Feb.) 1966.

Swick, M.: Personal communication to the author, 1968.

Voelcker, F., and Lichtenberg, A.: Pyelographie (Röntgenographie des Nierenbeckens nach Kollargolfüllung). München. med. Wchnschr. *53*:105 (Jan. 16) 1906.

von Lichtenberg, A.: The Principles of Intravenous Urography. J. Urol. *25*:249-257 (Mar.) 1931.

von Lichtenberg, A., and Swick, M.: Klinische Prüfung des Uroselectans. Klin. Wchnschr. *8*:2089-2091 (Nov. 5) 1929.

Ziegler, J., and Köhler, H.: Über perorale Pyelographie. Verhandl. deutsch. Gesellsch. Urol. *9*:344-345, 1929.

The Plain Film and Subsequent Parts

Abeshouse, B. S., Heller, E., and Salik, J. O.: Vasoepididymography and Vasoseminal Vesiculography. J. Urol. *72*:983-991 (Nov.) 1954.

Alyea, E. P., and Haines, C. E.: Intradermal Test for Sensitivity to Iodopyracet Injection, or "Diodrast." J.A.M.A. *135*:25-27 (Sept. 6) 1947.

Amplatz, K.: Two Radiographic Tests for Assessment of Renovascular Hypertension: A Preliminary Report. Radiology *79*:807-815 (Nov.) 1962.

Andersen, P. T.: On Tomography as an Adjunct to Urography. Acta radiol. *30*:225-236, 1948.

Andrews, J. R.: Planigraphy. I. Introduction and History. Am. J. Roentgenol. *36*:575-587 (Nov.) 1936.

Arata, J. A.: Personal communication to the authors.

Archer, V. W., and Harris, I. D.: An Ocular Test for Sensitivity to Diodrast Prior to Intravenous Urography. Am. J. Roentgenol. *48*:763-765 (Dec.) 1942.

Barnhard, H. J., and Barnhard, F. M.: The Emergency Treatment of Reactions to Contrast Media: Updated 1968. Radiology *91*:74-84 (July) 1968.

Bartelink, D. L.: Röntgenschnitte. Fortschr. a.d. Geb. d. Röntgenstrahlen. *47*:399-407, 1933.

Béclère, H., and Henry, R.: Quelques radiographies de rétrécissements de l'urètre. J. d'urol. *13*:417-424 (June) 1922.

Belfield, W. T.: Pus Tubes in the Male, and Their Surgical Treatment. J.A.M.A. *44*:1277 (Apr. 22) 1905.

Belfield, W. T.: Skiagraphy of the Seminal Ducts. J.A.M.A. *60*:800-803 (Mar. 15) 1913a.

Belfield, W. T.: Vasostomy—Radiography of the Seminal Duct. J.A.M.A. *61*:1867-1869 (Nov. 22) 1913b.

Benjamin, J. A., Joint, F. T., Ramsay, G. H., Watson, J. S., Weinberg, S., and Scott, W. W.: Cinefluorographic Studies of Bladder and Urethral Function. J. Urol. *73*:525-535 (Mar.) 1955.

Bergman, H., and Ellner, H.: Severe Reactions Following Previously Uneventful Intravenous Pyelograms. New York J. Med. *60*:105-106 (Jan. 1) 1960.

Bernstein, E. F., and Evans, R. L.: Low-Molecular-Weight Dextran. J.A.M.A. *174*:1417-1422 (Nov. 12) 1960.

Bersack, S. R., and Whitaker, T. E., Jr.: Effect of Diphenhydramine (Benadryl) on Side-Reactions in Intravenous Urography. A.M.A. Arch. Int. Med. *91*:618-625 (May) 1953.

Blackwood, J.: Presacral Perirenal Pneumography. Brit. J. Surg. *39*:111-119, 1951.

Bland, A. B.: A Simplified Apparatus for Presacral Carbon Dioxide Injection. J. Urol. *79*:171-172 (Jan.) 1958.

Bloom, J., and Richardson, J. F.: The Usefulness of a Contrast Medium Containing an Antibacterial Agent (Retrografin) for Retrograde Pyelography. J. Urol. *81*:332-334 (Feb.) 1959.

Boreau, J.: L'épididymographie. J. urol. *59*:416-423 (May 18) 1953.

Boreau, J., Elbim, A., Hermann, P., Vassel, B., and Fua, R.: L'épididymographie. Presse méd. *59*:1406-1407 (Oct. 24) 1951.

Boreau, J., Hermann, P., Vasselle, B., and Fua, R.: L'étude radiologique et radiomanométrique des voies génitales de l'homme appliquée à la clinique et à la physiologie. Semaine d. hôp. Paris *28*:1549-1556 (May 18) 1952.

Bunge, R. G.: Delayed Cystograms in Children. J. Urol. *70*:729-732 (Nov.) 1953.

Bunge, R. G.: Further Observations With Delayed Cystograms. J. Urol. *71*:427-434 (Apr.) 1954.

Burns, E.: Clinical Diagnosis of Tumors of Adult Renal Parenchyma. J. Urol. *70*:9-14 (July) 1953.

Cahill, G. F.: Air Injection To Demonstrate Adrenals by X-ray. J. Urol. *34*:238-243 (Sept.) 1935.

Cahill, G. F.: Roentgenography: Perirenal Insufflation. In Glasser, O.: Medical Physics. Chicago, Year Book Publishers, Inc., 1944, pp. 1309-1313.

Carelli, H. H.: Sur le pneumopéritoine et sur une méthode personelle pour voir le rein sans pneumopéritoine. Bull et mém. soc. méd. Hôp. Paris *45*:1409-1412, 1921.

Carelli, H. H., and Sordelli, E.: Un nuevo procedimiento para explorar el riñón. Rev. Asoc. méd. argent. *34*:424 (June) 1921.

Cattell, W. R., Fry, I. K., Spencer, A. G., and Purkiss, P.: Excretion Urography. 1—Factors Determining the Excretion of Hypaque. Brit. J. Radiol. *40*:561-571 (Aug.) 1967.

Cerny, J. C., Kendall, A. R., and Nesbit, R. M.: Subcutaneous Pyelography in Infants: A Reappraisal. J. Urol. *98*:405-409 (Sept.) 1967.

Chaoul, H.: Eine neue Röntgenuntersuchungsmethode in der Lungendiagnostik: Aufnakmen von Schnitten und Schichten der Lunge (Tomographie). Deutsche Med. Wchnschr. *61*:700-703 (May 3) 1935.

Cimmino, C. V.: The Problem of Compression in Intravenous Pyelography. (Editorial.) Am. J. Roentgenol. *93*:484-485 (Feb.) 1965.

Cobb, O. E., and Anderson, E. E.: Superimposition Cystography in the Diagnosis of Infiltrating Tumors of the Bladder. J. Urol. *94*:569-572 (Nov.) 1965.

Coleman, W. P., Ochsner, S. F., and Watson, B. E.: Allergic Reactions in 10,000 Consecutive Intravenous Urographies. South. M. J. *57*:1401-1404 (Dec.) 1964.

Cook, E. N., and Pool, T. L.: Urethral Diverticulum in the Female. J. Urol. *62*:495-497 (Oct.) 1949.

Cope, O., and Raker, J. W.: Cushing's Disease: The Surgical Experience in the Care of 46 Cases. New England J. Med. 253:165-172 (Aug. 4) 1955.

Cope, O., and Schatzki, R.: Tumors of the Adrenal Glands. I. A Modified Air Injection Roentgen Technic for Demonstrating Cortical and Medullary Tumors. Arch. Int. Med. 64:1222-1238 (Dec.) 1939.

Counseller, V. S.: Urethral Diverticulum in the Female: A Clinical Study. Am. J. Obst. & Gynec. 57:231-236 (Feb.) 1949.

Crepea, S. B., Allanson, J. C., and DeLambre, L.: The Failure of Antihistaminic Drugs to Inhibit Diodrast Reactions. New York J. Med. 49:2556-2558 (Nov. 1) 1949.

Culp, D. A., Van Epps, E. F., and Edwards, C. N.: Comparative Studies of Urographic Media. J. Urol. 78:493-495 (Oct.) 1957.

Cunningham, J. H., Jr.: The Diagnosis of Stricture of the Urethra by the Roentgen Rays. Tr. Am. A. Genito-Urinary Surgeons 5:369-371, 1910.

Daughtridge, T. G.: Ureteral Compression Device for Excretory Urography. Am. J. Roentgenol. 95:431-438 (Oct.) 1965.

Davis, H. J., and Cian, L. G.: Positive Pressure Urethrography: A New Diagnostic Method. J. Urol. 75:753-757 (Apr.) 1956.

Davis, H. J., and Telinde, R. W.: Urethral Diverticula: An Assay of 121 Cases. J. Urol. 80:34-39 (July) 1958.

Davis, L. A., Lich, R., Howerton, L., and Joule, W.: The Lower Urinary Tract in Infants and Children. Radiology 77:445-451 (Sept.) 1961.

Dean, A. L., Jr., Lattimer, J. K., and McCoy, C. B.: The Standardized Columbia University Cystogram. J. Urol. 78:662-668 (Nov.) 1957.

Detar, J. H., and Harris, J. A.: Venous Pooled Nephrograms: Technique and Results. J. Urol. 72:979-982 (Nov.) 1954.

Dolan, L. P.: Allergic Death Due to Intravenous Use of Diodrast: Suggestions for Possible Prevention. J.A.M.A. 114:138-139 (Jan. 13) 1940.

Doyle, O. W.: The Use of Chlor-Trimeton With Miokon in Intravenous Urography. J. Urol. 81:573-574 (Apr.) 1959.

Edling, N. P. G.: Urethrocystography in the Male With Special Regard to Micturition. Acta radiol. Suppl. 58, 1945, 144 pp.

Edling, N. P. G., Edvall, C. A., Helander, C. G., and Pernow, B.: Comparison of Urography With Selective Clearance as Tests of Renal Function. Acta radiol. 45:85-95 (Feb.) 1956.

Edling, N. P. G., and Helander, C. G.: Nephrographic Effect in Renal Angiography: An Experimental Study in Dogs. Acta radiol. 51:17-24 (Jan.) 1959.

Evans, J. A.: Nephrotomography in Investigation of Renal Masses. Radiology 69:684-689 (Nov.) 1957.

Evans, J. A., Dubilier, W., Jr., and Monteith, J. C.: Nephrotomography: A Preliminary Report. Am. J. Roentgenol. 71:213-223 (Feb.) 1954.

Eyler, W. R., Drew, D. R., and Bohne, A. W.: A Comparative Clinical Trial of Urographic Media: Renografin, Hypaque, and Urokon. Radiology 66:871-873 (June) 1956.

Feldman, M. I., Goade, W. J., Jr., Bouras, L., and Bargoot, F. J.: Total Urography by Rapid Intra-

venous Infusion. J. Urol. 99:220-222 (Feb.) 1968.

Finby, N., Evans, J. A., and Steinberg, I.: Reactions From Intravenous Organic Iodide Compounds: Pretesting and Prophylaxis. Radiology 71:15-17 (July) 1958.

Finby, N., Evans, J. A., and Steinberg, I.: Evaluation of Concentrated Contrast Media in Angiocardiography, Nephrotomography and Intravenous Aortography. Angiology 11:310-312 (June) 1960.

Fischer, H. W., and Cornell, S. H.: The Toxicity of the Sodium and Methylglucamine Salts of Diatrizoate, Iothalamate, and Metrizoate: An Experimental Study of Their Circulatory Effects Following Intracarotid Injection. Radiology 85:1013-1021 (Dec.) 1965.

Flocks, R. H.: The Roentgen Visualization of the Posterior Urethra. J. Urol. 30:711-736 (Dec.) 1933.

Friedenberg, M. J., and Carlin, M. R.: The Routine Use of Higher Volumes of Contrast Material to Improve Intravenous Urography. Radiology 83:405-413 (Sept.) 1964.

Fulton, R. E., Witten, D. M., and Wagoner, R. D.: Intravenous Urography in Renal Insufficiency. Am. J. Roentgenol. 106:623-634 (July) 1969.

Garrett, R. A., and Klatte, E. C.: Cineurography. J. Urol. 83:498-500 (Apr.) 1960.

Genereux, G. P.: The Collateral Vein Sign in Renal Neoplasia. J. Canad. Ass. Radiol. 19:46-55 (June) 1968.

Getzoff, P. L.: The Use of Histamine Antagonist in Intravenous Pyelography. New Orleans M. & S. J. 101:22-25 (July) 1948.

Getzoff, P. L.: Use of Antihistamine Drug Prophylaxis Against Diodrast Reactions. J. Urol. 65:1139-1142 (June) 1951.

Gilg, E.: The Influence of Diphenhydramine (Benadryl) on the Side-Effects of Diodone in Urography. Acta radiol. 39:299-307 (Apr.) 1953.

Glassman, I., Shapiro, R., and Robinson, F.: Air Embolism During Presacral Pneumography: A Case Report. J. Urol. 75:569-571 (Mar.) 1956.

Golji, H.: Clinical Value of Epididymo-vesiculography. J. Urol. 78:445-455 (Oct.) 1957.

Gronner, A. T., Arkoff, R. S., and Burhenne, H. J.: Routine High Dose Excretory Urography. California Med. 107:16-19 (July) 1967.

Grossmann, G.: Tomographie I (Röntgenographische Darstellung von Körperschnitten). Fortschr. a.d. Geb. d. Röntgenstrahlen. 51:61-80, 1935a.

Grossmann, G.: Tomographie II (Theoretisches über Tomographie). Fortschr. a.d. Geb. d. Röntgenstrahlen. 51:191-208, 1935b.

Gullmo, Å., and Sundberg, J.: A Method for Roentgen Examination of the Posterior Urethra, Prostatic Ducts and Utricle (Utriculography). Acta radiol. 48:241-247 (Oct.) 1957.

Hamm, F. C., Waterhouse, K., and Weinberg, S. R.: Dangers of Excretory Urography. J.A.M.A. 172:542-546 (Feb. 6) 1960.

Handek, M.: Zur Technik der Röntgenuntersuchung der Harnröhre. Wien. Med. Wchnschr. 71:490-491 (Mar. 12) 1921.

Hansen, L. K.: Micturition Cystourethrography With Automatic Serial Exposures. Acta radiol. Suppl. 207, 1961, 139 pp.

Harkins, H. N., and Harmon, P. H.: Embolism by

Air and Oxygen: Comparative Studies. Proc. Soc. Exper. Biol. & Med. 32:178-181, 1934.

Harrison, R. H., III, and Doubleday, L. C.: Roentgenologic Appearance of Normal Adrenal Glands. J. Urol. 76:16-22 (July) 1956.

Hart, L. E., Sachs, M. D., and Grabstald, H.: Comparative Study of Urographic Contrast Media. A.M.A. Arch. Surg. 77:75-78 (July) 1958.

Hartley, W.: Infusion Urography. Clin. Radiol. 17:237-241 (July) 1966.

Hemley, S. D., Gallagher, J., and Cusmano, J.: Large Bolus Injection With Compression in Routine Excretory Urography. J. Urol. 96:390-393 (Sept.) 1966.

Herbst, R. H., and Merricks, J. W.: Visualization and Treatment of Seminal Vesiculitis by Catheterization and Dilatation of Ejaculatory Ducts. J. Urol. 41:733-750 (May) 1939.

Herbst, R. H., and Merricks, J. W.: Transurethral Approach to the Diagnosis and Treatment of the Seminal Vesicles. Illinois M. J. 78:393-396 (Nov.) 1940.

Herbst, R. H., and Merricks, J. W.: Transurethral Drainage of the Seminal Vesicles in Seminal Vesiculitis. Illinois M. J. 86:190-195 (Oct.) 1944.

Hildreth, E. A., Pendergrass, H. P., Tondreau, R. L., and Ritchie, D. J.: Reactions Associated With Intravenous Urography: Discussion of Mechanisms and Therapy. Radiology 74:246-254 (Feb.) 1960.

Hinman, F., Jr., Miller, G. M., Nickel, E., and Miller, E. R.: Vesical Physiology Demonstrated by Cineradiography and Serial Roentgenography: Preliminary Report. Radiology 62:713-719 (May) 1954.

Hinman, F., Jr., Steinbach, H. L., and Forsham, P. H.: Preoperative Differentiation Between Hyperplasia and Tumor in Cushing's Syndrome. Tr. Am. A. Genito-Urinary Surgeons 48:97-106, 1956.

Hoffman, H. A., and de Carvalho, M. P.: Retrograde Pyelography and Use of Contrast Mediums Containing Neomycin. J.A.M.A. 172:236 (Jan. 16) 1960.

Hoffman, W. W., and Grayhack, J. T.: The Limitations of the Intravenous Pyelogram as a Test of Renal Function. Surg., Gynec. & Obst. 110:503-508 (Apr.) 1960.

Howard, T. L., and Buchtel, H. A.: Resection of Vesical Neck in Children: Indications and Results. J.A.M.A. 146:1202-1206 (July 28) 1951.

Izenstark, J. L., and Lafferty, W.: Medical Radiological Practice in New Orleans: Estimates and Characteristics of Visits, Examinations, and Genetically Significant Dose. Radiology 90:229-241 (Feb.) 1968.

Kieffer, J.: The Laminagraph and Its Variations: Applications and Implications of the Planigraphic Principles. Am. J. Roentgenol. 39:497-513 (Apr.) 1938.

Kjellberg, S. R., Ericsson, N. O., and Rudhe, U.: The Lower Urinary Tract in Childhood: Some Correlated Clinical and Roentgenological Observations. Chicago, The Year Book Publishers, Inc., 1957.

Knoefel, P. K.: The Nature of the Toxic Action of Radiopaque Diagnostic Agents. Radiology 71:13-14 (July) 1958.

Landes, R. R., and Ransom, C. L.: Technic for the Use of Carbon Dioxide in Presacral Retroperitoneal Pneumography. Surg., Gynec. & Obst. 105:268-272 (Sept.) 1957.

Landsteiner, K.: The Specificity of Serological Reactions. Springfield, Illinois, Charles C Thomas, 1936, 178 pp.

Landsteiner, K., Levine, P. H., and Van Der Scheer, J.: Anaphylactic Reactions Produced by Azodyes in Animals Sensitized With Azoproteins. Proc. Soc. Exper. Biol. & Med. 27:811-812 (May) 1930.

Lang, E. K., and Davis, H. J.: Positive Pressure Urethrography: Roentgenographic Diagnostic Method for Urethral Diverticula in the Female. Radiology 72:401-405 (Mar.) 1959.

Lasser, E. C.: Basic Mechanisms of Contrast Media Reactions. Radiology 91:63-65 (July) 1968.

Lasser, E. C., Lang, J. H., and Zawadzki, Z. A.: Contrast Media: Myeloma Protein Precipitates in Urography. J.A.M.A. 198:945-947 (Nov. 21) 1966.

Lattimer, J. K., Dean, A. L., Jr., and Furey, C. A.: The Triple Voiding Technique in Children With Dilated Urinary Tracts. J. Urol. 76:656-660 (Nov.) 1956.

Lefkovits, A. M.: Fatal Air Embolism During Presacral Insufflation of Air. J. Urol. 77:112-115 (Jan.) 1957.

Leucutia, T.: Multiple Myeloma and Intravenous Pyelography. (Editorial.) Am. J. Roentgenol. 85:187-189 (Jan.) 1961.

Levitt, J. I., Amplatz, K., and Loken, M. K.: Renovascular Hypertension: Correlation of Surgical Results With Certain Predictive Tests. Radiology 91:521-528 (Sept.) 1968.

Loew, E. R., and Kaiser, M. E.: Alleviation of Anaphylactic Shock in Guinea Pigs With Synthetic Benzhydryl Alkamine Ethers. Proc. Soc. Exper. Biol. & Med. 58:235-237 (Mar.) 1945.

Loew, E. R., Kaiser, M. E., and Moore, V.: Synthetic Benzhydryl Alkamine Ethers Effective in Preventing Fatal Experimental Asthma in Guinea Pigs Exposed to Atomized Histamine. J. Pharmacol. & Exper. Therap. 83:120-129 (Feb.) 1945.

Lowsley, O. S., and Kirwin, T. J.: Clinical Urology. Baltimore, Williams & Wilkins Company, 1956, p. 89.

MacEwan, D. W.: Improved Detail in Excretory Urography Using Twice the Amount of Contrast Agent. J. Canad. Ass. Radiol. 16:105-113 (June) 1965.

MacEwan, D. W., Dunbar, J. S., and Nogrady, M. B.: Intravenous Pyelography in Children With Renal Insufficiency. Radiology 78:893-903 (June) 1962.

Macht, S. H., Williams, R. H., and Lawrence, P. S.: Study of 3 Contrast Agents in 2,234 Intravenous Pyelographies. Am. J. Roentgenol. 98:79-87 (Sept.) 1966.

Mann, M. R.: The Pharmacology of Contrast Media. Proc. Roy. Soc. Med. 54:473-476 (June) 1961.

Marion, G.: Maladie du col vésical. In Joly, J. S.: Fifth Congress of the International Society of Urology. London, John Bale, Sons & Danielsson, Ltd., 1933, vol. 1, pp. 392-444.

Maxwell, M. H., Gonick, H. C., Wiita, R., and Kaufman, J. J.: Use of the Rapid-Sequence Intravenous Pyelogram in the Diagnosis of Renovascular

Hypertension. New England J. Med. 270:213-220 (Jan. 30) 1964.

McCarthy, J. F., Ritter, J. S., and Klemperer, P.: Anatomical and Histological Study of the Verumontanum With Especial Reference to the Ejaculatory Ducts. J. Urol. 17:1-16 (Jan.) 1927.

McMahon, S.: An Anatomical Study by Injection Technique of the Ejaculatory Ducts and Their Relations. J. Urol. 39:422-443 (Apr.) 1938.

Merricks, J. W.: The Modern Conception of the Diagnosis and Treatment of Infections of the Seminal Vesicles: With Roentgenographic Visualization of These Organs by Catheterization of Ejaculatory Ducts. New Internat. Clin. 2(n.s.3):193-199 (June) 1940.

Moore, S.: Body Section Roentgenography With the Laminagraph. Am. J. Roentgenol. 39:514-522 (Apr.) 1938.

Moore, T. D., and Sanders, N.: Reaction to Urographic Agents With and Without Antihistamines. J. Urol. 70:538-544 (Sept.) 1953.

Morales, O., and Romanus, R.: Urethrography in the Male With a Highly Viscous, Water-Soluble Contrast Medium, Umbradil-Viscous U. Acta radiol. Suppl. 95, 1952, pp. 9-91.

Morgan, C., Jr., and Hammack, W. J.: Intravenous Urography in Multiple Myeloma. New England J. Med. 275:77-79 (July 14) 1966.

Myers, G. H., Jr., and Witten, D. M.: Unpublished data.

Mygind, H. B.: Urogenital Tuberculosis in the Human Male: Vesiculographic and Urethrographic Studies. Danish Med. Bull. 7:13-18 (Feb.) 1960.

Narath, P. A.: Renal Pelvis and Ureter. New York, Grune & Stratton, Inc., 1951, 429 pp.

Naterman, H. L., and Robins, S. A.: Cutaneous Test With Diodrast to Predict Allergic Systemic Reactions From Diodrast Given Intravenously. J.A.M.A. 119:491-493 (June 6) 1942.

Neal, M. P., Jr., Howell, T. R., and Lester, R. G.: Contrast Infusion Nephropyelography. J.A.M.A. 193:1017-1020 (Sept. 20) 1965.

Nesbit, R. M.: The Incidence of Severe Reactions From Present Day Urographic Contrast Materials: A Report on Data Collected From Members of the Association. Tr. Am. A. Genito-Urin. Surgeons 50:148-151, 1958.

Nesbit, R. M.: The Incidence of Severe Reactions From Present Day Urographic Contrast Materials. J. Urol. 81:486-489 (Mar.) 1959.

Nesbit, R. M., and Nesbitt, T. E.: Experiences With High Concentration Urokon for Pyelography. Univ. Michigan M. Bull. 18:225-231 (Aug.) 1952.

Ochsner, S. F., Little, E., Buchtel, B., Giesen, A., and Morel, A.: Untoward Reactions Observed in 10,000 Consecutive Excretory Urographies. J. Louisiana M. Soc. 114:150-155 (May) 1963.

Olsson, O.: Antihistaminic Drugs for Inhibiting Untoward Reactions to Injections of Contrast Medium. Acta Radiol. 35:65-70 (Jan.) 1951.

Pasternack, B. S., and Heller, M. B.: Genetically Significant Dose to the Population of New York City From Diagnostic Medical Radiography. Radiology 90:217-228 (Feb.) 1968.

Pendergrass, E. P.: Excretory Urography as a Test of Urinary Tract Function. Radiology 40:223-246 (Mar). 1943.

Pendergrass, E. P., Hodes, P. J., Tondreau, R. L., Powell, C. C., and Burdick, E. D.: Further Consideration of Deaths and Unfavorable Sequelae Following the Administration of Contrast Media in Urography in the United States. Am. J. Roentgenol. 74:262-287 (Aug.) 1955.

Pendergrass, H. P., and Hodes, P. J.: Complications of Retroperitoneal Contrast Studies. Pennsylvania M. J. 60:1453-1456 (Nov.) 1957.

Pendergrass, H. P., Tondreau, R. L., Pendergrass, E. P., Ritchie, D. J., Hildreth, E. A., and Askovitz, S. I.: Reactions Associated With Intravenous Urography: Historical and Statistical Review. Radiology 71:1-12 (July) 1958.

Penfil, R. L., and Brown, M. L.: Genetically Significant Dose to the United States Population From Diagnostic Medical Roentgenology, 1964. Radiology 90:209-216 (Feb.) 1968.

Pereira, A.: Roentgen Interpretation of Vesiculograms. Am. J. Roentgenol. 69:361-379 (Mar.) 1953.

Peterson, A. P.: Retrograde Catheterization in Diagnosis and Treatment of Seminal Vesiculitis. J. Urol. 39:662-667 (Apr.) 1938.

Post, H. W. A., and Southwood, W. F. W.: The Technique and Interpretation of Nephrotomograms. Brit. J. Radiol. 32:734-738 (Nov.) 1959.

Powell, T., Lentle, B. C., Dew, B. T., ApSimon, H. T., and Pitman, R. G.: Intravenous Pyelography: A Comparative Trial of Ten Methods in Patients With Good Renal Function. Brit. J. Radiol. 40:30-37 (Jan.) 1967.

Pratt, A. D., Jr., and White, W. W.: Drip Infusion Pyelography. J.A.M.A. 202:206-207 (Nov. 6) 1967.

Ransom, C. L., Landes, R. R., and McLelland, R.: Air Embolism Following Retroperitoneal Pneumography: A Nation-Wide Survey. J. Urol. 76:664-670 (Nov.) 1956.

Rees, E. D., and Waugh, W. H.: Factors in the Renal Failure of Multiple Myeloma. Arch. Int. Med. 116:400-405 (Sept.) 1965.

Rhamy, R. K., Garrett, R. A., and Carr, J. R.: Cineradiographic Characteristics of Infravesical Obstruction. J. Urol. 88:696-699 (Nov.) 1962.

Riches, E. W., Griffiths, I. H., and Thackray, A. C.: New Growths of the Kidney and Ureter. Brit. J. Urol. 23:297-356 (Dec.) 1951.

Rivas, M. R.: Roentgenological Diagnosis: Generalized Subserous Emphysema Through a Single Puncture. Am. J. Roentgenol. 64:723-734 (Nov.) 1950.

Robb, G. P., and Steinberg, I.: Visualization of the Chambers of the Heart, the Pulmonary Circulation, and the Great Blood Vessels in Man: A Practical Method. Am. J. Roentgenol. 41:1-17 (Jan.) 1939.

Robertson, L. B., Jr., Anderson, E. E., and Glenn, J. F.: Retroperitoneal Contrast Studies: Simplified Bilateral Perirenal Carbon Dioxide Insufflation. J. Urol. 93:414-416 (Mar.) 1965.

Robins, S. A.: Hypersensitivity to Diodrast as Determined by Skin Tests. Am. J. Roentgenol. 48:766-769 (Dec.) 1942.

Roth, R. B., Kaminsky, A. F., and Hess, E.: A Bacteriocidal Additive for Pyelographic Media. J. Urol. 74:563-566 (Oct.) 1955.

St. Martin, E. C., Campbell, J. H., and Pesquier, C.

M.: Cystography in Children. J. Urol. 75:151-159 (Jan.) 1956.

Samellas, W., Biel, L., Jr., and Draper, J. W.: The Usefulness of Neomycin in Retrograde Pyelography. New York J. Med. 59:2570-2572 (July 1) 1959.

Sandström, C.: Secondary Reactions From Contrast Media and the Allergy Concept. Acta radiol. 44:233-242 (Sept.) 1955.

Sanger, M. D.: Further Observations With Antihistamines in Reducing Reactions in Intravenous Pyelography. Ann. Allergy 17:762-767 (Sept.-Oct.) 1959.

Schencker, B.: Drip Infusion Pyelography: Indications and Applications in Urologic Roentgen Diagnosis. Radiology 83:12-21 (July) 1964.

Schencker, B.: Further Experience With Drip Infusion Pyelography. Radiology 87:304-308 (Aug.) 1966.

Schencker, B., Marcure, R. W., and Moody, D. L.: Simplified Nephrotomography: The Drip Infusion Technique. Am. J. Roentgenol. 95:283-290 (Oct.) 1965.

Schreiber, M. H., Remmers, A. R., Sarles, H. E., and Smith, G. H.: The Normal Pyelogram Urea Washout Test: A Study of 33 Normotensive Controls. Am. J. Roentgenol. 98:88-95 (Sept.) 1966.

Schwartz, W. B., Hurwit, A., and Ettinger, Alice: Intravenous Urography in the Patient With Renal Insufficiency. New England J. Med. 269:277-283 (Aug. 8) 1963.

Sherwood, T., Breckenridge, A., Dollery, C. T., Doyle, F. H., and Steiner, R. E.: Intravenous Urography and Renal Function. Clin. Radiol. 19:296-302 (July) 1968.

Shopfner, C. E.: Cystourethrography: An Evaluation of Method. Am. J. Roentgenol. 95:468-474 (Oct.) 1965.

Simon, S. W., Berman, H. I., and Rosenblum, S. A.: Prevention of Reactions in Intravenous Urography. J. Allergy 25:395-399 (Sept.) 1954.

Smith, D. R., Steinbach, H. L., Lyon, R. B., and Stratte, P. B.: Extraperitoneal Pneumography. J. Urol. 68:953-959 (Dec.) 1952.

Spalding, C. K., and Cowing, R. F.: A Survey of Exposures Received by Hospitalized Patients During Routine Diagnostic X-ray Procedures. Radiology 82:113-119 (Jan.) 1964.

Staab, E. V., Amplatz, K., Stejskal, R., and Loken, M. K.: The Urea Wash-Out Test. Minnesota Med. 48:448-454 (Apr.) 1965.

Standen, J. R., Nogrady, ·M. B., Dunbar, J. S., and Goldbloom, R. B.: The Osmotic Effects of Methylglucamine Diatrizoate (Renografin 60) in Intravenous Urography in Infants. Am. J. Roentgenol. 93:473-479 (Feb.) 1965.

Steinbach, H. L., Hinman, F., Jr., and Forsham, P. H.: The Diagnosis of Adrenal Neoplasms by Contrast Media. Radiology 69:664-671 (Nov.) 1957.

Steinbach, H. L., Lyon, R. P., Smith, D. R., and Miller, E. R.: Extraperitoneal Pneumography. Radiology 59:167-175 (Aug.) 1952.

Steinbach, H. L., and Smith, D. R.: Extraperitoneal Pneumography in Diagnosis of Retroperitoneal Tumors. A.M.A. Arch. Surg. 70:161-172, 1955.

Steinberg, I., and Robb, G. P.: Mediastinal and Hilar Angiography in Pulmonary Disease: A Preliminary Report. Am. Rev. Tuberc. 38:557-569 (Nov.) 1938.

Stewart, C. M.: Delayed Cystograms. J. Urol. 70:588-593 (Oct.) 1953.

Stewart, C. M.: Delayed Cystography and Voiding Cystourethrography. J. Urol. 74:749-759 (Dec.) 1955.

Strain, W. H., and Rogoff, S. M.: Water-Soluble Radiopaques. In Medical Radiography and Photography: Radiologic Diagnostic Agents. Rochester, New York, Eastman Kodak Company, 1964, vol. 40, supplement, pp. 26-44.

Thornbury, J. R., and Immergut, M. A.: Polyview Voiding Cystourethrography in Children. Am. J. Roentgenol. 95:475-478 (Oct.) 1965.

Tristan, T. A., Murphy, J. J., and Schoenberg, H. W.: Cinefluorographic Investigation of Genitourinary Tract Function. Radiology 79:731-739 (Nov.) 1962.

Tucker, A. S., Yanagihara, H., and Pryde, A. W.: A Method for Roentgenography of the Male Genital Tract. Am. J. Roentgenol. 71:490-500 (Mar.) 1954.

Utz, D. C., and Thompson, G. J.: Evaluation of Contrast Media for Excretory Urography. Proc. Staff Meet., Mayo Clin. 33:75-80 (Feb. 19) 1958.

Vallebona, A.: Una modalità di tecnica per la dissociazione radiografica delle ombre applicata allo studio del cranio. Radiol. med. 17:1090-1097 (Sept.) 1930.

Vix, V. A.: Intravenous Pyelography in Multiple Myeloma: A Review of 52 Studies in 40 Patients. Radiology 87:896-902 (Nov.) 1966.

Voltz, P. W., Jr., Thaggard, A., Jr., O'Neill, F. E., Wiesner, J. J., and Douglass, C. F., Jr.: Large Dose Urography in Children. South. M. J. 59:519-524 (May) 1966.

Wall, B., and Rose, D. K.: The Clinical Nephrogram: Preliminary Report. J. Urol. 66:305-314 (Aug.) 1951.

Walter, R. C., and Goodwin, W. E.: Aortography and Pneumography in Children. J. Urol. 77:323-328 (Feb.) 1957.

Waterhouse, K.: Voiding Cystourethrography: A Simple Technique. J. Urol. 85:103-104 (Jan.) 1961.

Wechsler, H.: The Use of Benadryl to Decrease Reactions in Intravenous Urography. New York J. Med. 56:401-403 (Feb. 1) 1956.

Wechsler, H.: Further Studies of Reactions Due to Intravenous Urography. J. Urol. 78:496-497 (Oct.) 1957.

Weens, H. S., and Florence, T. J.: Nephrography. Am. J. Roentgenol. 57:338-341 (Mar.) 1947.

Weens, H. S., Olnick, H. M., James, D. F., and Warren, J. V.: Intravenous Nephrography: A Method of Roentgen Visualization of the Kidney. Am. J. Roentgenol. 65:411-414 (Mar.) 1951.

Wells, J. A., Morris, H. C., and Dragstedt, C. A.: Modification of Anaphylaxis by Benadryl. Proc. Soc. Exper. Biol. & Med. 61:104-106 (Feb.) 1946.

Wendth, A. J., Jr.: Drip Infusion Pyelography. Am. J. Roentgenol. 95:269-282 (Oct.) 1965.

Wesson, M. B., and Fulmer, C. C.: Influence of Ureteral Stones on Intravenous Urograms. Am. J. Roentgenol. 28:27-33 (July) 1932.

Wigh, R., Anthony, H. F., Jr., and Grant, B. P.: A

Comparison of Intravenous Urography, Urine Radiography, and Other Renal Tests. Radiology 78:869-878 (June) 1962.

Wilcox, L. F.: Kidney Function in Acute Calculous Obstruction of the Ureter: Some Observations of Kidney and Ureter Function in Acute Calculous Obstruction of the Ureter, Based on Excretory Urography. Am. J. Roentgenol. 34:596-605 (Nov.) 1935.

Wilhelm, S. F.: Vaso-seminal Vesiculography: Clinical and Experimental Application. J. Urol. 41:751-757 (May) 1939.

Wilhelm, S. F.: Gas Insufflation Through the Lumbar and Presacral Routes. Surg., Gynec. & Obst. 99:319-323 (Sept.) 1954.

Williams, D. I.: The Radiological Diagnosis of Lower Urinary Obstruction in the Early Years. Brit. J. Radiol. 27:473-481 (Sept.) 1954.

Witten, D. M., Greene, L. F., and Emmett, J. L.: An Evaluation of Nephrotomography in Urologic Diagnosis. Am. J. Roentgenol. 90:115-123 (July) 1963.

Witten, D. M., and Hirsch, F. D.: Unpublished data.

Witten, D. M., Hunt, J. C., Sheps, S. G., Greene, L. F., and Utz, D. C.: Excretory Urography in Renovascular Hypertension: Minute Sequence Filming and Osmotic Diuresis. Am. J. Roentgenol. 98:114-121 (Sept.) 1966.

Woodruff, M. W.: The Five Minute Intravenous Pyelogram as a Measure of Renal Function. Am. J. Roentgenol. 82:847-848 (Nov.) 1959.

Wright, F. W.: Intravenous Hydrocortisone in the Treatment of a Severe Urographic Reaction. Brit. J. Urol. 32:343-344 (May) 1959.

Young, B. W., Anderson, W. L., and King, G. C.: Radiographic Estimation of Residual Urine in Children. J. Urol. 75:263-272 (Feb.) 1956.

Young, H. H., and Waters, C. A.: X-ray Studies of the Seminal Vesicles and Vasa Deferentia After Urethroscopic Injection of Ejaculatory Ducts With Thorium: A New Diagnostic Method. Am. J. Roentgenol. 7:16-21 (Jan.) 1920.

Ziedses des Plantes, B. G.: Eine neue Methode zuer Differenzierung in der Röntgenographie (Planigraphie). Acta radiol. 13:182-192, 1932.

Ziedses des Plantes, B. G.: Planigraphie: Une méthode permettant en radiographie d'obtenu une image nette de la section d'un objet a un plan bien déterminé. J. Radiol. et d'electrol. 18:73-76, 1934.

CHAPTER 2

Techniques and Applications of Renal Angiography

By OWINGS W. KINCAID

GENERAL CONSIDERATIONS

In recent years, with the development and refinement of vascular catheterization techniques, the design and production of more sophisticated radiographic equipment, and the synthesis of safer contrast media, renal angiography has become an invaluable adjunct to urologic diagnosis. With modern angiographic techniques, the anatomy and gross pathology of the renal vessels and kidneys may be demonstrated in great detail.

Renal angiography may be performed by a variety of methods. These include (1) the percutaneous transfemoral catheterization method (Seldinger technique); (2) the translumbar method; (3) the percutaneous transaxillary catheterization method; and (4) the retrograde noncatheter brachial method.

The percutaneous transfemoral catheterization method has many important advantages over other methods of renal angiography, and is the technique of choice in virtually all patients. Other methods, however, must be resorted to on occasion, for in special circumstances one method may be feasible when other methods are not.

RADIOGRAPHIC EQUIPMENT AND TECHNIQUE

EQUIPMENT

Renal angiography requires the use of specialized, complex, and powerful x-ray equipment, and should be carried out in a completely equipped angiography suite or laboratory by a radiologist fully conversant with this equipment and with the basic principles of radiography and angiography.

The room for renal angiography should be of adequate size, certainly no smaller than 18 by 20 feet, with plenty of space for all x-ray equipment, a small instrument table, anesthesia equipment, a power injector, and other ancillary equipment (Fig. 2–1). Adequate storage space for needles, guide wires, catheters, sterile packs, contrast media, and other materials should be available.

A film changer, preferably capable of transporting four films per second, is a necessity. Three general types of film changers have been developed to meet the needs of angiography: (1) cassette changers, (2) cut-film changers, and (3) roll-film changers. Each type has its advantages and disadvantages.

Cassette changers are the least satisfactory. Because of the difficulties inherent in the rapid mechanical transport of heavy x-ray cassettes, such changers do not usually permit speeds in excess of two films per second.

Two film changers, both manufactured by Elema-Schonanader of Stockholm, one using cut-film and the other using roll-film, are ideal for renal angiography, as well as for many other angiographic examinations (Fig. 2–2). The cut-film changer is easier to load and unload and is somewhat more versatile than the roll-film changer. The cut-film changer is available as a single-plane or biplane

unit and is capable of making up to six film exposures per second. The roll-film changer is capable of making up to 12 exposures per second, and is available only as a biplane unit, but single-plane filming may be used if desired. The major advantage to the use of roll film lies in the fact that the individual frames do not get mixed up and out of order. This is a major advantage when large numbers of exposures are to be made, as in angiocardiography, but is not a significant advantage for renal angiography.

Powerful, three-phase, x-ray generators of at least 1,000-ma capacity and high-speed rotation 150-kv x-ray tubes are necessary if films of maximal quality are to be obtained.

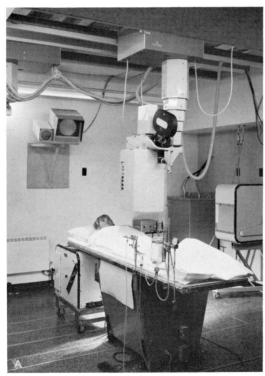 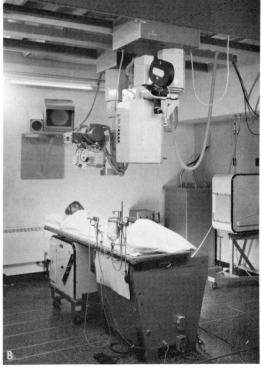

Figure 2–1. **A,** Room and equipment arrangement for renal angiography. Note wall-mounted television monitor and oscilloscope. Flushing system is mounted on table rail. **B,** Tabletop extended with patient centered over film changer. Radiographic tube in place for filming.

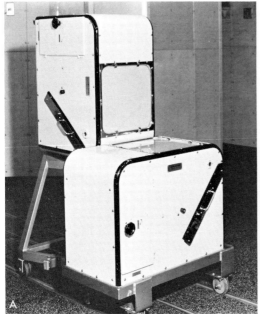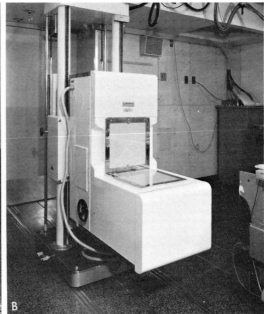

Figure 2–2. A, Cut-film changer manufactured by Elema-Schonanader of Stockholm. B, Roll-film changer, also manufactured by Elema-Schonanader.

RADIOGRAPHIC TECHNIQUE

Such equipment will permit exposure times as short as 7 msec. For renal angiography, 32 to 40 msec and a 36 to 40-inch target-film distance are usually employed. Image sharpness and film contrast will also be improved if the field is coned down so that only the kidneys and pertinent adjacent structures are included on the roentgenograms.

Appropriate grids of high quality are essential and some experimentation with various grids to be used with the equipment available will prove rewarding. We usually employ fine-line cross-hatch grids with a ratio of about 8 to 1.

One or two scout films made and viewed prior to angiography are necessary for proper choice of the exposure factors in each case.

The straight frontal projection is usually employed for renal arteriography. However, when the series of films made in this projection is viewed, a second series of films with rotation of the patient into the left or right oblique position may occasionally be indicated to eliminate overlapping of vessels and provide an unobscured view of important structures or lesions.

A minimum of three films per second is important for renal angiography. We most often expose four films per second during the period of injection and two per second for 1 to 2 seconds after completion of the injection, for visualization of the arterial phase. One film every 3 to 5 seconds is then exposed for the ensuing 15 to 20 seconds, during the nephrographic and venous phases of renal opacification.

SPECIAL TECHNIQUES

Stereoscopic Angiography

Some workers have employed two x-ray tubes, with alternate firing, in order to obtain stereoscopic arteriograms. Aside from the stereoscopic effect obtained, there is the added advantage of one being able to visualize the renal artery or other vessels from a slightly different angle on alternate films.

The equipment for stereoscopic angiography is rather expensive and complex and the value of this technique remains to be proved.

Direct Magnification Angiography

For magnification angiography, a mechanical design is necessary that will permit the patient to be positioned approximately midway between the target of the x-ray tube and the film. If the object is exactly at half the target-film distance, a twice normal magnification will be obtained. Some feel that diagnostic accuracy is improved by magnification technique, in that the renal vessels, as well as minute vessels barely visible on routine angiography, may be better visualized. An x-ray tube with a 0.3-mm or smaller focal spot is required for magnification angiography in order to reduce film unsharpness to a minimum.

Angiotomography

Prof. J. Frimann-Dahl of Oslo has described a technique in which tomography is combined with selective renal arteriography to produce tomograms of the kidney during the arterial phase of renal opacification (1964; 1966a). This promising new technique may be of considerable value in the differential diagnosis of renal mass lesions. For this technique, it is necessary that tomographic equipment be coupled to the angiographic table or that the patient be moved from the arteriographic table to the tomographic room after routine renal arteriography has been performed. A second selective injection is then made and tomography is carried out, three to five tomograms being made in rapid sequence.

RADIATION PROTECTION

As with other angiographic procedures, multiple x-ray exposures and large amounts of radiation are involved in the performance of renal arteriography. It is important that patient dosage be limited to the minimum necessary to obtain diagnostic studies. Of even greater importance is the protection of medical personnel who are exposed to radiation daily during the performance of angiography and other radiologic procedures.

The dose from fluoroscopy alone during catheterization procedures may pose a definite hazard, but these hazards can be considerably reduced if certain precautionary principles are adhered to. The smallest possible field size should be used for fluoroscopy and the primary field of radiation should never be permitted to extend outside the patient's body or outside the phosphor of the intensifying tube. The lowest possible level of radiation commensurate with adequate visualization of the catheter and pertinent anatomic structures should be employed, and the total time of fluoroscopy should be kept to a minimum. Protective leaded aprons should be worn by all personnel in the room. Whenever possible, all personnel should be out of the room or behind adequate protective barriers during the exposure of the films.

PREPARATION AND ANESTHESIA

The examiner should be certain that the patient has had no barium or other contrast medium for gastrointestinal examination within the past 3 or 4 days. If such has been given, 1 or 2 ounces of castor oil may be administered the day prior to arteriography in order to eliminate all contrast medium from the gastrointestinal tract.

The patient should be brought to the angiography room in a fasting state. Premedication is unnecessary if general anesthesia is to be employed. Moderate sedation should be given if the procedure is to be performed under local anesthesia.

Translumbar aortorenal arteriography may be carried out under local anesthesia. However, the discomfort of translumbar aortic puncture and the discomfort resulting from the intra-aortic injection of contrast medium with this technique make the use of local anesthesia unsatisfactory. We, therefore, employ general anesthesia for all patients undergoing translumbar aortography. Epidural anesthesia may be employed, but is quite time-consuming.

In the majority of patients, percutaneous transfemoral renal angiography may be carried out under local anesthesia. However, in patients under 16 years of age and in patients of any age who are apprehensive or uncooperative, general anesthesia is used. With modern-day anesthetic methods there is no appreciable hazard to general anesthesia, and we do not hesitate to employ it in patients undergoing renal arteriography. General anesthesia produces some reduction in cardiac output, which results in layering of the contrast medium in the renal arteries and in production of arteriograms of improved quality.

Reduction of blood pressure in severely hypertensive patients undergoing renal arteriography, utilizing ganglion-blocking agents, may be helpful in the prevention and control of bleeding from the aortic or femoral artery puncture site.

CONTRAST MEDIA

Ideally, contrast media used for renal arteriography should possess three essential qualities: high radiodensity, low toxicity, and low viscosity. Some of the more recently developed media are a distinct improvement over those used in the earlier days of angiography, particularly in regard to lower toxicity. The contrast media originally used were inorganic iodine compounds capable of causing serious renal damage. In recent years these have been replaced by organic iodine compounds, of which a large variety are available. (See discussion in Chapter 1.)

Hypaque-M (75%), Renovist (69%), and Renografin (76%) are excellent contrast media for renal angiography. All are mixtures of sodium and methylglucamine diatrizoate. Angio-Conray (sodium iothalamate) (80%) has a higher iodine content and is often preferable when translumbar aortography is employed.

Although the dosage of contrast medium may be varied somewhat with body weight, we generally employ 40 ml per injection for aortorenal arteriography and 10 to 15 ml for selective renal arteriography. Selective renal venography requires a larger dosage than selective arteriography, and 25 to 30 ml are usually employed.

PERCUTANEOUS TRANSFEMORAL CATHETERIZATION METHOD (SELDINGER TECHNIQUE)

Retrograde abdominal aortography with injection through an intra-aortic catheter was introduced by Fariñas in 1941. He cut down on and exposed the femoral artery, inserted a catheter, and passed it upward into the abdominal aorta. This method of aortography and visceral arteriography proved highly satisfactory but, since arteriotomy was required, was extremely time-consuming and difficult, requiring a certain amount of surgical experience and skill on the part of the physician performing the examination.

Peirce, in 1951, devised a method by which a catheter is passed into the aorta through a needle inserted percutaneously into the femoral artery. This technique, although it could be performed rapidly and did not require special surgical skills, did not prove highly satisfactory for angiography, owing to the small size of the catheter which can be inserted through the lumen of the femoral puncture needle.

This method of percutaneous catheterization was modified significantly in 1953 by Seldinger, who devised a means of percutaneous catheterization much more suitable for angiography since it permits the insertion of a much larger catheter than can be passed through a needle. In this technique, a guide wire is inserted through a small arterial puncture needle, the needle is removed, and the catheter passed into the artery over the guide wire. Catheterization of the femoral artery can be easily and rapidly accomplished with this technique. Indeed, almost any peripheral vessel can be so catheterized, and the technique has found many different applications in the field of angiography (Fig. 2-3).

The advantages of the percutaneous transfemoral catheterization technique for renal arteriography lie in the selectivity of the method (Edholm and Seldinger; Ödman; Olsson, 1961a). The injection of contrast medium may be made into the aorta at any chosen site relative to the origin of the renal arteries, or, by using a catheter with an appropriately curved tip, one or both renal arteries may be catheterized and selectively injected. By this selective technique, the renal arteries and the vascular architecture of the kidneys can be visualized in great detail and the problem of obscuration of the renal vessels by other opacified visceral arteries is avoided.

The percutaneous transfemoral method of renal angiography is the technique of choice in all patients except those with evidence of advanced aortoiliac atheromatous disease and those in whom transfemoral catheterization is unsuccessful, owing either to the presence of atheromatous disease or to extreme torsion of the iliac arteries.

Whereas the Seldinger technique of percutaneous transfemoral catheterization is impractical in young infants, it may be carried out with ease in older children.

Materials for Percutaneous Catheterization

Needles

Many physicians employ the Seldinger needle-cannula for percutaneous catheterization. This consists of a needle with an outer blunt-end cannula (Fig. 2-4). With this needle-cannula, the arterial puncture is performed without the use of a saline-filled syringe and connecting tubing. Most advocate that the artery be transfixed with the needle-cannula, the needle removed, and the cannula withdrawn until bleeding is obtained. The cannula is then threaded a short distance up the vessel and the guide wire inserted. Some believe that the use of the Seldinger needle-cannula reduces the chance that the guide wire will be passed upward in the wall of the artery rather than in the arterial lumen.

Many physicians, however, have found this rather complex needle-cannula difficult to use and a variety of needles of simpler design have been advocated. The author has found it convenient to employ a simple thin-walled needle with a removable wing adapter to facilitate handling during the insertion of the needle (Fig. 2-5). The needle may be used with or without the adapter. The puncture is carried out with a closed saline system, consisting of a saline-filled syringe and connecting tubing, attached to the needle. We have encountered no undue difficulties with intramural passage of the guide wire in using this needle.

Needles of different lumen diameter may be used, depending on the size of the guide wire and catheter to be employed. An 18-gauge needle, which will accommodate a standard 0.035-mm guide wire, is ordinarily employed.

Connecting Tubing and Syringe

The femoral puncture is best made, except when the Seldinger needle-cannula is used, with a saline system, consisting of a length of flexible tubing and a 10-ml syringe attached to the needle. We employ a 12-inch length of translucent nylon tubing with a stopcock at the syringe end and a simple glass adapter at the end to be attached to the needle. The puncture is made with the stopcock open and entry into the artery is signaled by the rush of blood back into the saline-filled tubing.

Guide Wires

The guide wire used for the Seldinger technique of percutaneous catheterization is of the "coil-spring" type with a very soft and flexible tip. This spring-guide must be of a size to slip easily through the arterial puncture needle and should just fit the lumen of the tip of the catheter to be used. It should be at least 10 cm longer than the catheter. Guide wires for percutaneous catheterization are available from several manufacturers in sizes designed to fit the various-sized catheter material which the manufacturer handles.

Catheters

Catheter materials for percutaneous catheterization include nonradiopaque polyethylene tubing, radiopaque polyethylene tubing, radiopaque polyfluoroethylene (Teflon) tubing, and radiopaque polyurethane (Ducor) tubing. Polyethylene tubing is available in rolls of various lengths from which catheters of any desired length and shape may be made. Polyethylene catheters are very suitable by reason of their thin walls and pliability. The major disadvantage of ordinary polyethylene catheters, however, is that they are not radiopaque and there-

fore cannot be observed fluoroscopically unless the guide wire is left in the catheter. The guide wire must be carefully measured ahead of time against the length of the catheter and marked so that the examiner may know the relationship of the tip of the guide wire to the tip of the catheter during placement.

Opaque catheter materials, particularly radiopaque polyethylene tubing and polyfluoroethylene tubing, are much more suitable for renal arteriography. These materials are supplied by a number of manufacturers. The tips of these catheters must be tapered and shaped and the necessary side holes placed by the user (Fig. 2–6). The radiopaque polyethylene catheters may be molded into any desired shape simply by emersion in hot water (above 75° C, but not boiling) and cooling in running cold water. Polyfluoroethylene catheter material will not retain its shape without autoclaving. The polyurethane catheter comes with a ready-prepared and preshaped tip.

We ordinarily employ a no. 7 polyfluoroethylene catheter for midstream aortorenal arteriography and replace this with a radiopaque polyethylene curved catheter for selective renal arteriography. The greater torque control of polyethylene catheters makes them more suitable for selective angiography than polyfluoroethylene catheters.

Technique of Percutaneous Catheterization

The inguinal region is prepared and draped, and the femoral artery is carefully palpated at and just below the level of the inguinal ligament. With a scalpel blade a small transverse slit is then made in the skin approximately 1 to 1½ inches distal to the site at which the needle will enter the artery. The slit so produced facilitates introduction of the needle and serves to permit free movement of the catheter through the skin.

With the saline-filled tubing and

syringe attached, the needle, with its bevel upward, is inserted through the skin slit and the femoral artery is punctured at an angle of approximately 50 to 55°. When good backflow of blood is obtained, the tubing and syringe are detached from the needle and the coil-spring guide wire is inserted through the needle and passed a short distance upward into the artery. The needle is then removed over the guide wire and the catheter is passed over the guide wire, through the skin, and into the artery. Except for slight resistance when the catheter passes through the arterial wall, no resistance should be encountered with passage of either the guide wire or the catheter. When the catheter tip has been passed upward a short distance within the artery, the guide wire is removed from the catheter and the catheter is attached to the flushing system. The catheter may now be advanced to any desired position under fluoroscopic control, utilizing the image intensifier. When the catheter has been properly positioned, the tabletop is extended and the patient's abdomen is appropriately centered over the film changer.

Flushing System

Although many prefer to attach the catheter to a saline-filled syringe from which saline can be periodically flushed through the catheter, we prefer to attach the catheter to a pressurized flush bottle mounted on the table rail (Fig. 2-7). The bottle is pressurized by means of a Tycos manometer bulb and gauge, and the pressure is maintained at a level above arterial pressure. The catheter may be flushed by simply turning a stopcock interposed in the flushing system. Furthermore, by interposing a strain gauge in the system, the arterial pulse curve and the flushes may be monitored on an oscilloscope (Kincaid, Mengis, and Fellows).

With this system, clotting in the catheter, lodging of its tip beneath an atheromatous plaque, or wedging of the tip in a small-sized renal artery or other vessel is signaled by some damping of the pulse curve and a slow return of the curve to the base line following flushing of the catheter. Heart rate and rhythm may also be determined continuously by observing the pulse curve on the oscilloscope.

Aortorenal Arteriography
(Midstream Aortic Injection)

A midstream aortic injection, or aortorenal arteriography, should be employed initially for visualization of the renal arteries. The series of films obtained with this injection will demonstrate the number of renal arteries present on each side and will permit the detection of atheromatous plaques or other lesions involving the renal artery ostia. In most instances, the renal arteries and their extrarenal and intrarenal branches will also be adequately visualized by this technique (Fig. 2-8). When the renal arteries are inadequately visualized, oblique views (Fig. 2-9) or selective arteriography may then be performed.

For aortorenal angiography a straight-tipped catheter is employed with four side holes distributed radially around the terminal 1 inch of the catheter. The side holes should be placed so that no two of them are opposite each other, as this tends to weaken the catheter at this point.

Under fluoroscopic control, the catheter is passed upward in the aorta until its tip lies approximately an inch below the anticipated level of origin of the renal arteries. If the injection is made at this level, rather than at or above the level of origin of the renal arteries, opacification of the renal arteries may often be obtained prior to, or without, opacification of the superior mesenteric artery and the celiac artery and its branches, thus

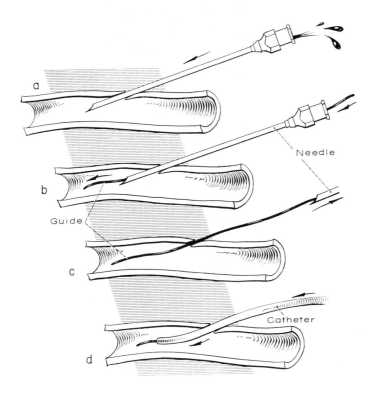

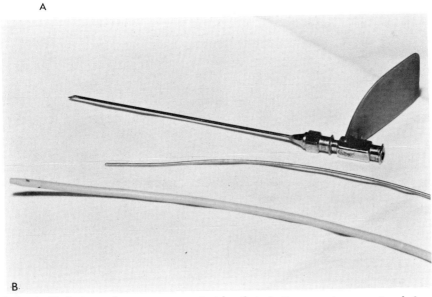

Figure 2–3. **A**, Technique of percutaneous arterial catheterization: *a*, artery punctured; *b*, guide wire inserted; *c*, needle removed over guide wire; *d*, catheter passed over guide wire into artery. **B**, Needle, guide wire, and catheter used for percutaneous catheterization. (From Kincaid, O. W., and Davis, G. D., 1961.)

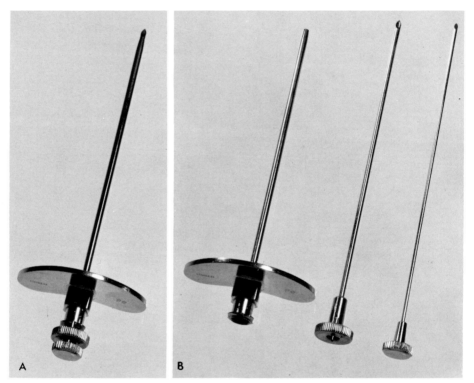

Figure 2–4. A, Seldinger needle-cannula assembled. B, Seldinger needle-cannula disassembled.

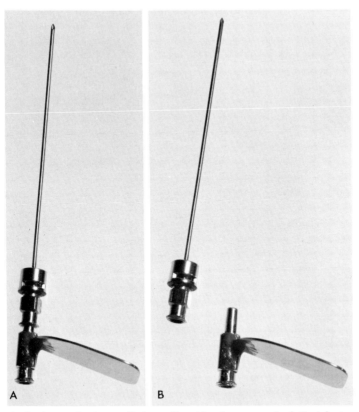

Figure 2-5. **A,** Author's simple thin-walled needle with adapter attached. **B,** Adapter, detached, fits all needles regardless of size.

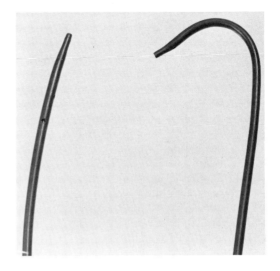

Figure 2-6. **Left,** Straight catheter for aortorenal arteriography. **Right,** Curved catheter for selective renal arteriography.

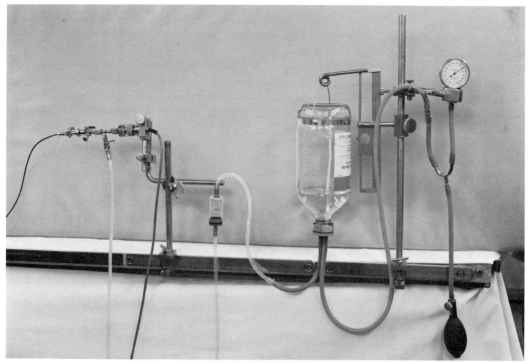

Figure 2–7. Flushing and pulse-pressure monitoring system attached to table rail. (From Kincaid, O. W., Mengis, J. L., and Fellows, J. L.)

permitting unobscured visualization of the renal vessels and kidneys.

When injection is made through a catheter into the aorta for visualization of the renal arteries, a mechanical injection syringe of some type must be employed (Fig. 2–10). The pressure of injection must be sufficient to permit delivery of at least 15 to 20 ml of contrast medium per second through the catheter.

Thirty to 40 ml of contrast medium are employed, this amount being delivered in approximately 1½ to 2 seconds.

Selective Renal Arteriography

Selective renal arteriography provides the ultimate in detailed visualization of the renal vessels and vascular architecture of the kidneys (Olsson, 1961a; Tillotson and Halpern) (Fig. 2–11). This technique avoids the superimposition of other visceral arteries often unavoidably opacified by aortorenal angiography, and

should always be performed in the study of renal mass lesions, as well as in other conditions when the intrarenal vasculature has not been adequately visualized by aortorenal technique (Fig. 2–12*A* and *B*).

As mentioned previously, aortorenal arteriography should always be performed initially to permit visualization of the aorta and the ostia of the renal arteries, and to permit determination of the number and position of the renal arteries present on each side. For selective arteriography, the guide wire is reinserted through the intra-aortic catheter until the tip of the guide wire protrudes several centimeters beyond the catheter tip. The catheter and guide wire are then withdrawn until the catheter tip is outside the skin. The catheter is then removed and replaced with a curved-tipped catheter, which is passed over the guide wire and into the femoral artery. The guide wire is then removed and the curved-tipped catheter is manipulated into the orifice of the renal artery.

For selective renal arteriography, most workers prefer a catheter with two side holes very near the tip, although some employ a catheter with no side holes. If the curved terminal portion of the catheter is made with a curve slightly wider than the anticipated width of the aorta, the catheter can usually be manipulated with ease into either renal artery (Fig. 2–6). The injection of 2 to 3 ml of contrast medium under fluoroscopic observation will permit the examiner to determine whether the tip is properly positioned in the renal artery.

Between 10 and 15 ml of contrast medium are injected manually from a 10 or 20-ml syringe, and filming is carried out as for aortorenal angiography. The manual injection must be carried out quite forcefully.

OTHER METHODS

In patients with clinical evidence of advanced aortoiliac atheromatous disease, and in those in whom transfemoral catheterization is unsuccessful due either to atheromatous narrowing in the aortoiliofemoral system or to extreme torsion of the iliac arteries, the examiner must resort to other methods of renal artery opacification. Three other techniques are available and will be considered briefly.

Percutaneous Transaxillary Catheterization Method

Percutaneous catheterization of the axillary artery, using the Seldinger technique, may be accomplished with ease in patients who are not obese and who have a palpable axillary pulse. The left axillary artery is used for easier access to the descending aorta. Once the catheter has been manipulated down the descending aorta, its tip is positioned just above the level of origin of the renal arteries and an intra-aortic injection made at this level.

Selective renal arteriography may also be performed by this route, although catheterization of the renal arteries is usually more difficult than with the transfemoral approach.

The brachial, rather than the axillary, artery may also be percutaneously catheterized. However, the brachial artery is a much smaller vessel than the axillary or femoral artery, making the procedure more difficult. Furthermore, due to the small size and greater mobility of the brachial artery, the likelihood of arterial complications is greater than with the axillary or femoral approach.

Translumbar Method

Translumbar aortography was first described in 1929 by dos Santos, Lamas, and Pereira Caldas, of Lisbon, Portugal. These authors, using this new technique, became the first to demonstrate the renal vessels angiographically. In this method, contrast medium is injected through a needle inserted percutaneously through the left lumbar paraspinal tissues into the abdominal aorta. The technique is simple and rapid, and, when performed with care, fewer complications are encountered than with other methods of renal arteriography.

Because of the small size of the needle employed and the nonselectivity of the method, visualization of the renal arteries is not nearly as good as that obtained with catheterization techniques (Fig. 2–12C and D). Nevertheless, translumbar aortography constitutes an important alternative means of renal arteriography in those cases in which percutaneous catheterization of the aorta cannot be accomplished.

The procedure is carried out with the patient in a prone position over the film changer. The needle, a 6-inch 18-gauge thin-walled needle with stylet in place, is introduced through the skin over the left flank at a point just below the inferior margin of the left twelfth rib and 8 cm or approximately 4 fingerbreadths lateral to the midline (spinous processes). The needle is advanced obliquely cephalad, medially and ventrally through the left lumbar paraspinal tissues at an angle which will permit entry into the aorta at the desired level (Fig. 2–13).

The puncture is made with a saline-filled syringe and connecting tubing attached to the needle. Entry into the aorta is signaled by the rush of blood back into the saline-filled tubing and, by alternately injecting saline and observing the backflow of blood into the tubing, free position of the needle tip within the aortic lumen is ascertained.

The saline-filled syringe is replaced with one containing 30 to 40 ml of contrast medium. The injection is made manually as rapidly as possible and serial films are exposed by means of the automatic film changer (Fig. 2–14).

The injection may be made into the aorta just above the level of origin of the celiac artery or at any other level at or proximal to the level of origin of the renal arteries (Fig. 2–15). We always employ a test injection to determine the level of the aortic puncture and to be certain that the needle is not in such a position that undue opacification of the celiac or mesenteric artery occurs. In such an event, it may be necessary to reinsert the needle at a slightly different level and repeat the test injection.

Percutaneous Noncatheter Brachial Method

This technique is an adaptation of the technique of countercurrent thoracic aortography first described by Castellanos and Pereiras. The technique entails the forceful injection of contrast medium through a needle-cannula inserted percutaneously into the left brachial artery immediately above the elbow. The use of this technique for visualization of the renal arteries was first described by Karras and his associates (1963a and b).

A 17-gauge needle-cannula is employed to transfix the left brachial artery just above the brachial bifurcation. When the artery has been transfixed, the pointed obturator is removed from the cannula and the cannula withdrawn until its tip lies within the artery. The tip of the cannula is then threaded up the artery for a distance of about 3 cm and the cannula is connected through a length of tubing to an automatic injector.

The injection is made at a pressure which will deliver at least 25 to 30 ml of contrast medium per second.

Filming is carried out over the abdomen at the rate of three or four exposures per second, the first film being exposed just before completion of the injection.

The renal arteries may be opacified adequately by this method. However, the technique is completely nonselective and is to be employed only when other methods have failed.

VENOGRAPHY

Renal venography has not been extensively employed, but is a technique of considerable importance in the evaluation of patients with suspected renal vein obstruction.

The technique employed is almost identical to that used for percutaneous transfemoral renal arteriography. Needle puncture of the femoral vein, which lies just medial and slightly deep to the femoral artery, is first accomplished and a catheter is inserted via the Seldinger technique.

Since some patients with renal vein thrombosis have associated inferior vena caval thrombosis, or complete thrombosis of the renal vein, we perform inferior vena cavography initially. With the catheter tip lying in the common iliac vein, 30 to 40 ml of contrast medium are injected at a pressure permitting the injection of 20 to 30 ml per second (Fig. 2–16).

If the inferior vena cava is patent,

selective renal venography is then carried out on the side in question, or bilaterally. The catheter tip should have a somewhat longer curve than that used for renal arteriography, and a larger dose of contrast medium must be employed to insure good visualization of the renal vein and its tributaries. We employ 25 to 35 ml of contrast medium, delivering at least 20 ml per second with a power injector.

The main renal veins and their primary and secondary tributaries may be readily visualized by this technique (Fig. 2–17). Venous backflow, however, even with high pressure injection, is usually not adequate to opacify smaller intrarenal tributaries.

Inferior vena cavography, and renal venography when the inferior vena cava is patent, may also be of value in the study of renal tumors in that renal vein invasion and retroperitoneal metastases may be identified.

(Text continued on page 120.)

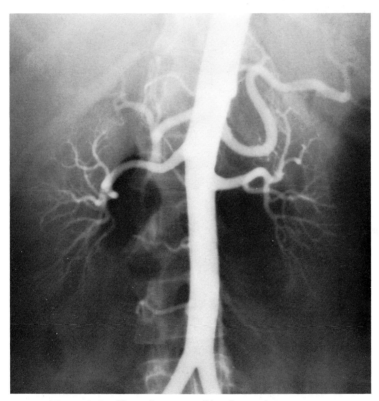

Figure 2–8. Normal *aortorenal (midstream) arteriogram.*

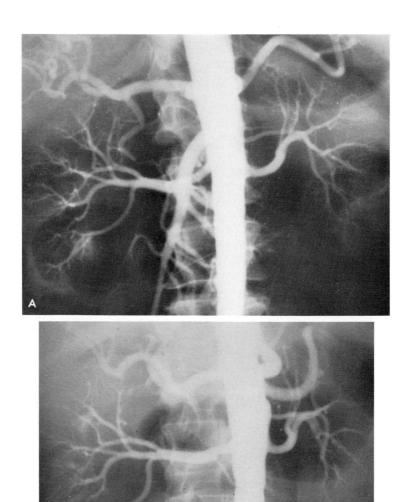

Figure 2–9. *Aortorenal arteriograms.* **A,** Superior mesenteric artery obscures portion of right renal artery. **B,** Left anterior oblique projection provides unobscured view of right renal artery. Superior mesenteric artery, which in frontal projection had obscured stenotic lesion of renal artery, now overlies aorta.

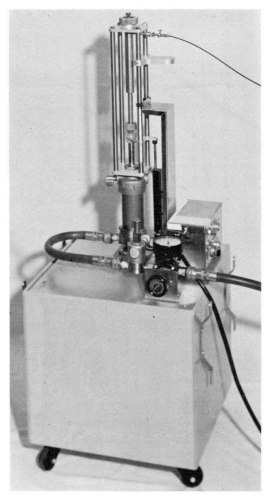

Figure 2–10. Air-driven injector designed and made by Section of Engineering, Mayo Clinic. Although not commercially available, a number of different injectors are available and suitable for renal angiography.

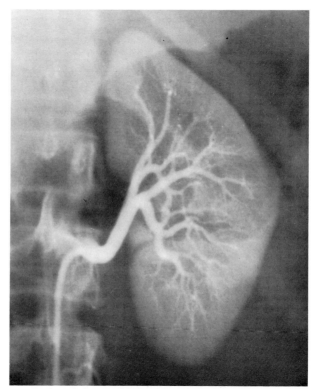

Figure 2–11.   Normal *selective left renal arteriogram.*

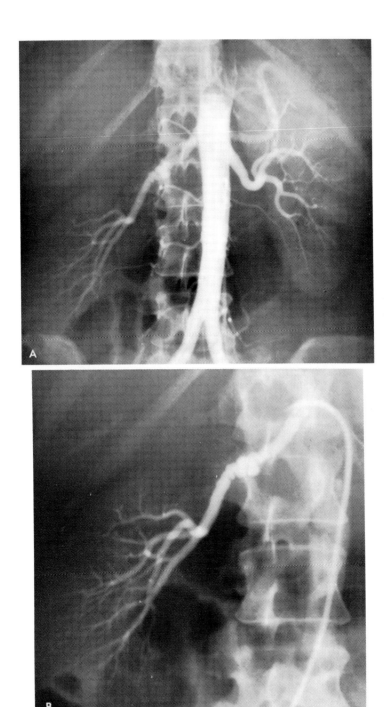

Figure 2–12. A and B, Comparison of midstream and selective renal arteriograms. **A,** *Aortorenal (midstream) arteriogram* shows poor definition of lesion of right renal artery. **B,** Selective *right renal arteriogram* of same patient clearly shows **fibromuscular dysplasia** involving midportion of right renal artery.

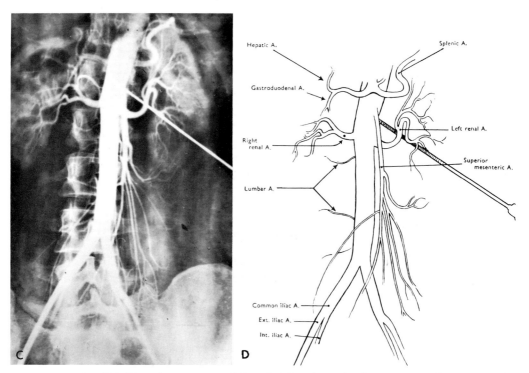

Figure 2–12. C and D, Normal aortogram with key. C, Normal translumbar aortogram showing opacification of all aortic branches, including renal arteries. D, Key. (From Stirling, W. B.)

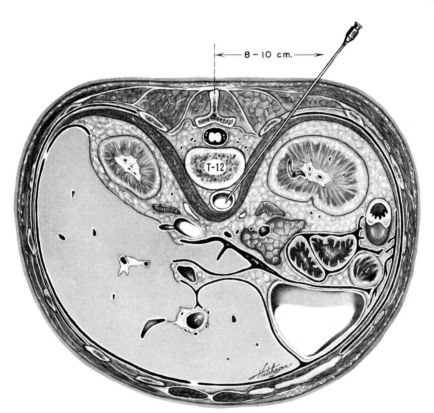

Figure 2–13. Drawing of transverse section of prone patient illustrating left lumbar approach to abdominal aorta.

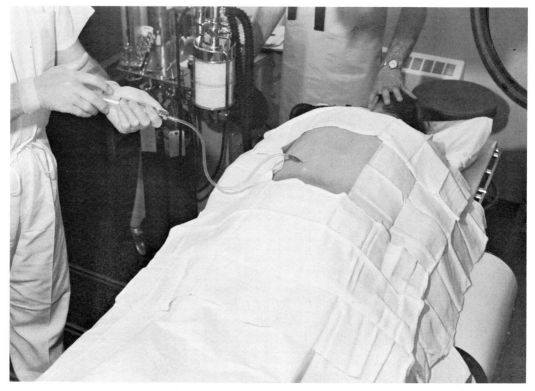

Figure 2–14. Patient positioned over film changer and injection being made for translumbar aortorenal arteriogram.

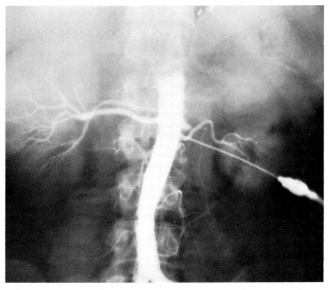

Figure 2–15. *Translumbar aortorenal arteriogram* of patient with two renal arteries supplying each kidney. On left, **occlusion of superiormost renal artery** 1 cm distal to its orifice is seen.

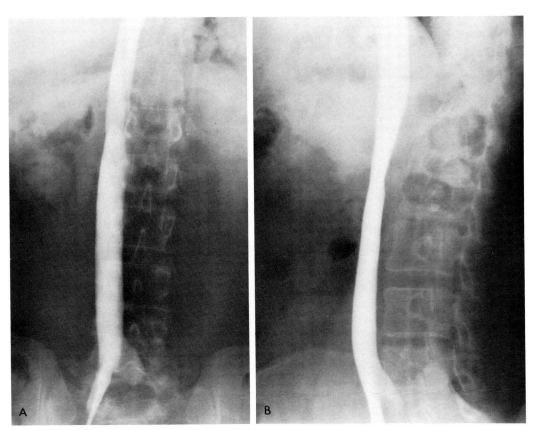

Figure 2–16. Normal *inferior vena cavograms*. **A**, Frontal projection. **B**, Left anterior oblique projection.

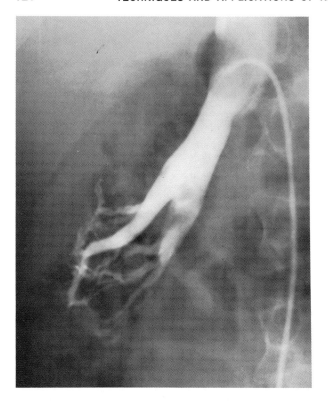

Figure 2–17. Normal *selective right renal venogram.*

HAZARDS

Renal angiography is not without risk. Although complications are quite infrequent, they may on rare occasions be extremely serious. Therefore, as with all angiographic procedures, renal angiography should not be undertaken by those without adequate training and experience. The urologist and internist have the very important responsibility of requesting such studies only when the information to be obtained is likely to prove of definite benefit to the patient. The risks should be explained to the patient before the procedure is scheduled.

Many, though by no means all, complications are due to faults of technique. As pointed out by Sutton, many angiographic techniques which superficially appear simple can prove technically very difficult. Experience is one of the most vital factors in reducing the incidence of complications, and there is much to be said for referral of patients to centers where sufficient numbers of examinations are performed to enable the examiners to gain adequate skill.

Complications Due to Contrast Media

Allergic Reactions

Reactions due to the injection of contrast media have been discussed in Chapter 1. Such reactions may be occasionally encountered whenever iodine-containing contrast media are injected into the vascular system for any purpose. Allergic reactions are most commonly manifested by urticaria, coughing, or wheezing. This type of reaction, in most instances, may be readily controlled by the intravascular administration of antihistamine preparations. Minor allergic reactions to angiography are very difficult to assess. Faintness, nausea, or transient hypotension may occur on an allergic basis, but probably more often they represent a vasovagal or psychosomatic response.

Rarely, shock and sudden death may occur following the injection of radiopaque media. The allergic nature of all such reactions, however, is open to some question. It seems possible that these deaths often represent some type of neurovascular reaction to the injection of medium.

Although there is much question as to the value of sensitivity testing, we always employ a 1-ml intravascular test injection whenever a history of previous allergic response is elicited. Deaths have been reported following angiography when such a sensitivity test has been negative. Furthermore, deaths have occurred, particularly in children, from 1-ml intravascular test doses.

When there is a history of severe allergy, angiography should be avoided unless the examination is absolutely necessary.

Red blood cell agglutination has been shown to occur as the result of the injection of hypertonic contrast media and may be responsible for some reactions to angiography (Read and associates).

Renal Damage

In renal angiography the kidneys are subjected to the effect of contrast medium in high concentration. The effect of contrast medium on the kidneys has been studied experimentally by several investigators (Idbohrn and Berg; Mullady and associates). From these studies it seems probable that transitory subclinical renal insufficiency results much more frequently from renal angiography than had been generally assumed. Renal insufficiency, when severe, most often appears 24 to 72 hours after angiography. Albuminuria, hematuria, oliguria, and increase in blood urea are commonly found when renal damage has occurred (Miller, Wylie, and Hinman). In 12 cases reviewed by McAfee in which death resulted from renal damage, the patients died in uremia 12 hours to 13 days following angiography.

Although there is great individual variation in the susceptibility of the kidney to the effect of contrast medium, the risk of damage is definitely related to the amount and concentration of medium reaching the renal tissues.

It should be pointed out, however, that the majority of cases of renal insufficiency following renal arteriography or abdominal aortography occurred with older types of contrast media, particularly with iodopyracet (Diodrast) and acetrizoate (Urokon). Since the advent of newer media (diatrizoates), renal damage due to the effect of contrast media has been rare. Nevertheless, the amount of contrast medium used for renal arteriography should be kept to the minimum consistent with adequate visualization of the renal arteries. Repeat injections should not be performed unless absolutely necessary.

Neurologic Complications

Although neurologic damage does not occur as a complication of selective renal arteriography, spinal cord damage has been reported as a complication of abdominal aortography. Killen and Foster, in 1960, collected reports of 38 cases of spinal cord damage following aortography performed at various centers.

Although in some cases the neurologic damage has been transient, all too often it has been permanent. Paralysis may involve only one lower extremity or may be confined to muscles supplied by the sciatic or obturator nerves. In a few cases, transient or permanent foot drop has been the only result. A number of cases have been reported in which transverse myelitis and paraplegia have resulted from aortography.

Neurologic damage is evidently attributable to the direct toxic action of the contrast medium on the spinal cord, which receives its major blood supply from the aorta by way of the radicular arteries. The major radicular artery, which is the principal vessel supplying the cord, usually arises from a left lumbar artery, most often at the level of the second lumbar vertebra, but occasionally as high as the eighth thoracic or as low as the fourth lumbar vertebra. It has been shown that the risk of neurologic complications is in part related to the quantity of contrast medium entering the radicular arteries.

Fortunately, neurologic complications have occurred with extreme rarity since the advent of newer contrast media. We have observed no instance of neurologic damage in more than 4,000 abdominal aortographic procedures done for various purposes and by various techniques.

Vascular Complications

Percutaneous Catheterization Techniques

A survey study of the complications of percutaneous catheterization has been reported by Lang. In 11,402 percutaneous aortographic procedures reported by 142 radiologists, urologists, and vascular surgeons, there were 7 deaths, 81 serious complications, and 325 minor complications.

A frequent complication is hematoma formation at the femoral catheterization site. Bleeding almost always occurs within the first 24 hours following percutaneous catheterization. Although small hematomas commonly occur, massive bleeding into the thigh is a rare complication. We have observed three cases of massive hematoma formation occurring from 2 to 24 hours following percutaneous femoral catheterization. All three of these patients were hypertensive. In one, surgical evacuation of the hematoma was required.

Arterial thrombosis at the site of arterial puncture and catheterization is also a rare occurrence, but is a complication of extreme importance. Such thrombosis is usually evident immediately on completion of the procedure and removal of the catheter from the artery. Anticoagu-

lant therapy should be started in such cases as soon as possible. If ischemia of the extremity persists and viability of the limb seems threatened, thromboendarterectomy should be performed without delay.

The guide wire and catheter used for percutaneous catheterization may be passed subintimally without encountering much resistance. Such intramural passage of a catheter rarely results in complications unless the intramural position of the catheter is not recognized and a high pressure injection of contrast medium is made (Fig. 2–18). Aortic rupture has been reported as a result of such injections. Therefore, fluoroscopic observation of a small test injection prior to renal arteriography is wise.

Elevation and dislodgment of an atheromatous plaque by the needle, guide wire, or catheter are frequently mentioned as a hazard of percutaneous catheterization. This, somewhat surprisingly, occurs with extreme rarity.

A number of other complications of percutaneous catheterization have been reported. These include breakage of the tip of the guide wire within an artery, perforation of a vessel wall by the guide wire, formation of an aneurysm or arteriovenous fistula at the site of the arterial puncture, damage to a peripheral nerve, and infection of the skin and subcutaneous tissues of the groin.

Translumbar Technique

Translumbar aortography, although often an inadequate technique for renal arteriography, has an extremely low incidence of complications.

The most important complication of translumbar aortography is hemorrhage from the aortic puncture site. McAfee found only 13 cases of serious bleeding from the aortic puncture site in his survey of 12,832 translumbar aortograms. In five of these the bleeding was massive and fatal. Of these 13 patients, 7 were hypertensive, and in 3 the bleeding followed direct puncture of an aortic aneurysm. In our experience of approximately 3,000 translumbar aortograms, massive retroperitoneal bleeding has been known to occur in 4 patients. In each case, a large retroperitoneal hematoma was discovered at later operation, the bleeding having been clinically unrecognized. No fatalities have occurred.

Dislodgment of an atheromatous plaque by translumbar needle has been reported, but to the author's knowledge this complication has not occurred in Mayo Clinic experience.

Subintimal aortic dissection occasionally occurs with translumbar aortography as the result of the intramural injection of contrast medium (Gaylis and Laws; Wolfman and Boblitt). This occurs when the bevel of the puncture needle lies partly within the aortic lumen and partly overrides the aortic wall. Although subintimal dissection is commonly observed with this technique, its deleterious effects are extremely rare.

Isolated cases of pneumothorax, accidental spinal puncture, and retroperitoneal sepsis have also been reported.

THE NORMAL RENAL ANGIOGRAM

Description of the anatomy of the renal vessels and the many variations of this anatomy is beyond the scope of this chapter, the purpose of which is to consider the techniques and applications of renal angiography. Technique, however, relates importantly to anatomy, and the following comments are concerned with the visualization of the essential structures in the angiogram.

The renal angiogram consists of an arterial, a nephrographic, and a venous phase (Fig. 2–19).

Arterial Phase

It is essential that the anatomy of the renal arteries and their number, course, and arborization be visualized in great detail on the renal angiogram. Rapid serial filming at three to four films per second is required for adequate visualization of this anatomy.

The renal arteries typically arise from the anterolateral aspects of the aorta between the midportion of the first lumbar vertebral body and the upper third of the second vertebral body. In many instances, however, they may arise from the lateral aspect of the aorta or, less frequently, from its posterolateral aspect. The right renal artery most commonly arises at a slightly higher level than does the left one. The two renal arteries are usually of equal size, although the right renal artery is often somewhat longer than the left.

The branching of the main renal artery is quite variable. The most common type of division is into two branches which have been called anterior or ventral and posterior or dorsal branches. Occasionally, however, the main renal artery divides into three or even four branches rather than two. These branches enter the renal hilus where further branching occurs, so that from three to seven branches may be visualized as the vessels enter the renal sinus.

The arborization pattern of the smaller segmental arteries is readily visible in the renal arteriogram, but arterioles are not visible by conventional angiographic techniques.

Many variations in the number and division of the renal arteries may be encountered.* One or both kidneys may be supplied by multiple renal arteries with separate aortic origins (Figs. 2–20 and 2–21). Multiple renal arteries (more than one to each kidney) have been shown to occur in approximately 25% of the population. So-called aberrant renal arteries may arise from the aorta anywhere between the level of the eleventh thoracic and the level of the fourth lumbar vertebra, and sometimes from the iliac artery. When there is more than one renal

---

*(Boijsen; Davis, Kincaid, and Hunt; Graves, 1954; 1956; 1957; Hollinshead; Ljungqvist; Merklin and Michels; Olsson, 1961b; 1962)

artery supplying a kidney, there is no communication between the branches of these separate arteries, each artery providing the sole arterial supply to its own segment of the renal parenchyma.

In the performance of renal arteriography it is necessary to carry out a midstream aortic injection prior to consideration of selective arteriography, in order to define the number, size, levels of origin, and distribution of the renal arteries.

Nephrographic Phase

Approximately 6 to 8 seconds after the intra-arterial injection of contrast medium, dense homogeneous opacification of the kidneys occurs due to the presence of contrast medium in the renal capillaries and renal excretory system (Olsson, 1961b). This period of renal opacification is known as the nephrographic phase, and the roentgenograms obtained at this time may be called nephrograms. This opacifi-cation may last for several seconds or even minutes, depending upon the renal blood flow. During the later phases of the nephrogram, the renal pyramids may be clearly visualized as contrasted to the fat in the renal sinus.

Films made during the nephrographic phase of renal opacification should be obtained in every renal arteriographic examination. A normal nephrogram implies a considerable degree of integrity of the intrarenal circulation and offers a means of evaluating the comparative function of the two kidneys. The size and outline of the kidneys may also be accurately evaluated on these films. The nephrogram, of course, is highly important in the differential diagnosis of renal mass lesions and renal infarction.

Venous Phase

Approximately 12 seconds after the beginning of the rapid intra-arterial injection of contrast medium, the renal veins

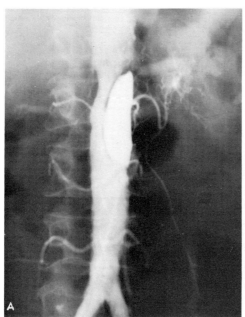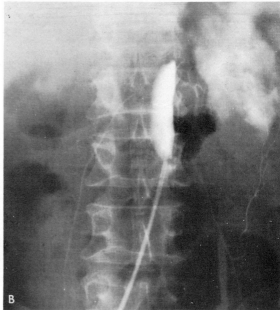

Figure 2–18. A, Contrast-medium **dissection of aortic wall** occurring with percutaneous transfemoral catheterization technique. B, Film made 8 seconds later showing some contrast medium lingering in wall of aorta.

become opacified. Opacification of the veins is usually maximal at 18 to 20 seconds after the beginning of the injection (Olsson, 1961b).

In contrast to the renal arteries, the renal veins have no segmental arrangement, and there is free anastomosis of the veins throughout the kidney (Hollinshead).

Usually there is a single vein from each kidney, but occasionally two or even three veins are present. The left renal vein is often more than twice as long as the right.

Detailed opacification of the renal veins may be obtained only by means of selective renal venography (Fig. 2–22).

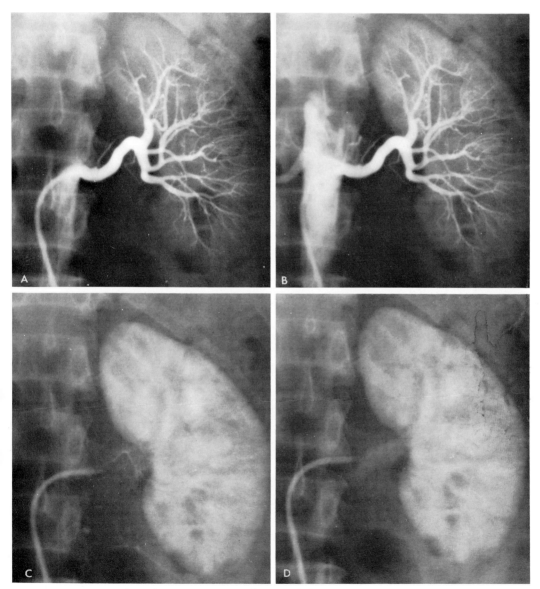

Figure 2–19. Normal *renal angiograms*. **A,** Early arterial phase. **B,** Late arterial phase. **C,** Nephrographic phase. **D,** Venous phase.

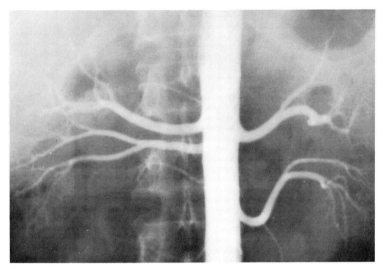

Figure 2–20.   Multiple renal arteries. Two renal arteries of approximately equal size supplying right kidney and two arteries of widely separated origins supplying left kidney.

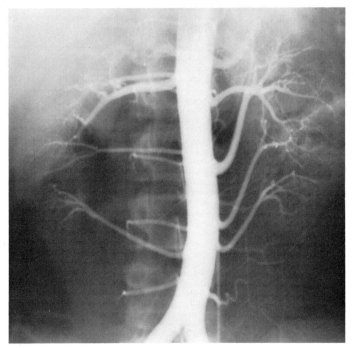

Figure 2–21.   Multiple renal arteries with four arteries supplying each kidney.

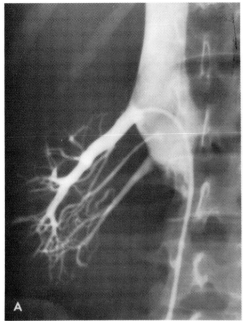 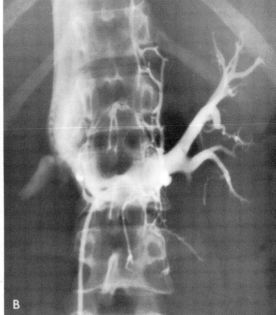

Figure 2–22. **A,** *Selective right renal venogram* in patient with **three renal veins** communicating with inferior vena cava. Intrarenal and extrarenal venous anastomoses are visualized and two lower renal veins are opacified via these anastomoses. Multiple renal veins occur in about 14% of kidneys and are far more common on right than on left. **B,** *Selective left renal venogram.* Left renal vein is usually much longer than right.

APPLICATIONS OF RENAL ANGIOGRAPHY

No attempt will be made in this chapter to cover in detail the diagnostic findings in the many renal and renal vascular lesions for which renal angiography is employed. Instead, only a few representative angiograms will be used to illustrate in general some of the many useful applications of the technique of renal angiography. Other angiographic material has been supplied for use throughout the book, under discussion of various disease processes.

RENAL VASCULAR DISEASES

The importance of renal vascular lesions lies principally in the fact that such lesions commonly result in secondary hypertension (Dustan, Page, and Poutasse; Goldblatt and associates). Since the advent of renal angiography and of surgical techniques permitting reestablishment of blood flow distal to stenotic lesions of the renal arteries, renal vascular lesions have become diagnosable and potentially curable lesions (see Chapters 13 and 14).

The renal arteries are subject to involvement by a variety of pathologic conditions, both intrinsic and extrinsic.* An outline of the various conditions which may compromise renal blood flow and result in renal vascular hypertension is shown in Table 2–1.

Atherosclerosis and fibromuscular dysplasia are the two most common primary lesions of the renal arteries resulting in renal artery stenosis. The two conditions have rather characteristic arteriographic manifestations and, in most instances, can be readily differentiated.

Atherosclerosis, in the vast majority of

*(Eyler and associates; Hunt and associates; Kincaid and Davis, 1961; Kincaid and associates, 1968; McCormack, Hazard, and Poutasse; Palubinskas and Wylie; Sutton; Sutton and associates; Utz and Kincaid; Yuile)

Table 2–1. **Causes of Renovascular Hypertension***

Intrinsic Renal Vascular Lesions
  Atherosclerosis
  Fibromuscular dysplasia
  Renal artery aneurysm
  Renal arteriovenous fistula
  Embolism
  Thrombosis (usually secondary to other renal artery lesions)
  Miscellaneous arteritides
    Takayasu's disease
    Syphilitic arteritis
    Thromboangiitis
    Periarteritis nodosa
  Renal vein thrombosis

Extrinsic Lesions
  Atherosclerotic or dissecting aneurysm of the aorta
  Extrinsic fibrous or musculotendinous bands
  Trauma
  Renal tumor
  Other intra-abdominal tumor or cyst
  Coarctation of aorta

*Pyelonephritis and other renal parenchymal diseases not considered here.

cases, involves the ostium or proximal 1 to 2 cm of the main renal artery (Figs. 2–23 and 2–24). Although often occurring as isolated lesions of the renal artery, very commonly atherosclerotic stenosis results from involvement of the ostium and proximal main renal artery by atherosclerotic plaques of aortic origin.

Fibromuscular dysplasia virtually always involves the middle or distal third of the renal artery, involvement of the proximal 1 to 2 cm of the main renal artery being quite rare. Extension into one or more primary renal artery branches occurs in approximately one third of the cases.

Fibromuscular dysplasia may present angiographically and pathologically as multifocal, focal, or tubular stenosis (Figs. 2–25 through 2–28) (Harrison, Hunt, and Bernatz; Kincaid and associates, 1968). In the multifocal form, the so-called string-of-beads appearance is highly characteristic.

In stenotic lesions of the renal arteries, collateral circulation to the kidney may often be demonstrated by angiography.

True renal artery aneurysms are rare, but are of importance in that approximately 75% of cases are associated with hypertension. Furthermore, spontaneous rupture of the aneurysm has been reported to occur in from 5% to 30% of cases. Such aneurysms are often multiple and bilateral. False aneurysms and dissecting aneurysms of the renal artery are extremely rare. Renal arteriography provides the only means of diagnosis (Figs. 2–28 and 2–29) (Boijsen and Köhler, 1963; Olsson, 1963; Poutasse; Utz and Kincaid). Another important vascular lesion read-

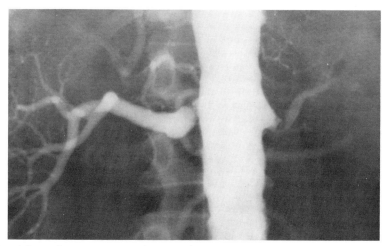

Figure 2–23. **Atherosclerotic stenosis** of proximal portion of both renal arteries. There is poststenotic dilatation on right. Left renal artery is almost completely obstructed.

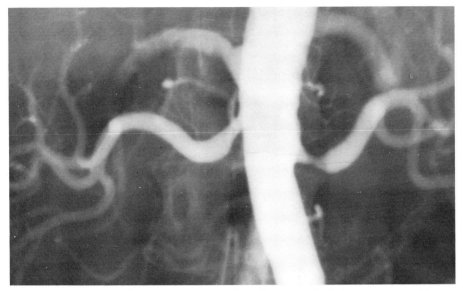

Figure 2–24.   Bilateral atheromatous stenosis of renal artery with slight poststenotic dilatation.

ily diagnosable by renal arteriography is renal arteriovenous fistula (Fig. 2–30) (Boijsen and Köhler, 1962; Scheifley and associates). Hypertension is an outstanding feature of these lesions and is present in the majority of cases.

Renal vein thrombosis is also an impor-tant vascular lesion requiring renal angiog-raphy for diagnosis. A definite diagnosis cannot be made by renal arteriography, inferior vena cavography and selective re-nal venography being the necessary pro-cedures when renal vein thrombosis is suspected (Fig. 2–31).

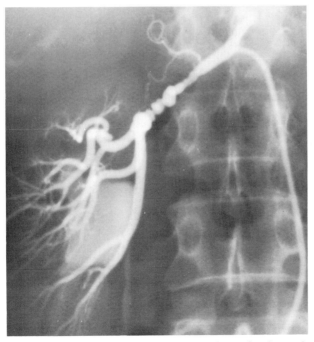

Figure 2–25.   Multifocal type of fibromuscular dysplasia involving distal two thirds of right main renal artery. Note characteristic "string-of-beads" appearance of involved portion of vessel.

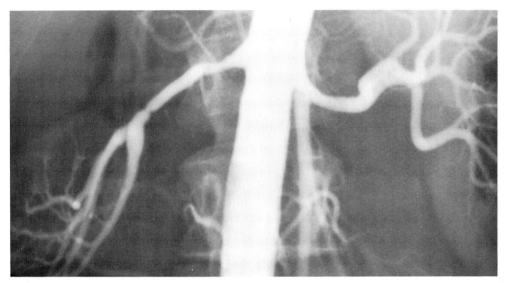

Figure 2–26. Tubular form of **fibromuscular dysplasia** involving both main renal arteries. There is also an area of **focal stenosis** in distal right main renal artery.

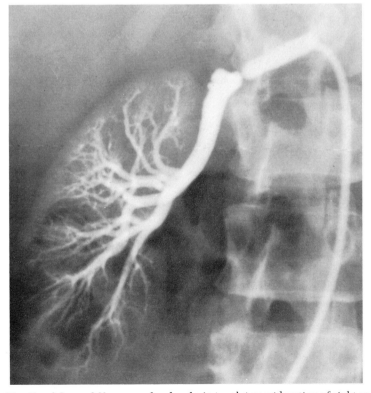

Figure 2–27. Focal form of **fibromuscular dysplasia** involving midportion of right renal artery.

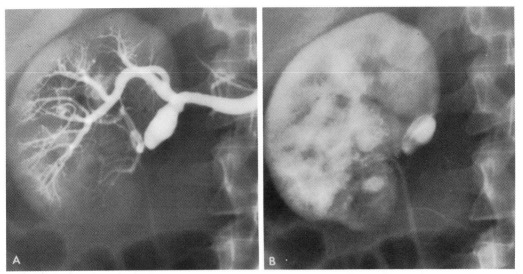

Figure 2–28. **A,** **Fibromuscular dysplasia** involving distal right renal artery and its anterior primary branch. There is intramural **dissection** of anterior branch with high-grade **stenosis** distally and **infarction** of lower pole of kidney. **B,** *Nephrographic phase* in same case shown in **A.** Contrast medium lingers in wall of dissected branch and infarcted lower pole is well demonstrated.

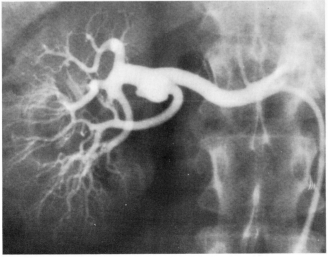

Figure 2–29. Aneurysm arising at bifurcation of right renal artery.

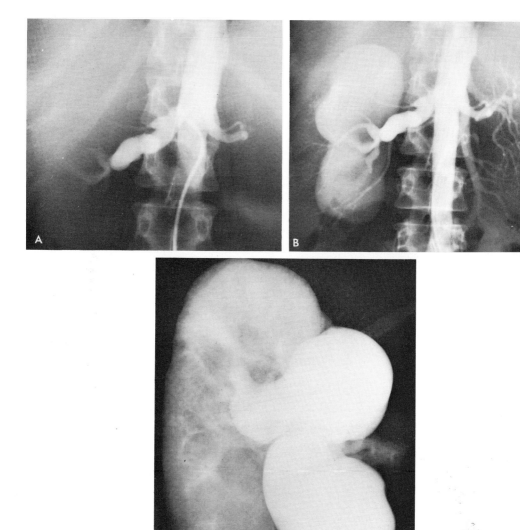

Figure 2–30. Arteriovenous fistula, believed due to rupture of renal artery aneurysm into renal vein, involving right renal vessels: **A**, *Early arterial phase* showing marked dilatation of right renal artery and beginning opacification of fistulous communication. **B**, *Later arterial phase.* Fistulous communication is visualized as indistinct jet of contrast medium just lateral to renal artery bifurcation. Large densely opacified saccular structure proved to be markedly **dilated renal vein**. Renal artery branches are seen to extend well beyond dilated vein. **C**, Injected specimen from case shown in **A** and **B**. More densely opacified structure is extremely **dilated renal vein**.

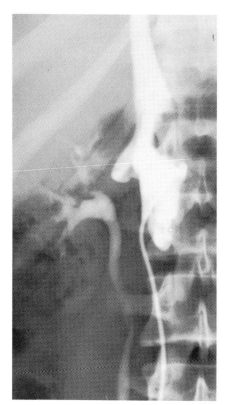

Figure 2–31. Thrombosis of left renal vein. *Inferior vena caval injection* shows thrombus protruding from orifice of left renal vein into inferior vena cava.

RENAL MASS LESIONS

The differentiation of renal tumors and cysts represents one of the more useful applications of renal angiography (Boijsen and Folin; Frimann-Dahl, 1964, 1966a; Olsson, 1962). Selective renal arteriography should be performed for this purpose whenever possible, for accurate diagnosis depends upon very detailed visualization of the intrarenal vascular architecture.

The differentiation between tumors and cysts depends principally upon the difference in vascularity of these two types of lesions (Figs. 2–32, 2–33, and 2–34). (See discussion in Chapters 9 and 10.) The vast majority of renal tumors are highly vascu-lar, whereas renal cysts are completely nonvascular. Unfortunately, in a small percentage of cases neoplasms of the kidney may be avascular and may be mistaken for cysts. In approximately 95% of renal masses the visualization of tumor vessels or the very sharp demarcation of a cyst against the surrounding normal parenchyma will permit the correct diagnosis to be made with certainty. In other cases, however, positive diagnosis must be made by either cyst puncture or surgical exploration.

Tumors of the renal pelvis may yield no abnormal findings on renal arteriography and are extremely difficult to diagnose by this means. Unless distinct tumor vessels can be visualized on the arteriogram, all such lesions should probably be explored.

Renal angiography is also quite useful in the diagnosis of adrenal tumors.

OTHER APPLICATIONS

Renal angiography has important applications in the diagnosis of a variety of other conditions.

In abdominal trauma, renal angiography may serve importantly to define the presence and extent of renal or renal artery injury, providing an invaluable guide to the surgeon in such cases (Halpern; Olsson and Lunderquist) (see Chapter 15).

Hydronephrosis may on occasion present a perplexing problem in diagnosis when the kidney functions poorly and when marked obstruction is present, in which case urography and pyelography may provide little diagnostic information (Frimann-Dahl, 1966b).

The arteriographic changes in renal inflammatory diseases such as chronic pyelonephritis, glomerulonephritis, renal papillary necrosis, and renal tuberculosis have been described by many authors (Frimann-Dahl, 1966c; Olsson, 1963). In general, however, renal arteriography does not offer significant advantage over conventional diagnostic methods in the diagnosis of most types of renal parenchymal disease.

Renal anomalies can usually be diagnosed by urography. However, in some instances renal angiography may be quite useful in the diagnosis of renal malformations, such as unilateral renal agenesis, renal hypoplasia, renal ectopia, and fusion malformations (Olsson and Wholey) (see Chapter 12).

One of the very important applications of renal angiography is in the evaluation of the renal vessels and kidneys following various operative procedures, particularly following those procedures performed for the reestablishment of blood flow distal to stenotic lesions of the renal arteries (Figs. 2–35, 2–36, and 2–37). Whether the procedure consists of endarterectomy, segmental resection and reanastomosis of the renal artery, reimplantation of the renal artery, bypass grafting, or splenorenal anas-

tomosis, the question arises on occasion as to the postoperative status of the renal vessels and the kidney. If hypertension persists postoperatively in patients on whom such surgical procedures have been performed, restudy of the patient by angiography is indicated.

Renal angiography also finds important use in the evaluation of patients who have undergone kidney transplantation and in whom the possibility of mechanical narrowing or thrombosis of the anastomosed renal artery is clinically suspected. The rejection phenomenon may also be recognized on renal angiography. (See Renal Transplantation in Chapter 17.)

All prospective renal donors should, of course, have a renal arteriogram for delineation of the renal vascular anatomy. The presence of multiple renal arteries or of other vascular anomalies, such as very early prehilar branching, may make one or both kidneys unsuitable for transplantation.

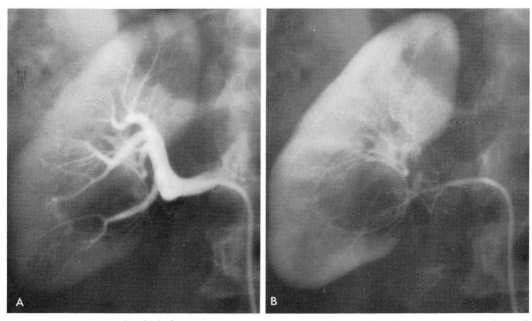

Figure 2–32. Cyst of right kidney. **A,** *Arterial phase.* **B,** *Nephrographic phase.* Cyst is avascular and renal artery branches are stretched around it.

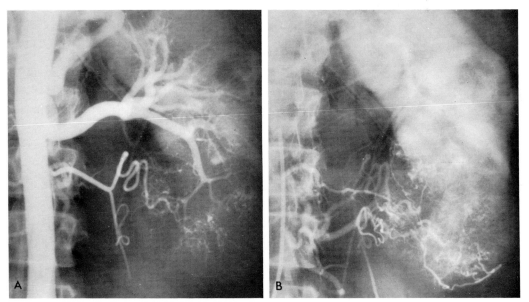

Figure 2–33. **A** and **B,** Large vascular **hypernephroma** involving lower portion of left kidney. Tumor is supplied by branches of left main renal artery and also by branches of lower polar aberrant artery. It also receives branches from capsular artery.

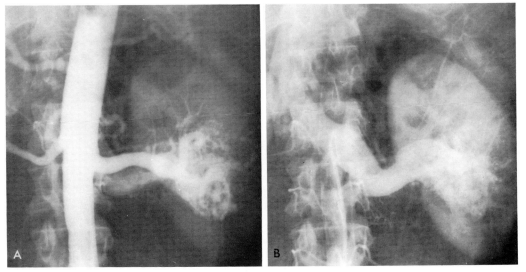

Figure 2–34. **Hypernephroma** of left kidney. **A,** *Arterial phase* showing highly vascular renal mass. Tumor growth has resulted in arteriovenous communications. Note early opacification of left renal vein. **B,** *Nephrographic phase* showing dense opacification of left renal vein and inferior vena cava.

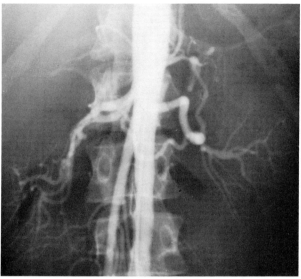

Figure 2–35. *Postoperative aortorenal arteriogram* of patient with bilateral fibromuscular dysplasia, showing well-functioning left splenorenal anastomosis.

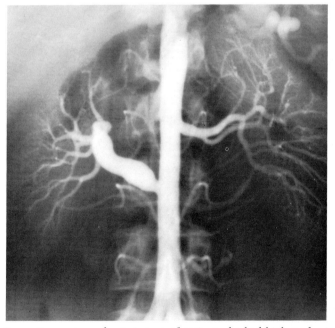

Figure 2–36. *Postoperative aortorenal arteriogram* of patient who had high-grade stenosis of right renal artery. Right aortorenal vein graft is well functioning.

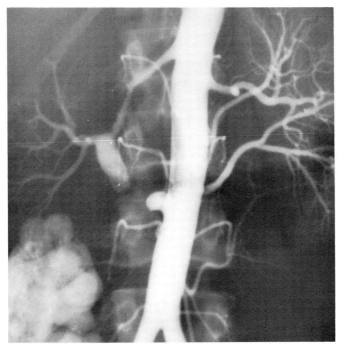

Figure 2–37. *Postoperative aortorenal arteriogram* showing **thrombotic obstruction of right aortorenal vein graft.**

ACKNOWLEDGMENT

The author wishes to thank the Year Book Medical Publishers, Inc., Chicago, Illinois, for permission to reproduce the following figures from Kincaid, O. W.: Renal Angiography, 1966: Figures 2-2, 2-4, 2-5, 2-6, 2-8, 2-10, 2-12, 2-13, 2-18, 2-19, 2-23, 2-27, 2-29, 2-30A and B, and 2-35.

REFERENCES

Boijsen, E.: Angiographic Studies of the Anatomy of Single and Multiple Renal Arteries. Acta radiol., Suppl. 183, 1959, pp. 1-135.

Boijsen, E., and Folin, J.: Angiography in the Diagnosis of Renal Carcinoma. Radiologe *1*:173-191 (Sept.) 1961.

Boijsen, E., and Köhler, R.: Renal Arteriovenous Fistulae. Acta radiol. 57:433-445, 1962.

Boijsen, E., and Köhler, R.: Renal Artery Aneurysms. Acta radiol. [Diagn.] *1*:1077-1090 (Sept.) 1963.

Castellanos, A., and Pereiras, R.: Retrograde or Counter-Current Aortography. Am. J. Roentgenol. 63:559-565 (Apr.) 1950.

Davis, G. D., Kincaid, O. W., and Hunt, J. C.: Roentgenologic Evaluation of Multiple Renal Arteries. Am. J. Roentgenol. 90:583-592 (Sept.) 1963.

dos Santos, R., Lamas, A., and Pereira Caldas, J.: L'artériographie des membres de l'aorte et de ses branches abdominales. Bull. et mém. Soc. nat. de chir. 55:587-601 (May 4) 1929.

Dustan, Harriet P., Page, I. H., and Poutasse, E. F.: Renal Hypertension. New England J. Med. *261*:647-653 (Sept. 24) 1959.

Edholm, P., and Seldinger, S. I.: Percutaneous Catheterization of the Renal Artery. Acta radiol. *45*:15-20 (Jan.) 1956.

Eyler, W. R., Clark, M. D., Garman, J. E., Rian, R. L., and Meininger, D. E.: Angiography of the Renal Areas Including a Comparative Study of Renal Arterial Stenoses in Patients With and Without Hypertension. Radiology 78:879-891 (June) 1962.

Fariñas, P. L.: A New Technique for the Arteriographic Examination of the Abdominal Aorta and Its Branches. Am. J. Roentgenol. *46*:641-645 (Nov.) 1941.

Frimann-Dahl, J.: Tumours of the Kidneys and Suprarenals. IV. Radiology in Renal Cysts, Particularly on the Left Side. Brit. J. Radiol. *37*:146-153 (Feb.) 1964.

Frimann-Dahl, J.: Angiography in Renal Tumors and Cysts. In Kincaid, O. W.: Renal Angiography. Chicago, Year Book Medical Publishers, Inc., 1966a, pp.171-208.

Frimann-Dahl, J.: Angiography in Hydronephrosis. In Kincaid O. W.: Renal Angiography. Chicago, Year Book Medical Publishers, Inc., 1966b, pp. 209-229.

Frimann-Dahl, J.: Angiography in Renal Inflammatory Diseases. In Kincaid, O. W.: Renal Angiography. Chicago, Year Book Medical Publishers, Inc., 1966c, pp. 230-252.

Gaylis, H., and Laws, J. W.: Dissection of Aorta as a Complication of Translumbar Aortography. Brit. M. J. 2:1141-1146 (Nov. 17) 1956.

Goldblatt, H., Lynch, J., Hanzal, R. F., and Summerville, W. W.: Studies on Experimental Hypertension. I. The Production of Persistent Elevation of Systolic Blood Pressure by Means of Renal Ischemia. J. Exper. Med. 59:347-379 (Mar. 1) 1934.

Graves, F. T.: The Anatomy of the Intrarenal Arteries and Its Application to Segmental Resection of the Kidney. Brit. J. Surg. 42:132-139 (Sept.) 1954.

Graves, F. T.: The Anatomy of the Intrarenal Arteries in Health and Disease. Brit. J. Surg. 43:605-616 (May) 1956.

Graves, F. T.: The Aberrant Renal Artery (Synopsis). Proc. Roy. Soc. Med. 50:368-369, 1957.

Halpern, M.: Angiography in Renal Trauma. In Kincaid, O. W.: Renal Angiography. Chicago, Year Book Medical Publishers, Inc., 1966, pp. 253-264.

Harrison, E. G., Jr., Hunt, J. C., and Bernatz, P. E.: Morphology of Fibromuscular Dysplasia of the Renal Artery in Renovascular Hypertension. Am. J. Med. 43:97-112 (July) 1967.

Hollinshead, W. H.: Anatomy for Surgeons. Volume II. The Thorax, Abdomen, and Pelvis. New York, Paul B. Hoeber, Inc., 1956, 934 pp.

Hunt, J. C., Harrison, E. G., Jr., Kincaid, O. W., Bernatz, P. E., and Davis, G. D.: Idiopathic Fibrous and Fibromuscular Stenoses of the Renal Arteries Associated With Hypertension. Proc. Staff Meet., Mayo Clin. 37:181-216 (Mar. 28) 1962.

Idbohrn, H., and Berg, N.: On the Tolerance of the Rabbit's Kidney to Contrast Media in Renal Angiography: A Roentgenologic and Histologic Investigation. Acta radiol. 42:121-140 (Aug.) 1954.

Karras, B. G., Cannon, A. H., and Ashby, R. N.: Percutaneous Left Brachial Aortography. Am. J. Roentgenol. 90:564-570 (Sept.) 1963a.

Karras, B. G., Cannon, A. H., and Sokol, J. K.: Percutaneous Left Brachial Renal Angiography. J. Urol. 89:101-105 (Jan.) 1963b.

Killen, D. A., and Foster, J. H.: Spinal Cord Injury as a Complication of Aortography. Ann. Surg. 152:211-230 (Aug.) 1960.

Kincaid, O. W., and Davis, G. D.: Abdominal Aortography. New England J. Med. 259:1017-1024 (Nov. 20); 1067-1073 (Nov. 27) 1958.

Kincaid, O. W., and Davis, G. D.: Symposium on Hypertension Associated With Renal Artery Disease: Renal Arteriography in Hypertension. Proc. Staff Meet., Mayo Clin. 36:689-701 (Dec. 20) 1961.

Kincaid, O. W., Davis, G. D., Hallermann, F. J., and Hunt, J. C.: Fibromuscular Dysplasia of the Renal Arteries: Arteriographic Features, Classification, and Observations on Natural History of the Disease. Am. J. Roentgenol. 104:271-282 (Oct.) 1968.

Kincaid, O. W., Mengis, J. L , and Fellows, J. L.: A Combined Flushing and Pulse-Pressure Monitoring System for Percutaneous Catheterization and Angiography. Am. J. Roentgenol. 101:234-237 (Sept.) 1967.

Lang, E. K.: A Survey of the Complications of Percutaneous Retrograde Arteriography: Seldinger Technic. Radiology 81:257-263 (Aug.) 1963.

Ljungqvist, A.: The Intrarenal Arterial Pattern in the Normal and Diseased Human Kidney: A Microangiographic and Histologic Study. Acta med. scandinav., Suppl. 401, 1963, pp. 1-38.

McAfee, J. G.: A Survey of Complications of Abdominal Aortography. Radiology 68:825-838 (June) 1957.

McCormack, L. J., Hazard, J. B., and Poutasse, E. F.: Obstructive Lesions of the Renal Artery Associated With Remediable Hypertension. (Abstr.) Am. J. Path. 34:582 (May-June) 1958.

Merklin, R. J., and Michels, N. A.: The Variant Renal and Suprarenal Blood Supply With Data on the Inferior Phrenic, Ureteral and Gonadal Arteries: A Statistical Analysis Based on 185 Dissections and Review of the Literature. J. Internat. Coll. Surgeons 29:41-76 (Jan.) 1958.

Miller, G. M., Wylie, E. J., and Hinman, F., Jr.: Renal Complications From Aortography. Surgery 35:885-896 (June) 1954.

Mullady, T. F., Wakim, K. G., Hunt, J. C., and Kincaid, O. W.: Effects of Diatrizoate Sodium on Kidney Function in Dogs. J.A.M.A. 184:716-718 (June 1) 1963.

Ödman, P.: Percutaneous Selective Angiography of the Main Branches of the Aorta (Preliminary Report). Acta radiol. 45:1-14 (Jan.) 1956.

Olsson, O.: Techniques and Hazards of Renal Angiography. In Abrams, H. L.: Angiography. Boston, Little, Brown & Company, 1961a, vol. 2, pp. 539-543.

Olsson, O.: Anatomic and Physiologic Considerations. In Abrams, H. L.: Angiography. Boston, Little, Brown & Company, 1961b, vol. 2, pp. 545-548.

Olsson, O.: Roentgen Examination of the Kidney and the Ureter. In Encyclopedia of Urology. V/1. Diagnostic Radiology. Berlin, Springer-Verlag, 1962, pp. 1-365.

Olsson, O.: Renal Angiography in Vascular and Inflammatory Disease of the Kidney. Congressus Radiologicus Cechoslovacua (Karlovy vary). 44, 1963.

Olsson, O., and Lunderquist, A.: Angiography in Renal Trauma. Acta radiol. N.S. 1:1-21 (Jan.) 1963.

Olsson, O., and Wholey, M.: Vascular Abnormalities in Gross Anomalies of Kidneys. Acta radiol. N.S. 2:420-432 (Sept.) 1964.

Palubinskas, A. J., and Wylie, E. J.: Roentgen Diagnosis of Fibromuscular Hyperplasia of the Renal Arteries. Radiology 76:634-639 (Apr.) 1961.

Peirce, E. C., II: Percutaneous Femoral Artery Catheterization in Man With Special Reference of Aortography. Surg., Gynec. & Obst. 93:56-74 (July) 1951.

Poutasse, E. F.: Renal Artery Aneurysm: Report of 12 Cases, Two Treated by Excision of the Aneurysm and Repair of Renal Artery. J. Urol. 77:697-708 (May) 1957.

Read, R. C., Johnson, J. A., Vick, J. A., and Meyer, M. W.: Vascular Effects of Hypertonic Solutions. Circulation Res. 8:538-548 (May) 1960.

Scheifley, C. H., Daugherty, G. W., Greene, L. F., and Priestley, J. T.: Arteriovenous Fistula of the Kidney: New Observations and Report of Three Cases. Circulation 19:662-671 (May) 1959.

Seldinger, S. I.: Catheter Replacement of the Needle in Percutaneous Arteriography: A New Technique. Acta radiol. 39:368-376, 1953.

Stirling, W. B.: Aortography: Its Application in Urology and Some Other Conditions. London, E. & S. Livingstone, Ltd., 1957.

Sutton, D.: Arteriography. Edinburgh, E. & S. Livingstone, Ltd., 1962, 322 pp.

Sutton, D., Brunton, F. J., Foot, E. C., and Guthrie, J.: Fibromuscular, Fibrous and Non-atheromatous Renal Artery Stenosis and Hypertension. Clin. Radiol. *14*:381-391, 1963.

Tillotson, P. M., and Halpern, M.: Selective Renal Arteriography. Am. J. Roentgenol. *90*:124-134 (July) 1963.

Utz, D. C., and Kincaid, O. W.: Renal Vascular Disease and Renal Hypertension: Miscellaneous Vascular Lesions Affecting the Urinary Tract. In Emmett, J. L.: Clinical Urography: An Atlas and Textbook of Roentgenologic Diagnosis. Ed. 2, Philadelphia, W. B. Saunders Company, 1964, vol. 2, pp. 1076-1123.

Wolfman, E. F., Jr., and Boblitt, D. E.: Intramural Aortic Dissection as a Complication of Translumbar Aortography. A.M.A. Arch. Surg. *78*:629-638 (Apr.) 1959.

Yuile, C. L.: Obstructive Lesions of the Main Renal Artery in Relation to Hypertension. Am. J. M. Sc. *207*:394-404 (Mar.) 1944.

CHAPTER 3

The Plain Film of the Urinary Tract (KUB)

TERMINOLOGY

Since the inception of roentgenographic studies of the urinary tract there has been considerable confusion in nomenclature. Nowhere has this been more apparent than in the failure to choose a suitable name for the plain film of the urinary tract taken before any contrast medium has been introduced. Among the terms suggested have been *plain film; flat film; roentgenogram of the kidney, ureter, and bladder area; KUB; scout film; simple film of the abdomen; preliminary roentgenogram; and urinary tract roentgenogram.* Because of its brevity, the term *KUB* has been much used in common urologic parlance. It is obviously an unscientific and inaccurate term, however, and its use can hardly be countenanced in formal writing. Other terms, though more proper and accurate, are cumbersome, especially when repetition is necessary. In the absence of a better term and in an effort to maintain accuracy, we shall employ the term *plain film* to mean the preliminary roentgenogram made of the region of the kidneys, ureters, and bladder before the introduction of contrast medium by any route whatsoever.

METHOD OF EXAMINING THE PLAIN FILM

As in any type of roentgenographic interpretation, one must adopt a fairly routine method of examining roentgenograms to avoid overlooking points of importance. There is, of course, no wrong or right method. Each physician sooner or later adopts a method best suited to himself. To the beginner some such method as the following may prove acceptable.

The two roentgenograms (upper and lower) are first scanned hastily to be sure that the upper roentgenogram has been taken high enough to include the suprarenal area and the lower roentgenogram low enough to include the prostatic area well below the pubic arch (Fig. 3-1A and B). If the patient is short enough, one roentgenogram may include the entire area (Fig. 3-2).

The physician then turns his attention to the upper roentgenogram. In a good roentgenogram the outlines of both kidneys stand out quite clearly (Fig. 3-3). In a normal person the center of the kidney is approximately opposite the transverse process of the second lumbar vertebra. Often the borders of the liver and spleen are well outlined. Both renal areas are

141

observed to be sure that no shadows are present which could be calculi. Next, both ureteral areas, the spinal column, and the outlines of the psoas muscles are observed. Scoliosis of the spinal column or obliteration of the normal psoas muscle shadows or both may be suggestive of perirenal inflammation or of a retroperitoneal mass and should not be overlooked. The region of the sacrum must be examined carefully, as small calculi, and even larger ones of moderate opacity, may be overlooked when they overlie bone (see Fig. 3-130).

The lower roentgenogram is then closely examined for shadows in the region of the bladder. Phleboliths (see Fig. 3-21) are very common in this location and their shadows are often suggestive of ureteral stone. The commonest error in interpretation is the failure to examine the prostatic area carefully for shadows of calculi or calcification. If the shadows are located behind the pubic ramus, they may be easily overlooked. Also, if the roentgenogram is not taken low enough to visualize an area at least 2 cm below the pubic ramus, prostatic calculi may be missed. Because of the overlying pubic bones, small prostatic calculi or prostatic calcification of poor density may be overlooked. For an unobstructed view of the prostate, the patient should be turned face down on the table and the x-ray tube angled upward to project the rays upward and toward the table. This will project the image of the prostate entirely above the symphysis pubis (Fig. 3-4A and B). Finally, one must carefully observe the bony structure of the spinal column and pelvis for evidence of injury, infection, metabolic disease, or metastasis from malignant tumors.

IMPORTANCE OF THE PLAIN FILM (KUB) AS A PRELIMINARY PROCEDURE IN ALL UROGRAPHIC DIAGNOSIS

It is absolutely imperative that a plain film be made as a preliminary procedure before any urographic study is undertaken. In spite of the fact that this principle is generally understood, one still encounters attempts to make a diagnosis from urograms in cases in which no preliminary roentgenogram has been taken. Although this subject has already been discussed in Chapter 1 (see Figs. 1-2A and B and 1-3A and B), it is of sufficient importance to be reemphasized here. A few illustrations of the errors that may be made by such slipshod diagnostic practices may prove to be a timely warning against this practice. In Figures 3-5A and B and 3-6A and B, one sees the plain films and urograms of patients with stones in renal pelves. If no preliminary roentgenogram had been made, the stones would have been missed, as the opaque medium obscures them completely. Often an opaque catheter or contrast medium in the ureter in a retrograde pyelogram or excretory urogram may obscure a small ureteral stone completely and leave no deformed area to permit its recognition (see Figure 1-4A and B). If a preliminary roentgenogram had not been made in this case, the stone could have been completely overlooked. Small calculi in the renal calyces may be missed if no preliminary roentgenogram is made (Fig. 3-7A and B).

The errors described in the preceding paragraph may be classified as the overlooking of pathologic lesions which are present. It is quite as easy to err in the opposite manner; namely, to make a diagnosis of pathologic lesions that are not present. In Figure 3-8A a beginner might be led to believe that stones were present in the upper portions of both ureters. The preliminary roentgenogram (Fig. 3-8B), however, shows no shadow to be present, a fact which enables the physician to know that the apparent "stone" is nothing more than a kink in the ureter where the ureter folds back on itself and produces the increased density of medium at this point. Minor calyces may point in a peculiar anteroposterior direction, affording a relatively deep column of medium, to cast a considerably denser shadow than the other calyces. The area of increased density could easily be mistaken for a stone if no preliminary roentgenogram had been available for comparison.

IMPORTANCE OF MAKING TECHNICALLY GOOD FILMS

Diagnostic Errors Caused by Films of Poor Quality

ERRORS IN TECHNIQUE

In Chapter 1 thorough preparation of the patient and careful roentogenographic technique were stressed as being necessary if one is to obtain satisfactory roentgenograms. *A poor roentgenogram is no doubt the greatest single source of error in urologic diagnosis.* It is impossible to overemphasize this statement. No matter how expert one may become in urographic interpretation, mistakes will be made from placing too much reliance on roentgenograms of poor quality.

Among the commonest errors in technique is improper exposure of the film. Figure 3-9 shows the results of overexposure. Figure 3-10 demonstrates a film which has been underexposed. Improper placing of the cassette often is responsible for the complete overlooking of a pathologic lesion. Artifacts are most often the result of dirty cassettes and careless handling of the x-ray film. Cassettes must be kept scrupulously clean at all times. Motion or breathing of the patient during exposure of the film results in poor, blurred roentgenograms that are of little or no diagnostic value. One must keep the Bucky diaphragm in good working order because, if it sticks while the film is being exposed, a shadow of the lead grid may appear on the roentgenogram, or the roentgenogram may be blurred and "fuzzy" instead of clear, with sharp detail. As a result important shadows may be overlooked.

FECAL MATERIAL, GAS, OR AIR IN THE GASTROINTESTINAL TRACT

No doubt the commonest cause of poor films is fecal material, gas, or air in the gastrointestinal tract. Swallowed air in the stomach casts a characteristic shadow (Fig. 3-11). Gas in the bowel is, of course, the commonest problem, the large intestine being a more common offender than the small intestine. One can usually tell by the pattern of the gas shadows which bowel is involved (Fig. 3-12). Fecal material in the colon may cast a fairly dense shadow which may be erroneously interpreted as residual barium (Fig. 3-13).

(Text continued on page 152.)

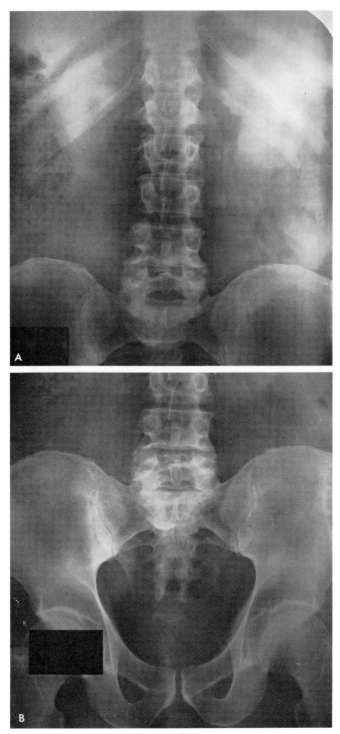

Figure 3–1. **A,** *Plain film, upper.* Shows both renal and adrenal area. **B,** *Plain film, lower.* Shows vesical and prostatic areas.

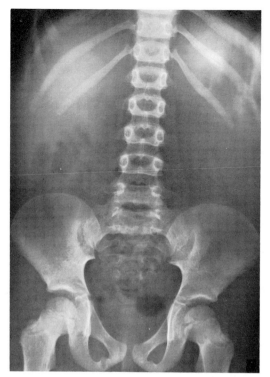

Figure 3–2. *Plain film* of child, showing that it is possible to include adrenal, renal, vesical, and prostatic areas in one roentgenogram.

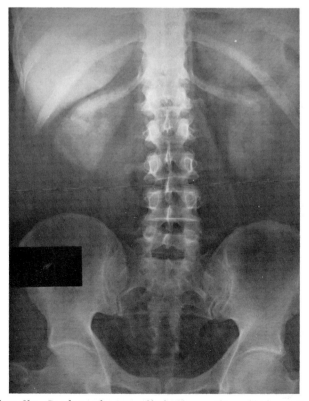

Figure 3–3. *Plain film.* Good visualization of soft-tissue outline of kidneys, liver, and spleen.

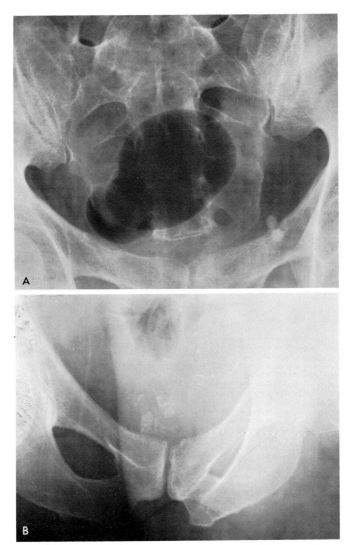

Figure 3–4. Demonstration of how prostatic calculi may be missed because of poor technique. **A,** *Plain film.* Prostatic area only partially shown. Prostatic calculi completely obscured by pubic bones and gas in rectum. **B,** Same case. Prostatic area projected above pubic bones by *having patient lie prone and directing tube from below upward.* **Multiple prostatic calculi** easily visible.

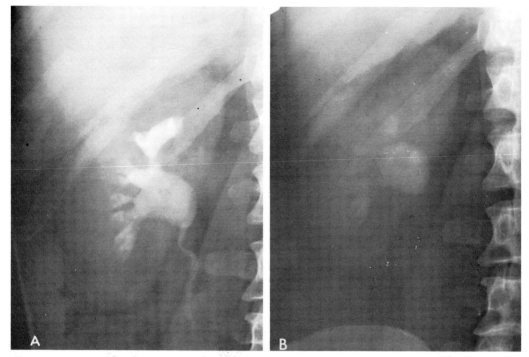

Figure 3–5. Example of importance of preliminary plain film. **A,** *Excretory urogram.* **Apparent pyelectasis** graded 1 in right kidney. One might not suspect presence of calculi. **B,** *Plain film.* **Branched calculus** which completely fills pelvis and most of calyces.

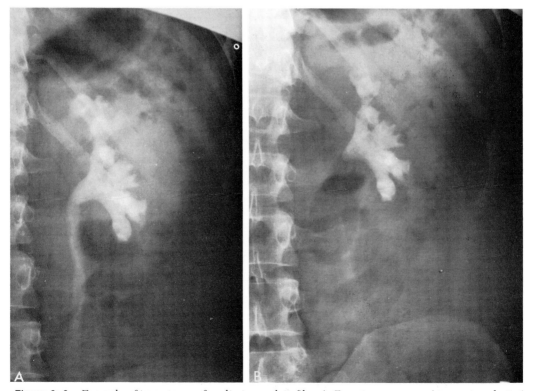

Figure 3–6. Example of importance of preliminary plain film. **A,** *Excretory urogram.* **Apparent pyelectasis** graded 1 in left kidney. One might not suspect presence of calculus. **B,** *Plain film.* **Branched calculus** which completely fills pelvis and most of calyces.

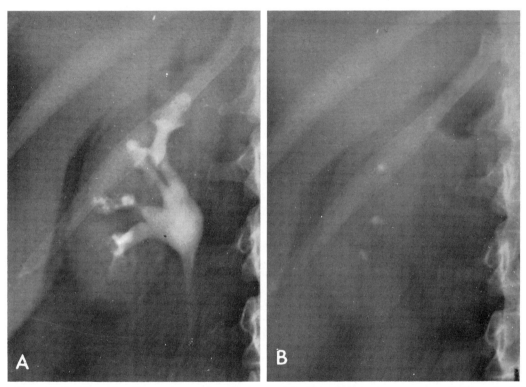

Figure 3–7. Example of importance of preliminary plain film. **A,** *Excretory urogram.* Outline of what appear to be fairly normal renal pelvis and calyces. Renal calculi might not be suspected from urogram. **B,** *Plain film.* Calculi in tips of several calyces.

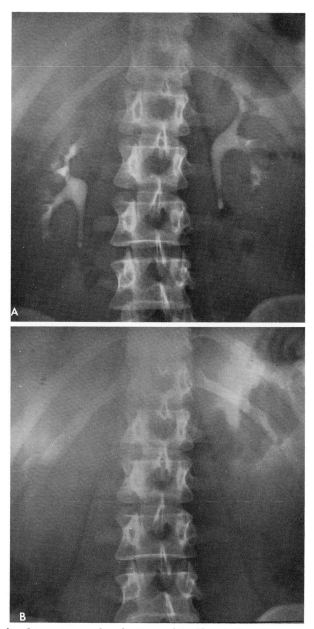

Figure 3–8. Example of importance of preliminary plain film. **A,** *Excretory urogram.* **Suggests bilateral ureteral stones** situated 3 or 4 cm below level of each ureteropelvic juncture. **B,** *Plain film.* **No stone present.** Apparent shadows suggesting stones in **A** are caused by kinks in ureters.

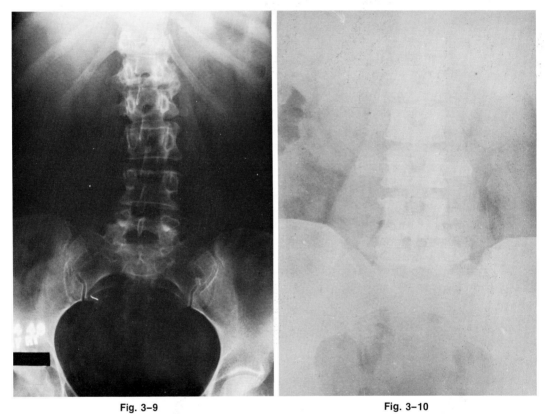

Fig. 3–9   Fig. 3–10

Figure 3–9.   *Plain film.* Results of òverexposure.
Figure 3–10.   *Plain film.* Results of underexposure.

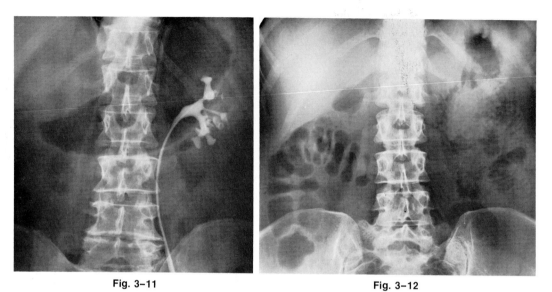

Fig. 3–11   Fig. 3–12

Figure 3–11. *Retrograde pyelogram.* Stomach outlined with air.
Figure 3–12. *Plain film.* Gas in intestine shows characteristic pattern of both large and small bowel.

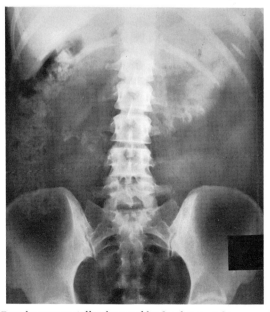

Figure 3–13. *Plain film.* Renal areas partially obscured by fecal material in ascending and transverse colon.

CONFUSING EXTRA-URINARY SHADOWS

Opaque Shadows Simulating the Density of Calcific Material, Contrast Media, or Bone

SHADOWS OF COSTAL CARTILAGES AND TRANSVERSE PROCESSES OF LUMBAR VERTEBRAE

Calcification of costal cartilages causes much confusion in urographic diagnosis because the shadows are so often projected over the renal areas. When the calcification is fragmentary, irregular, and scattered, it may simulate renal calculi and require a plain film made in the oblique projection or occasionally even urographic examination for identification (Fig. 3-14). Complete dense calcification causes less confusion but may obscure a kidney almost completely (Fig. 3-15). Occasionally the density of the tip of a transverse process of a lumbar vertebra may be increased sufficiently to cast a shadow suggestive of a ureteral stone (see Figs. 6-112 and 6-113).

SHADOWS ORIGINATING FROM SURFACE OF BODY, BANDAGES, CLOTHING, AND OTHER SOURCES

Shadows arising from the skin, body wall, clothing, or bandages can prove embarrassing to the physician interpreting films if he is not familiar with their appearance and does not keep them in mind. Among some commonly encountered items are colonic and ileal stomas (Figs. 3-16 and 3-17), nevi or warts, adhesive tape, bandages, buckles, and buttons. More unusual are umbilical hernias (Fig. 3-18) and skin folds in obese patients (Figs. 3-19 and 3-20).

CALCIFICATION OF BLOOD VESSELS

Calcification in the walls of both veins and arteries is not infrequently encoun-tered and must be recognized. By far the commonest are phleboliths of the pelvic veins, which appear roentgenographically in the region of the bladder and lower part of the ureteral regions (Dovey). Their presence is extremely common after middle age and the shadows that they produce may be the source of much confusion in urographic diagnosis. As a general rule phleboliths are round and regular in outline. Close inspection will reveal that in most cases the central part of the shadow is less dense than the periphery (Fig. 3-21). Ureteral calculi, on the other hand, are usually not so completely circular and regular in outline. They tend to assume more irregular shapes, the oval predominating. They usually are of more or less uniform density as contrasted to the phleboliths with centers of poor density.

Shadows arising from calcification of the iliac arteries provide difficulty in interpretation only if the calcification is fragmentary. If the vessel wall is uniformly calcified, the vessel stands out clearly in the roentgenograms (Figs. 3-22 and 3-23). When there are only small fragmentary areas of calcification in the vessels, however, the shadows may be easily confused with ureteral calculi by the uninitiated. The position of the calcification adds to the confusion in diagnosis because in the majority of cases the shadows lie just below the sacro-iliac joints in line with the ureters (Figs. 3-24A and B and 3-25). After one has had considerable experience in urographic diagnosis, these shadows can be identified without urography.

Calcification of the *aorta* and *renal* and *splenic vessels*, as well as aneurysms of these vessels, must be readily recognized by the urologist (Figs. 3-26 through 3-34). Not only are such shadows sometimes confused with urinary calculi, but abnormalities of these vessels may contribute to pathologic changes within the urinary tract.

(Text continued on page 161.)

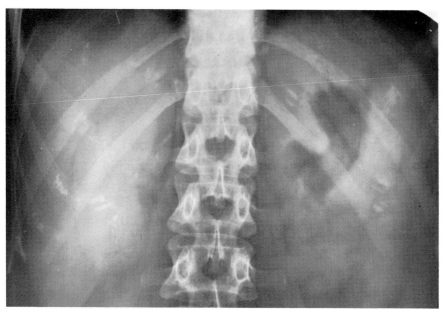

Figure 3–14. *Plain film.* **Calcified costal cartilages** overlying right kidney suggest possible renal calculi.

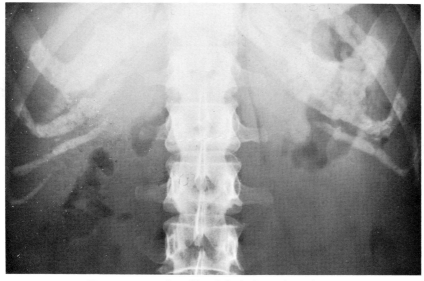

Figure 3–15. *Plain film.* Calcified costal cartilages.

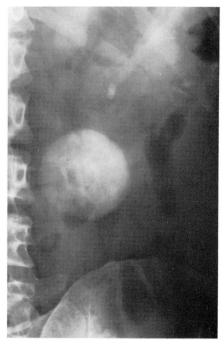

Figure 3–16. *Plain film.* Soft-tissue outline of **colonic stoma.**

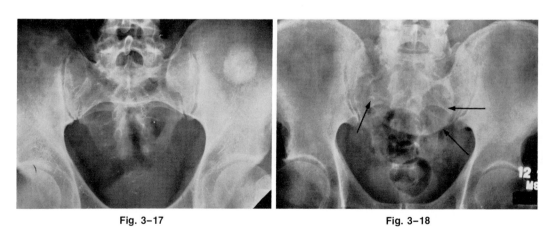

Fig. 3–17   Fig. 3–18

Figure 3–17. *Plain film.* **Colostomy.**
Figure 3–18. *Plain film.* Soft-tissue shadow of **umbilical hernia** (*arrows*) overlying sacrum.

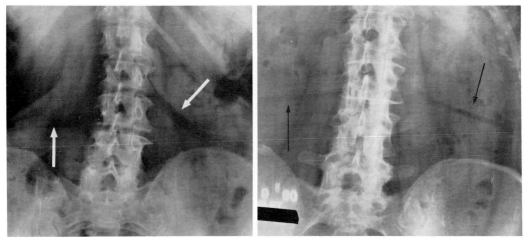

Fig. 3–19   Fig. 3–20

Figure 3–19. *Plain film.* **Obese abdominal wall** casting transverse negative shadows (*arrows*) from folds of skin.

Figure 3–20. *Plain film.* Transverse negative shadows (*arrows*) from folds of skin of obese patient.

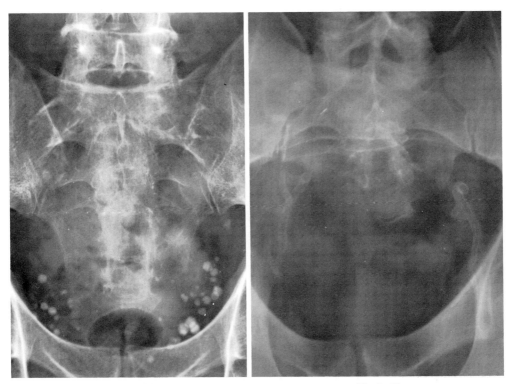

Fig. 3–21   Fig. 3–22

Figure 3–21. *Plain film.* **Multiple phleboliths** on both sides of bony pelvis, illustrating circular outline, with dense periphery and less dense center.

Figure 3–22. *Plain film.* **Calcification of iliac arteries.**

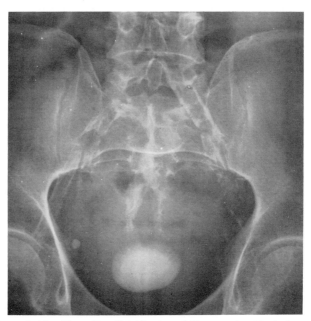

Figure 3–23. *Plain film.* Calcification of iliac arteries. Vesical stone.

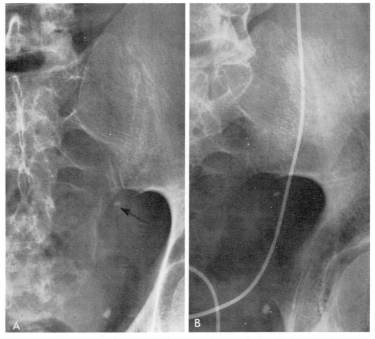

Figure 3–24. **A,** *Plain film.* Fragmentary calcification of artery below left sacro-iliac joint. Could be mistaken for ureteral calculus. **B,** *Plain film.* Lead catheter in left ureter, roentgenogram in oblique position: shadows excluded from ureter.

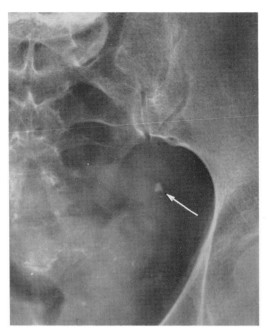

Figure 3–25. *Plain film.* Fragmentary calcification of artery below left sacro-iliac joint, which could be confused with ureteral calculus.

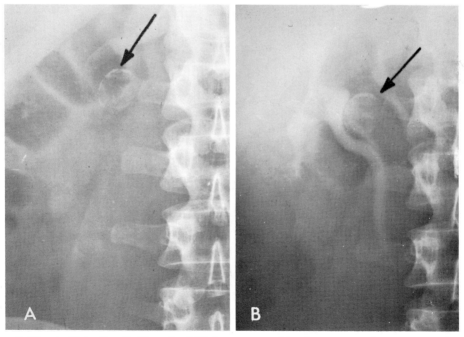

Figure 3–26. **A,** *Plain film.* Outline of calcified aneurysm of renal artery on right. **B,** *Excretory urogram.* Deformity of medial border of pelvis and adjacent ureter from aneurysm.

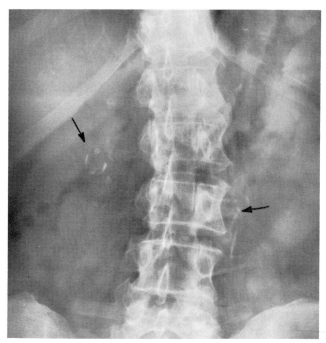

Figure 3-27. *Plain film.* Calcific shadows of **aneurysms of renal artery** (right side) and **abdominal aorta** (*arrows*).

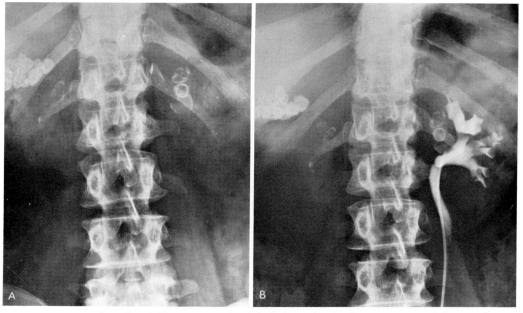

Figure 3-28. A, *Plain film.* **Gallstones** on right. **Calcified renal and splenic arteries** on left. B, *Left retrograde pyelogram.* Localization of vascular shadows.

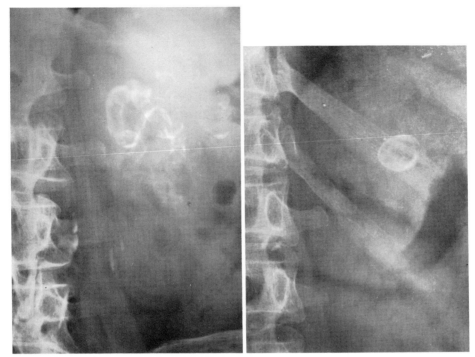

Fig. 3–29   Fig. 3–30

Figure 3–29. *Plain film.* Calcification of splenic artery and aorta.
Figure 3–30. *Plain film.* Calcified aneurysm of splenic artery.

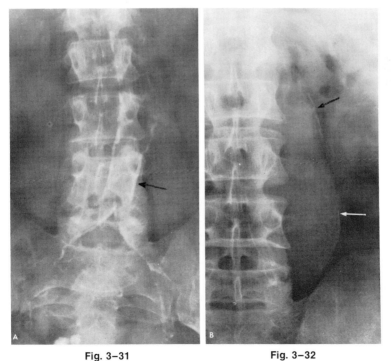

Fig. 3–31   Fig. 3–32

Figure 3–31. *Plain film.* Calcification of aorta (*arrow*) and iliac arteries.
Figure 3–32. *Plain film.* Calcification of aneurysm of abdominal aorta (*arrows*).

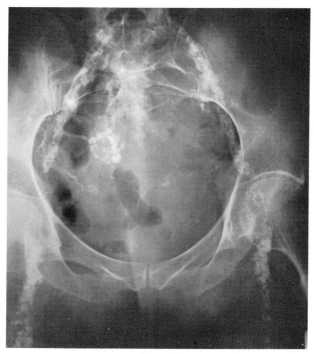

Figure 3–33. *Plain film.* Extensive calcification of iliac and femoral arteries.

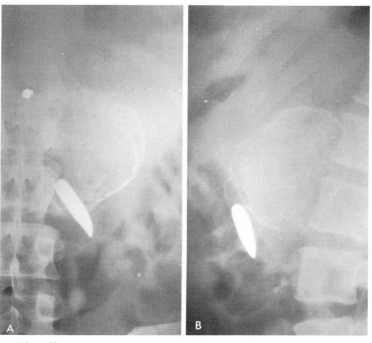

Figure 3–34. **A,** *Plain film, anteroposterior view.* Calcification of aneurysm between vena cava and aorta caused by gunshot wound. Bullet still present. **B,** *Lateral roentgenogram* showing aneurysm and bullet.

As a result of disease, it is possible to find calcification in almost any organ in the abdominal cavity. The organs most commonly involved are the spleen, adrenal glands, liver, pancreas, and mesentery (McCullough and Sutherland).

Liver and Spleen

Calcification in the spleen is usually miliary in type or it involves the capsule. In the liver it may be of miliary variety or the result of calcification in a chronic abscess cavity or cyst (Figs. 3-35 through 3-38).

Biliary Tract

Gallstones usually are easily recognized roentgenographically because of their laminated structure and faceted appearance (Figs. 3-39 through 3-42). Some gallstone shadows, however, are neither laminated nor faceted and may closely resemble those of renal calculi (Figs. 3-43 and 3-44A and B). Conversely, renal calculi occasionally are laminated and faceted and suggest gallstones until their true identity is disclosed by means of a urogram (Fig. 3-45A and B).

If only the periphery of the gallstone is calcified, the resulting shadow may simulate a calcified artery or aneurysm (Fig. 3-46). A calcified psoas abscess may simulate a gallbladder filled with contrast medium (Fig. 3-47).

In rare cases a high calcific content of the bile in the gallbladder (milk or calcium bile) may completely outline the gallbladder and appear as a large gallstone on a cholecystogram (Fig. 3-48). A neglected empyematous gallbladder also may exhibit calcification in its walls (Fig. 3-49). Stones in the common bile duct only occasionally calcify sufficiently for visualization in the plain films (Fig. 3-50).

Pancreas

Calcification of the pancreas and pancreatic calculi present a typical appearance that the urologist must learn to recognize so that he will not confuse them with renal calculi or calcified mesenteric glands. The location of the pancreas varies somewhat according to the patient's habitus, but usually the head of the pancreas is visualized just to the right of, or overlies the body of, either the first or second lumbar vertebra. The body and tail are situated somewhat higher and project to the left side of the spinal column. Calcification in the tail of the pancreas has been visualized as high as the eleventh thoracic and as low as the third lumbar vertebra (Pugh).

Calcifications of the pancreas usually appear as densely radiopaque, small, round, discrete shadows, but in occasional cases may appear to be strand-like and irregular. It is impossible to distinguish parenchymal pancreatic calcifications from pancreatic calculi in the duct system. If the calcification overlies the vertebra, it may be overlooked unless oblique or lateral films are made (Figs. 3-51 through 3-55). Calcification also may occur in the wall of a pancreatic cyst (Fig. 3-56).

Mesenteric and Retroperitoneal Lymph Nodes

Calcified mesenteric lymph nodes are extremely common and, fortunately, are of such characteristic appearance that they rarely cause confusion in diagnosis. They vary greatly in size and consistency, usually occur in groups, and tend to change their position in relation to each other, as well as to the skeleton, in subsequent roentgenograms. Often they overlie the vertebral column and are not observed until in a subsequent roentgenogram their position has shifted away from the bony structures. Although urographic examination usually is not necessary for their identification, mistakes occasionally can be made if the physician is not careful (Figs. 3-57 through 3-60).

Tuberculous Peritonitis; Histoplasmosis. Extensive calcification of mesenteric and retroperitoneal nodes is occasionally seen in patients who have had tuberculous peritonitis. Histoplasmosis (reticuloendothelial cytomycosis) is another cause of this advanced calcific process (Fig. 3-61).

Adrenal Glands

Calcification of an adrenal gland is recognized chiefly by the location and shape of the gland. The adrenal glands are situated immediately above and adjacent to each kidney and usually close to the spinal column. Calcification of the adrenal glands is seen in cases of tuberculosis of the adrenal glands (Addison's disease), adrenal cyst, and tumor. It is seen also in patients who apparently are normal, that is, without any demonstrable disease of the adrenals (Figs. 3-62A and B and 3-63).

(Text continued on page 174.)

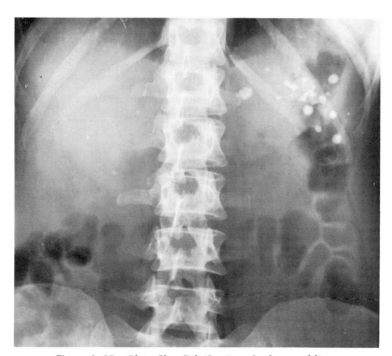

Figure 3–35. *Plain film.* Calcification of spleen and liver.

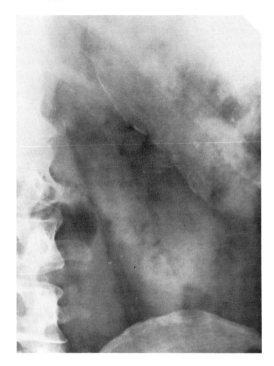

Figure 3–36. *Plain film.* Calcification of splenic capsule.

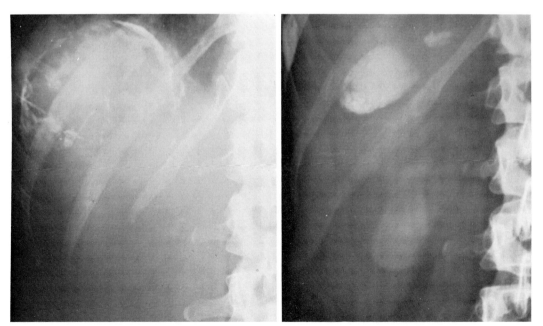

Fig. 3–37   Fig. 3–38

Figure 3–37. *Plain film.* **Echinococcus cyst of liver with calcification.** (From Bartholomew, L. G., Cain, J. C., Davis, G. D., and Bulbulian, A. H.: Unpublished portion of exhibit.)

Figure 3–38. *Plain film.* **Calcified abscess of liver.** Gallbladder (below) is outlined by opaque medium. (From McCullough, J. A. L., and Sutherland, C. G.)

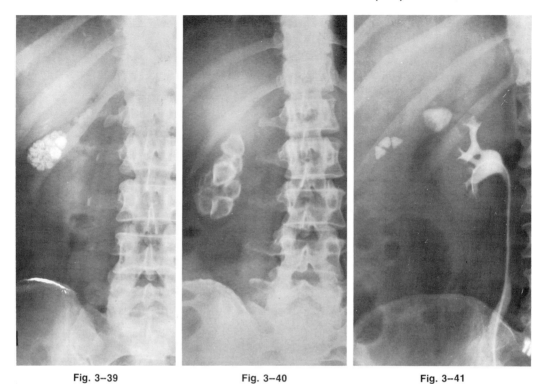

Fig. 3–39   Fig. 3–40   Fig. 3–41

Figures 3–39 and 3–40. *Plain films.* Multiple faceted gallstones.
Figure 3–41. *Right retrograde pyelogram.* Three faceted gallstones and one large, irregular gallstone excluded from urinary tract with pyelogram in oblique position.

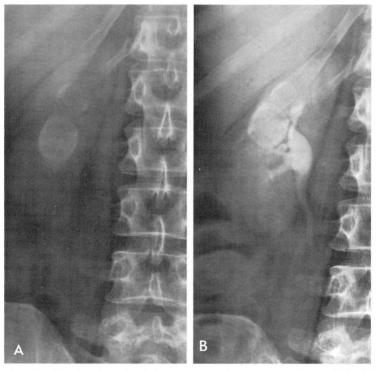

Figure 3–42. A, *Plain film.* Laminated gallstones. B, *Excretory urogram.* Laminated gallstones overlying kidney.

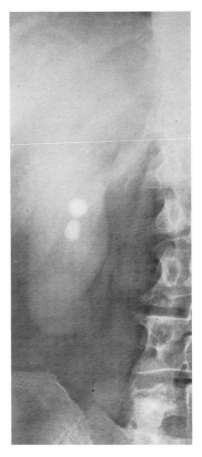

Figure 3–43. *Plain film.* **Gallstones** which are neither laminated nor faceted and could be mistaken for renal calculi if no urogram were made.

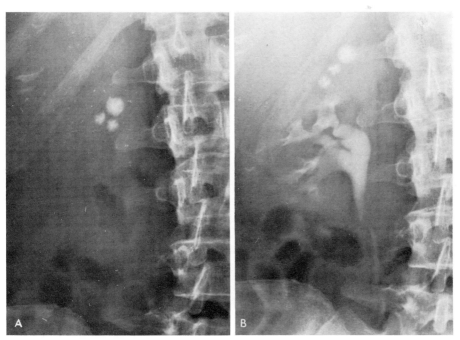

Figure 3–44. Gallstones. **A,** *Plain film.* Gallstones simulate renal calculi. **B,** *Excretory urogram.* Shadows shown to be extrarenal.

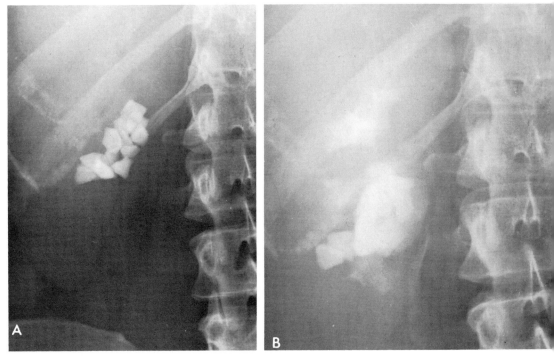

Figure 3–45. **A,** *Plain film.* **Laminated, faceted calculi** which appear to be gallstones. **B,** *Excretory urogram.* Shadows are identified as being **renal calculi** filling pelvis and one of lower calyces of right kidney.

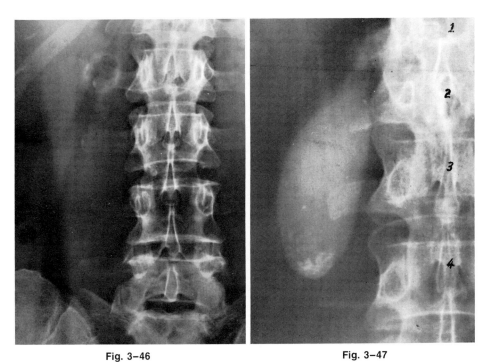

Fig. 3–46   Fig. 3–47

Figure 3–46. *Plain film.* **Gallstone** simulating calcified aneurysm of renal artery.
Figure 3–47. *Plain film.* **Calcified psoas abscess** simulating dye in gallbladder.

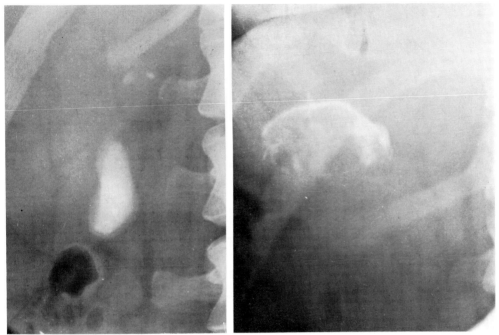

Fig. 3–48   Fig. 3–49

Figure 3–48. *Plain film.* Gallbladder outlined with milk of calcium. (From Bartholomew, L. G., Cain, J. C., Davis, G. D., and Bulbulian, A. H.)

Figure 3–49. *Plain film.* Empyema of gallbladder with calcification of wall. (From Bartholomew, L. G., Cain, J. C., Davis, G. D., and Bulbulian, A. H.: Unpublished portion of exhibit.)

Figure 3–50. *Excretory urogram.* C-shaped calcific shadow is stone impacted in common duct (*arrow*). Gallbladder is outlined by milk of calcium bile. Normal kidney is outlined by excretory urogram. (From McCullough, J. A. L., and Sutherland, C. G.)

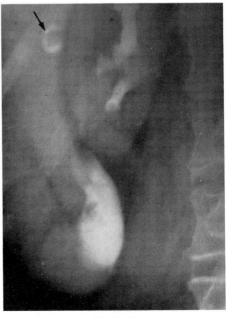

Fig. 3–50

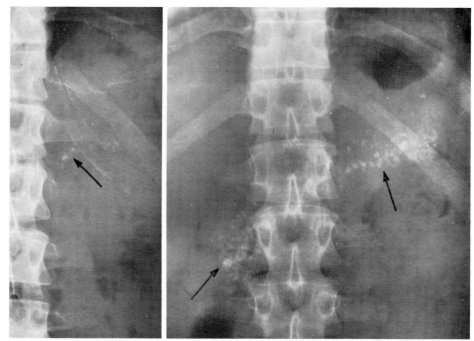

Fig. 3–51   Fig. 3–52

Figures 3–51 and 3–52.   *Plain films.* Calcification of pancreas.

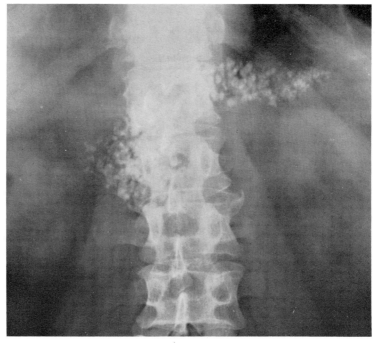

Figure 3–53.   *Plain film.* Calcification of pancreas. (From Bartholomew, L. G., Cain, J. C., Davis, G. D., and Bulbulian, A. H.)

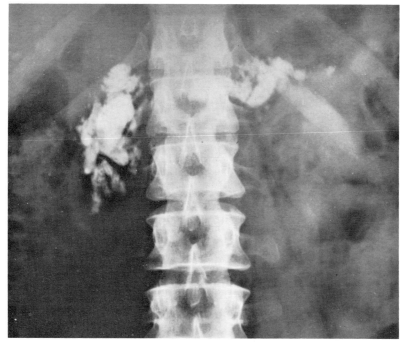

Figure 3–54. *Plain film.* Pancreatic calculi.

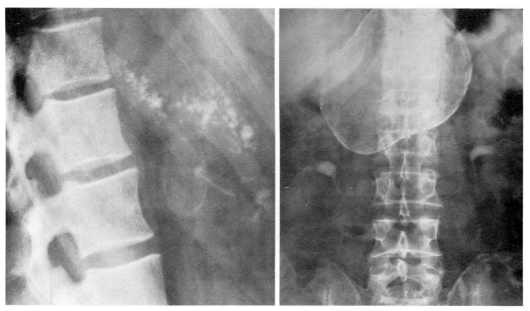

Fig. 3–55   Fig. 3–56

Figure 3–55. *Plain film, lateral view.* Pancreatic calculi. Cyst of pancreas is also outlined by fine deposit of calcium in its walls. (From McCullough, J. A. L., and Sutherland, C. G.)

Figure 3–56. *Plain film.* Calcified cyst of pancreas. (From Bartholomew, L. G., Cain, J. C., Davis, G. D., and Bulbulian, A. H.)

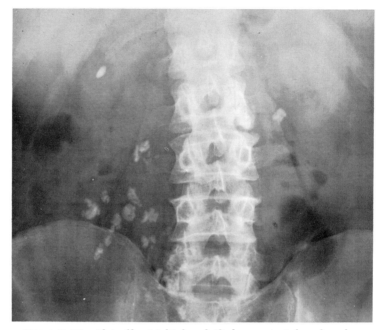

Figure 3–57. *Plain film.* Multiple calcified mesenteric lymph nodes.

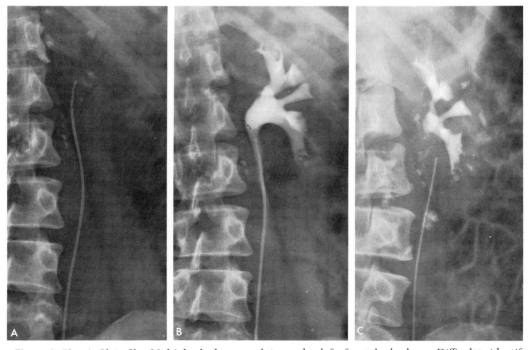

Figure 3–58. A, *Plain film.* Multiple shadows overlying and to left of vertebral column. Difficult to identify in this roentgenogram. B, *Left retrograde pyelogram, anteroposterior view.* Some of the shadows are definitely excluded and are **mesenteric lymph nodes.** C, *Oblique retrograde pyelogram.* More of the shadows are excluded and apparently all are **mesenteric lymph nodes.**

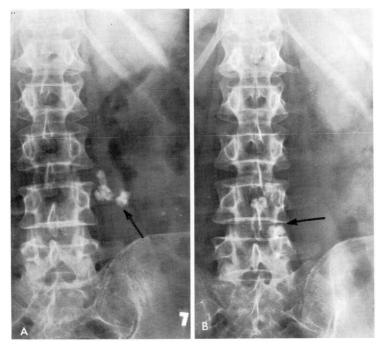

Figure 3–59. A, *Plain film.* Calcified mesenteric lymph nodes to left of fourth lumbar vertebra. B, *Plain film.* Lymph nodes (*arrow*) have moved over lumbar vertebrae and easily could be missed.

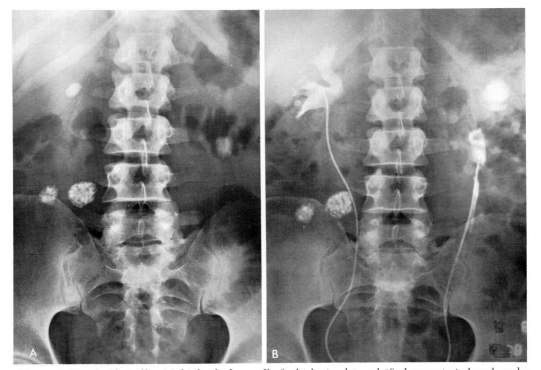

Figure 3–60. A, *Plain film.* Multiple shadows, all of which simulate calcified mesenteric lymph nodes. B, *Bilateral retrograde pyelogram.* Two shadows over right renal area are demonstrated to be **stones in kidney.** Large shadow to left of third lumbar transverse process is **large ureteral stone with hydronephrosis** above. Other shadows on right are definitely **mesenteric lymph nodes.**

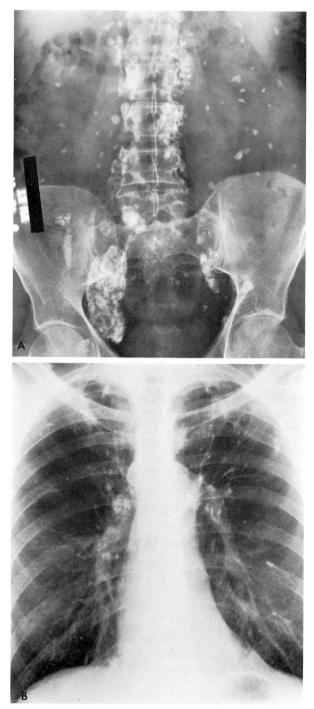

Figure 3–61. A, *Plain film.* Histoplasmosis with extensive calcification of retroperitoneal and mesenteric lymph nodes. B, *Roentgenogram of thorax* in same case, showing fibrosis and calcification in both upper lobes.

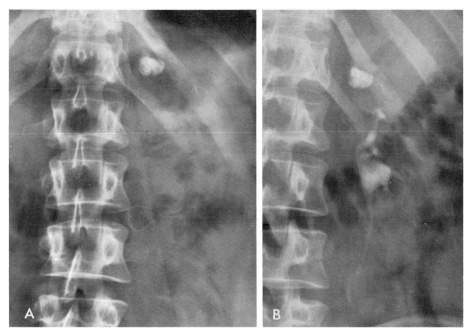

Figure 3–62. A, *Plain film.* **Calcific shadow** in region of upper pole of left kidney. B, *Excretory urogram.* Shadow demonstrated to be well above upper calyx, apparently above upper pole of kidney. Apparently **calcified adrenal gland.** (Not proved by operation.)

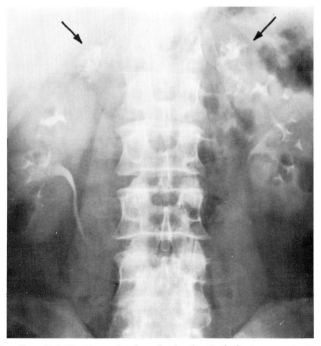

Figure 3–63. *Plain film.* **Calcification of adrenal glands.** Pathologic examination revealed extensive deposits of calcium in otherwise normal left adrenal gland. (Gland removed with left kidney because of carcinoma of ureter.)

BONES OF FETUS IN PREGNANT WOMAN

Visualization of the fetal parts in pregnant women should give little trouble in interpretation unless the pregnancy is in its early stages so that only one or two bones are sufficiently calcified to cast a shadow. In such a case one might confuse the shadow or shadows with calcification or calculi in the urinary tract (Figs. 3-64 and 3-65).

MISCELLANEOUS CALCIFIC SHADOWS

Calcification can be the result of disease or trauma of almost any intra-abdominal organ. Calcification of a malignant tumor of the appendix, calcification in a retroperitoneal hematoma, and the end result of failure of resorption of a nonviable extrauterine fetus (a mummified lithopedion) are shown in Figures 3-66, 3-67, and 3-68.

OPACITY OF GALLBLADDER FROM PREVIOUS CHOLECYSTOGRAM

It may seem superfluous here to mention the possibility of a cholecystogram causing confusion in urologic diagnosis. This, however, is not an uncommon situation encountered in a clinic type of practice where a patient is undergoing investigation for several conditions in the space of only a few days. If the cholecystogram has been done only recently, or if there is delay in the emptying time of the gallbladder, the shadow may persist when the urologic roentgenograms are made. Very often this shadow lies over the right renal area and may be misinterpreted if the examiner does not keep the possibility in mind (Figs. 3-69A and B and 3-70A and B).

RESIDUUM FROM SUBCUTANEOUS AND INTRAMUSCULAR MEDICATION

Injections of salts of heavy metals such as bismuth (from previous treatment of syphilis or other diseases) or injections of iodized oil for myelography may leave residua that cast characteristic shadows. Most of these are encountered in the gluteal areas where the appearance is typical. The physician will have little trouble in recognizing them (Figs. 3-71 and 3-72). Intragluteal injections of medicaments that do not cast shadows may set up local fibrotic reactions (injection granulomas) which may cast a shadow on the film. Such shadows may cause diagnostic errors if their true nature is not suspected (Fig. 3-73).

OPAQUE MATERIAL IN BOWEL

Lead shot sometimes are observed in the alimentary tract (Fig. 3-74). When present in the appendix, they give the appearance of a short strand of beads. Residual barium in the bowel (Figs. 3-75 and 3-76) after either a barium meal or a barium enema is one of the most common causes of poor, obscured urologic roentgenograms. Undissolved pills in the stomach or intestine (Fig. 3-77) may result in an error in roentgenographic interpretation unless the examiner is alert to their appearance. Enteric-coated pills are especial offenders. In case of question, a later film will show the shadows to have moved or disappeared.

SHADOWS RESULTING FROM PREVIOUS OPERATIVE PROCEDURES

When unusual shadows appear in a film, the possibility of their resulting from previous operative procedures must be borne in mind. Surgical fusion of the spinal column (Figs. 3-78 and 3-79) must be recognized, as well as the characteristic roentogenographic appearance of iodized oil remaining in the spinal canal after a spinogram (Fig. 3-80). Gold seeds containing radon or other radioactive isotopes, especially those implanted into tumors of the urinary bladder, are commonly seen in urologic practice (Fig. 3-81). Their appearance is so characteristic that they usually cause no confusion in interpretation. At times metal clips or nonabsorbable sutures used in general, neurologic, or orthopedic surgery may confuse urographic interpretation, unless the physician is well acquainted with their characteristic appearance (Figs. 3-82, 3-83, and 3-84). A peculiar regrowth of bone from the remaining periosteum may follow resection of a rib (Fig. 3-85).

Nephrostomy tubes (Fig. 3-86) and splinting urethral catheters left after operation on the urinary tract cause no trouble in interpretation. Tantalum wire mesh used in the repair of extensive hernias has a rather dramatic appearance (Fig. 3-87; see also Fig. 3-84).

SHADOWS ARISING FROM FEMALE PELVIS AND GENITAL TRACT

Pessaries, Tampons, Powder, and Residuum of Tubal Insufflation

Pessaries (Figs. 3-88 and 3-89) or vaginal tampons (Figs. 3-90 and 3-91) may be the cause of rather disturbing shadows if the examiner is unfamiliar with them. Powder in the vagina (Fig. 3-92) used by gynecologists in the treatment of such vaginal conditions as *Trichomonas vaginalis* may produce confusing shadows unless the physician is aware of this possibility. Residual contrast medium in the female pelvis following diagnostic insufflation of the fallopian tube may present a bizarre appearance (Figs 3-93 and 3-94).

Fibroid Tumors of the Uterus

Fibromatous tumors of the uterus occasionally become calcified. They appear as spheroid masses with calcification arranged in irregular whorls. They also have been described as resembling the print of a sponge after it has been dipped in a solution of barium. When located in the commonest site within the bony pelvis (in the midline or to either side), they present no diagnostic problem (Figs. 3-95 through 3-98). In cases in which the uterus is greatly enlarged, however, these calcific shadows may assume unusual and bizarre positions, even lying so high that they are confused with gallstones or renal calculi (Fig. 3-99).

CARCINOMA OF THE OVARY

Figure 3-100 shows calcification from bilateral carcinoma of the ovaries with extensive abdominal metastasis.

DERMOID CYSTS OF THE OVARY

More than 95% of the dermoid cysts arise from the ovary (see "Sacral and Presacral Tumors" later in this chapter). The capsule of the cyst is fairly radiopaque and the oily fluid inside is radiolucent. This combination gives a roentgenologic appearance of calcification of the cyst wall. A derivative of any ectodermal structure, such as hair or teeth, may be present in the cyst and may indicate its true identity (Figs. 3-101 through 3-104).

(Text continued on page 189.)

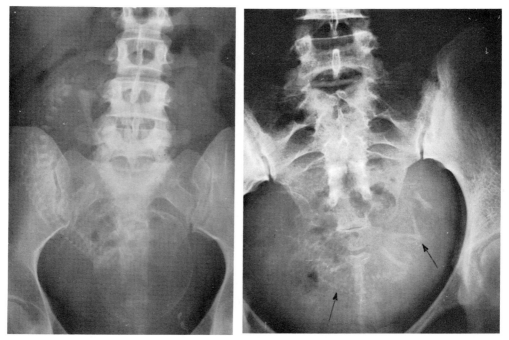

Fig. 3-64   **Fig. 3-65**

Figures 3-64 and 3-65. *Plain films.* Shadow of fetal parts in pregnant woman.

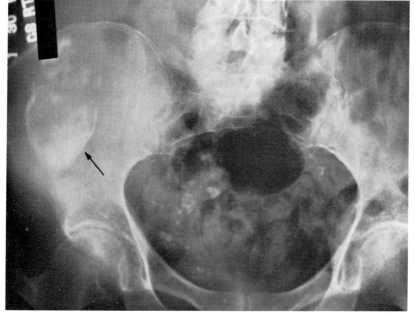

Figure 3-66. *Plain film.* **Calcified malignant tumor of appendix** simulates calcified pericecal abscess. (From Bartholomew, L. G., Cain, J. C., Davis, G. D., and Bulbulian, A. H.)

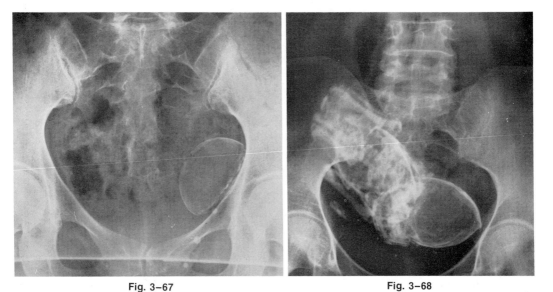

Fig. 3–67   Fig. 3–68

Figure 3–67. *Plain film.* Calcified retroperitoneal hematoma. (From Bartholomew, L. G., Cain, J. C., Davis, G. D., and Bulbulian, A. H.)

Figure 3–68. *Plain film.* Lithopedion. (From Bartholomew, L. G., Cain, J. C., Davis, G. D., and Bulbulian, A. H.)

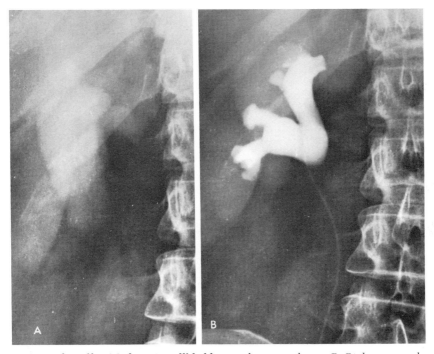

Figure 3–69. **A,** *Plain film.* **Medium in gallbladder** overlying renal area. **B,** *Right retrograde pyelogram.* Demonstrates that shadow is distinct from pelviocalyceal system and represents remains of medium in gallbladder.

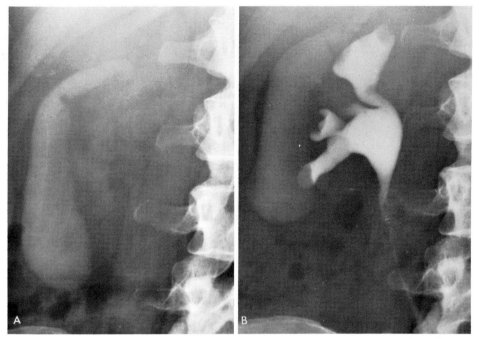

Figure 3–70.   Residual contrast medium in gallbladder. **A,** *Plain film.* **B,** *Retrograde pyelogram.*

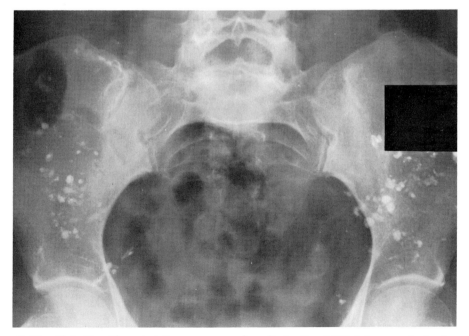

Figure 3–71.   *Plain film.* Characteristic appearance of result of antisyphilitic intramuscular treatment with salts of heavy metals.

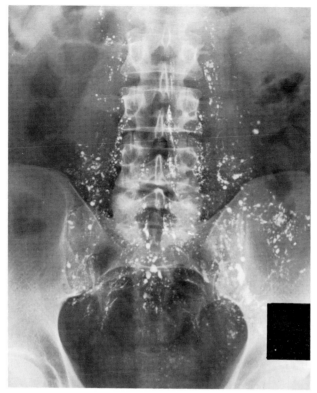

Figure 3–72. *Plain film.* **Iodized oil** scattered throughout the muscles.

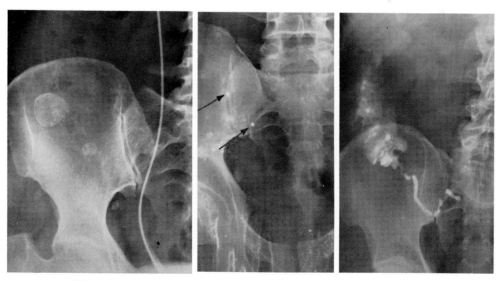

Fig. 3–73   Fig. 3–74   Fig. 3–75

Figure 3–73. *Plain film.* **Fibromas in right buttock** from previous intramuscular injections of penicillin. Opaque catheter in right ureter.
Figure 3–74. *Plain film.* Appearance of **lead shot in alimentary tract.**
Figure 3–75. *Excretory urogram.* **Residual barium in bowel.** Appendix is outlined.

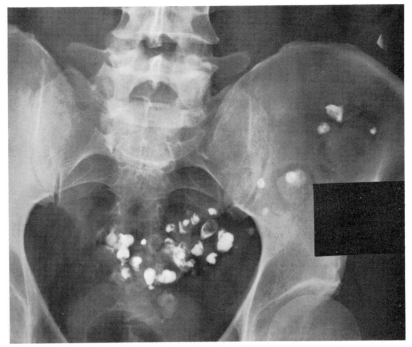

Figure 3–76. *Plain film.* Residual barium in bowel in case of diverticulosis of sigmoid.

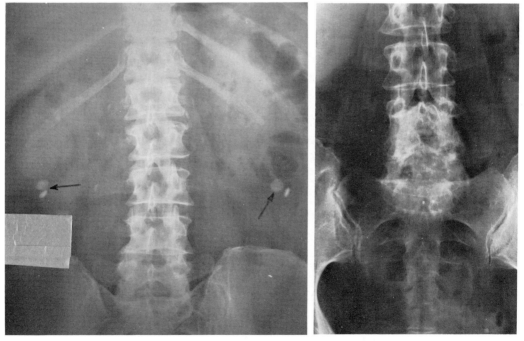

Fig. 3–77   Fig. 3–78

Figure 3–77. *Plain film.* Undissolved pills in alimentary tract.
Figure 3–78. *Plain film.* Previous surgical fusion of lumbosacral vertebrae.

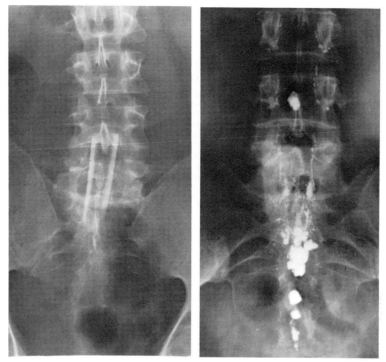

Fig. 3–79   Fig. 3–80

Figure 3–79. *Plain film.* Bone graft in lumbosacral portion of spinal column.
Figure 3–80. *Plain film.* Iodized oil remaining in spinal canal.

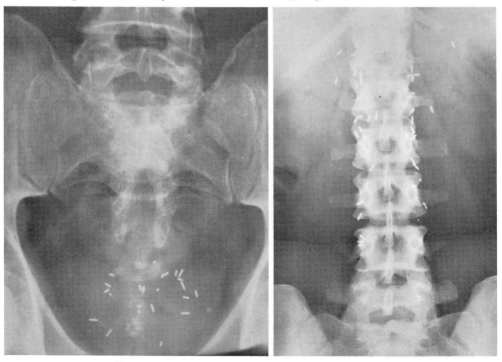

Fig. 3–81   Fig. 3–82

Figure 3–81. *Plain film.* **Radon seeds** implanted into bladder.
Figure 3–82. *Plain film.* **Metal clips** employed in abdominal surgery.

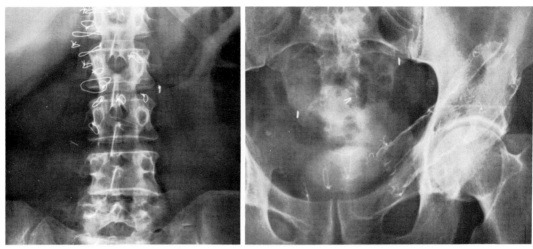

Fig. 3–83   Fig. 3–84

Figure 3–83. *Plain film.* Wire surgical sutures.

Figure 3–84. *Plain film.* Nonabsorbable surgical sutures and silver clips. Also tantalum wire mesh used in repair of left inguinal hernia.

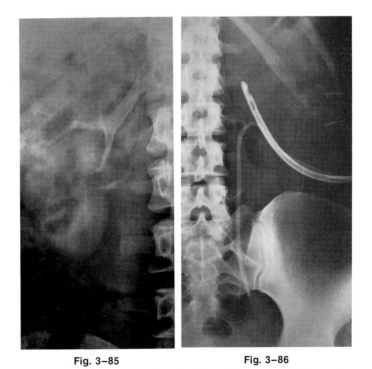

Fig. 3–85   Fig. 3–86

Figure 3–85. *Plain film.* Previously resected 12th rib. Peculiar regrowth of bone from remaining periosteum.

Figure 3–86. *Plain film.* Nephrostomy tube and catheter used as ureteral splint.

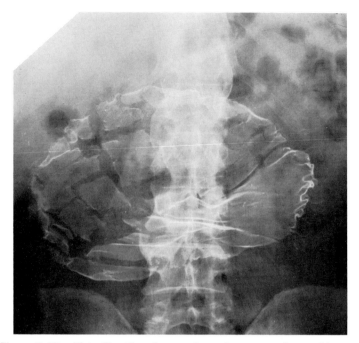

Figure 3–87. *Plain film.* Tantalum mesh used in repair of ventral hernia.

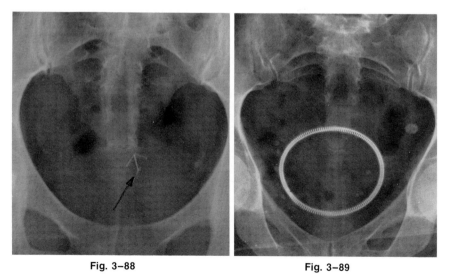

Fig. 3–88   Fig. 3–89

Figure 3–88. *Plain film.* Contraceptive pessary in uterine cervix.
Figure 3–89. *Plain film.* Vaginal pessary in place.

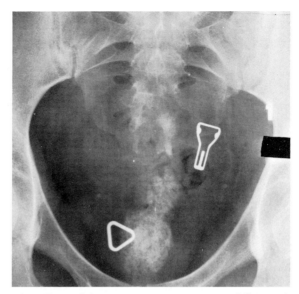

Figure 3–90. *Plain film.* Iodoform gauze sponge in vagina, following biopsy of cervix.

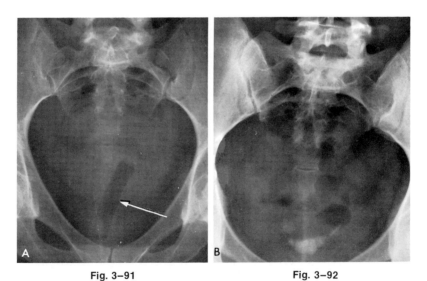

Fig. 3–91   Fig. 3–92

Figure 3–91. *Plain film.* Negative shadow cast by **tampon in vagina.**
Figure 3–92. *Plain film.* **Powder remaining in vagina,** which has been used in treatment of *Trichomonas vaginalis* infection.

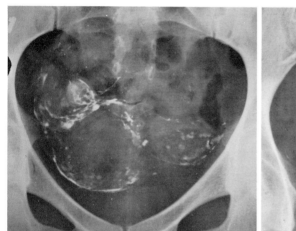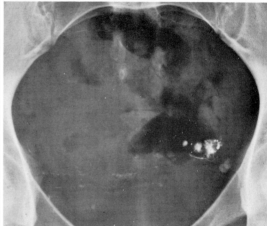

Fig. 3–93   Fig. 3–94

Figure 3–93. *Plain film.* Residual contrast medium from tubular insufflation.
Figure 3–94. *Plain film.* Residual contrast medium from previous diagnostic tubular insufflation.

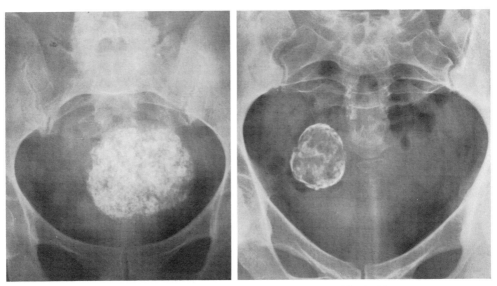

Fig. 3–95   Fig. 3–96

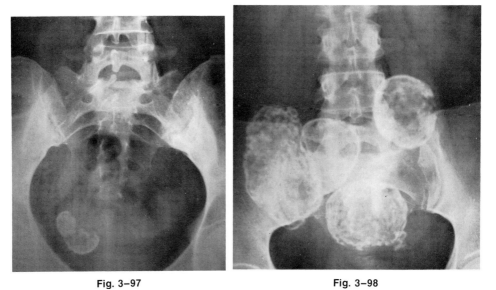

Fig. 3–97   Fig. 3–98

Figures 3–95, 3–96, and 3–97. *Plain films.* Calcified uterine fibroids in three women.

Figure 3–98. *Plain film.* **Multiple large calcified fibroid tumors of uterus.** (From McCullough, J. A. L., and Sutherland, C. G.)

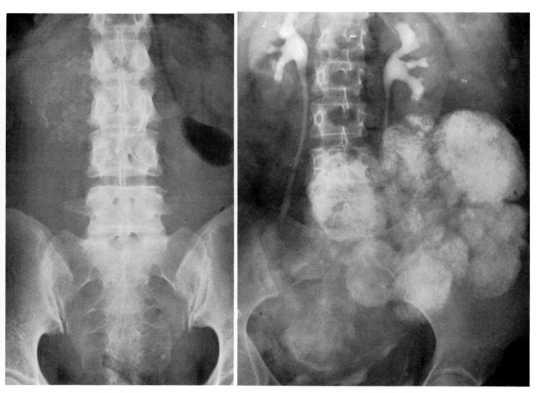

Fig. 3–99   Fig. 3–100

Figure 3–99. *Plain film.* Calcification in uterine fibromyoma, medial to and below lower pole of right kidney. Huge uterus extends to this level. (From Bartholomew, L. G., Cain, J. C., Davis, G. D., and Bulbulian, A. H.)

Figure 3–100. *Excretory urogram.* Bilateral carcinoma of ovaries, with extensive abdominal metastasis and calcification. There is little if any renal displacement, in spite of extensive abdominal lesion. (See text.)

Fig. 3–101   Fig. 3–102

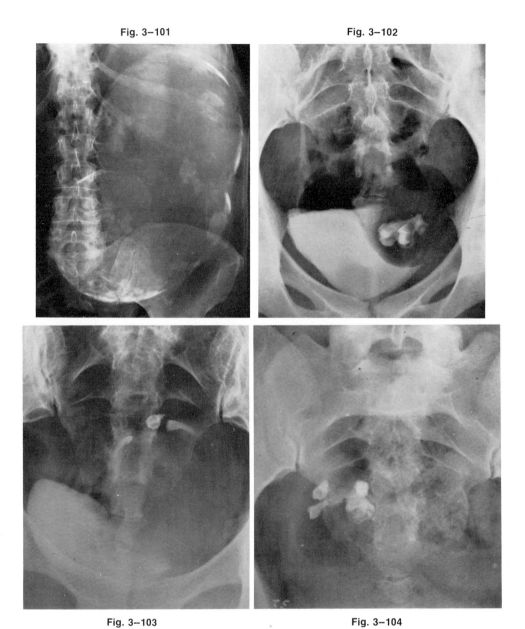

Fig. 3–103   Fig. 3–104

Figure 3–101.   *Plain film.* **Large ovarian dermoid cyst.** (From Bartholomew, L. G., Cain, J. C., Davis, G. D., and Bulbulian, A. H.)

Figure 3–102.   *Excretory cystogram.* **Dermoid cyst of ovary, containing teeth.** Left wall of bladder is displaced by cyst.

Figure 3–103.   *Excretory urogram.* Displacement of bladder downward and to right from **dermoid cyst of left ovary.** Note three teeth easily seen in upper margin of soft-tissue mass. At operation cyst was found to contain components of all three germ layers, including teeth, hair, and sebaceous material.

Figure 3–104.   *Plain film* showing **teeth in dermoid cyst of right ovary.**

SHADOWS ARISING FROM THE MALE PELVIS AND GENITAL TRACT

Calcification of the Spermatic Tract (Vasa Deferentia, Ampullae, and Seminal Vesicles)

Calcification of the seminal vesicles and vasa is not common. The earliest reports (Clement, 1830; Duplay, 1855; Orth, 1893; Chiari, 1903; and George, 1906) were from routine necropsies. The first roentgenologic demonstration of calcification of the seminal vesicle was reported by Kretschmer in 1922 and that of the vasa by Bianchini in 1930.

Lowsley and Riaboff in 1942 reviewed the literature up to 1939. They found 31 cases and included 1 of their own. They found that calcification of the vasa deferentia (including the ampullae) was considerably commoner than calcification of the seminal vesicle. Data on the 32 cases are given in Table 3-1.

Earlier authors have mentioned the chief causes of calcification of the spermatic tract as degenerative changes and tuberculosis (see Figs. 8-22, 8-25, 8-82, and 8-83). In the last few years attention has been called to the frequency with which calcification of the vas deferens is found in patients with diabetes of long standing. The largest series of cases was reported by Wilson and Marks in 1951. In 56 of the 60 cases that they reported, diabetes was present. They noted that calci-

fication was confined to the intrapelvic portion of the vas in approximately 80% of cases and that in all of these the calcification in the vas was confined to an area medial to the point at which the vas crosses the ureter (Figs. 3-105 through 3-111). (See also Figures 1-50 and 1-51 for an anatomic demonstration of the relation of vasa deferentia, ampullae, and seminal vesicles.) In the absence of inflammatory reaction and stricture of the vas they found that the calcification involves the muscular wall of the vas. It is considered a degenerative process somehow related to the diabetic state. A report of four cases by Camiel also emphasizes the role of diabetes as an etiologic factor.

Prostatic Calcification

Calcification in the region of the prostate gland usually represents ordinary prostatic calculi, although tuberculous prostatic calcification does occur (see Fig. 8-82). Prostatic calculi are considered in Chapter 6 (see Figs 6-198 through 6-205). Attention has been called in this chapter to the importance of projecting the prostatic area upward so that it will not be obscured by the symphysis pubis (see Fig. 3-4).

PAPILLARY MUCOUS CYSTADENOCARCINOMA (PSEUDOMYXOMA PERITONAEI)

Papillary mucous cystadenocarcinomas arise principally from the *ovaries* and in rare instances from the *appendix* in both men and women. More rarely they occur in *other structures* such as a *urachal cyst of the bladder.* These tumors produce encapsulated gelatinous masses of mucin which has an affinity for calcium. The calcium appears to be dispersed in a fine granular form throughout the tumor. The roentgenologic appearance is that of multiple, calcium-bearing, finely granular, globular masses (Figs. 3-112, 3-113, and

Table 3-1. **Calcification of Vasa Deferentia, Vasa Ampullae, and Seminal Vesicles: Lesions in 32 Cases Summarized From Lowsley and Kirwin**

	UNILATERAL	BILATERAL
Vas deferens	5	3
Ampulla	2	8
Seminal vesicle	2	7
Vas and seminal vesicle	0	2
Ampulla and seminal vesicle	0	1
Vas and ampulla	0	2

3-114). These tumors tend to rupture, and when this occurs the tumor may be implanted onto almost every part of the peritoneal cavity. In such cases the globular masses may involve most of the abdominal cavity.

Nonopaque Soft-Tissue Shadows of Both Urinary and Extra-urinary Organs

UPPER PART OF ABDOMEN

Although it is of interest to speculate on the identity of shadows produced by soft tissue, one should remember that any conclusion drawn may be erroneous. In many roentgenograms the outlines of such organs as the *kidneys, spleen, liver, pancreas, gallbladder,* and so forth are quite distinct (Figs. 3-115, 3-116, and 3-117). Only too often, however, when one thinks it is possible to discern the outline of a kidney in relation to the outline of some adjacent soft tissue mass, a urogram will reveal the fallacy of the diagnosis and the outline thought to be that of a kidney will be shown to be caused by something entirely different. For the sake of accuracy, therefore, one must usually check findings in the plain film by means of excretory or retrograde urography.

This warning should not serve to discourage careful examination of the plain films for evidence of significant changes in the shape of the so-called soft tissues. In every roentgenogram the *renal outline* should be carefully observed for evidence of *asymmetry, hypoplasia* or *hyperplasia,* *irregularity* (as in renal tumor, cyst, hydronephrosis, or polycystic disease), or evidence of *ectopia* or *fusion* (Figs. 3-118, 3-119, and 3-120).

Massive hemorrhage, retroperitoneal tumor, or an extensive inflammatory process in and around a kidney may appear in the plain film as a large, diffuse area of increased density involving almost the entire half of the abdomen and obliterating the normal outline of the abdominal organs on the involved side (Figs. 3-121 and 3-122). Of especial importance is the *obliteration of the shadow of the psoas muscle* associated with scoliosis of the spinal column, which is often seen in cases of perinephric abscess (Fig. 3-123). This condition will be more completely discussed under the subject of infection of the renal cortex and perinephric abscess (Chapter 7).

LOWER PART OF ABDOMEN AND PELVIS

Soft-tissue shadows should be carefully looked for in the region of the pelvis. In some cases the outline of the urinary bladder can be determined accurately in the plain film. This apparently is due to an increase in density of the viscus when filled with urine (Fig. 3-124). It is unwise to rely on this information, however, if there is any question with regard to the integrity of this organ. *Pelvic tumors* in women, even in the absence of calcification, may at times cast a sufficient shadow to suggest the diagnosis (Figs. 3-125 and 3-126).

(Text continued on page 199.)

Fig. 3–105

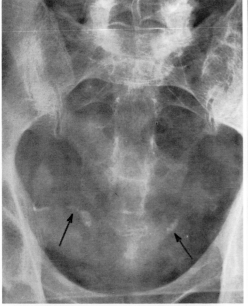

Fig. 3–106

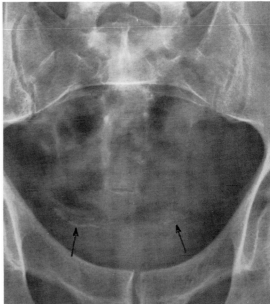

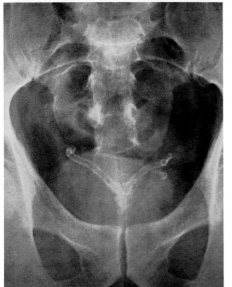

Fig. 3–107

Figure 3–105. *Plain film.* Calcification of vasa deferentia and ampullae.

Figure 3–106. *Plain film.* Calcification of ampullae of vasa.

Figure 3–107. *Plain film.* Calcification of vasa deferentia and ampullae. Probably also some calcification in left seminal vesicle.

Fig. 3–108

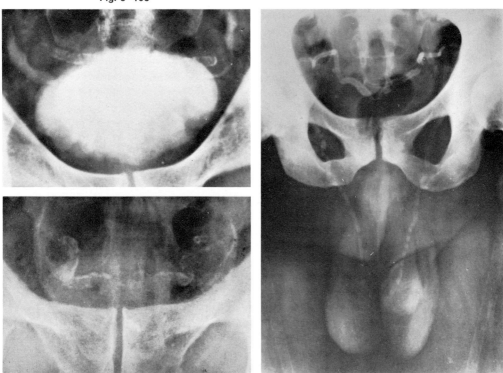

Fig. 3–109   Fig. 3–110

Figure 3–108. *Excretory urogram.* Calcification of vasa deferentia in diabetic. Relation of vasa to ureters is illustrated. Note that calcification is medial to ureters. (From Camiel, M. R.)

Figure 3–109. *Plain film.* Calcified vasa deferentia in diabetic. (From Camiel, M. R.)

Figure 3–110. *Plain film.* Calcification of vasa deferentia in patient, 44 years of age, who had had diabetes for 5 years. This case is unusual in that entire lengths of both ducts are calcified. (From Wilson, J. L., and Marks, J. H.)

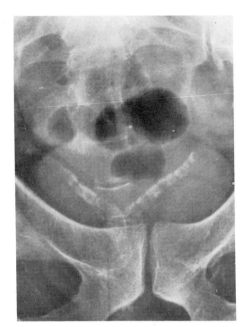

Figure 3–111. *Plain film.* Plaque-like calcification of walls of vasa deferentia in diabetic. (From Culver, G. J., and Tannenhaus, J.)

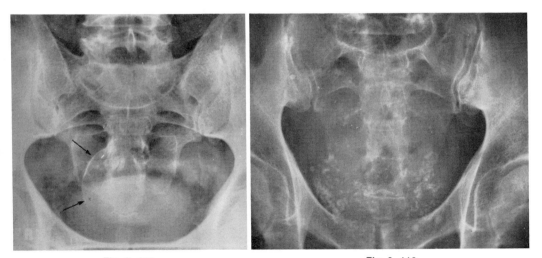

Fig. 3–112   Fig. 3–113

Figure 3–112. *Plain film.* Calcified cyst of urachus containing grade 1 mucus-producing adenocarcinoma with metastatic pseudomyxoma peritonaei (*arrows*).

Figure 3–113. *Plain film.* Calcification in grade 1 mucus-producing adenocarcinoma (pseudomyxoma peritonaei) which originated in appendix.

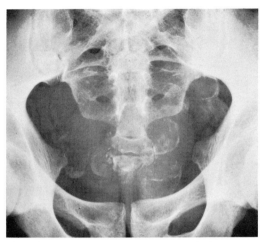

Figure 3–114. *Plain film.* **Pseudomyxoma peritonaei.** (From Bartholomew, L. G., Cain, J. C., Davis, G. D., and Bulbulian, A. H.)

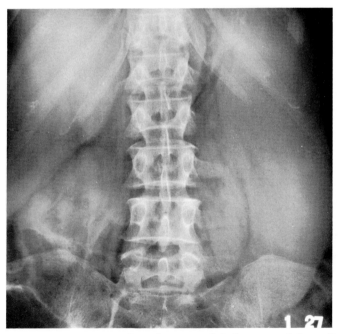

Figure 3–115. *Plain film.* **Splenomegaly.** Spleen extends below crest of ilium. (Splenectomy.)

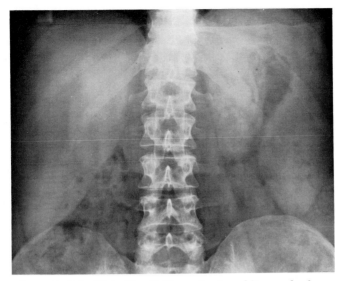

Figure 3–116. *Plain film.* Outlines of enlarged liver and spleen.

Figure 3–117. *Excretory urogram.* Distended gallbladder due to stones obstructing both cystic and common ducts (proved surgically) has caused medial displacement and malrotation of kidney.

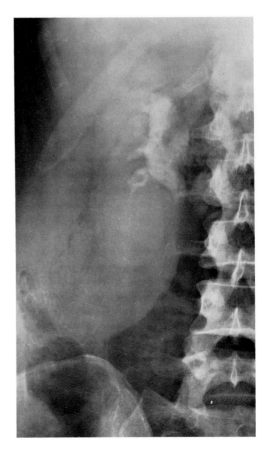

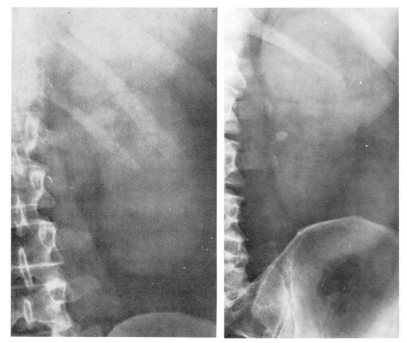

Fig. 3–118   Fig. 3–119

Figure 3–118.   *Plain film.* Irregular outline of lower pole of left kidney, produced by **simple cyst.**
Figure 3–119.   *Plain film.* Irregularity of soft-tissue outline of upper pole of left kidney, caused by **hyper-nephroma.** Calcific shadow above third lumbar transverse process. **Tumor and stone** in same kidney.

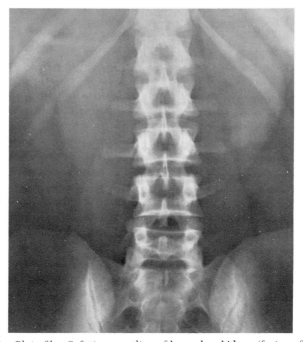

Figure 3–120.   *Plain film.* Soft-tissue outline of **horseshoe kidney** (fusion of lower poles).

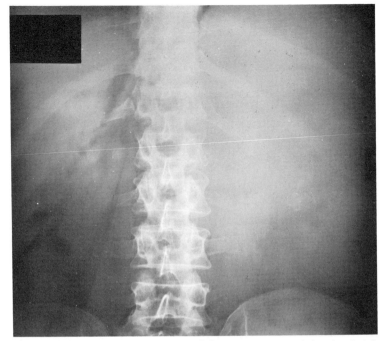

Figure 3–121. *Plain film.* Diffuse area of increased density occupying left side of abdomen, caused by retroperitoneal tumor.

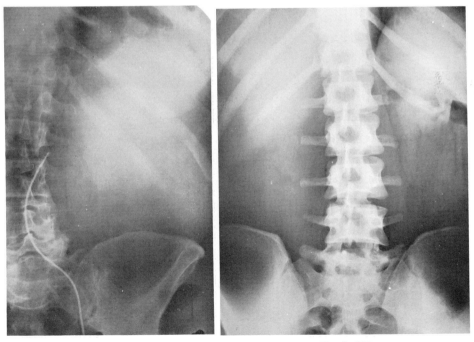

Fig. 3–122   Fig. 3–123

Figure 3–122. *Plain film.* Large area of increased density occupying left side of abdomen and displacing left ureter; also obliterating outline of left psoas muscle. **Retroperitoneal tumor.**

Figure 3–123. *Plain film.* Obliteration of outline of right psoas muscle and concavity of spinal column toward right, resulting from **perinephric abscess of right kidney.**

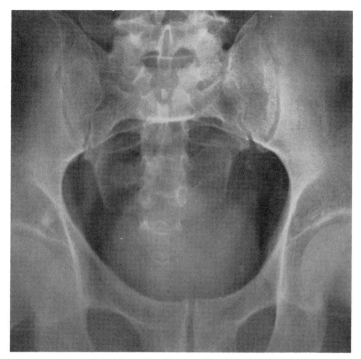

Figure 3–124. *Plain film.* Urinary bladder filled with urine.

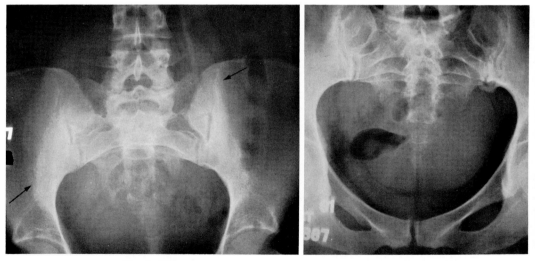

Fig. 3–125   Fig. 3–126

Figure 3–125. *Excretory urogram.* Soft-tissue outline of **large ovarian cyst** (*arrows*). (Proved surgically.)
Figure 3–126. *Plain film.* Soft-tissue outline of **large fibroid uterus.** Note encroachment on bladder, which is compressed and flattened below uterus.

OPAQUE SHADOWS ORIGINATING WITHIN THE URINARY TRACT

Dense shadows in or about the urinary tract are, in nearly all cases, the result of a deposition of calcium found in stones or calcification in soft tissues such as the kidneys, lymph nodes, and so forth. In a smaller number of cases, foreign bodies encrusted with calcium or composed of metal may be responsible.

Calcific Deposits

CALCULI IN KIDNEYS AND URETERS

By far the most common shadows encountered in the urinary tract are calculi. In the case of *renal calculi* it often is possible to determine the location of the stone if it has formed a cast of the pelvis or calyces, as is seen in the case of a *branched calculus* (Fig. 3-127) or a stone assuming the contour of a terminal calyx (Fig. 3-128). Other types of calculi, however, usually require a urogram to establish their position (Fig. 3-129). One should always be hesitant to attempt to state the position of a stone by simply observing its position in relation to the soft-tissue outlines of the kidney. *Ureteral calculi* always must be identified by a urogram or a roentgenogram made after the introduction of an opaque ureteral catheter, since opaque objects such as *phleboliths* and small *calcified lymph nodes* along the course of the ureter may be sources of error in diagnosis (see Fig. 6-120A and *B)*. Attention is called again to the importance of carefully examining areas where the ureter lies over bony structures. Ureteral stones in this location are easily overlooked (Figs. 3-130, 3-131, and 3-132).

CALCIFICATION OF KIDNEYS AND URETERS

Calcification in a kidney or ureter or both is of special diagnostic importance and must be looked for in every roentgenogram. It appears in a variety of conditions, most important of which are tuberculosis (Fig. 3-133; see also Figs. 8-3 through 8-19), nephrocalcinosis (Fig. 3-134), chronic pyelonephritis, renal tumor (Fig. 3-135), and calcified cysts (Figs. 3-136 and 3-137). It will be discussed more fully under each of these subjects.

VESICAL CALCULI

Of all urinary calculi, those in the bladder are most easily overlooked, because vesical calculi frequently are only slightly radiopaque and, therefore, cast either a dim shadow or none at all. When such stones are lying over the sacrum or are somewhat obscured by shadows from gas in the bowel, they may not be suspected until cystoscopic examination is performed. After they have been found cystoscopically, reexamination of the roentgenogram usually will disclose their presence, although in some instances the density of the stone is so slight that it does not cast a visible shadow (Fig. 3-138A and *B*). Shadows cast by vesical calculi of good opacity usually yield excellent roentgenograms which in most cases require no further urologic investigation (Fig 3-139). A stone in a vesical diverticulum, however, may be situated so far to one side of the midline that the examiner may not suspect it of being a vesical calculus (Fig. 3-140).

URETHRAL CALCULI

Urethral calculi are not very commonly observed. Although one occasionally encounters a case in which a primary calculus has formed in a urethral diverticulum, most urethral calculi are either ureteral or vesical calculi which have been passed and have caught in the urethra.

Foreign Bodies

The variety of foreign bodies that may be encountered both inside and outside of the urinary tract is endless. They may be foreign bodies resulting from penetrating wounds, such as bullets (see Fig. 3-34A and B), shrapnel, and knives, or objects left in wounds after surgical procedures, such as sponges, needles, and forceps (Figs. 3-141 through 3-146). The most unusual foreign bodies, however, are those that are manipulated into the urethra and bladder by the patient (Figs. 3-147 through 3-151).

(Text continued on page 210.)

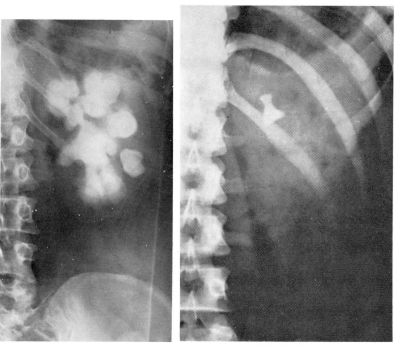

Fig. 3–127   **Fig. 3–128**

Figure 3–127. *Plain film.* Branched calculi in left kidney.
Figure 3–128. *Plain film.* Renal stone forming cast of upper calyces.

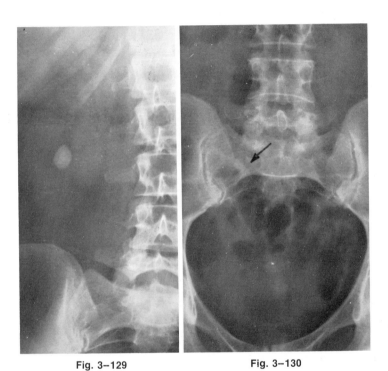

Fig. 3–129　　　　　　　　　Fig. 3–130

Figure 3–129. *Plain film.* **Renal calculus;** position in relation to pelvis and calyces cannot be determined without urogram.

Figure 3–130. *Plain film.* Shadow of **ureteral calculus overlying right side of sacrum** (*arrow*) might easily be missed if roentgenograms were not carefully scrutinized.

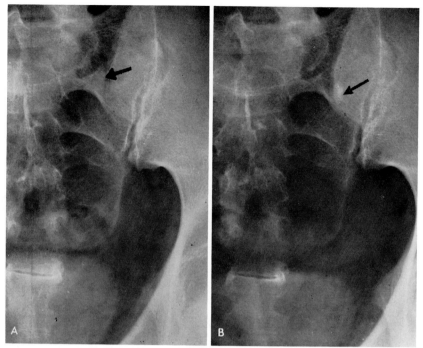

Figure 3–131.   *Plain films.* **A,** Ureteral stone overlying left sacro-iliac joint (*arrow*) almost impossible to see because of bone shadow. **B,** Same case. Stone shadow now well visualized.

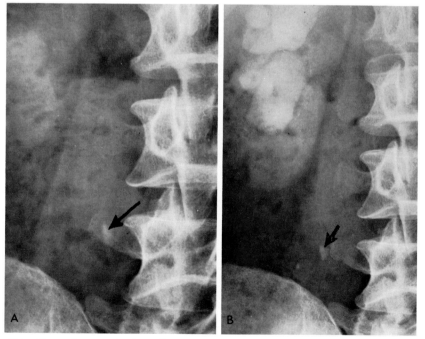

Figure 3–132.   Ureteral stone. **A,** *Plain film.* Stone (*arrow*) is partially obscured by transverse process of fourth lumbar vertebra on right. **B,** *Excretory urogram.* **Stone** (*arrow*) is projected lateral to transverse process and is now easily seen. Note **pyelectasis.**

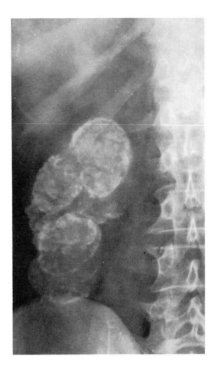

Figure 3–133. *Plain film.* Tuberculous calcification of non-functioning kidney (autonephrectomy).

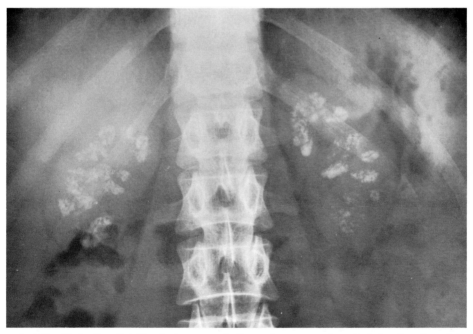

Figure 3–134. *Plain film.* Calcific shadows over both renal areas are characteristic of **nephrocalcinosis.**

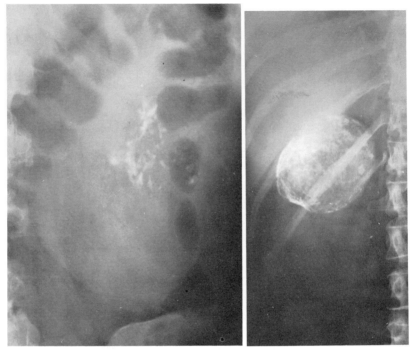

Fig. 3–135   Fig. 3–136

Figure 3–135. *Plain film.* Reticular zone of calcification in hypernephroma. (From Bartholomew, L. G., Cain, J. C., Davis, G. D., and Bulbulian, A. H.)

Figure 3–136. *Plain film.* Calcification in renal cyst.

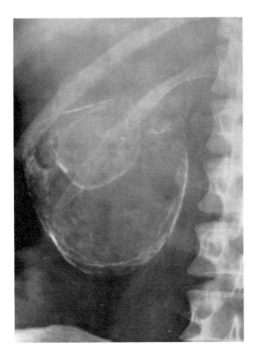

Figure 3–137. *Plain film.* Echinococcus cyst of kidney. (From McCullough, J. A. L., and Sutherland, C. G.)

Fig. 3–137

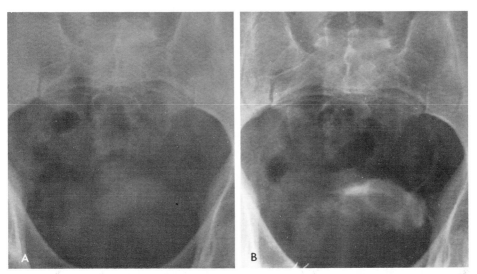

Figure 3–138. *A, Plain film.* **Vesical calculi** of poor density. **B,** *Excretory cystogram.* **Vesical calculi** produce negative shadows in cystogram.

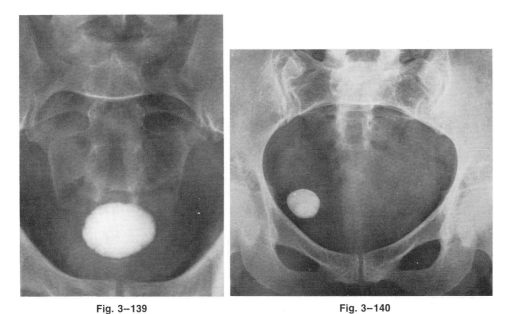

Fig. 3–139   Fig. 3–140

Figure 3–139. *Plain film.* **Vesical calculus** of good density.
Figure 3–140. *Plain film.* **Stone in vesical diverticulum** is so far to side that one might not consider possibility of vesical calculus. (From Bartholomew, L. G., Cain, J. C., Davis, G. D., and Bulbulian, A. H.)

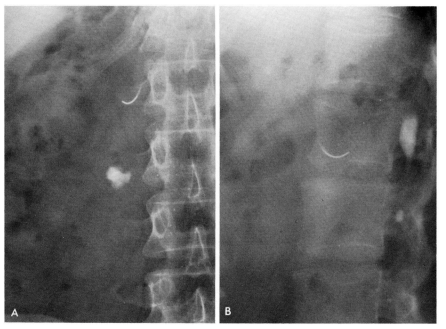

Figure 3–141. *Plain films.* **Fragment of surgical needle** remaining after nephrectomy many years previously. **A,** *Anteroposterior view.* **B,** *Lateral view.*

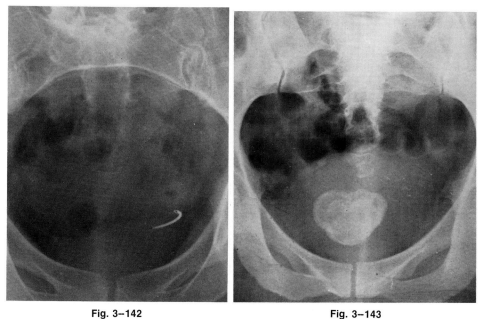

Fig. 3–142   **Fig. 3–143**

Figure 3–142. *Plain film.* Surgical needle in pelvis.
Figure 3–143. *Plain film.* Calcified sponge in bladder.

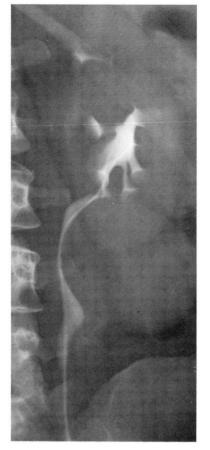

Figure 3–144. Gauze sponge left at time of operation on left kidney. *Left retrograde pyelogram.* **Bifid pelvis with postoperative deformity.** Marked medial displacement of upper third of ureter, which seems to skirt around circular soft-tissue mass in region of lower pole of kidney. Exploration revealed gauze sponge which had been left in wound at previous operation.

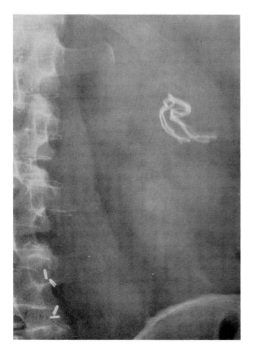

Figure 3–145. *Plain film.* **Surgical sponge containing radiopaque threads** left in operative site during resection of aortic aneurysm.

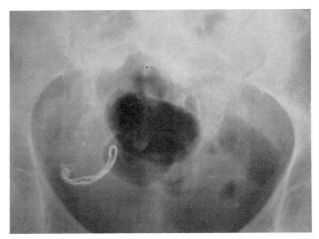

Figure 3–146. *Plain film.* **Surgical sponge** left in wound following ureterolithotomy. Threads in sponge cast opaque shadow.

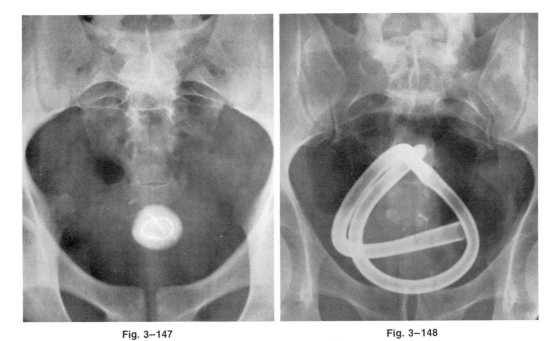

Fig. 3–147   Fig. 3–148

Figure 3–147. *Plain film.* Stone in bladder, nucleus of which was copper wire.
Figure 3–148. *Plain film.* Urethral catheter coiled in bladder.

Fig. 3–149

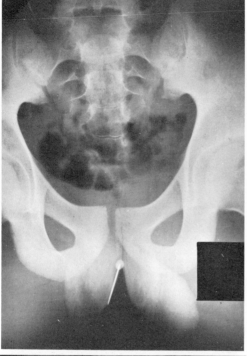

Fig. 3–151

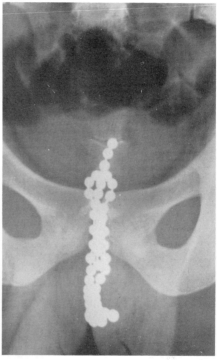

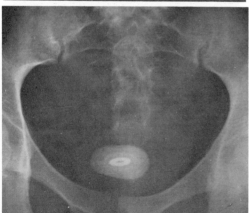

Fig. 3–150

Figure 3–149. *Plain film.* Hatpin in bulbomembranous urethra in male patient.

Figure 3–150. *Plain film.* Steel washer acting as nidus for formation of vesical calculus. (From Cristol, D. S., and Greene, L. F.)

Figure 3–151. *Plain film.* String of beads in posterior urethra and bladder of man. (Courtesy of Dr. J. M. Pace.)

LESIONS ORIGINATING IN, OR INVOLVING SECONDARILY, THE LUMBAR VERTEBRAE AND BONY PELVIS

The urologist who reads films of the genitourinary tract frequently encounters lesions of the lumbar vertebrae and pelvis. Some of these may bear directly on the urologic problem and require recognition by the urologist. Others may have no urologic implication but may be of greater importance than the urologic problem under investigation. If the urologist is moderately familiar with such lesions, he will be of great service to the patient by recognizing them and requesting orthopedic or other consultation. Early recognition of such lesions before symptoms arise may provide the important factor that assures successful treatment.

Inflammatory Lesions

ANKYLOSING (RHEUMATOID) SPONDYLITIS (DIFFERENTIATION FROM ASYMPTOMATIC OSTEOARTHRITIS AND PHYSIOLOGIC CALCIFICATION OF VERTEBRAL LIGAMENTS)

Probably the commonest bony abnormalities encountered by the urologist reading urograms are arthritic changes in the spinal column and pelvis. *Rheumatoid spondylitis* involves chiefly the sacro-iliac and the apophyseal joints. Roentgenographically the earliest changes are seen in the sacro-iliac joints and consist of blurring and irregularity of the articular markings caused by patchy decalcification of subchondral bone at the margins of the joint. Marginal sclerosis of both the sacral and iliac borders of the joint then ensues, the degree of density varying with the extent and duration of the inflammatory process. In advanced cases, complete obliteration and ankylosis of the joints may be the end result (Polley; Wholey, Pugh, and Bickel).

As the disease progresses, calcification of the longitudinal spinal ligaments occurs. The typical appearance of a calcified spinal ligament is a thickening of homogeneous density superimposed on the surface of the vertebra and spanning a normal intervertebral space. (Intervertebral disks usually are not involved by rheumatoid spondylitis.) The calcified ligament is in close apposition to the vertebra, but close inspection of the film will show that it is superimposed on, rather than an integral part of, the vertebra (Figs. 3-152, 3-153, and 3-154). This distinguishes it from the more or less asymptomatic osteoarthritis with spur formation.

As rheumatoid spondylitis progresses, osteoporosis of the vertebrae develops, which in advanced states has been described as "bamboo spine" (Figs. 3-155, 3-156, and 3-157). This appearance is due to the contrast of the calcified intervertebral ligaments against the "ghost-like" outline of the osteoporotic vertebrae.

Spondylitic calcification of the spinal ligaments must be distinguished from asymptomatic physiologic calcification of vertebral ligaments. This condition occurs as a degenerative or aging process rather than as an inflammatory one (Smith, Pugh, and Polley); it is distinguished from rheumatoid spondylitis in that it occurs in older persons, is asymptomatic, and usually is *not* associated with arthritic changes in the sacro-iliac joints (Fig. 3-158).

Osteoarthritis is also a more or less benign, relatively asymptomatic condition which yields rather dramatic-appearing roentgenograms. It is characterized by "spur" formation, which is an outgrowth of the vertebral body. This first appears as a "lipping" and may proceed to "bridging" of the vertebrae (Figs. 3-159, 3-160, and 3-161).

TUBERCULOSIS

A tuberculous lesion of the spinal column is most often apparent as a destructive process which involves one or more vertebral bodies associated with narrowing or obliteration of the intervening intervertebral disks. This concomitant destruction of intervertebral disks differentiates the condition from destructive lesions due to metastatic carcinoma or injury which do not usually affect the intervertebral disks (Figs. 3-162 through 3-166).

OSTEOMYELITIS OF VERTEBRAE

Osteomyelitis of vertebrae is of especial interest to the urologist because it is not infrequently the result of a blood-borne infection originating in an inflammatory lesion in the urinary tract (Henson and Coventry). It may follow operative procedures on the prostate, bladder, kidneys, or ureters, or it may arise as a manifestation of a severe urinary infection. The lesion may be extremely painful and disabling and in the early stages may not be apparent in the x-ray films. The earliest bony changes are rarefaction and loss of trabecular detail. Later, fuzziness may develop along the upper and lower bony plates, followed by partial or complete collapse of the vertebra with angulation. *The intervertebral disk is involved early in the process,* and as it disintegrates, the x-ray appearance is that of rapid narrowing of the disk, or it may actually protrude into the diseased vertebra (Fig. 3-167A and B). Diagnosis may be confirmed by needle biopsy with culture.

OSTEITIS PUBIS

Osteitis pubis is the name given to a painful and disabling clinical syndrome manifested by pain in the region of the symphysis pubis, pelvis, and adductor region of one or both thighs. It may extend into the perineum and involve the lower abdominal muscles and ischial tuberosities. In the acute stage the patient may be bedridden, because any movement, such as turning, walking, sitting, and climbing stairs, brings on excruciating pain. In the more chronic stage the patient limps with a waddling type of gait, which is partly from pain and partly from a stiff tight feeling in the adductor muscles. The condition has received its greatest attention in the urologic literature (Warwick); it was reported for the first time in the United States by Beer, a urologic surgeon, in 1924. Urologically, it has usually followed open prostatectomy or surgical procedures on the bladder or lower part of the ureters, but it also has followed transurethral prostatic resection. In women it may follow pregnancy or pelvic operations. Trauma has been considered the etiologic factor in some cases. In many cases no predisposing factor can be found, but in nearly all, urinary infection is present and is thought to be a contributing factor. In some of these cases, urethral instrumentation with sounds, cystoscopes, or catheters had been performed and has been suspected of being a precipitating factor. The average interval between operation (or urethral instrumentation) and onset of symptoms is about 6 weeks.

Roentgenologic changes include rarefaction and destructive changes in the bone with widening of the symphysis. As healing occurs, sclerosis of bone, with narrowing and even ankylosis of the symphysis, may result. Roentgenographic changes may not be demonstrable until 2 to 4 weeks or more after onset of symptoms. Usually the first changes noted are widening of the symphysis, loss of definition of the margins of the symphysis, with a "fraying" of the periosteum, and fuzziness of the borders caused by erosion and progressive decalcification. More advanced changes show rarefaction or "washing out" of the bony trabeculae and woolly or moth-eaten destruction resulting in loss of both bone and cartilage. Subluxation may occur. This stage usually lasts from 4 to 6 weeks but may continue as long as 8 to 12 months before regenerative changes begin. As healing progresses, sclerosis of the involved bone occurs with an irregular callus and the symphysis narrows and again becomes stable. The regenerative process may progress to actual ankylosis.

It should be emphasized that osteitis pubis is a clinical entity diagnosed by symptoms and clinical findings. Roentgenographic changes are only incidental to diagnosis, and in some cases they are never demonstrated. Also, in countless cases evidence of changes consistent with those of osteitis pubis are reported by the roentgenologist in routine films of the abdomen although the patient has never had symptoms suggestive of the disease. The commonest finding in such cases is, of course, sclerosis of the pubic bones adjacent to the symphysis pubis.

The disease though self-limiting is often protracted and discouraging. Conservative treatment has included antibiotics, sulfonamides, and steroids. X-ray therapy has been reported to be effective, and local injection of hydrocortisone has been used. Corsets and body casts have been tried. Obturator neurectomy has given relief in some very disabling cases. Quadrangular and wedge resections of the symphysis pubis have been employed, usually in the more chronic cases when healing does not occur (Figs. 3-168 through 3-171).

(*Text continued on page 224.*)

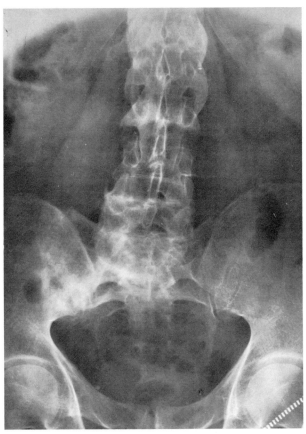

Figure 3–152. *Plain film.* Clearly marked **sacro-iliac arthritis on right** in patient who had had **ankylosing spondylitis** for 10 years. **Calcification of spinal ligaments in lumbar region.** (From Polley, H. F., and Slocumb, C. H.)

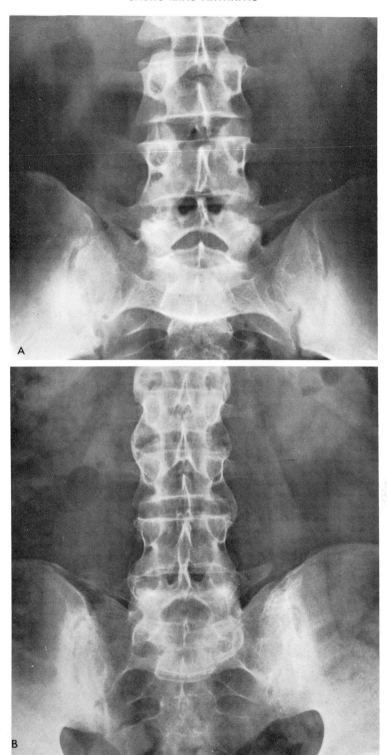

Figure 3–153. *Plain films.* Bilateral sacro-iliac arthritis characteristic of ankylosing spondylitis. **A,** On admission, Oct. 16, 1933. **B,** Ten years later. Marked progression. There is also evidence of ligamentous calcification in lumbar region. Sacro-iliac joints are nearly obliterated. (From Polley, H. F., and Slocumb, C. H.)

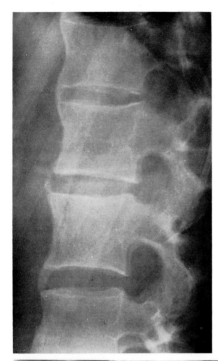

Figure 3–154. *Plain film.* Calcification of anterior spinal ligament.

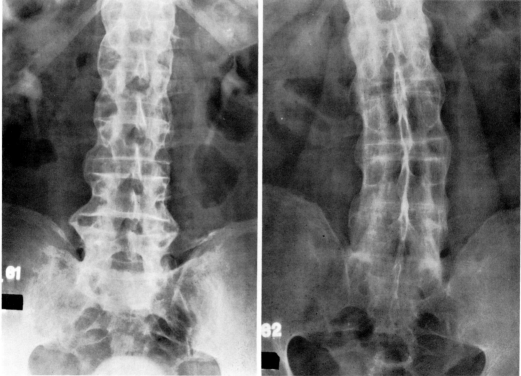

Fig. 3–155   Fig. 3–156

Figure 3–155. *Excretory urogram.* **Moderately advanced spondylitis** showing calcification of vertebral ligaments and moderate osteoporosis characteristic of bamboo spine. Note obliteration of sacro-iliac joints.

Figure 3–156. *Plain film.* **Advanced spondylitis** showing calcification of vertebral ligaments and moderate osteoporosis characteristic of bamboo spine. Note obliteration of sacro-iliac joints.

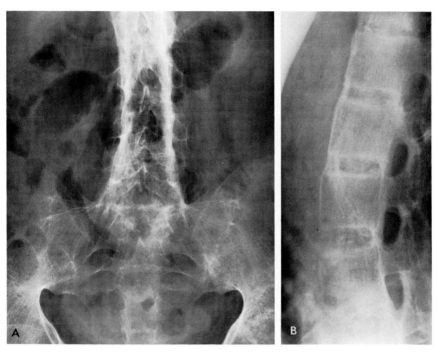

Figure 3–157. *Plain films of lumbar spine.* **A,** *Anteroposterior view.* Advanced spondylitis (bamboo spine) with marked osteoporosis. **B,** *Lateral view.* Calcification of intervertebral ligaments with fusion of vertebral bodies and lateral facets.

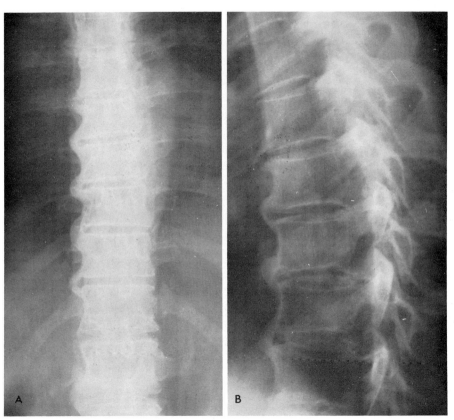

Figure 3–158. Physiologic vertebral ligamentous calcification. **A,** *Anteroposterior view*, showing thick tortuous and calcified lateral longitudinal ligaments. Costovertebral joints appear normal. **B,** *Lateral view.* Calcification of anterior longitudinal ligament. Note that calcification is homogeneous and distinct from anterior margins of vertebrae. (From Smith, C. F., Pugh, D. G., and Polley, H. F.)

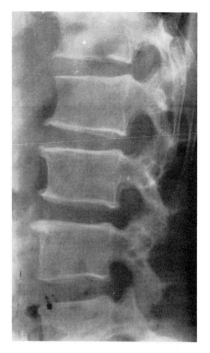

Figure 3–159. Osteophytes (lipping) in osteoarthritis of lumbar portion of spinal column.

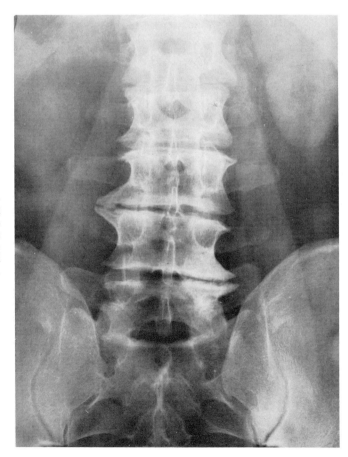

Figure 3–160. *Plain film.* Osteoarthritis of lumbar spine with lipping (osteophytic spurs). Degenerative changes in intervertebral disks with narrowing of intervertebral spaces between third and fourth and fourth and fifth lumbar vertebrae are apparent.

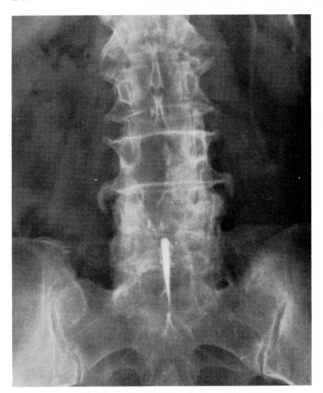

Figure 3–161. Osteoarthritis (hypertrophic arthritis) with lipping and bridging. Residuum of Lipiodol in spinal canal. Degenerative changes of intervertebral disks.

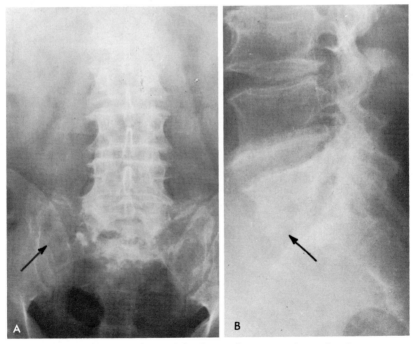

Figure 3–162. *Plain films.* Tuberculosis of lumbosacral portion of spinal column. A, *Anteroposterior view.* B, *Lateral view.* (See text.)

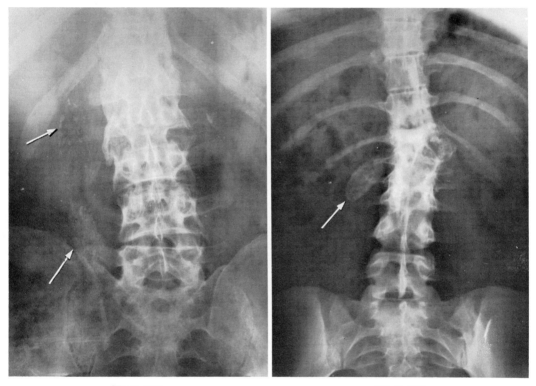

Fig. 3–163   Fig. 3–164

Figure 3–163. *Plain film.* Tuberculosis of 12th thoracic and first lumbar vertebrae and calcified tuberculous psoas abscess on right (*arrows*). (See text.)

Figure 3–164. *Plain film.* Tuberculosis of spinal column and calcified tuberculous psoas abscess (*arrow*).

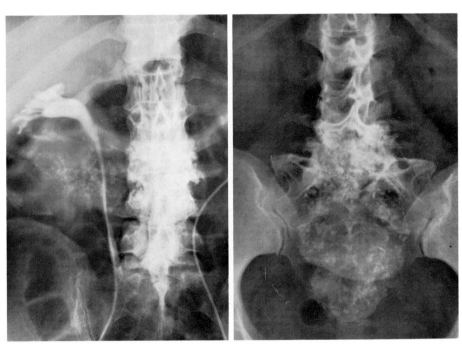

Fig. 3–165　　　　　　　　　　　　　　**Fig. 3–166**

Figure 3–165. *Excretory urogram.* Old tuberculous lesion of lumbar vertebrae (Pott's disease) in man 39 years of age, for which fusion had been done. Old psoas abscess with calcification which displaces right kidney upward and laterally. No definite tuberculous involvement of calyces can be seen, and no pus cells were found in ureteral specimen of urine, but results of inoculating guinea pig were positive, and there was moderate degree of tuberculous cystitis. No gross evidence of genital involvement. Antimicrobial treatment given.

Figure 3–166. Tuberculosis of lumbar part of spinal column and sacrum (Pott's disease) and right renal tuberculosis in man 20 years of age. Destruction of lumbar vertebrae with collapse of lower three vertebrae. Destruction of sacrum and possibly old tuberculous abscess anteriorly.

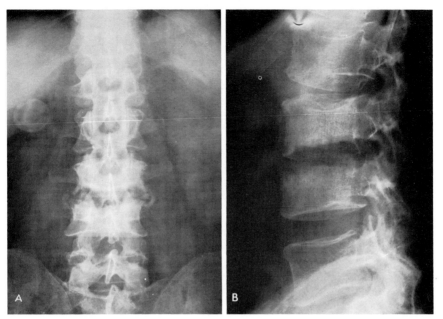

Figure 3–167. *Plain films.* **Osteomyelitis of second and third lumbar vertebrae. A,** *Anteroposterior view.* Note **gallstone also. B,** *Lateral view.* (From Henson, S. W., Jr., and Coventry, M. B.)

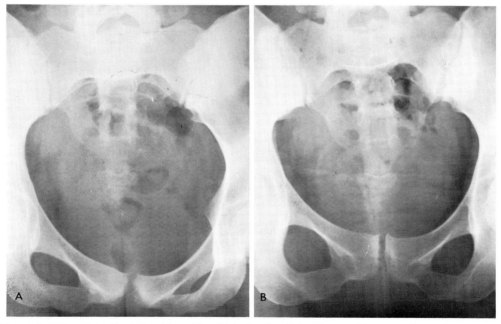

Figure 3–168. *Plain films.* **Osteitis pubis** which developed in 23-year-old woman 1 month post partum. **A, Acute process** 6 months after onset. **B,** Ten years later. **Normal pubic symphysis.** (From Coventry, M. B., and Mitchell, W. C.)

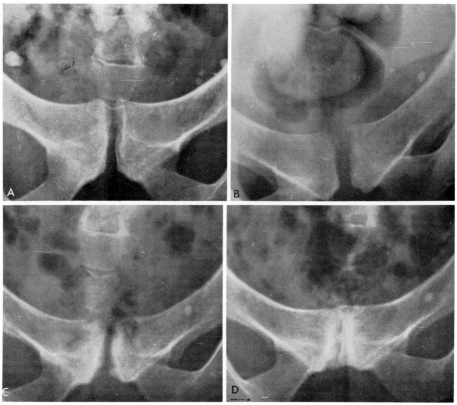

Figure 3–169. Osteitis pubis following retropubic prostatectomy. **A,** Preoperative film. **B,** Ten weeks after operation. Note widening of symphysis pubis, bilateral erosion of bone, and fraying of periosteum. **C,** Healing. Filling in of symphysis with callus. **D,** Healing complete. Symphysis almost completely obliterated by bony fusion. (Courtesy of Dr. R. O. Pearman.)

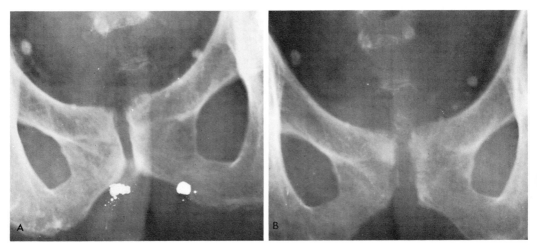

Figure 3–170. Osteitis pubis following retropubic prostatectomy. **A,** Early stage (7 weeks after operation). Widening of symphysis, irregularity of margins of pubis, beginning erosion of bone. **B,** Active stage (15 weeks after operation). Increased widening of symphysis with erosion, "fraying" of periosteum, and osteoporosis. (Courtesy of Dr. C. K. Pearlman.)

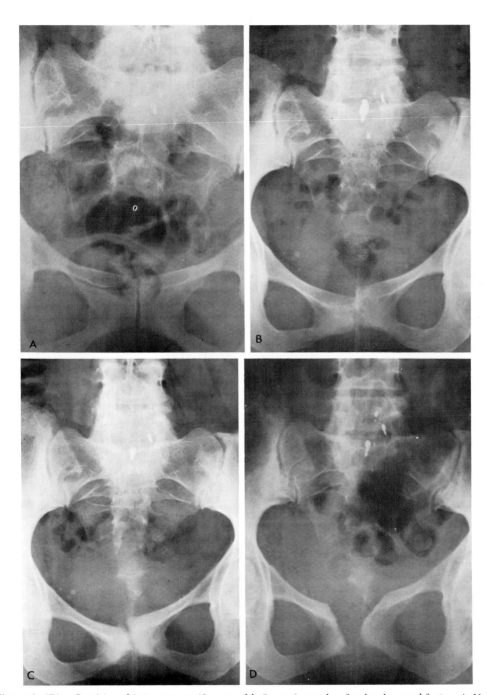

Figure 3–171. **Osteitis pubis** in woman 40 years old. Onset 2 months after lumbosacral fusion. **A,** Normal symphysis prior to onset of symptoms. **B,** Fifteen months after onset of symptoms with subluxation and early rarefaction apparent. **C,** Twenty-one months after **B.** Disabling symptoms still present. **D,** Three and one-half months following posterior wedge-type resection of symphysis. No pain remaining; only mild instability. (From Coventry, M. B., and Mitchell, W. C.)

Congenital and Degenerative Lesions

SCOLIOSIS

Angulation between vertebral bodies is now throught to be due principally to muscle weakness or imbalance, muscle spasm, or ligamentous relaxation plus muscle spasm. Two main groups of cases are recognized: (1) those resulting from residual paralysis of poliomyelitis, and (2) those of an idiopathic or a metabolic deficiency type.

In the presence of such angulation, growth is unopposed on the convex side; thus, this side of the vertebra becomes thicker than the concave side. When such structural changes become well-established, little can be done therapeutically. In the lumbar portion of the spinal column, owing to the posterior position of the articular facets, scoliosis is also associated with vertebral rotation (Fig. 3-172).

SPONDYLOLISTHESIS

Spondylolisthesis is a condition in which the body of the fifth lumbar vertebra (and the spinal column above it) slips forward over the base of the sacrum (Sullivan and Bickel). To be a true spondylolisthesis, there must be a definite break in the contour of the anterior wall of the spinal canal demonstrated by lateral films. Neither a sharply angulated sacrum nor a fifth lumbar vertebra that projects to some degree in front of the first piece of the sacrum is sufficient basis for the diagnosis of spondylolisthesis. This condition, formerly regarded as of congenital origin, more recently has been considered the result of injury in which there is a "break in the normal arch" that permits the forward dislocation. The roentgen

appearance is typical and, in some cases, can be suspected with the anteroposterior film (Fig. 3-173). A lateral film, however, is necessary for absolute confirmation (Figs. 3-174 and 3-175).

EXSTROPHY OF THE BLADDER

Exstrophy of the bladder is always associated with a wide separation of the symphysis pubis, which has a typical and characteristic appearance, and is almost never confused with any other lesion (Fig. 3-176). This abnormality is usually accompanied by epispadias.

SPINA BIFIDA AND ANOMALIES OF THE SACRUM

Spina bifida, a congenital defect of the spinal column, results from failure of fusion of the dorsal walls of the primitive neural canal. It is nearly always situated dorsally and nearly always located in the lumbosacral region. In extremely rare cases, the defect may be a ventral one. (See the discussion of presacral tumors further on in this chapter.) There is no correlation between the type or degree of spina bifida and the incidence of a neurologic deficit. This is illustrated by the fact that in routine x-ray examinations of the lumbosacral region, some defect in closure of the laminae is apparent in at least one third of the cases. The defect varies from involvement of only the lower sacral segments ("open neural arch") to wide separation of the lamina of all the sacral and many of the lumbar vertebrae (Figs. 3-177 through 3-180). In severe cases, the sacrum may be badly deformed and partially or totally absent (Figs. 3-181, 3-182, and 3-183).

(Text continued on page 230.)

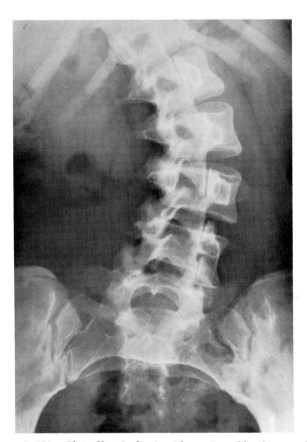

Figure 3–172. *Plain film.* Scoliosis with rotation of lumbar vertebrae.

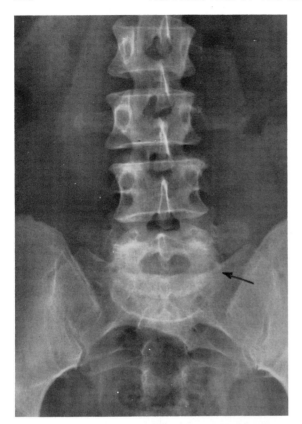

Figure 3–173. *Plain film.* Spondylolisthesis.

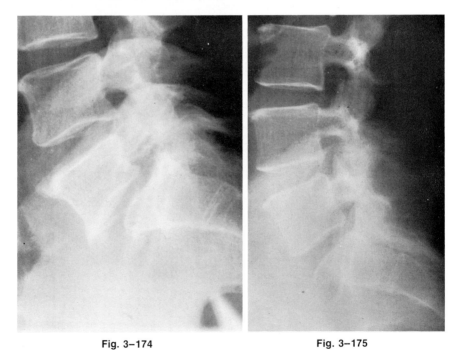

Fig. 3–174   Fig. 3–175

Figure 3–174. *Lateral view of lumbosacral part of spinal column.* Spondylolisthesis of lumbosacral articulation.

Figure 3–175. *Lateral view of lumbosacral portion of normal spinal column* for comparison.

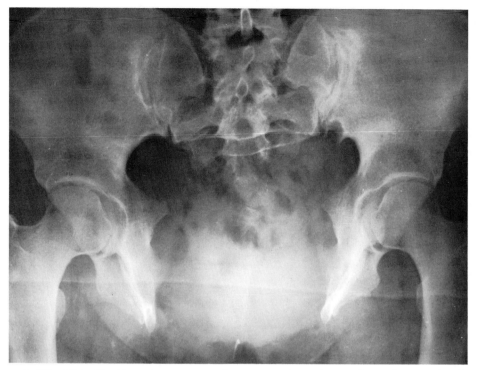

Figure 3–176. *Plain film.* Typical appearance of separation of symphysis pubis with exstrophy of urinary bladder.

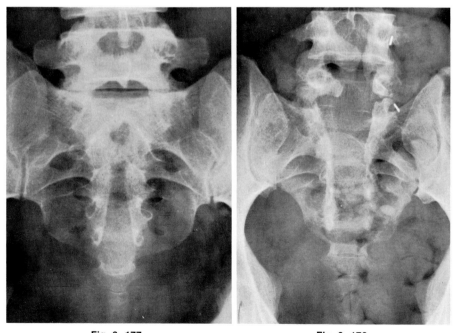

Fig. 3–177   **Fig. 3–178**

Figure 3–177. *Plain film.* **Normal sacrum.** Sacral hiatus is prominent. This should not be confused with spina bifida of lower sacral segments.

Figure 3–178. *Plain film.* **Spina bifida.** Note two surgical clips on left.

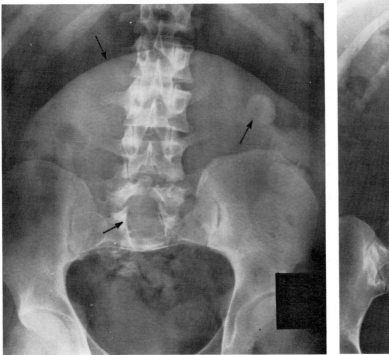

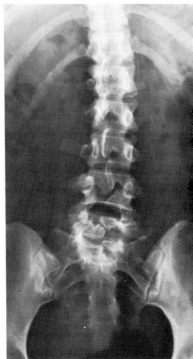

Fig. 3–179   **Fig. 3–180**

Figure 3–179.   *Plain film.* Spina bifida occulta, large meningomyelocele, and hairy mole. Partial absence of sacrum.

Figure 3–180.   *Plain film.* Spina bifida occulta.

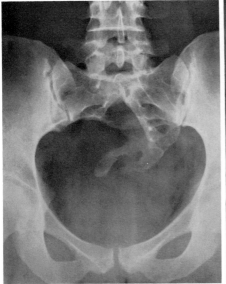

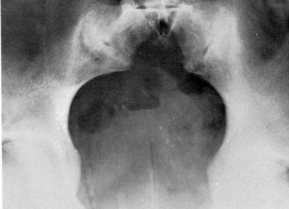

Fig. 3–181   **Fig. 3–182**

Figure 3–181.   *Plain film.* Congenital deformity of sacrum.

Figure 3–182.   *Plain film.* Congenital absence of sacrum in girl, 16 years of age, with **myelodysplasia** and involvement of bladder, intestines, and lower extremities.

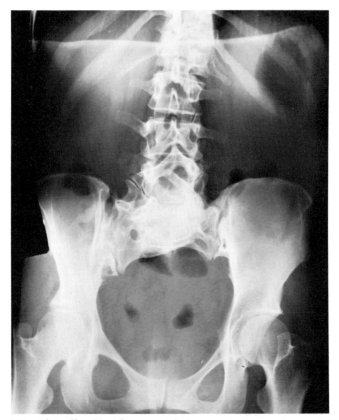

Figure 3–183. *Plain film.* Partial congenital absence of sacrum with myelodysplasia.

Neoplasms (Primary)

CARTILAGINOUS TUMORS: OSTEOCHONDROMA, CHONDROSARCOMA, AND ENCHONDROMA

When these tumors originate in the bones of the pelvis, they usually present as a mass felt by the patient or by pain in the pelvis or leg. There may be weakness of the leg with a definite limp. Occasionally the tumors may be of sufficient size to cause urinary symptoms such as difficult micturition or urethral discharge.

It is difficult to distinguish a benign osteochrondroma from a malignant chondrosarcoma, by either roentgenographic or microscopic examination of tissue (Coley and Higinbotham; Kunkel, Dahlin, and Young). From a roentgenographic point of view, the chief characteristics of the tumor are destruction of bone and secondary mottled calcification of the tumor mass. Generally speaking, the benign osteochondroma has a rather uniform outline. When it undergoes malignant transformation, it tends to lose its uniformity, its regular borders being replaced by a more or less densely calcified tumor (Figs. 3-184, 3-185, and 3-186).

MULTIPLE MYELOMA

Multiple myeloma is a highly malignant tumor of the bone marrow (Ghormley and associates, 1942). Microscopically the tumors are made up predominantly of cells which closely resemble plasma cells. The myeloid tissue and fat spaces seen in normal marrow are not encountered, however. Symptoms are diverse and frequently unrelated; backache is by far the most common symptom. Loss of strength and progressive weakness are characteristic. Bence Jones protein is present in the urine in about 60% of cases. *Renal function is impaired in many cases, apparently the result of tubular damage.* Anemia is common. The characteristic roentgenographic appearance consists of small punched-out areas of destruction in the long bones, vertebrae, pelvis, ribs, and skull (Figs. 3-187 and 3-188A and B). Diagnosis can usually be made by aspiration of bone marrow.

SACRAL AND PRESACRAL TUMORS

The most commonly encountered tumors in this region are chordomas, ependymomas, and teratomas. Other tumors formed there include dermoid cysts, ganglioneuromas, neurofibromas, fibrosarcomas, Ewing's tumors, and giant cell tumors (Brindley; Camp and Good; MacCarty and associates).

Chordoma

Chordoma is the commonest tumor arising from the sacrum in adults. In a series of presacral tumors reported by Adson, Moersch, and Kernohan from the Mayo Clinic, 27.5% were chordomas. This neoplasm occurs chiefly in middle or later life and is more common in males than in females. It rarely is found in children. It arises from remnants of the notochord. Roentgenologically, its most characteristic feature is expansion of the sacrum, especially in its anteroposterior dimension. It is definitely a malignant tumor and destroys the sacrum by both erosion and invasion. In some cases, remnants of bone are seen to be free in the large soft mass of the tumor. The density of these remnants may be increased so that in the plain film they may appear to be sequestra or calcification (Figs. 3-189 and 3-190A and B). They are difficult to remove completely at operation.

Ependymoma

Ependymomas arise from ependymal cells, which in the early embryo form a large part of the neural tube. They occur chiefly in young adults well before middle life. In contrast to the chordoma, the ependymoma is essentially a benign lesion which enlarges the sacrolumbar canal and erodes the bone from pressure rather than invasion (Fig. 3-191). It can usually be enucleated completely on extensive laminectomy. Prognosis is good with regard to life, but the preoperative neurogenic deficit (vesical, rectal, sensory, and reflex disturbance) is usually not improved.

Teratoma

Teratomas are composite masses possessing more than one germinal layer. Some, however, may be formed almost entirely of cells from only one germinal layer. They may be benign or malignant. They occur most commonly in infants and children, more frequently in females than males, and vary in size from small (1 to 2 cm in diameter) to huge lesions that may be so large that they interfere with delivery. The tumors may grow ventrally into the hollow of the sacrum or inferiorly or posteriorly to protrude from the perineum, sacrum, or buttocks. The pelvic organs are usually displaced rather than invaded. The tumor nearly always is attached to the coccyx. In contrast to ependymoma there is rarely any neurologic deficit present. (See discussion in Chapter 10.) In Gross, Clatworthy, and Meeker's series of 40 cases, the coccyx was involved and partially destroyed in only 2 cases. Calcification in the tumor was demonstrated in 16 (40%) of their cases.

Dermoid Cyst

Dermoid cysts are ectodermal in origin and are lined with epithelium which is constantly secreting and desquamating. They are filled with an oily radiolucent fluid and may contain ectodermal derivatives such as hair and teeth. The capsule is fairly radiopaque, which, in contrast to the radiolucent fluid inside, imparts a rather peculiar roentgenographic appearance to the tumor, as though it had a calcified capsule. Erosion of bone caused by pressure of the cyst is most unusual (Fig. 3-192). (See also discussion in Chapter 10.)

More than 95% of dermoid cysts arise from the ovary. In males they are principally found in the testes. A few, however, arise from the retroperitoneal and presacral areas.

Neurofibroma and Spina Bifida Cystica

Among other lesions in the sacral area which may cause bony absorption are neurofibroma (Fig. 3-193) and the rare spina bifida cystica (Fig. 3-194), which extends anteriorly into the pelvis rather than posteriorly.

Cyst of Sacral Nerve Root

Cysts of the spinal nerve roots may cause pressure erosion of the vertebral bodies or laminae as they lie within the spinal canal. In Figure 3-195 a cyst of the second sacral nerve root has eroded the sacrum.

(Text continued on page 238.)

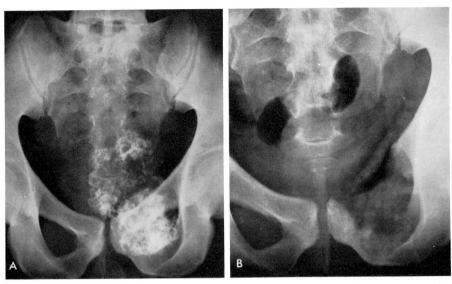

Figure 3–184. *Plain films.* **A,** **Osteochondroma** which has caused urethral drainage in male patient. **B,** Same case, 1 month after removal of tumor. (From Ghormley, R. K., Meyerding, H. W., Mussey, R. D., Jr., and Luckey, C. A.)

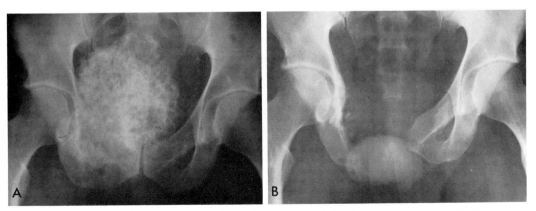

Figure 3–185. *Plain films.* **A,** **Osteochondroma** that has caused slowing of urinary stream. **B,** Recurrence of tumor 11 months after operation. (From Ghormley, R. K., Meyerding, H. W., Mussey, R. D., Jr., and Luckey, C. A.)

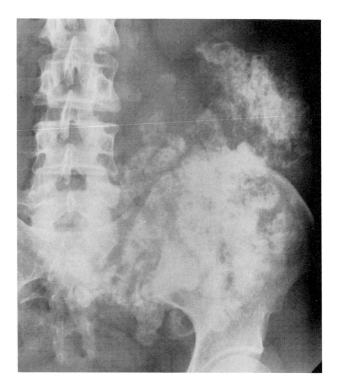

Figure 3–186. *Plain film.* **Chondro-sarcoma of left ilium,** exhibiting extensive calcification. (From Dahlin, D. C., and Henderson, E. D.)

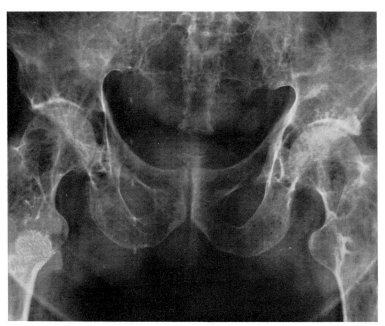

Figure 3–187. *Plain film.* **Multiple myeloma.** Characteristic small punched-out areas of destruction in pelvis and vertebrae. (From Ghormley, R. K., and Pollock, G. A.)

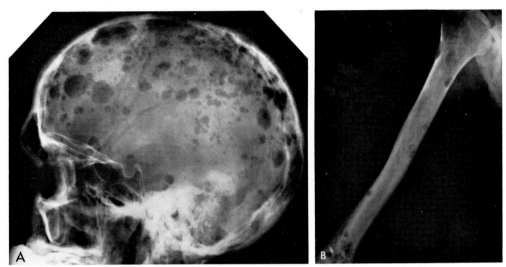

Figure 3–188. Multiple myeloma. Characteristic small punched-out areas of destruction. **A,** Skull. **B,** Humerus. (From Ghormley, R. K., and Pollock, G. A.)

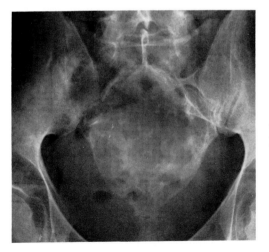

Figure 3–189. *Plain film.* **Destruction of sacrum by chordoma.** (From Adson, A. W., Moersch, F. P., and Kernohan, J. W.)

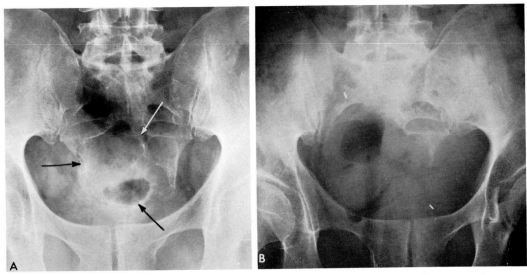

Figure 3–190. *Plain films.* **A,** Erosion of sacrum from chordoma. **B,** After resection of lower part of sacrum.

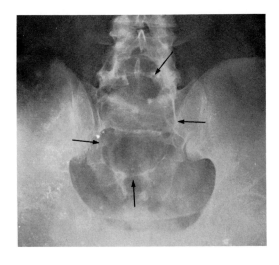

Figure 3–191. *Plain film.* Erosion of sacrum and lumbar vertebrae by pressure from ependymoma. (From Adson, A. W., Moersch, F. P., and Kernohan, J. W.)

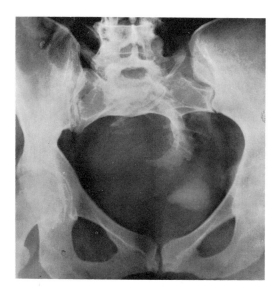

Figure 3–192. *Plain film.* Erosion of sacrum by extensive dermoid cyst of pelvis. (From Adson, A. W., Moersch, F. P., and Kernohan, J. W.)

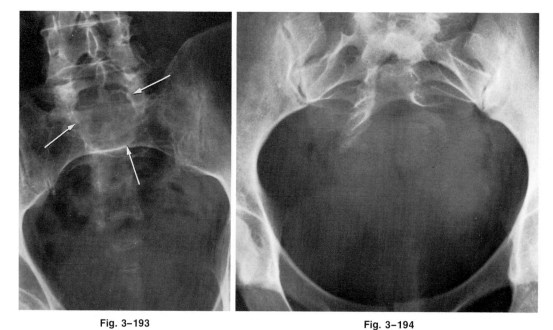

Fig. 3–193   Fig. 3–194

Figure 3–193. *Plain film.* Neurofibroma of lumbosacral canal, producing definite bony absorption of fifth lumbar and first and second sacral segments (*arrows*). (From Adson, A. W., Moersch, F. P., and Kernohan, J. W.)

Figure 3–194. *Plain film.* Malformation of sacrum, associated with spina bifida cystica that originated in sacral region and extended into pelvis. (From Adson, A. W., Moersch, F. P., and Kernohan, J. W.)

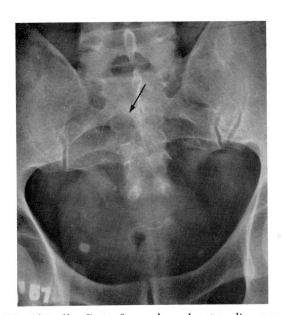

Figure 3–195. *Plain film.* Cysts of second sacral root eroding sacrum (*arrow*).

Metastasis to Bone From Carcinoma of Prostate and Other Tumors: Differential Diagnosis From Osteitis Deformans (Paget's Disease)

OSTEOLYTIC VERSUS OSTEOPLASTIC METASTASIS

Metastatic lesions of bone are of two principal varieties; namely, osteolytic (or melted-ice type) and osteoplastic. The former is the most commonly seen, as it is produced by carcinoma of almost all organs (including the urinary tract). This type of lesion produces destruction of bone. When seen in the pelvis and lumbar portion of the spinal column, the characteristic image may vary from multiple small punctate regions of varying size, from which bone has "disappeared" (commonly described as the "melted-ice" appearance), to large lesions in which whole areas of bone have disappeared (Figs. 3-196 through 3-201).

OSTEOPLASTIC METASTASIS

Of most importance to the urologist is the *osteoplastic* type of metastasis. In the male, this almost entirely results from carcinoma of the prostate gland; in the female, it usually results from metastatic carcinoma of the breast. It is occasionally seen with carcinoma of the stomach or the thyroid gland and in rare instances with a variety of other tumors. Sutherland described the general picture of this condition as "a background of bone destruction with concomitant hyperplasia of the bone tissue." In the average case the process of "proliferation or hyperplasia" keeps pace with the process of destruction, so that the general picture is one of sclerosis and increased density, which simulates a reaction of bone and eventually results in homogeneous eburnation. The lesions involve any part of the bony skeleton but on urographic films are most frequently seen in the pelvis, the lumbar vertebrae, and the upper portion of the femora (Figs. 3-202 through 3-209). Early lesions may be most difficult to recognize. The lesion may begin as an area of increased density in the inner margin of one or both ilia under the overlapping wing of the sacrum, in which case it could be easily mistaken for an early form of rheumatoid spondylitis. In other cases it may begin as a single area or multiple discrete areas (or splotches) of increased density which may simulate bone islands. In early cases it may not be possible (without the opportunity of making subsequent progress roentgenograms) to distinguish the osteoplastic type of metastatic malignant lesion from bone islands (Fig. 3-210) unless clinical data are sufficient. It should be stated parenthetically here that the origin and etiology of "bone islands" are not known. Such lesions do not change in appearance, or at most enlarge very slowly, and apparently are benign processes of no clinical significance.

Although in most cases the proliferative and hyperplastic process more than keeps pace with the destruction of bone, in occasional cases the reverse may be true. This will result in roentgenographic images in which both osteolytic and osteoplastic lesions are present simultaneously. The most characteristic roentgenographic image in this situation is that of the stippled, "punched-out" areas interspersed with multiple discrete areas of bony sclerosis (Figs. 3-211 and 3-212; see also Fig. 3-196). In rare cases the proliferative phase seems to be nonexistent, so that a typical osteolytic lesion results.

Advanced osteoplastic metastasis from carcinoma of the prostate presents most dramatic roentgenograms (Fig. 3-209B). Replacement of the normal bone by large irregular "splotches" of increased density or complete eburnation of bone is not uncommonly seen. Such a process, even though extensive, may be confined to one innominate bone or to one or more lumbar vertebrae (Fig. 3-213A, B, and C). In rare instances, diffuse bony sclerosis from agnogenic myeloid metaplasia or ingestion of large amounts of fluoride (Fig. 3-214) may mimic metastasis from carcinoma of the prostate.

Therapeutic Effect of Castration

The therapeutic effect of estrogenic treatment for carcinoma of the prostate is occasionally demonstrated by dramatic regression of metastatic lesions in bone following castration (Figs. 3-215 through 3-218).

PULMONARY METASTASIS FROM CARCINOMA OF THE PROSTATE

Clinical evidence of pulmonary metastasis is distinctly uncommon as compared to that of metastasis to bone. Bolton has reported that 5.7% of 298 patients with carcinoma of the prostate had roentgenographic and clinical evidence for pulmonary metastasis. In other studies, the reported incidence of clinically suspected metastasis has ranged from 4.9% to 10% (Alyea and Henderson; Bumpus; Mintz and Smith). At autopsy pulmonary metastasis is found much more frequently, Bolton recording an incidence of 25% in his series.

Roentgenographically, metastases may present as diffuse lymphangitic type infiltrates (Fig. 3-219) with few if any discrete deposits of tumor, or they appear as multiple bilateral discrete nodular deposits (Fig. 3-220). There are no roentgenographic characteristics which differentiate these lesions from metastasis to lung from cancer originating in other organs. In some cases, dramatic improvement of pulmonary metastasis has been demonstrated after orchiectomy or endocrine therapy (Bolton) (Figs. 3-221A through D).

OSTEITIS DEFORMANS (PAGET'S DISEASE)

Paget's disease is of concern to the urologist because differentiating it from the metastatic lesions of carcinoma of the prostate is sometimes a most difficult diagnostic problem. Paget's disease most frequently involves the bony pelvis and femur. These are also the common sites for metastatic involvement from carcinoma of the prostate.

Paget's disease as usually seen in the pelvis combines two phases: (1) the sclerotic phase and (2) the combined phase. A third almost purely destructive or lytic phase is also seen in rare cases and is known as osteoporosis circumscripta. The sclerotic phase is characterized by a homogeneous increase in density of bone, which makes the detail of the cancellous trabeculae no longer perceptible. In the combined phase, nonhomogeneous alterations in the density of bone occur. Areas of osteoporosis and osteosclerosis are present, and cysts may be demonstrable. In the osteoporotic areas, the cancellous trabeculae may be much coarser than normal, and their contour may be distorted. **Generally speaking, however, the trabecular elements of bone are maintained or increased to a greater extent than in metastatic lesions** as they are destroyed in metastatic lesions (Figs. 3-222 through 3-228).

In Paget's disease there is often a definite increase in the dimensions of the involved bones, which is not seen in metastatic disease from prostatic cancer. This is thought to result from subperiosteal deposition of bony tissue. In some films of the lumbar vertebrae and pelvis it may be impossible to distinguish Paget's disease from an osteoplastic metastatic lesion. In such cases, demonstration of Paget's disease of the skull or long bones or of both may help to settle the diagnosis. In the *skull, long bones,* and rarely the *pelvis,* early lesions appear as localized or diffuse areas of finely mottled osteoporosis

(osteoporosis circumscripta) (Fig. 3-229A). Later the sclerotic process ensues; it produces multiple shadows of increased density with woolly margins scattered throughout a thickened calvarium (Fig. 3-229B). Ultimately the outlines of the diploë become obliterated. The contour of the inner table of bone remains distinct, but identification of the external table becomes difficult (Fig. 3-230). The skull becomes thickened so that in some cases it may reach a thickness of 1½ inches (3.8 cm). In the *long bones*, the early phase is manifested by areas of osteoporosis in the upper and lower ends of the bone (Fig. 3-231). Later the sclerotic process takes over much the same as was described for the skull and pelvis. The diseased portion of the bone usually has a greater circumference than the uninvolved parts (Fig. 3-232). In rare instances osteogenic sarcoma arises in lesions of Paget's disease.

(References begin on page 264.)

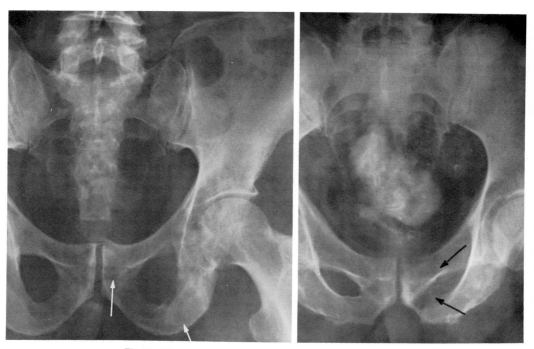

Fig. 3–196   Fig. 3–197

Figure 3–196. *Plain film.* Osteoplastic and osteolytic metastasis involving ischium and pubis from carcinoma of bladder.

Figure 3–197. *Excretory urogram.* Osteolytic metastasis to left pubis from carcinoma of bladder after total cystectomy and implantation of ureters to bowel. Note contrast medium in rectum.

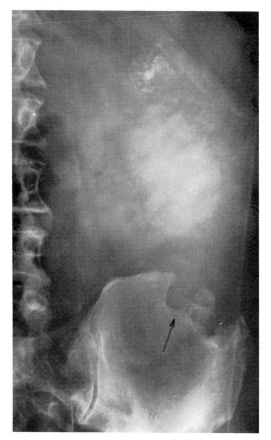

Figure 3–198. *Plain film.* Osteolytic metastasis involving left ilium, from hypernephroma of left kidney.

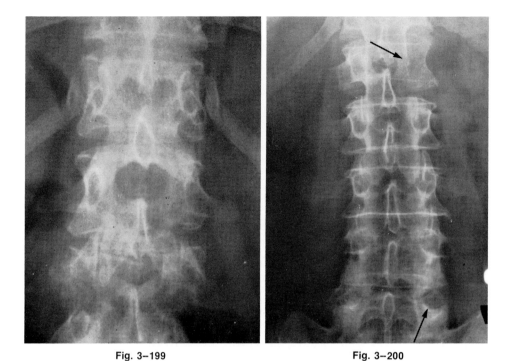

Fig. 3–199   Fig. 3–200

Figure 3–199. *Plain film.* **Osteolytic metastasis to vertebra,** with destruction of left pedicle of first lumbar vertebra and bilateral destruction of pedicles of second lumbar vertebra. Primary lesion was **carcinoma of breast.**

Figure 3–200. **Osteolytic metastatic lesions from hypernephroma.** Destruction of (left) pedicles and transverse processes of first and fifth lumbar vertebrae.

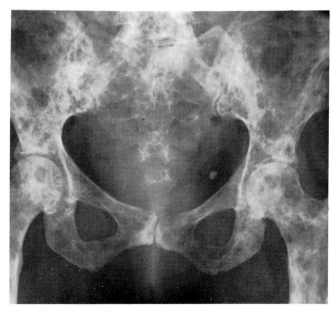

Figure 3–201. *Plain film.* Advanced osteolytic metastasis to pelvis from primary lesion in breast.

Fig. 3–202

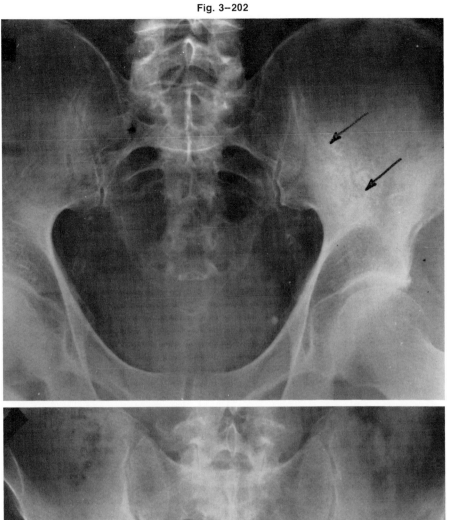

Fig. 3–203

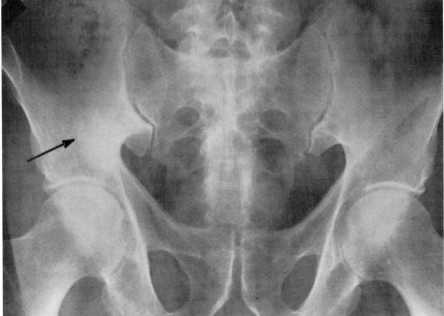

Figure 3–202. *Plain film.* Carcinoma of prostate with osteoplastic metastasis; minimal lesions involving left innominate bone. (See text.)

Figure 3–203. *Plain film.* Carcinoma of prostate with osteoplastic metastasis; minimal lesions involving right innominate bone. (See text.)

Fig. 3–204

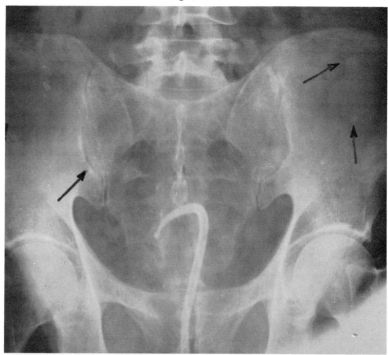

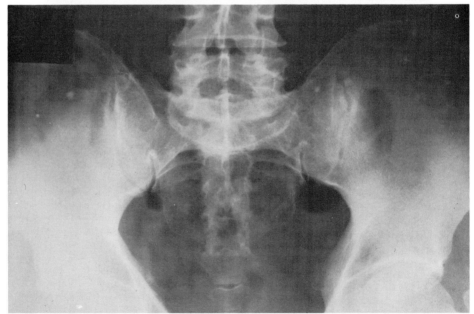

Fig. 3–205

Figure 3–204.   *Plain film.* Carcinoma of prostate with osteoplastic metastasis. Small, early, "spotty" lesions involving both innominate bones. (See text.)

Figure 3–205.   *Plain film.* Carcinoma of prostate with osteoplastic metastasis. Small, early, "spotty" lesions involving both innominate bones. (See text.)

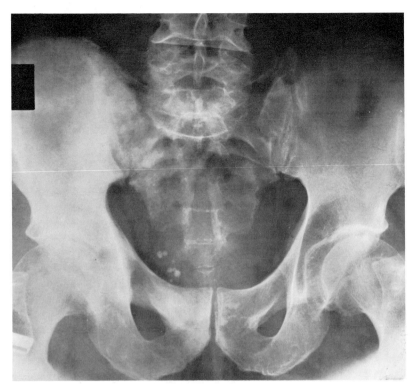

Figure 3–206. *Plain film.* Carcinoma of prostate with osteoplastic involvement of right innominate bone only. (See text.)

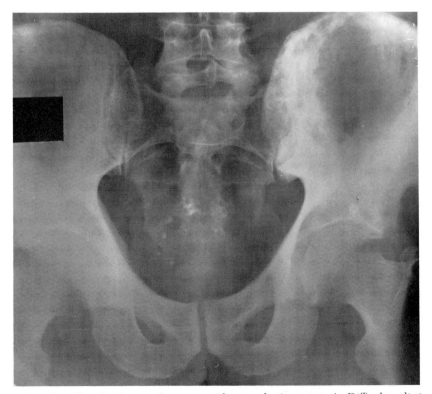

Figure 3–207. *Plain film.* Carcinoma of prostate with osteoplastic metastasis. Difficult to distinguish from Paget's disease. (See text.)

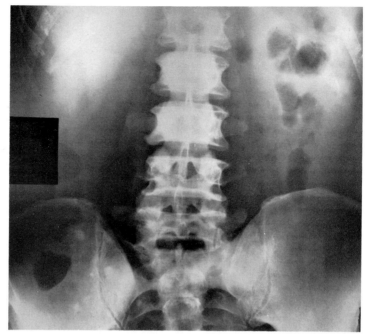

Figure 3–208. *Plain film, anteroposterior view.* **Osteoplastic metastasis from carcinoma of prostate involving lumbar portion of spinal column and pelvis.** Second and third lumbar bodies principally involved. Note spotty involvement of right innominate bone.

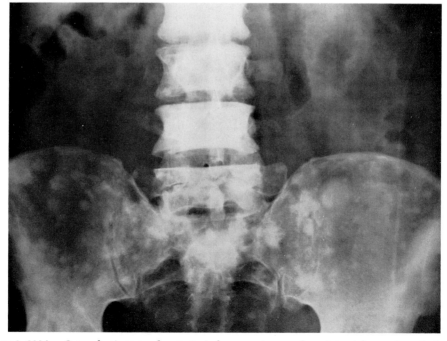

Figure 3–209A. Osteoplastic type of metastasis from carcinoma of prostate. Advanced spotty lesion.

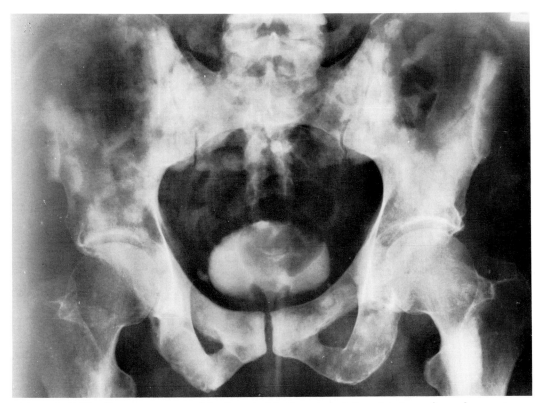

Figure 3–209B.   *Excretory urogram.* **Massive osteoblastic metastasis in pelvic bones** from adenocarcinoma of prostate gland. (Courtesy of Dr. H. W. ten Cate.)

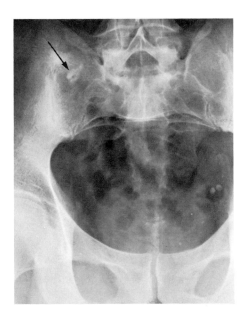

Figure 3–210. *Plain film.* Island of nonmalignant bony sclerosis in right sacrum.

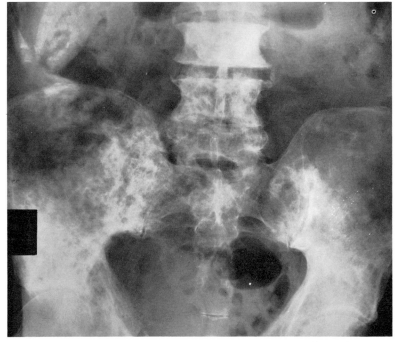

Figure 3–211. *Plain film.* Carcinoma of prostate, with both osteoplastic and osteolytic types of metastasis. Difficult to distinguish from osteolytic type of metastasis. (See text.)

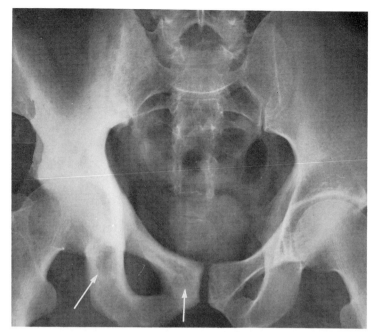

Figure 3–212. *Plain film.* Mixed osteolytic (*arrows*) and osteoplastic metastatic lesions involving right innominate bone. Patent has bladder tumor.

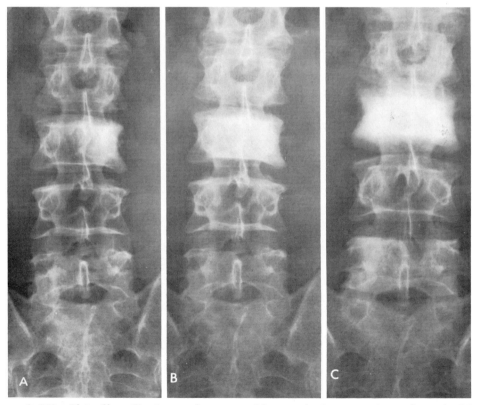

Figure 3–213. *Plain films.* Carcinoma of prostate with osteoplastic metastasis involving third lumbar vertebra. Gradual progression of lesion. **A,** Roentgenogram dated May 7, 1942, showing minimal involvement of third lumbar vertebra. **B,** Roentgenogram dated Mar. 17, 1943, showing increased involvement. **C,** Roentgenogram dated May 5, 1944, showing still greater involvement of third lumbar vertebra, with beginning involvement of fifth lumbar vertebra. (See text.)

249

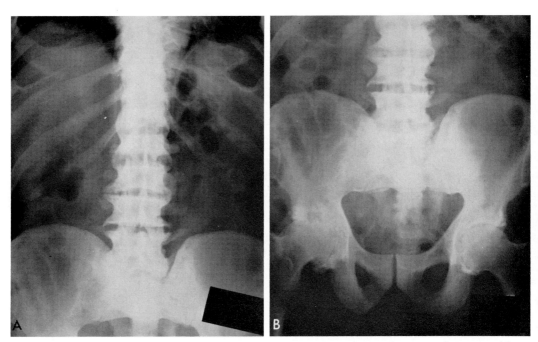

Figure 3–214. *Plain films.* **Fluoride osteosclerosis simulating carcinoma of prostate. A,** Increased bone density with hypertrophic changes of lumbar spinal column. Note even distribution and ground-glass appearance. **B,** Increased density of entire lumbar spinal column and pelvis with bilateral calcification of sacrospinous ligament. (From Gilbaugh, J. H., Jr., and Thompson, G. J.)

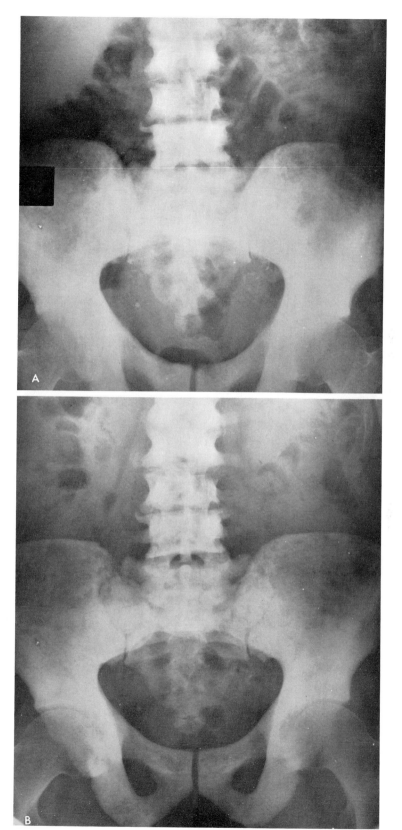

Figure 3–215. Beneficial effect of castration on bony metastasis from carcinoma of prostate. *Plain films.* **A,** Extensive osteoplastic metastasis from carcinoma of prostate. **B,** Eight months later. Moderate regression following bilateral orchiectomy. (See text.)

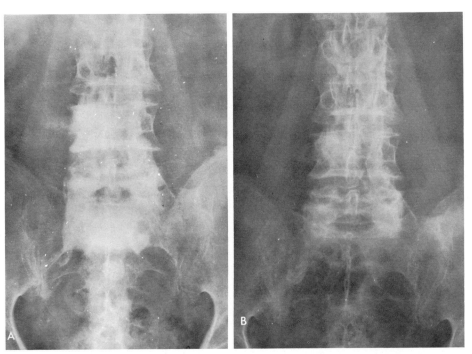

Figure 3–216.   Beneficial effect of castration on bony metastasis from carcinoma of prostate. *Plain films.*
A, Carcinoma of prostate with **osteoplastic metastasis involving lumbosacral portion of spinal column.**
B, Marked regression 3 years following orchiectomy. (See text.)

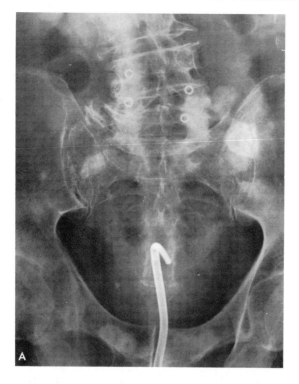

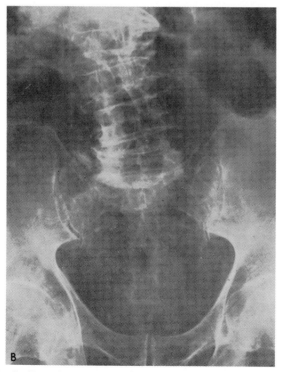

Figure 3–217. Beneficial effect of castration on bony metastasis from carcinoma of prostate. *Plain films.* A, Carcinoma of prostate, with **extensive osteoplastic metastasis of "spotty" type. B,** Roentgenogram made 2 years after orchiectomy; lesions have almost disappeared. (Defects in roentgenogram are artifacts.) (See text.)

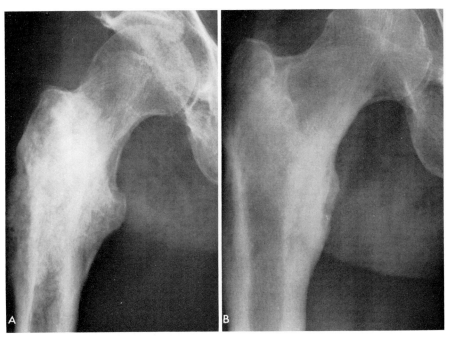

Figure 3–218. *Plain films.* Beneficial effects of castration on bony metastasis from carcinoma of prostate. **A,** Metastasis to intertrochanteric portion of right femur from carcinoma of prostate. **B,** Twenty months after bilateral orchiectomy. Marked healing.

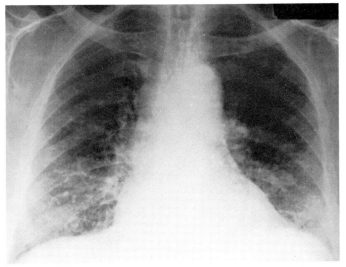

Figure 3–219. Lymphangitic type of metastasis from carcinoma of prostate. Diffuse infiltrate with no discrete deposits of tumor is present throughout both lungs.

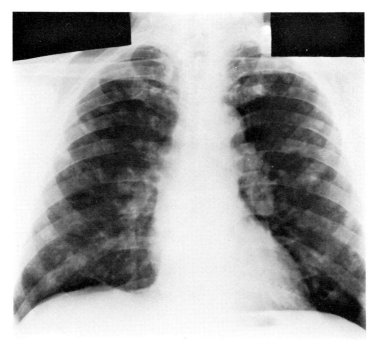

Figure 3–220. Pulmonary metastasis from carcinoma of prostate. Nodular metastases are present throughout both lungs.

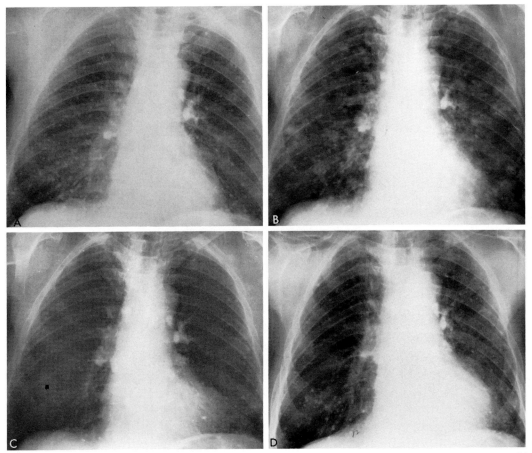

Figure 3–221. A, Pulmonary metastasis from carcinoma of prostate; regression following estrogens. Old calcified granular lesions 5 years before diagnosis of carcinoma of prostate in man, age 65. B, Multiple soft infiltrative metastatic lesions in both lung fields at time of diagnosis of carcinoma of prostate (1957). (Transurethral resection done and stilbestrol, 5 mg three times a day, prescribed.) C, Regression of metastatic nodules 4 months later. D, Metastases have disappeared 6 years after beginning of treatment. (From Bolton, B. H.)

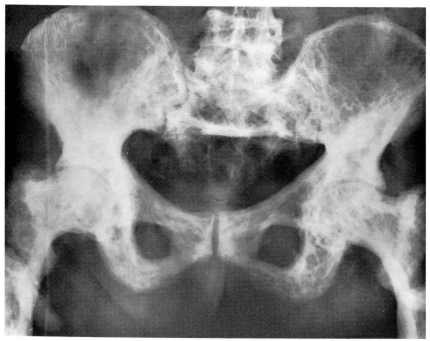

Figure 3–222. *Plain film.* **Paget's disease.** Areas of osteosclerosis and "cysts" which represent the combined phase of osteitis deformans. (From Dickson, D. D., Camp, J. D., and Ghormley, R. K.)

Fig. 3–223

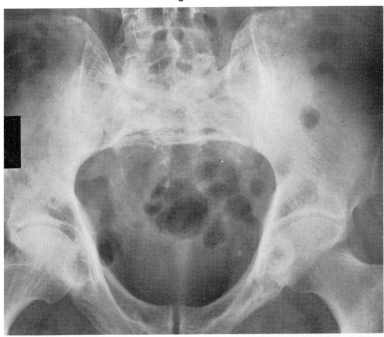

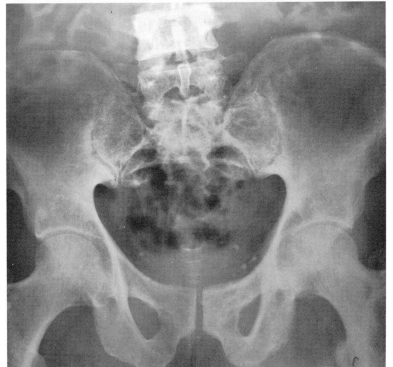

Fig. 3–224

Figure 3–223. *Plain film.* Paget's disease of lumbar portion of spinal column and pelvis. (See text.) Note that *bony trabeculae are maintained* (in contradistinction to osteoplastic metastatic carcinoma).

Figure 3–224. *Plain film.* Paget's disease involving principally the left innominate bone, left ischium, fourth lumbar vertebra, and head and neck of left femur. (See text.) Note that *bony trabeculae are well maintained* and that there is typical thickening of femora due to subperiosteal deposition of bone.

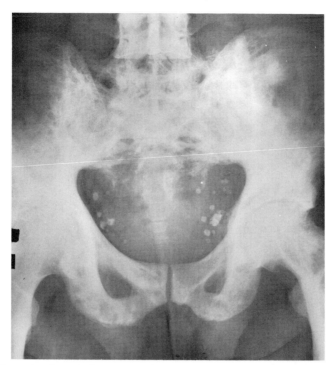

Figure 3–225. Extensive Paget's disease involving lumbar portion of spinal column, pelvis, and both femora. (See text.) Homogeneous increase of density of bone with loss of detail of cancellous trabeculae represents sclerotic phase of Paget's disease. Difficult to distinguish from osteoplastic metastasis from carcinoma of prostate.

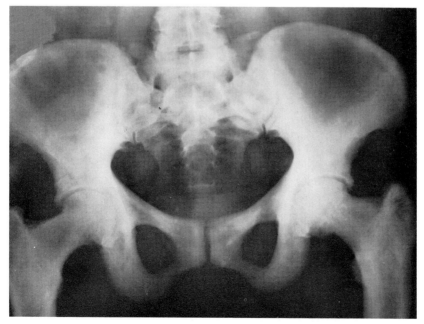

Figure 3–226. *Plain film.* Homogeneous increase in density of bone, with loss of detail of cancellous trabeculae; this represents **sclerotic phase of osteitis deformans.** (From Dickson, D. D., Camp, J. D., and Ghormley, R. K.)

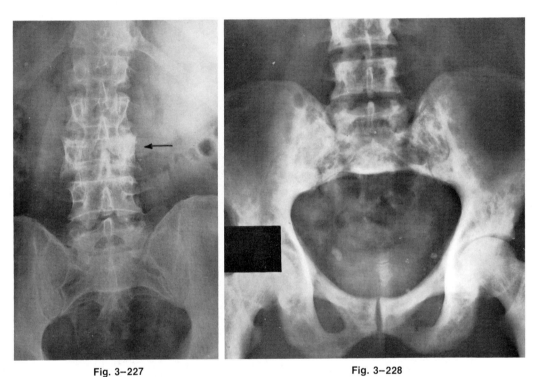

Fig. 3–227   Fig. 3–228

Figure 3–227. *Plain film.* Paget's disease involving third lumbar vertebra. (See text.)

Figure 3–228. Extensive Paget's disease involving lumbar portion of spinal column, pelvis, and both femora. (See text.) Homogeneous increase of density of bone with loss of detail of cancellous trabeculae represents **sclerotic phase of Paget's disease**. Difficult to distinguish from osteoplastic metastasis from carcinoma of prostate.

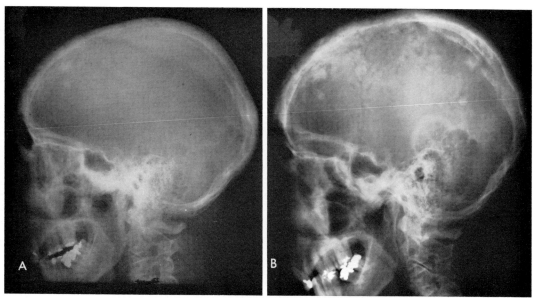

Figure 3–229. Paget's disease. Lateral views of skull showing osteoporosis. **A,** Extension and sharply defined regions of osteoporosis with thickening and opacities, particularly in frontal region. **B,** Same skull 4²/₃ years later, showing further extension of the osteoporotic zone and typical osteitis deformans, with increased density of bone and woolly margins. (From Dickson, D. D., Camp, J. D., and Ghormley, R. K.)

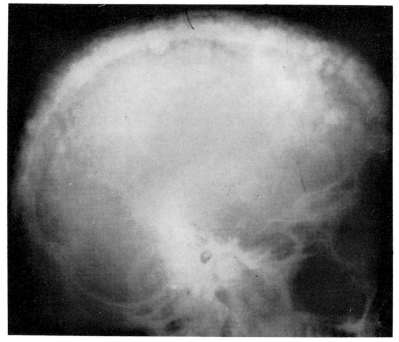

Figure 3–230. Advanced Paget's disease of skull.

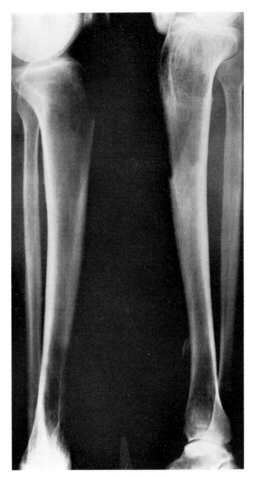

Figure 3–231. Early phase of Paget's disease (osteitis deformans). Zones of osteoporosis in upper and lower ends of both tibias. Diseased portion of bone has greater circumference than uninvolved parts have. (From Dickson, D. D., Camp, J. D., and Ghormley, R. K.)

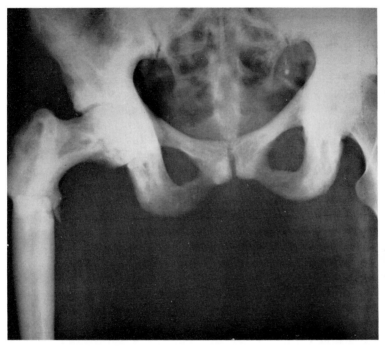

Figure 3–232. Extensive Paget's disease of femur and bony pelvis with pathologic fracture of neck of femur. (From Dickson, D. D., Camp, J. D., and Ghormley, R. K.)

REFERENCES

Adson, A. W., Moersch, F. P., and Kernohan, J. W.: Neurogenic Tumors Arising From the Sacrum. Arch. Neurol. & Psychiat. 41:535-555 (Mar.) 1939.

Alyea, E. P., and Henderson, A. F.: Carcinoma of the Prostate: Immediate Response to Bilateral Orchiectomy; Clinical and X-ray Evidence. J.A.M.A. 120:1099-1102 (Dec. 5) 1942.

Bartholomew, L. G., Cain, J. C., Davis, G. D., and Bulbulian, A. H.: Misleading Calcific Shadows in the Abdomen. Postgrad. Med. 30:51-66 (July) 1961.

Beer, E.: Periostitis of the Symphysis and Descending Rami of the Pubes Following Suprapubic Operations. Internat. J. Med. & Surg. 37:224 (May) 1924.

Bianchini, A.: Su di un caso di calcificazione quasi totale delle vie deferenziali. Arch. di radio. 6:228-233, 1930.

Bolton, B. H.: Pulmonary Metastases From Carcinoma of the Prostate: Incidence and Case Report of a Long Remission. J. Urol. 94:73-77 (July) 1965.

Brindley, G. V.: Sacral and Presacral Tumors. Ann. Surg. 121:729 (May) 1945.

Bumpus, H. C., Jr.: Carcinoma of the Prostate: A Clinical Study of One Thousand Cases. Surg., Gynec. & Obst. 43:150-155 (Aug.) 1926.

Camiel, M. R.: Calcification of Vas Deferens Associated With Diabetes. J. Urol. 86:634-636 (Nov.) 1961.

Camp, J. D., and Good, C. A., Jr.: The Roentgenologic Diagnosis of Tumors Involving the Sacrum. Radiology 31:398-403 (Oct.) 1938.

Chiari, H.: Ueber senile Verkalkung der Ampullen der Vasa Deferentia und der Samenblasen. Ztschr. f. Heilk. 24:283-292, 1903.

Clement: Dissertation sur les maladies des organes générateurs de l'homme. Thèse de Montpellier, 1830. Quoted by Lowsley and Riaboff.

Coley, B. L., and Higinbotham, N. L.: Secondary Chondrosarcoma. Ann. Surg. 139:547-557 (May) 1954.

Coventry, M. B., and Mitchell, W. C.: Osteitis Pubis: Observations Based on a Study of 45 Patients. J.A.M.A. 178:898-905 (Dec. 2) 1961.

Cristol, D. S., and Greene, L. F.: Vesical Calculi in Women. S. Clin. North America 987-992 (Aug.) 1945.

Culver, G. J., and Tannenhaus, J.: Calcification of the Vas Deferens in Diabetes. J.A.M.A. 173:648-651 (June 11) 1960.

Dahlin, D. C., and Henderson, E. D.: Chondrosarcoma: A Surgical and Pathological Problem. J. Bone & Joint Surg. 38-A:1025-1038 (Oct.) 1956.

Dickson, D. D., Camp, J. D., and Ghormley, R. K.: Osteitis Deformans: Paget's Disease of the Bone. Radiology 44:449-470 (May) 1945.

Dovey, P.: Pelvic Phleboliths. Clin. Radiol. 17:121-125 (Apr.) 1966.

Duplay, A.: Recherches sur les changements et les altérations que présente chez les vieillards l'appareil sécréteur et excréteur du sperme: Canaux déférents. Arch. gén. de méd. 96:428-443, 1855.

George, S.: Calcification of the Vas Deferens and the Seminal Vesicles. J.A.M.A. 47:103-105 (July 14) 1906.

Ghormley, R. K., Meyerding, H. W., Mussey, R. D., Jr., and Luckey, C. A.: Osteochondromata of the Pelvic Bones. J. Bone & Joint Surg. n.s. 28:40-48 (Jan.) 1946.

Ghormley, R. K., and Pollock, G. A.: Multiple Myeloma. Surg., Gynec. & Obst. 69:648-655 (Nov.) 1939.

Ghormley, R. K., Pollock, G. A., Hall, B. E., and Beizer, L. H.: Multiple Myeloma. Surg., Gynec. & Obst. 74:242-244 (Feb.) 1942.

Gilbaugh, J. H., Jr., and Thompson, G. J.: Fluoride Osteosclerosis Simulating Carcinoma of the Prostate With Widespread Bony Metastasis: A Case Report. J. Urol. 96:944-946 (Dec.) 1966.

Gross, R. E., Clatworthy, H. W., Jr., and Meeker, I. A., Jr.: Sacrococcygeal Teratomas in Infants and Children: A Report of 40 Cases. Surg., Gynec. & Obst. 92:341-354 (Mar.) 1951.

Henson, S. W., Jr., and Coventry, M. B.: Osteomyelitis of the Vertebrae as the Result of Infection of the Urinary Tract. Surg., Gynec. & Obst. 102:207-214 (Feb.) 1956.

Kretschmer, H. L.: Calcification of the Seminal Vesicles. J. Urol. 7:67-71 (Jan.) 1922.

Kunkel, M. G., Dahlin, D. C., and Young, H. H.: Benign Chondroblastoma. J. Bone & Joint Surg. 38-A:817-826 (July) 1956.

Lowsley, O. S., and Riaboff, P. J.: Calcification of the Vasa Deferentia. J. Urol. 47:293-298 (Mar.) 1942.

MacCarty, C. S., Waugh, J. M., Mayo, C. W., and Coventry, M. B.: The Surgical Treatment of Presacral Tumors: A Combined Problem. Proc. Staff Meet., Mayo Clin. 27:73-84 (Feb. 13) 1952.

McCullough, J. A. L., and Sutherland, C. G.: Intraabdominal Calcification: The Interpretation of Its Roentgenologic Manifestations. Radiology 36:450-457 (Apr.) 1941.

Mintz, E. R., and Smith, G. G.: Autopsy Findings in 100 Cases of Prostatic Cancer. New England J. Med. 211:479-487 (Sept. 13) 1934.

Orth, J.: Lehrbuch der speciellen pathologischen Anatomie. Berlin, A. Hirschwald, 1893, pp. 309-310.

Polley, H. F.: The Diagnosis and Treatment of Rheumatoid Spondylitis. M. Clin. North America 509:528 (Mar.) 1955.

Polley, H. F., and Slocumb, C. H.: Rheumatoid Spondylitis: A Study of 1035 Cases. Ann. Int. Med. 26:240-249 (Feb.) 1947.

Pugh, D. G.: The Roentgenologic Aspects of Pancreatic Calcification. Proc. Staff Meet., Mayo Clin. 24:437-441 (Aug. 17) 1949.

Smith, C. F., Pugh, D. G., and Polley, H. F.: Physiologic Vertebral Ligamentous Calcification: An Aging Process. Am. J. Roentgenol. 74:1049-1058 (Dec.) 1955.

Sullivan, C. R., and Bickel, W. H.: The Problem of Traumatic Spondylolysis. Am. J. Surg. 100:698-708 (Nov.) 1960.

Sutherland, C. G.: The Roentgenographic Image of Bone Lesions. Internat. Clin. n.s. 2:99-111 (June) 1939.

Warwick, R. T. T.: The Pathogenesis and Treatment of Osteitis Pubis. Brit. J. Urol. 32:464-472 (Dec.) 1960.

Wholey, M. H., Pugh, D. G., and Bickel, W. H.: Localized Destructive Lesions in Rheumatoid Spondylitis. Radiology 74:54-56 (Jan.) 1960.

Wilson, J. L., and Marks, J. H.: Calcification of the Vas Deferens: Its Relation to Diabetes Mellitus and Arteriosclerosis. New England J. Med. *245:* 321-325 (Aug. 30) 1951.

Osteitis Pubis

Adams, R. J., and Chandler, F. A.: Osteitis Pubis of Traumatic Etiology. J. Bone & Joint Surg. *35-A:* 685-696 (July) 1953.

Beneventi, F. A., and Spellman, R.: Unsuccessful Attempts To Produce Osteitis Pubis in Dogs. J. Urol. *69:*405-406 (Mar.) 1953.

Cibert, J.: Post-operative Osteitis Pubis: Causes and Treatment. Brit. J. Urol. *24:*213-215 (Sept.) 1952.

Daw, W. J., and Funke, A. H.: Osteitis Pubis Treated by Cortisone. J. Urol. *69:*686-691 (May) 1953.

Goldstein, A. E., and Rubin, S. W.: Osteitis Pubis Following Suprapubic Prostatectomy: Results With Deep Roentgen Therapy. Am. J. Surg., *74:*480-487 (Oct.) 1947.

Hoffman, C. A., and Erhard, R. F.: Cortisone Therapy in Osteitis Pubis. J. Urol. *72:*247-250 (Aug.) 1954.

Kirz, E.: Osteitis Pubis After Suprapubic Operations on Bladder, With Report of 10 Cases. Brit. J. Surg. *34:*272-276 (Jan.) 1947.

Kleinberg, S.: Osteitis Pubis, With Report of Case in Woman. J. Urol. *48:*635-641 (Dec.) 1942.

Klinefelter, E. W.: Osteitis Pubis: Review of the Literature and Report of a Case. Am. J. Roentgenol. *63:*368-371 (Mar.) 1950.

Lame, E. L., and Chang, H. C.: Pubic and Ischial Necrosis Following Cystostomy and Prostatectomy (Osteitis Pubis). Am. J. Roentgenol. *71:*193-212 (Feb.) 1954.

Lavalle, L. L., and Hamm, F. C.: Osteitis Pubis: Diagnosis and Treatment. J. Urol. *61:*83-95 (Jan.) 1949.

Legueu and Rochet: Les cellulitis périvésicales et pelviennes: Après certaines cystostomies ou prostatectomies suspubiennes. J. d'urol. *15:*1-11 (Jan.) 1923.

Leucutia, T.: Osteitis Pubis and Its Treatment by Roentgen Irradiation. Am. J. Roentgenol. *66:*385-404 (Sept.) 1951.

Marshall, V. F.: Osteitis Pubis Treated With Adrenocorticotrophic Hormone. J. Urol. *67:*364-369 (Mar.) 1952.

Mortensen, H.: Osteitis Pubis. J. Urol. *66:*412-417 (Sept.) 1951.

Muschat, M., Leventhal, G. S., and Krause, J.: Obturator Crush for Osteitis Pubis. J. Urol. *68:* 532-533 (Aug.) 1952.

Nugent, J. J.: Osteitis Pubis Treated With Cortisone. J. Urol. *70:*940-942 (Dec.) 1953.

Pearlman, C. K.: Osteitis Pubis Following Retropubic Prostatectomy. J. Urol. *67:*117-120 (Jan.) 1952.

Stähler, V. H.: Osteitis Pubis. Zentralbl. f. Chir. *84:*933-939, 1959.

Steinbach, H. L., Petrakis, N. L., Gilfillan, R. S., and Smith, D. R.: The Pathogenesis of Osteitis Pubis. J. Urol. *74:*840-846 (Dec.) 1955.

Stutter, B. D.: The Complications of 'Osteitis Pubis': Including a Report of a Case of Sequestrum Formation Giving Rise to Persistent Purulent Urethritis. Brit. J. Surg. *42:*164-171 (Sept.) 1954.

Thornley, R.: Some Uses of Cortisone in Urology With Special Reference to Osteitis Pubis. Brit. J. Urol. *27:*1-10 (Mar.) 1955.

CHAPTER 4

The Normal Urogram

THE KIDNEYS AND URETERS

Anatomy

An important requisite for exact urographic interpretation is the ability to recognize the normal urogram in its many variations. Probably the most serious, if not the most common, error made by the uninitiated is the erroneous diagnosis of pathologic conditions from urograms made of patients with normal urinary tracts. The most difficult part of one's urographic training is to learn the many variations in normal urograms and to be able to recognize them readily. Difficulty in recognizing normal urograms usually is due to the failure of the student to visualize the urogram in terms of the anatomy of the kidney and of the renal pelvis.

For instance, one is likely to lose sight of the fact that renal pyramids may often be composite, so that they have more than one papilla. The minor calyx serving multiple papillae may, therefore, assume rather bizarre outlines. Also, one is likely to forget that there are usually two rows of pyramids, the calyces which serve them projecting in different planes. This accounts for the unusual appearance of some urograms when reviewed in one plane only.

Again, it is not unusual in man to observe occasionally a reversion of the pelvis or calyces to the types found in the lower animals. As a basis, therefore, for the study of the normal urogram, a few pertinent anatomic facts need review.

Anatomic Relation of the Kidneys

The position of the kidneys varies in different individuals. The variation is so great that it is difficult to assert dogmatically just which is the normal position. The following description is that given in Cunningham's *Anatomy* for the position of the kidneys in the average anatomic specimen.

The upper limit of the kidney is indicated by a line drawn transversely across the loin opposite the eleventh thoracic spine, the lower limit by a line on a level with the third lumbar spine. The upper pole reaches to the eleventh rib; the lower, which lies immediately lateral to the tip of the transverse process of the third lumbar vertebra, is ½ in. to 2 in. above the iliac crest. About a third of the kidney lies above the lower margin of the twelfth rib. The left kidney is usually about ½ in. higher than the right. The most lateral point of the lateral border is 4 in. from the median plane while the hilum lies 1½ or 2 in. lateral to the median plane in front of the interval between the tips of the transverse processes of the first and second lumbar vertebrae.

There is so much variation in position of the kidneys, however, that it is difficult to state when the degree of variation is sufficient to be classed as a pathologic condition. This will be completely discussed under the subject of nephroptosis.

The relation of the posterior surface of the kidney to the soft tissues is common to both kidneys. The upper portion of the kidney rests against the diaphragm, while the remainder (from medial to lateral border) is in contact with the psoas, the quadratus lumborum, and the tendons of the transversus abdominis muscles. The *relation* of the *anterior surfaces of kidneys* varies in each kidney. The *right kidney* (from above down) is in contact with the right adrenal gland, liver, second portion of the duodenum, and the hepatic flexure of the colon. In the same order but for the *left kidney,* the organs in apposition to its anterior surface are: the left adrenal gland, stomach, pancreas, and on the extreme lateral margin, the spleen and splenic flexure of the colon.

Anatomic Relation of the Ureters

The ureters are flattened tubes about 25 to 29 cm long and with lumens about 3 mm in diameter. They consist essentially of *two portions,* the *abdominal ureter* and the *pelvic ureter.* The abdominal portion begins at the renal pelvis at a point approximately at the level of the second lumbar vertebra and about 1½ inches (about 4 cm) lateral to the median line of the body. From this point it courses down on the anterior surface of the psoas muscle almost parallel to the median line but inclining a little inward and crosses the brim of the pelvis at the bifurcation of the common iliac artery, at which point it becomes the pelvic ureter. At this point it curves abruptly backward and outward, following closely the contour of the pelvis. Its most lateral aspect is reached when it crosses the obliterated hypogastric artery opposite the ischial spine. It then runs mesially and forward to enter the bladder. There are three natural points of narrowing of the ureter: (1) at the ureteropelvic juncture, (2) where the ureter crosses the pelvic brim, and (3) at its entrance into the bladder.

Relation of Pelvis and Calyces to Architecture of the Kidney

Before describing the character of the renal pelvis it is necessary to describe the architecture of the kidney which it serves. It will be recalled that when a kidney is sectioned longitudinally it presents a very characteristic appearance. From such a section it is apparent that the peripheral portion of the kidney consists of a reddish granular substance called the *cortex,* while the inner portion consists of a lighter, striped substance called the *medulla* (Fig. 4–1). The medullary substance is arranged in several pyramidal portions, separated from each other by a downgrowth of columns of cortical tissue. The bases of the *pyramids* point toward the periphery of the kidney, while the apexes project into the renal sinus. The number of pyramids present in each kidney varies from 4 to 18, while the average number is about 8. The pyramids arrange themselves either anterior or posterior to an imaginary line which bisects the kidney longitudinally into an anterior and a posterior half. (A downgrowth of a thin column of cortical tissue is responsible for this separation.) Pyramids may be *single or composite.* The latter type may be double, triple, or quadruple, and is usually found near a pole of the kidney. In the case of composite pyramids, each division has a papilla of its own, so that *double, triple, or quadruple papillae* are present, requiring an unusual composite type of minor calyx to serve them.

The cortex of the kidney contains both glomeruli and uriniferous tubules, while the medulla contains only tubules. As the larger collecting tubules in the pyramid approach the apex (papilla), they coalesce into larger papillary ducts, which pierce the tip of the papilla and open into a receptacle called a minor calyx. The number of papillary ducts piercing each papilla varies from 7 to 50. The average papilla contains from 10 to 24. The papillae which form the apexes of the renal pyramids project into the renal sinus to be received by the renal pelvis and its projections, the major and minor calyces. Together these structures form a closed drainage system which permits urine to flow from the papillae, via the renal pelvis and ureter, into the urinary bladder.

The *relation of the pelvis and calyces to the kidney* can be best visualized in the longitudinal section of a kidney (Figs. 4–1 and 4–2). It will be observed that, in the hilum of the kidney, the infundibula of the minor calyces and part or all of the renal pelvis are separated from the adjacent parenchyma by a space containing various amounts of loose fatty tissue, which is known as the *renal sinus*. The renal sinus is continuous with the perirenal fat and is lined by an invagination of the renal capsule. It contains, in addition to fat and loose fibrous areolar tissue, the renal arteries, veins, nerves, and lymphatics. Within the kidney, a *minor calyx* is formed by the projection of a papilla into the calyx, much as one would poke a finger into the resilient surface of a rubber ball. The portion of the minor calyx projecting upward around the sides of the papilla is called the *fornix of the calyx*. In the upper pole of the kidney one may observe a *double pyramid with two papillae* requiring the presence of double fornices in a minor calyx to receive them. In *composite pyramids* with multiple papillae, multiple fornices may require that a minor calyx be so large that it may be larger than the pelvis and assume almost any unusual contour. Openings of other calyces may be seen going to the uncut portion of the kidney, illustrating that the papillae and pyramids lie in different planes, thereby requiring the calyces to point in divergent directions.

Description of the Pelviocalyceal System of an Average Normal Human Kidney

As mentioned previously, there is so much variation in contour of the renal pelvis that no one form can be considered as the true normal. Nevertheless, for the purpose of description, one must arbitrarily choose a pelvis in which are incorporated most of the features that one finds in the normal renal pelvis. The following description will serve to represent such a composite form:

The *normal renal pelvis* is triangular or pyramidal. The base is inside the renal sinus and usually parallels the long axis of the kidney. The triangle bends downward so that its apex points downward and medially to join the ureter. This bending requires that both borders of the pelvis be curved in a medial direction, the upper medial border being convex, the lower lateral border being concave. The capacity of the normal pelvis varies widely, usually averaging from 3 to 10 ml.

Arising from the pelvis are divisions known as the *major calyces*. These may vary in number from two to four. Anatomically one recognizes usually but two major calyces, whereas in the urogram three major calyces usually appear. From the lateral edge of the kidney, as drawn in Figure 4–3, it may be seen that the *minor calyces*, which branch from the major calyces, tend to arrange themselves into two distinct rows (one row in the anterior half of the kidney and one in the posterior half), which point in divergent directions. The reason for this is quite obvious after one has read the anatomic description of the kidney given previously. The usual number of minor calyces is 6, 7, or 8, although the number may vary from 4 to 12, depending on the number of renal pyramids or papillae present. It must be remembered, however, that there may be more papillae than minor calyces, as one minor calyx may receive a double, triple, or quadruple papilla. It will also be noticed from Figure 4–3 that the minor calyces of one row are usually not on the same level as those of the opposite row, so that they are not superimposed in a urogram made in only one plane. Superimposition does occur frequently, however, giving rise to erroneous conclusions if urograms are not properly interpreted.

Anatomic Variations in Contour of Pelvis and Calyces. The variations in outline of the normal renal pelvis can best be shown subsequently by means of urograms. One of the greatest difficulties, however, in the interpretation of urograms is to be able to form a mental picture in three dimensions of the pelvic outline in the urogram, which is projected only in one plane. One great help in teaching in this regard is to make stereoscopic pyelograms and view them in a specially constructed stereoscopic viewbox. This type of teaching will do more to acquaint the student with the actual contour of the renal pelvis than any other method. As stereoscopic vision is impossible to reproduce in a book, the next best procedure has been employed; namely, three-dimensional drawings of casts of various types of renal pelves. The ability to project a urogram mentally in three dimensions will simplify many apparently unusual deformities of the pelvis or calyces.

To illustrate the great variety of forms which the normal renal pelvis may assume, three-dimensional drawings of several varieties (after Hauch) are presented in Figure 4–4. It will be noticed that there is no regularity of the size, number, or arrangement of the major or minor calyces. When observing the urogram of an unusual type of pelvis, the physician must always remember that the burden of proof rests on him if he states that the condition is abnormal or pathologic.

It is of interest that the contours of both renal pelves in an individual may be alike, or symmetrical (Figs. 4–5 and 4–6). It is well to remember this, since the knowledge of this fact may prevent many embarrassing situations from arising. For instance, if one is undecided whether a pyelogram of a kidney shows a pathologic or only an atypical form of normal pelvis, comparison with a pyelogram taken of the opposite kidney will often make the decision easy.

COMPARATIVE ANATOMY OF KIDNEYS AND RENAL PELVES

To assist the student to understand better the variations in form of human renal pelves, a few words concerning the *types of renal pelvis found in animals* may be helpful. The comparative anatomy of the kidneys has been considered in detail by Hinman. He divided the kidneys of mammals into two groups: (1) multipapillary and (2) unipapillary. The multipapillary variety occurs in such mammals as the cow (Fig. 4–7), seal (Fig. 4–8), bear, pig, and man. The unipapillary type is found in the rabbit (Fig. 4–9), dog, and monkey (Fig. 4–10). The difference between these two types depends on the "method and manner of the branching ureteral bud in the metanephrogenic mother substance and of reabsorption of certain orders of subdivisions to form a common cavity." This is not difficult to understand when one remembers that embryologically the ureter, pelvis, calyces, and collecting tubules arise from the wolffian duct and grow up to meet and join with the metanephros, which forms the remainder of the kidney. It is easy to visualize the many possible configurations that could result from the multiple branching of the ureter to form the calyces, papillary ducts, and collecting tubules. There is a distinct tendency for human renal pelves to revert occasionally more or less to types seen in some of these lower animals. Although one never encounters a human kidney with as many papillae as that of the seal, it is not uncommon to see a human kidney with the "ramifying type of ureter" common to the cow. A unipapillary kidney probably never occurs in the human, yet at times one encounters pyelograms in which it is difficult to distinguish more than two minor calyces.

(*Text continued on page 275.*)

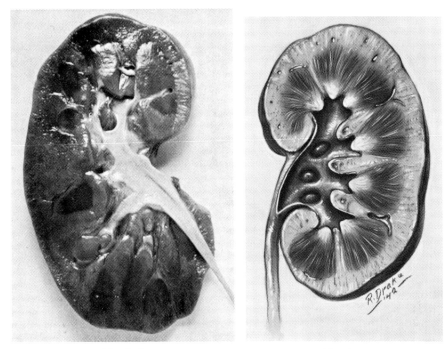

Fig. 4–1   Fig. 4–2

Figure 4–1. *Longitudinal section* of normal kidney.
Figure 4–2. *Diagrammatic longitudinal section of kidney,* showing cortex, medulla, renal papillae, and pelviocalyceal collecting system.

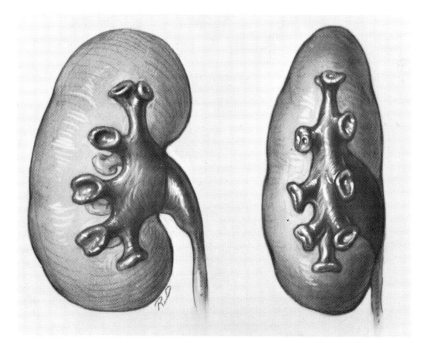

Figure 4–3. *Three-dimensional drawing of kidney:* anteroposterior and lateral views. Calyces arrange themselves in two distinct rows, which point in divergent directions. (From Kelly, H. A., and Burnam, C. F.: Diseases of the Kidneys, Ureters and Bladder, With Special Reference to the Diseases in Women. New York, D. Appleton and Company, 1914.)

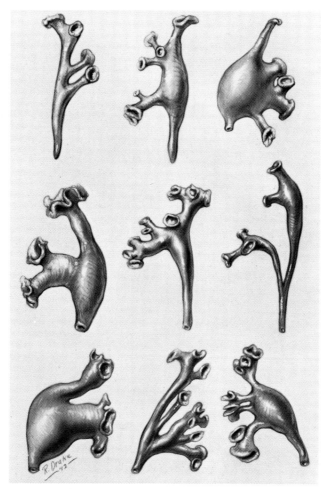

Figure 4–4. *Three-dimensional drawing* illustrating **few of many variations in contour of normal renal pelvis** (after Hauch). (From Kelly, H. A., and Burnam, C. F.: Diseases of the Kidneys, Ureters and Bladder, With Special Reference to the Diseases in Women. New York, D. Appleton and Company, 1914.)

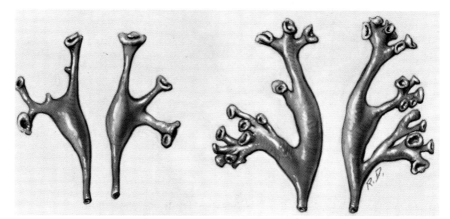

Figure 4–5. *Three-dimensional drawing* illustrating **tendency to symmetry of renal pelves** in same individual (after Hauch). (From Kelly, H. A., and Burnam, C. F.: Diseases of the Kidneys, Ureters and Bladder, With Special Reference to the Diseases in Women. New York, D. Appleton and Company, 1914.)

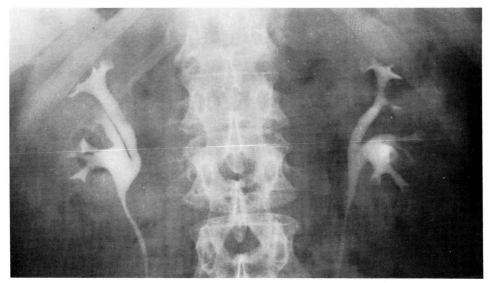

Figure 4–6. *Bilateral retrograde pyelogram.* **Tendency to symmetry of renal pelves** in same individual.

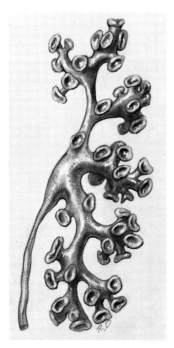

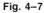

Fig. 4–7

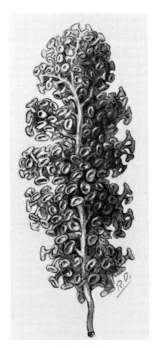

Fig. 4–8

Figure 4–7. **Multipapillary pelvis of cow** (after Hyrtl). (From Kelly, H. A., and Burnam, C. F.: Diseases of the Kidneys, Ureters and Bladder, With Special Reference to the Diseases in Women. New York, D. Appleton and Company, 1914.)

Figure 4–8. **Multipapillary pelvis of seal** (after Hyrtl). (From Kelly, H. A., and Burnam, C. F.: Diseases of the Kidneys, Ureters and Bladder, With Special Reference to the Diseases in Women. New York, D. Appleton and Company, 1914.)

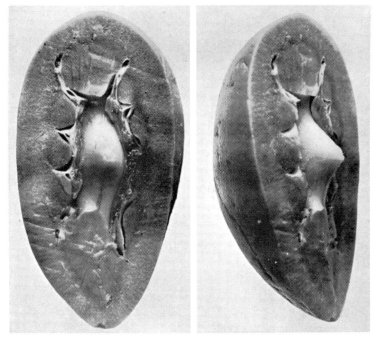

Figure 4–9. Unipapillary type of pelvis found in rabbit. (From Hinman, F.)

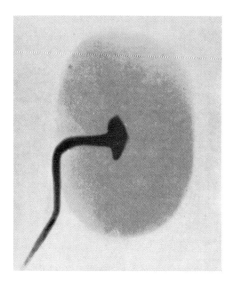

Figure 4–10. *Pyelogram of kidney of monkey,* showing unipapillary type of kidney. (From Hinman, F.)

Urography

Excretory Urograms Valuable in All Age Groups

As mentioned in Chapter 1, excretory urography may be used for patients of any age. Figures 4–11, 4–12, and 4–13 (also, see Fig. 1–20) are examples of normal excretory urograms of infants and children. Figures 4–14 and 4–15 are examples of normal excretory urograms of adults.

Position of Kidneys in Relation to Transverse and Longitudinal Axes of Body

In the average normal case the right renal pelvis is located opposite the transverse process of the second lumbar vertebra. The left kidney is ordinarily about 2 cm higher than the right. Occasionally one encounters cases in which one or both kidneys lie considerably higher than this (Fig. 4–16). More frequently, however, one finds the position of the kidneys lower than the average just described. Just how low a kidney may be situated and still be regarded as normal is questionable. *Every normal kidney possesses a certain amount of mobility*, which may be easily demonstrated roentgenologically by making roentgenograms in the erect and supine positions. A valuable rule of thumb which works well in clinical diagnosis specifies that an excursion of not more than the length of one lumbar vertebra may be considered within normal limits. A kidney which will descend to a level where its pelvis is below the level of the lower border of the third lumbar vertebra is usually considered abnormal. This subject will be more completely discussed under the heading of nephroptosis.

Concerning the position of the kidney with respect to the transverse axis of the body, the most medial border of the renal pelvis is usually just lateral to the tips of the transverse processes of the lumbar vertebrae. Normal kidneys may be seen in more lateral or medial situations than this, but when the departure from normal is too great, the possibility of displacement of the kidney by some pathologic process must be considered (Fig. 4–17).

Position of Kidneys in Relation to Anteroposterior Axis of Body; the Lateral Pyelogram

Study of the kidney and ureter in relation to the anteroposterior axis of the abdomen may be an informative adjunct to routine urography. In order to employ the lateral pyelogram in the diagnosis of pathologic conditions, however, the physician must be familiar with its variations in the normal.

The kidney to be studied should be *down* – closer to the Bucky diaphragm and film (Fig. 4–18A and B). To study the left kidney, therefore, the patient should be lying on his left side; to study the right kidney, he should be lying on his right side. If the reverse position is used and the kidney to be studied is up (away from the film), it will fall forward (away from the vertebral column and toward the anterior abdominal wall) thereby supplying inaccurate information (Fig. 4–19A and B). For a true lateral pyelogram, there should be no more than 1 inch (2.5 cm) of rotation; this can best be assured by making certain that the iliac crests are superimposed on the film. If rotation is more than minimal, the relationship between the kidney, pelvis, and vertebral bodies will be distorted. Only one kidney should be studied at a time; therefore, retrograde pyelography is preferable to the excretory urography. The lateral pyelogram shows the vertical position of the kidney, its relationship to the anteroposterior axis of the abdomen, and the degree of rotation of the kidney on its longitudinal and transverse axes.

The normal lateral pyelogram has been well described by Mertz, Mertz and Hamer, and Dell and Barnwell. The paper of

Dell and Barnwell indicated that when the kidney is in a normal position so that the tip of the lower calyx lies above the lower margin of the body of the second lumbar vertebra, none of the renal pelvis or calyces lies anterior to the anterior border of the vertebral column (Fig. 4-18A and B). The axis of the renal pelvis is almost parallel to the longitudinal axis of the vertebral column. The posterior border of the upper calyx is 2 to 3 cm posterior to the posterior border of the lower calyx.

As the kidney descends, the pelvis is projected further forward and the upper pole of the kidney is tipped backward (rotation on its transverse axis). When the pelvis reaches the level of fourth and fifth lumbar vertebrae, the pelvis and calyces may be situated completely anterior to the anterior margin of the vertebrae (Fig. 4-20A and B). A common normal variant is a mild degree of rotation of the kidney on its longitudinal axis so that the calyces tend to point posteriorly and are well outlined in profile in the lateral film. The ureter in the lateral pyelogram follows the anterior border of the vertebral bodies and is lost from view at the brim of the sacrum.

THE NORMAL RENAL PELVIS

The type of renal pelvis regarded as the classic example of the true normal is found in a definite minority of "normal" kidneys. Nevertheless, it serves to illustrate the cardinal features of the normal renal pelvis. The normal pelvis is described as being triangular with the base of the triangle parallel with the long axis of the body. The axis of the pelvis points downward and medially, a fact which requires that both sides of the triangle be moderately curved. The upper, inner border of the triangular pelvis, therefore, is convex, while the lower, lateral border is concave. The apex of the pelvis blends gradually with the ureter at the ureteropelvic junction (Fig. 4-21).

Variations in Shape: Intrarenal and Extrarenal Varieties

Although the majority of normal renal pelves will coincide with this description, many are encountered in which the axis of the pelvis points in an entirely different direction. Pelves are seen in which the axis is almost horizontal (Fig. 4-22), whereas in some the axes are almost vertical and caudad in direction (Fig. 4-23). In most cases the pelvis blends with the ureter almost imperceptibly like a funnel, but occasionally one sees rather bizarre types of ureteropelvic junctions (Figs. 4-24, 4-25, and 4-26). In some cases one might be inclined to describe the ureteropelvic junction as distinctly abnormal; yet a normal renal pelvis above it and the absence of retention and symptoms suggest that the deformity is probably of no clinical significance (Fig. 4-27). The contour of the proximal portion of the ureter is subject to wide variation and often makes the ureteropelvic junction appear abnormal when in reality it is normal. The subject is more fully discussed subsequently in this chapter under the heading "The Ureters: Variations in Caliber."

The *shape of the normal renal pelvis* varies widely. Among the factors which may have a part in determining the shape of the pelvis is its position in relation to the renal sinus. *An intrarenal type of pelvis* which lies almost completely within the renal sinus is usually rather short and small (Fig. 4-28), whereas a typical extrarenal type of pelvis is likely to be large and associated with long major calyces (Fig. 4-29). Among the more common variations is the square type of pelvis (Fig. 4-30). An oddity which has not been entirely explained is the pelvis with a very straight medial border (Fig. 4-31), which is thought to be the result of pressure exerted by the psoas muscle. Oval and globular pelves are not uncommon and at times it may be difficult to distinguish them from an early stage of pyelectasis (Figs. 4-32 and 4-33). It has been observed that the size of the renal pelves and calyces varies with the size of the individual. A large man may have exceedingly large kidneys with pelves and calyces that are in proportion, whereas a small woman may have small kidneys.

Another variation is the elongated pelvis. This type of pelvis, usually extrarenal, may assume many forms and is often erroneously described as indicative of pyelectasis (Figs. 4–34 and 4–35). It may be associated with elongated calyces, most of which project at right angles to the long axis of the pelvis and present a bizarre appearance which has been described by the term *spider-leg pelvis*. The latter may be confused with elongated calyces observed with renal neoplasm.

Borderline States: Normal Large Pelvis Versus Minimal Pyelectasis; the Flabby Pelvis

As in any type of study in which standards representing the normal state are subject to considerable variation and are difficult to determine accurately, borderline situations are likely to cause confusion in diagnosis. This is especially applicable to the renal pelvis when one is trying to decide whether a certain urogram represents an unusually large normal pelvis or a pathologic early pyelectasis. Figures 4–33, 4–34, and 4–35 represent rather large pelves which we should be inclined to describe as "normal pelves of generous size" rather than abnormal pyelectasis. In this category may be mentioned the condition that Dr. John Crenshaw has described as a "flabby" pelvis (Fig. 4–36). It gives the appearance of a large pelvis that may not be completely filled and, in some cases, this appearance may be the correct explanation. Many physicians have described such films as indicative of "chronic pyelonephritis," but opinions of experienced urologists and roentgenologists may vary considerably in the interpretation of such roentgenograms. If one were confronted with such a situation, it might be necessary to consider additional factors, such as symptoms, evidence of infection, and the presence or absence of urinary retention, to aid one in making an intelligent decision. If the urogram has been made by the retrograde method or in some cases where a ureteral compression device is used, the possibility of overdistention of the pelvis by the urographic medium must be considered (Figs. 4–32 and 4–33). Although there are no definite earmarks which will distinguish this condition, the tense appearance of the pelvis and the associated moderate dilatation of the calyces should make one suspect that the condition exists.

Diminutive Types

Just as there are pelves which appear larger than the average, so are there unusually small pelves (Fig. 4–37). These have been described by various terms such as *diminutive* and *rudimentary* and have also been likened to the "branching ureter" type of pelvis seen in the lower animals. In this variety, combined capacity of the calyces usually exceeds that of the pelvis.

Bifid and Trifid Types

The basis of an almost endless variety of pelvic contours is the partial division of the pelvis into segments or branches. The most common type is the *bifid* or *duplex* pelvis (Fig. 4–38). When three divisions are present, the pelvis is called a *trifid pelvis* (Fig. 4–39A, B, and C). These conditions are an abortive attempt at complete duplication or triplication of the pelvis and ureter.* Owing to the arrangement of the calyces, it may be difficult at times to decide whether a condition is a bifid pelvis or merely a peculiar arrangement or elongation of the major calyces associated with a rudimentary pelvis (Fig. 4–39D). For a true bifid pelvis or trifid pelvis one should be able to identify definite major calyces arising from each of the pelvic divisions.

---

*See "Anomalies," Chapters 11 and 12.

(*Text continued on page 289.*)

Fig. 4–11   Fig. 4–12

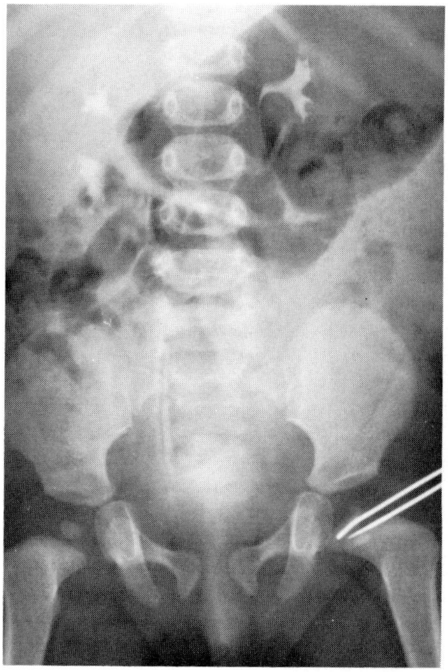

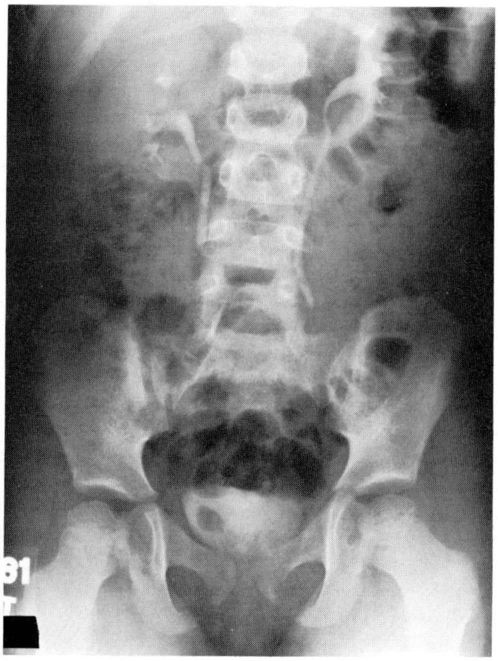

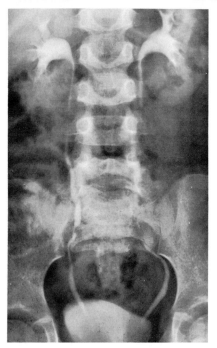

Fig. 4–13

Figure 4–11. *Excretory urogram* of girl, 9 months of age. **Normal on left; duplication on right.** Note outline of stomach filled with gas overlying left kidney.

Figure 4–12. *Excretory urogram* of girl, 4 years of age. Normal.

Figure 4–13. *Excretory urogram* of girl, 5 years of age. Normal.

Fig. 4–14

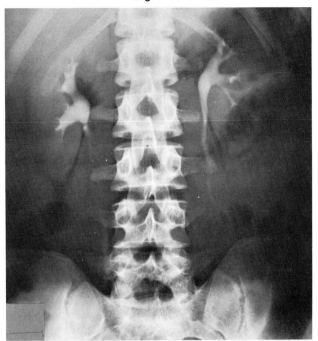

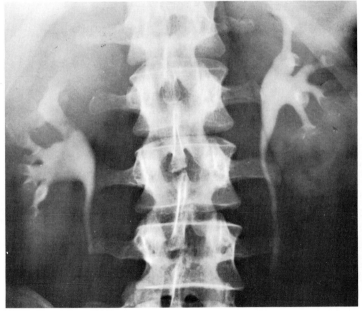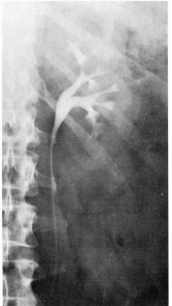

Fig. 4–15   Fig. 4–16

Figure 4–14. *Excretory urogram in an adult.* **Normal.** Right kidney opposite second lumbar transverse process; left kidney opposite first lumbar transverse process. Illustrates most common relative positions of kidneys.

Figure 4–15. *Excretory urogram in an adult.* **Normal renal pelves.** Both kidneys are lower than usual, right being opposite third and left opposite second lumbar vertebra.

Figure 4–16. *Left retrograde pyelogram in an adult.* **Normal.** Kidney is higher than usual. Pelvis is opposite 12th thoracic vertebra.

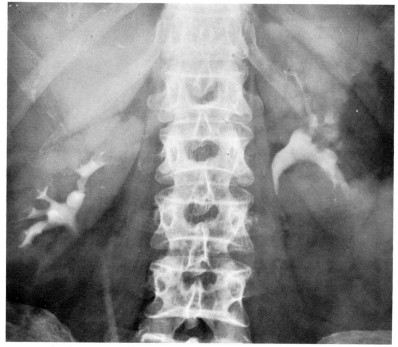

Figure 4–17. *Excretory urogram.* **Normal.** Right kidney is more lateral than usual.

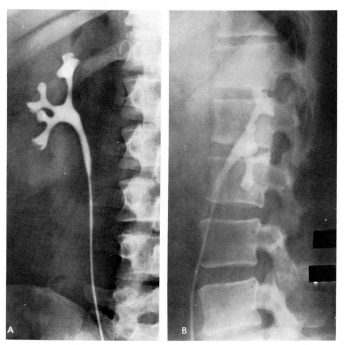

Figure 4–18. Normal. **A,** *Right retrograde pyelogram.* Pelvis opposite first lumbar interspace. **B,** Lateral view, illustrating that no part of pelvis and calyces is projected beyond anterior surface of vertebra when kidney is situated at its normal level.

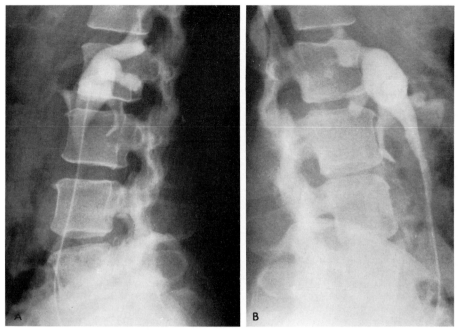

Figure 4–19. Normal right kidney. *Lateral pyelograms.* A, Right side down (against cassette). B, Left side down. Kidney and ureter are thrown forward anterior to spine.

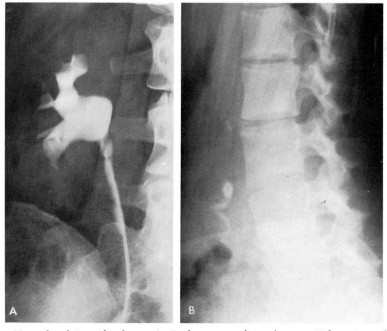

Figure 4–20. Normal pelvis and calyces. A, *Right retrograde pyelogram.* Kidney is at abnormally low level. B, Lateral film, illustrating that when kidney is situated at lower level, pelvis and calyces may be projected anterior to anterior surface of vertebra.

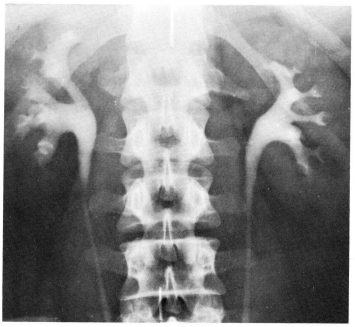

Figure 4–21. *Excretory urogram.* Triangular contour of normal pelvis, with concave lateral and convex medial borders. (See text.)

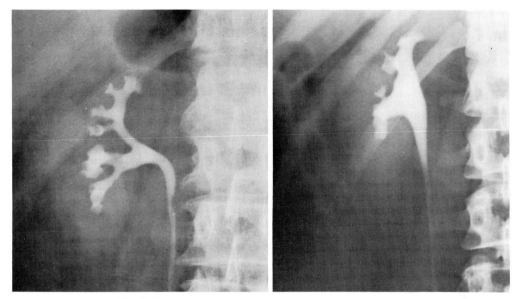

Fig. 4–22   Fig. 4–23

Figure 4–22.   *Right retrograde pyelogram.* **Normal pelvis and calyces.** Axis of pelvis is horizontal.
Figure 4–23.   *Right retrograde pyelogram.* **Normal.** Axis of pelvis is vertical.

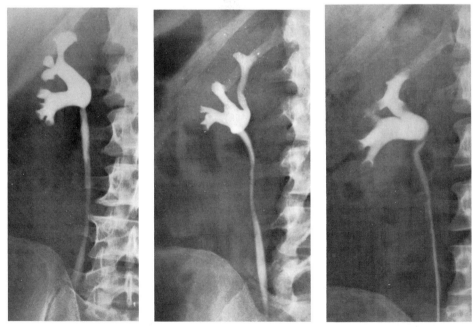

Fig. 4–24   Fig. 4–25   Fig. 4–26

Figures 4–24, 4–25, and 4–26.   *Retrograde pyelograms.* **Atypical insertion of ureter into renal pelvis.** This problem represents abnormal ureteropelvic juncture, yet absence of dilatation (there is mild overdistention present in all) justifies their inclusion as "normal" kidneys.

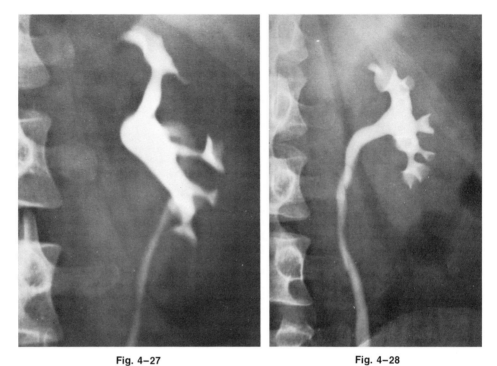

Fig. 4–27   Fig. 4–28

Figure 4–27. *Left retrograde pyelogram.* **Normal.** Atypical insertion of ureter into pelvis.
Figure 4–28. *Left retrograde pyelogram.* **Normal.** Intrarenal type of pelvis.

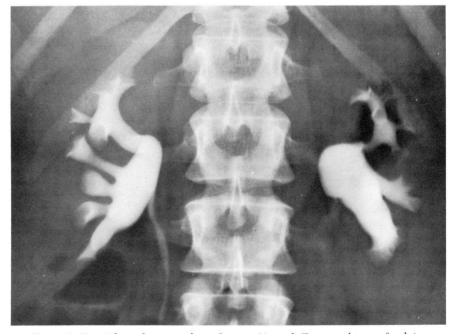

Figure 4–29. *Bilateral retrograde pyelogram.* **Normal.** Extrarenal type of pelvis.

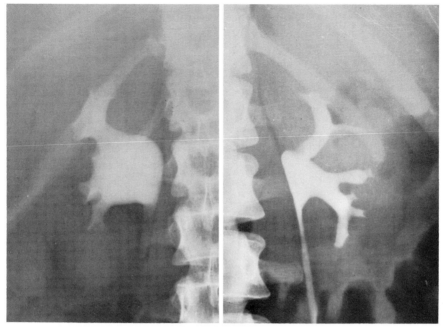

Fig. 4–30   Fig. 4–31

Figure 4–30. *Right retrograde pyelogram.* **Normal.** Square type of pelvis.
Figure 4–31. *Left retrograde pyelogram.* **Normal.** Straight medial border of pelvis, apparently caused by pressure from psoas muscle.

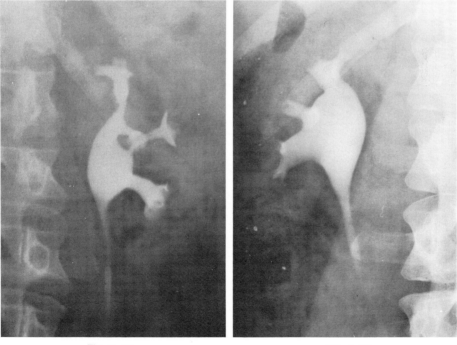

Fig. 4–32   Fig. 4–33

Figure 4–32. *Left retrograde pyelogram.* Oval type of normal pelvis.
Figure 4–33. *Right retrograde pyelogram.* **Normal** pelvis overdistended with medium.

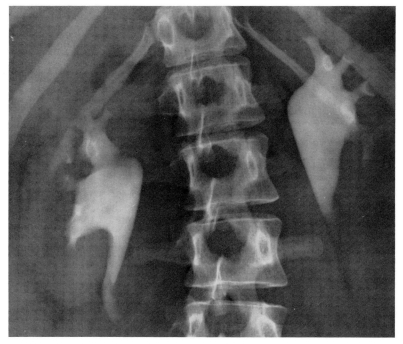

Figure 4–34. *Excretory urogram.* Large (borderline) pelves.

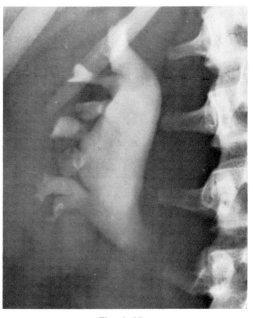

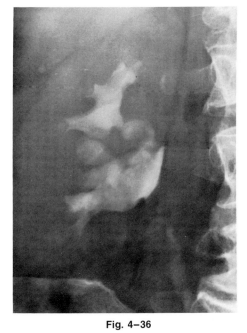

Fig. 4–35   Fig. 4–36

Figure 4–35. *Right retrograde pyelogram.* Normal. Extrarenal type of elongated pelvis.
Figure 4–36. *Excretory urogram.* Flabby type of pelvis. **Normal pelvis or pyelonephritis (?).**

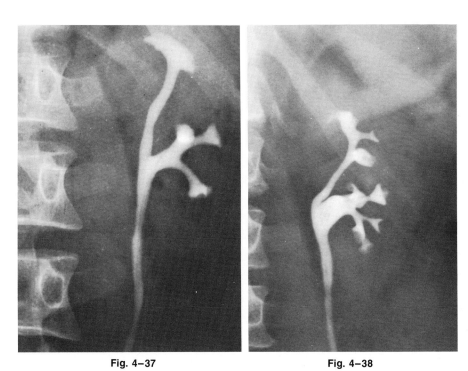

Fig. 4–37   Fig. 4–38

Figure 4–37. *Left retrograde pyelogram.* "Branching ureter" type of **normal renal pelvis.**
Figure 4–38. *Left retrograde pyelogram.* **Normal.** Bifid pelvis.

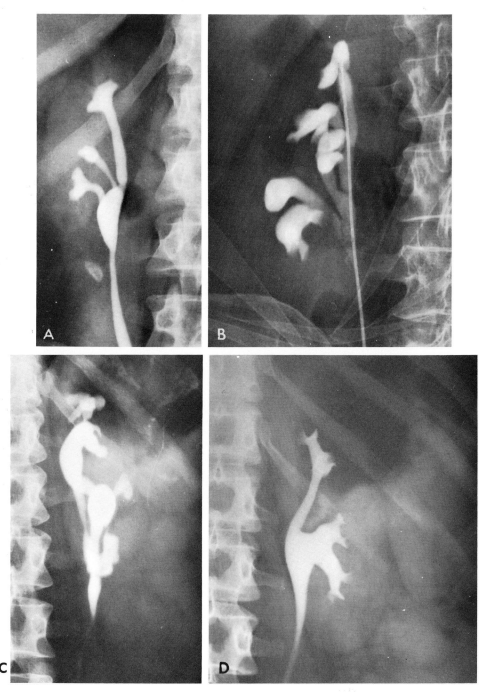

Figure 4-39. A through **D,** *Retrograde pyelograms of different kidneys.* **A,** Trifid pelvis. **B** and **C,** Trifid pelvis with malrotation. **D, Normal.** Attempt at duplication. Difficult to say if pyelogram represents bifid pelvis or simply elongated upper calyx.

Distortion of Pelvic Outline Caused by Incomplete Filling With Contrast Medium

Incomplete filling of a normal pelvis and calyces is also capable of producing unusual configurations which may be erroneously considered as pathologic lesions; with better filling the pyelogram will usually show normal conditions (Figs. 4–40A and B and 4–41A and B). Probably the most common situation encountered in this category is the problem of the negative "filling defect" that suggests such lesions as tumors of the renal pelvis (and calyces) or nonopaque stones (Figs. 4–41C and D through 4–44).

Arterial Impressions on Renal Pelvis Simulating "Negative Filling Defects." Urograms frequently are seen in which gross indentations of the margins of the renal pelvis suggest pressure from an extrapelvic structure (Fig. 4–45). In another peculiar variant one portion of the pelvis (usually the lateral) fills only with difficulty while the distal portion fills readily. If the film is an excretory urogram, a late film may demonstrate adequate filling, or a retrograde pyelogram may be necessary to secure sufficient filling to exclude a filling defect from a tumor or nonopaque stone. Kreel and Pyle, Baum and Gillenwater, as well as others have shown that most of these deformities result from impressions of normal renal arteries or their branches as they cross the renal pelvis or calyces, but a large vein crossing the infundibulum of the superior calyx may also produce a filling defect which tends to be horizontal, wide, and smooth and is readily distinguished from the defect produced by the renal artery (Meng and Elkin). When the condition was suspected from the excretory urogram, Kreel and Pyle obtained an aortogram to outline the renal arteries and their branches. By making a second aortogram (combined angiopyelogram) a few minutes after the first, when the pelvis and calyces were well filled with contrast medium from the first injection, they demonstrated dramatically the relationship of the pelvic defects to the overlying arteries (Figs. 4–46, 4–47, and 4–48). They also have demonstrated other varieties of apparent filling defects from this cause (Fig. 4–49). There is no doubt that in the past many patients with such urographic aberrations have undergone needless exploratory operations to exclude intraluminal lesions such as an epithelial tumor or nonopaque stone. In rare instances, however, obstruction of the calyx may result from pressure of the artery (Fraley, 1966), and operations have been devised to correct this condition (Fraley, 1969). (See discussion in Chapter 5, Figs. 5-56 and 5-57.)

(Text continued on page 296.)

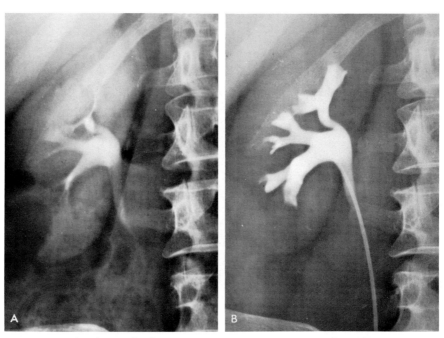

Figure 4–40. Normal pelvis and calyces. **A,** *Excretory urogram.* Incomplete filling suggests crescentic deformity of upper calyx. **B,** *Retrograde pyelogram.* Good filling. Calyx normal.

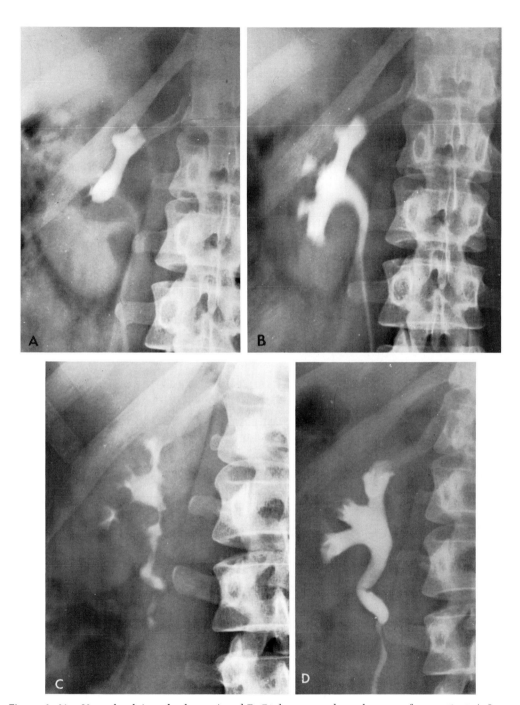

Figure 4–41.   Normal pelvis and calyces. A and **B**, *Right retrograde pyelograms* of one patient. **A**, Incomplete visualization; only upper calyx outlined. Suggests pathologic lesion in lower pole of kidney. **B**, Completely filled kidney. Pelvis and calyces normal. **C** and **D**, Another patient. **C**, *Excretory urogram.* Incomplete filling of pelvis and calyces suggests possible filling defect in kidney and ureter. **D**, *Right retrograde pyelogram.* Pelvis, calyces, and ureter well filled and normal.

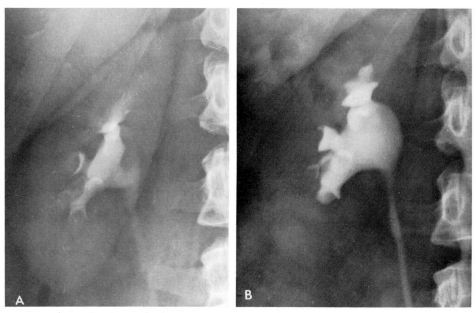

Figure 4–42.   Normal pelvis and calyces. **A,** *Excretory urogram.* Incomplete filling; suggests filling defect in pelvis of right kidney. **B,** *Right retrograde pyelogram.* Completely filled. Pelvis and calyces normal. Normal renal outline.

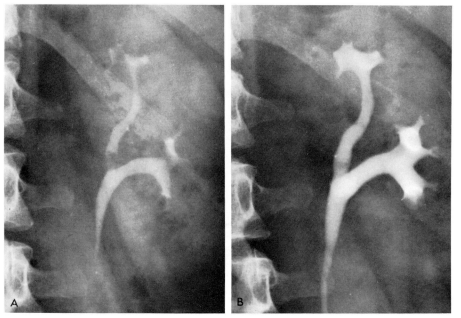

Figure 4–43.   Bifid pelves. **A,** *Excretory urogram.* Negative filling defect in upper division of pelvis. **B,** *Retrograde pyelogram.* Better filling. Filling defect no longer apparent.

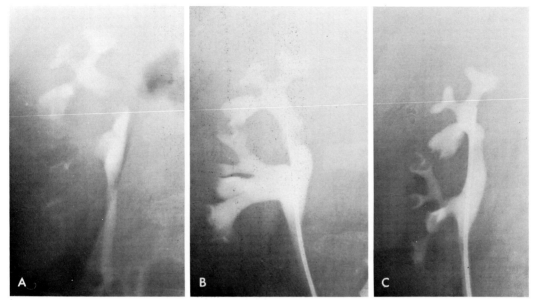

Figure 4–44. Normal calyces. A, *Excretory urogram.* Negative filling defect in infundibulum of upper calyx. Suggests possible transitional cell epithelioma of renal pelvis or soft stone. **B**, and **C**, *Retrograde pyelograms* made in anteroposterior and oblique positions. Infundibulum now better filled, suggesting that filling defect is result of pressure from either anomalous blood vessel or some anatomic variation in plane of infundibulum which makes filling with contrast medium difficult.

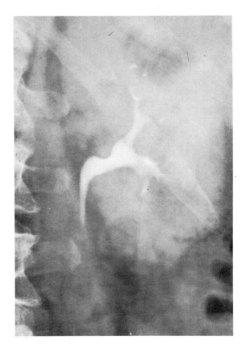

Figure 4–45. *Excretory urogram.* Indentation on upper margin of renal pelvis from external pressure, most likely branch of renal artery.

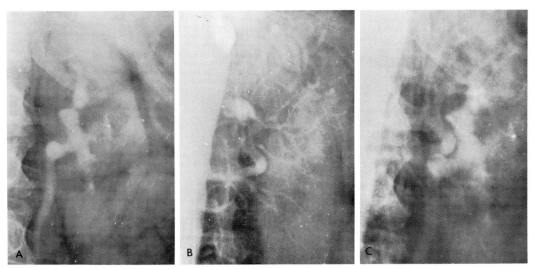

Figure 4–46.   Distortion of renal pelvis. A, *Excretory urogram.* Identations on medial margin of renal pelvis. **B** and **C,** *Aortogram and combined angiopyelogram* show that tortuous renal artery pressing against renal pelvis is cause of deformity. (From Kreel, L., and Pyle, R.)

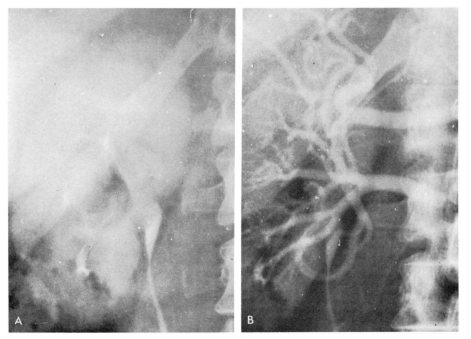

Figure 4–47.   Distortion of renal pelvis. A, *Excretory urogram.* Poor filling of proximal (lateral) part of renal pelvis with sharp pelvic "cutoff"; good filling distal to this. **B,** *Combined angiopyelogram* shows large artery crossing pelvis at this point. Apparently this is cause of deformity. (From Kreel, L., and Pyle, R.)

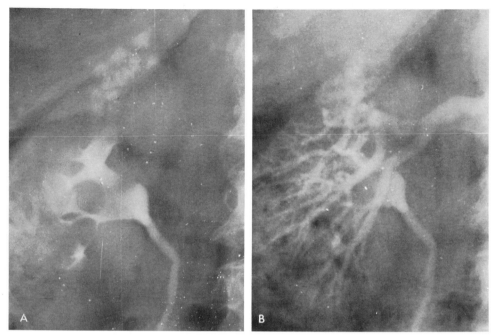

Figure 4–48. Distortion of renal pelvis. **A,** *Excretory urogram,* 20-minute film. Incomplete filling of lateral half of renal pelvis and adjacent part of upper calyx suggests indentation or possible filling defect. **B,** *Combined angiopyelogram.* Area of indentation coincides with large branch of renal artery which is pressing against it. (From Kreel, L., and Pyle, R.)

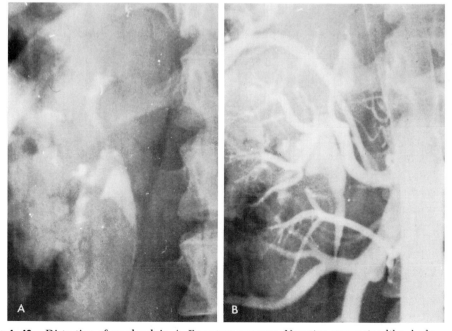

Figure 4–49. Distortion of renal pelvis. **A,** *Excretory urogram.* Negative serpentine-like shadow or filling defect, crossing pelvis and dividing it into lateral half and medial half. **B,** *Combined angiopyelogram* shows that filling defect is result of large branch of renal artery compressing pelvis. (From Kreel, L., and Pyle, R.)

THE NORMAL CALYCES

The Major Calyces

Calyces may be divided into two segments; namely, major and minor (Fig. 4-50A; see also Fig. 4-21). In the typical normal case the major calyx is the larger. It begins at the periphery of the pelvis and extends to its junction with the minor calyces. Each major calyx may be divided into three parts: the *base*, which is adjacent to the pelvis; the *isthmus* or *infundibulum*, which is the long tubular portion; and the *apex* or terminal portion, from which one or more minor calyces project. The form and size of the major calyces are subject to wide variation. As mentioned before, although anatomically the renal pelvis in most instances appears to have only two major calyces (Fig. 4-50B), from a urographic standpoint a third or middle calyx is usually apparent and in some cases a fourth or even more major calyces may be seen (Figs. 4-51 through 4-54; see also Fig. 4-21).

The Minor Calyces

The minor calyces arise from the terminal portion (apex) of a major calyx. Each minor calyx consists of two parts, the *calyx proper,* which is the short tubular projection beginning at the apex of the major calyx, and the *fornix,* which is the portion that surrounds the conical renal papilla. The *number of minor calyces* which arise from each major calyx is extremely variable, and there may be more fornices than minor calyces. This subject has been discussed previously. As has been explained elsewhere, a minor calyx is formed by the conical renal papilla projecting down into a calyx, much as one would poke the end of a finger into a rubber ball. It is apparent, therefore, that the urographic appearance of the normal minor calyx will depend on the plane in which it is viewed. In the urogram of the typical normal renal pelvis most of the calyces are projected laterally so that minor calyces are seen in profile. When viewed from this angle, the tip or fornix of a minor calyx appears as a small, hollowed-out pyramidal depression fashioned to receive the conical papilla. The periphery of this depression is formed by the contrast medium in the fornix of the calyx and the characteristic appearance is spoken of as the *terminal irregularity of the calyx* (see Figs. 4-16, 4-21, 4-26, 4-28, 4-50, 4-54, 4-58, and 4-64).

Inasmuch as the minor calyces project in different planes, not all of the minor calyces can be viewed in profile in any one urogram. It will be observed (Figs. 4-55 and 4-56) that some minor calyces appear as perfectly round areas of contrast medium with no hollowed-out area visible. The reason for this is apparent, since such calyces are viewed "head on" parallel to their long axis. Therefore, one sees the shadow cast by the contrast medium, which outlines the entire circumference of the fornix, as well as the calyx itself.

The tendency to variation in the size, shape, and number of the major and minor calyces is extremely marked. This wide variation is chiefly responsible for the difficulty in learning to recognize the many types of normal urograms. For this reason a large selection of normal urograms has been included in this chapter.

Difficulties in Distinguishing Major From Minor Calyces

Though one speaks quite positively of major and minor calyces, it is at times rather difficult to distinguish one from the other (Figs. 4-57 and 4-58). The reason for this is the multitude of variations in size, shape, and type of branching of the calyces found in the normal kidney.

In discussing the normal major calyx, it would be of help if one could ascribe to it certain definite dimensions. If such were the case, one could say that calyces which were larger or smaller than this were definitely pathologic. Unfortunately, this is

not possible. In Figure 4–59 is seen a urogram of a kidney with calyces almost
twice as broad as those seen in Figure
4–51, yet it is apparent from the normal
terminal calyces that there has been no
obstruction to produce dilatation. Occasionally a case is seen with only two ab-
breviated major calyces and with minor
calyces so small that they are visualized
only with difficulty (Fig. 4–60). Such a
urogram suggests a pathologic lesion, until it is examined more carefully. In some
cases, partial or complete obliteration of
the major calyces gives the impression
that the minor calyces come directly off
the pelvis (Figs. 4–61, 4–62, and 4–63). At
times one is confronted by a pelvis similar
in type to that seen in lower animals in
which only a pelvis seems to be present,
with no major calyces and very short minor calyces attached directly to the pelvis.

Long Extrarenal Type of Calyces. Excessively long major calyces are not uncommon (Fig. 4–64). The upper calyx is

most often the one involved and in some
instances may be regarded as forming a
bifid pelvis (Fig. 4–65). Elongated calyces
are very likely to be confused with the
pathologic lengthening found in cases of
renal tumor. The difference is that normal
minor calyces arise from the tips of the
calyces in the normal case (Fig. 4–66) but
not in the case of renal tumor. Elongated
major calyces, especially when they arise
from an elongated type of pelvis, often
assume the characteristic formation called
spider-leg pelvis.

Bridging of Calyces. When a major calyx is tortuous, it may cause some confusion as it crosses or recrosses other calyces. The apparent "bridging of the calyces" or "anastomosis of the calyces"
(Fig. 4–67) is explained by the crossing of
calyces in different planes. Large major
calyces which seem to replace the renal
pelvis, as found in the "branching of the
ureter" of the lower animals, have been
previously described.

(*Text continued on page 304.*)

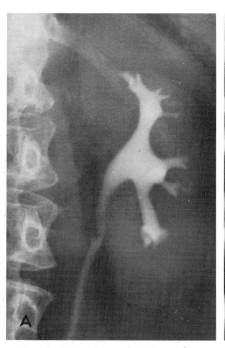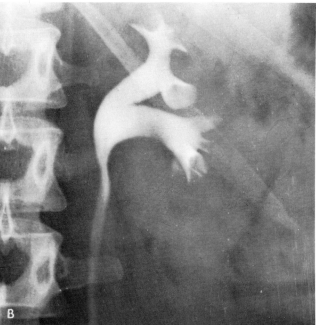

Figure 4–50. Normal major and minor calyces. **A** and **B**, *Left retrograde pyelograms.* Only two major
calyces are present.

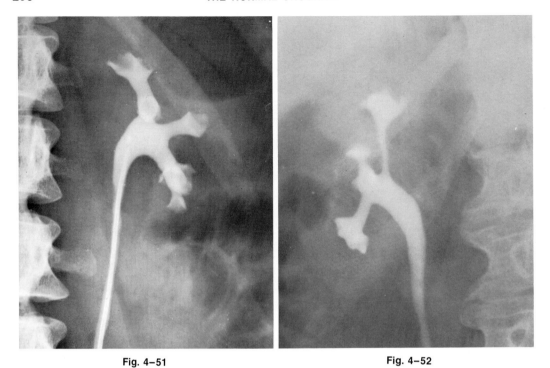

Fig. 4–51   Fig. 4–52

Figure 4–51. *Left retrograde pyelogram.* **Normal.** Three definite major calyces.
Figure 4–52. *Right retrograde pyelogram.* Oblique view. **Middle calyx somewhat rudimentary and** projected in posteroanterior plane.

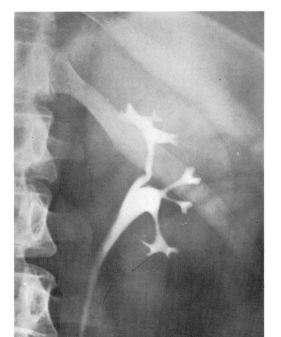

Figure 4–53. *Left retrograde pyelogram.* **Normal.** Might be interpreted as having four major calyces.

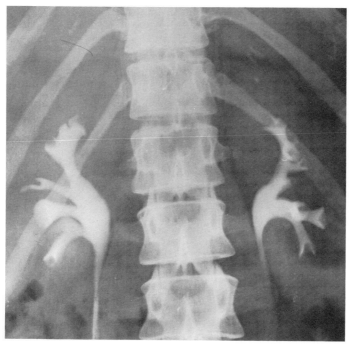

Figure 4–54. *Bilateral retrograde pyelogram.* **Asymmetry of kidneys.** Right kidney might be interpreted as having four major calyces.

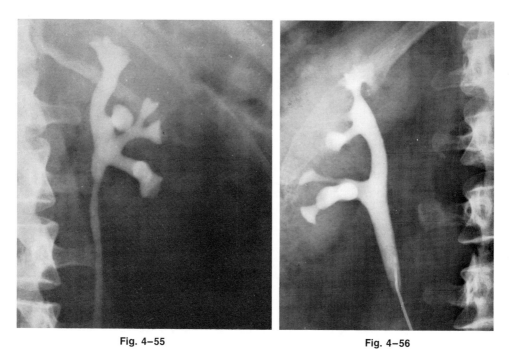

Fig. 4–55   Fig. 4–56

Figure 4–55. *Left retrograde pyelogram.* **Normal minor calyces** seen both in profile and "head-on." They are of broad, flaring type.

Figure 4–56. *Retrograde pyelogram.* **Normal.** Some of minor calyces seen "head-on."

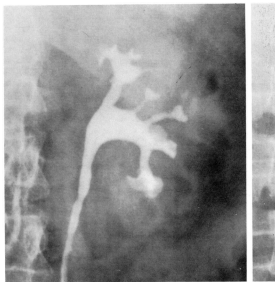

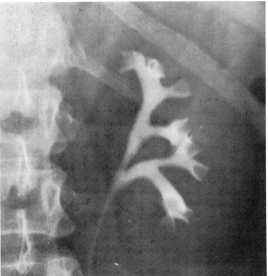

Fig. 4-57
Fig. 4-58

Figures 4-57 and 4-58. *Left retrograde pyelograms.* **Normal.** Difficult to distinguish major from minor calyces.

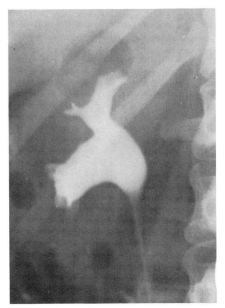

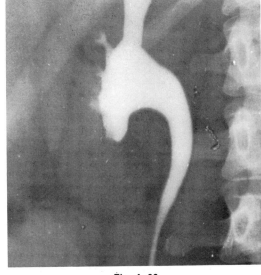

Fig. 4-59
Fig. 4-60

Figure 4-59. *Right retrograde pyelogram.* **Normal.** Broad major calyces.
Figure 4-60. *Right retrograde pyelogram.* **Normal.** Rudimentary or diminutive type of lower and middle major calyces.

Fig. 4–61

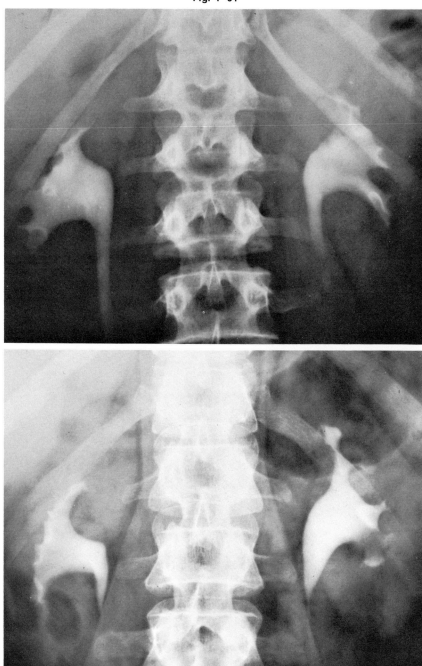

Fig. 4–62

Figures 4–61 and 4–62. *Excretory urograms.* Difficult to make out definite major calyces, especially in right kidneys. Minor calyces appear to come directly off pelvis.

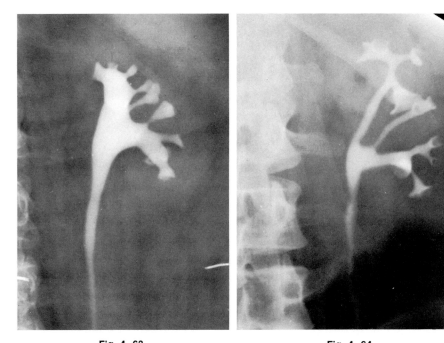

Fig. 4–63   **Fig. 4–64**

Figure 4–63. *Left retrograde pyelogram.* **Normal.** Diminutive type of calyces.
Figure 4–64. *Left retrograde pyelogram.* **Normal.** Unusually long major calyces.

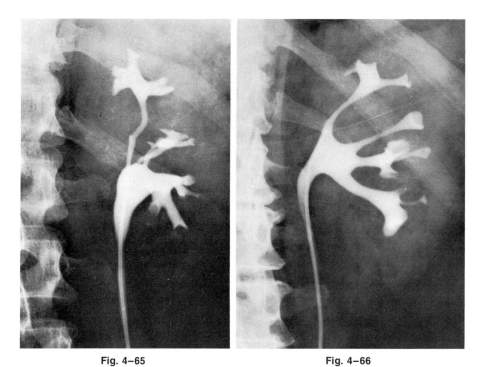

Fig. 4–65   **Fig. 4–66**

Figure 4–65. *Retrograde pyelogram.* **Normal.** Long upper calyx can be regarded as attempt at duplication. Note bridging of middle calyces.
Figure 4–66. *Retrograde pyelogram.* **Extrarenal pelvis with excessively long calyces.** Picture might be confused with renal tumor. Presence of normal terminal irregularities of all minor calyces demonstrates that calyces are normal.

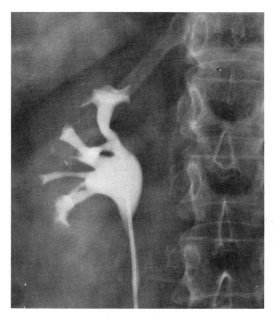

Figure 4–67. *Right retrograde pyelogram.* **Normal.** Overlapping calyces give impression of bridging of calyces.

Composite Type of Minor Calyces. Variations in the urographic appearance of the minor calyces no doubt cause more confusion in interpretation than does any other factor. In the section discussing the anatomy of the kidney, it was pointed out that the number of minor calyces may vary from 4 to 12. Some minor calyces receive more than one papilla, so that more than one fornix is necessary. Therefore, there may be more fornices than minor calyces. Composite pyramids with multiple papillae are most commonly found in the poles of the kidney. The average number of minor calyces seen in a kidney is 6 to 8. Occasionally kidneys are seen with only 3 or 4 minor calyces. On the other hand, kidneys with an excessive number of minor calyces are occasionally seen (Fig. 4–68). When a composite pyramid with multiple papillae is encountered, the minor calyx serving it may be of considerable size. Such an arrangement may give rise to the *T-shaped or flaring calyx* containing multiple fornices (Figs. 4–69 and 4–70). In most cases the fornices arising from the various parts of the minor calyx may be quite easily recognized. In other cases, however, it may be extremely difficult to demonstrate the position of the fornices, a fact which evidently results from the peculiar plane in which the fornices project. At times a minor calyx serving multiple papillae may be so large that it presents the largest cavity in the entire kidney. In such a case it may be difficult at times to distinguish a normal calyx from a pathologic calycectasis (Figs. 4–71 through 4–74).

Widely Cupped Minor Calyces. Even though a minor calyx is single and serves only one papilla, its form may vary widely in different kidneys. The typical "terminal irregularity" of the minor calyx has been previously described. The most common departure from the typical normal variety is the large cupped calyx which suggests the presence of large, broad papillae (Figs. 4–75 through 4–78). This "cupping" is usually increased if the calyx is overdistended. If "cupping" is exaggerated, a *trumpet or bell type of calyx* is produced (Figs. 4–79, 4–80, and 4–81).

Calyces Obscuring Each Other; Calyces Projected in Anteroposterior Plane Seen "Head-On." It is not always possible in a single urogram to visualize all of the minor calyces. This is because the calyces are projected in different planes and may be partially obscured by the contrast medium in the pelvis or in other calyces (Figs. 4–82 through 4–85). It is usually not necessary, however, to resort to supplementary urograms taken at different angles, for in most cases a satisfactory diagnosis can be made if the urograms are carefully studied. One of the most common causes of error in interpretation of urograms is to make a diagnosis of calycectasis, when in reality one is observing a normal calyx projected "head-on."

In the usual urogram not all of the minor calyces are clearly outlined, some appearing more or less rounded and indefinite in shape, with none of the characteristic terminal irregularities. This is no doubt due to such factors as the amount of medium that the fornix is able to hold, whether or not the fornix is incompletely filled or overdistended, and the plane in which the calyx is projecting. As a general rule, however, one can tell from the appearance of the well-visualized minor calyces whether or not the others are within normal limits.

Renal Sinus Lipomatosis (Renal Fibrolipomatosis). As was pointed out earlier in this chapter, small to moderate amounts of loose fatty and fibrous tissue are always present in the renal sinus surrounding the pelvis and calyces in the renal hilum. In some instances, however, the accumulation of excessive amounts of fat in the renal sinus produces a condition known as *renal sinus lipomatosis* (Faegenburg, Bosniak, and Evans; Olsson and Weiland; Simril and Rose). This condition may be a normal variant associated with extrarenal pelvis and anomalous elongated calyces (Fig. 4–86), but it is most often encountered in obese individuals (Fig. 4–87). In other instances, especially in older patients, it is associated with loss of renal parenchyma from arteriosclerotic ischemia, infection, or infarction. In these instances it has been referred to as *fibrolipomatosis* (Olsson and Weiland) since fibrosis may be a prominent feature (Fig. 4–88). The importance of this condition results from its frequent simulation of multiple peripelvic masses, owing to the elongation and flaring of the calyces (Fig. 4–89). Occasionally, the deposition of fat simulates a solitary peripelvic mass (Fig. 4–90). Renal sinus lipomatosis can be differentiated from renal tumor by nephrotomography (Fig. 4–91) and renal arteriography, but it is often difficult to distinguish this condition from multiple small peripelvic cysts.

(Text continued on page 315.)

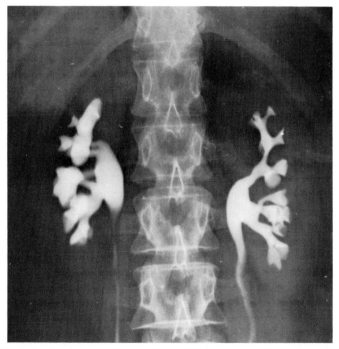

Figure 4–68.   *Bilateral retrograde pyelogram.* **Normal.** Excessive number of minor calyces. (Also called *multiplicity of calyces.*) Overdistention of right renal pelvis.

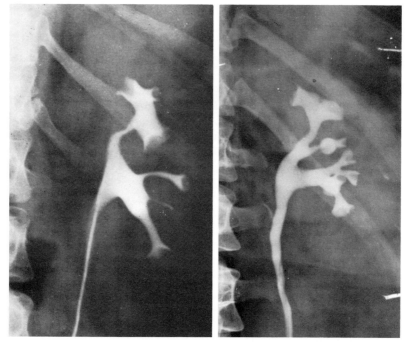

Fig. 4–69   Fig. 4–70

Figures 4–69 and 4–70. *Left retrograde pyelograms.* **Normal.** Composite, T-shaped upper calyx.

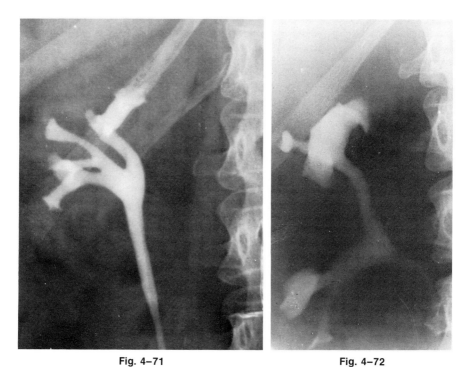

Fig. 4–71   Fig. 4–72

Figure 4–71. *Right retrograde pyelogram.* Unusual variation of composite, T-shaped upper calyx. It is impossible to demonstrate position of fornices.

Figure 4–72. *Right retrograde pyelogram.* **Normal.** Composite upper calyx larger than renal pelvis.

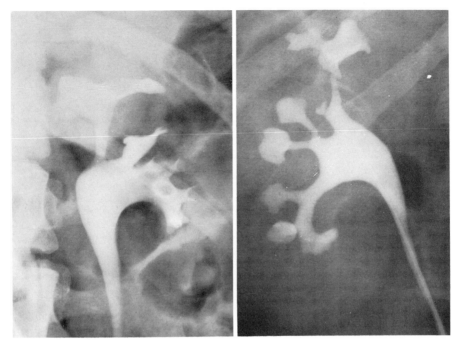

Fig. 4–73   Fig. 4–74

Figures 4–73 and 4–74. *Retrograde pyelograms.* Composite T-shaped upper calyx.

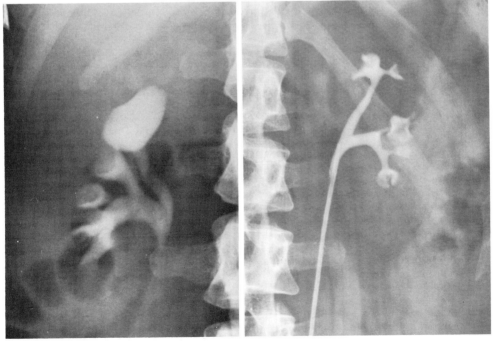

Fig. 4–75   Fig. 4–76

Figure 4–75. *Excretory urogram.* Normal. Composite upper calyx of right kidney, which could be interpreted as calycectasis, but probably is due to multiple broad papillae being served by one composite calyx.
Figure 4–76. *Left retrograde pyelogram.* Normal. Large calyces, produced by broad papillae.

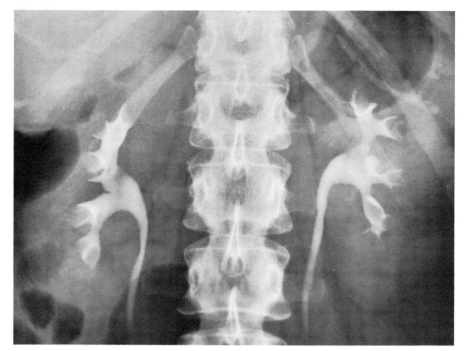

Figure 4–77. *Excretory urogram.* Broad cupped calyces.

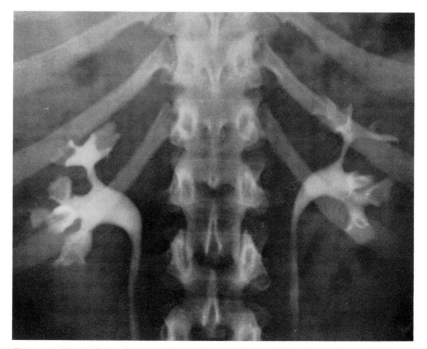

Figure 4–78. *Bilateral retrograde pyelogram.* Normal. Broad cup-shaped calyces.

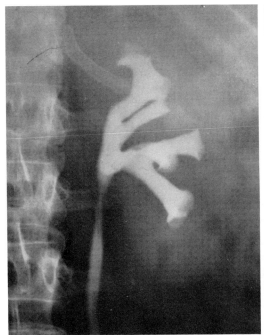

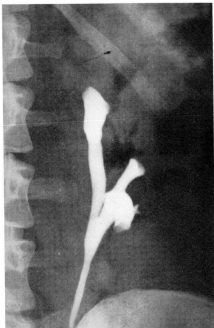

Fig. 4–79   Fig. 4–80

Figures 4–79 and 4–80. *Left retrograde pyelograms.* **Normal.** Exaggerated cupped calyces, which have been described as *trumpet* or *bell* calyces.

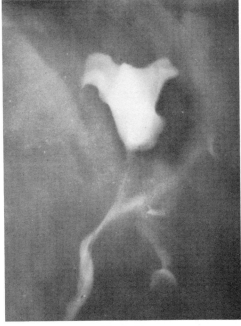

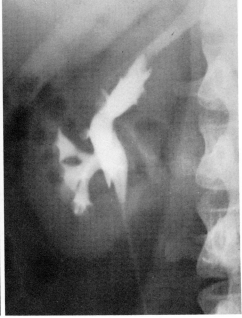

Fig. 4–81   Fig. 4–82

Figure 4–81. *Left retrograde pyelogram.* **Composite type of calyx,** having appearance of flower.
Figure 4–82. *Right retrograde pyelogram.* **Normal.** Some calyces are projected in anteroposterior plane, so that they are obscured by pelvis and other calyces.

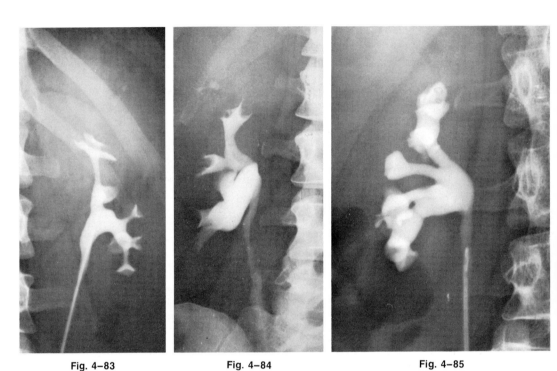

| Fig. 4–83 | Fig. 4–84 | Fig. 4–85 |

Figure 4–83. *Left retrograde pyelogram.* Some calyces are in anteroposterior plane and are obscured by major calyx.

Figure 4–84. *Right retrograde pyelogram.* **Normal.** Calyces overlying other calyces and pelvis, which causes confusion in interpretation.

Figure 4–85. *Right retrograde pyelogram.* **Normal.** Unusual variations of cupped calyces. Minor calyces tend to overlie each other and major calyces, so that delineation is not perfect.

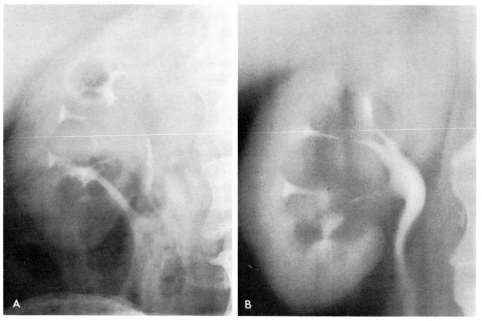

Figure 4–86. Renal sinus lipomatosis. **A,** *Excretory urogram.* Extrarenal pelvis with elongated and distorted calyces suggesting peripelvic mass. **B,** *Nephrotomogram.* Large collection of radiolucent fat is present in renal sinus.

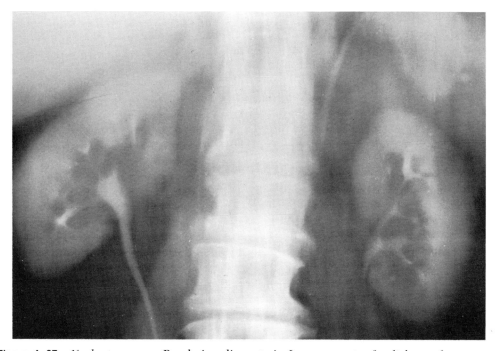

Figure 4–87. *Nephrotomogram.* **Renal sinus lipomatosis.** Large amounts of radiolucent fat are present in renal sinuses of both kidneys of obese patient weighing 220 lb.

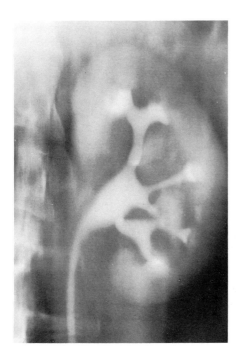

Figure 4–88. *Nephrotomogram.* **Renal sinus lipomatosis.** Calyces are somewhat anomalous. Renal cortex is thinned and considerable fat is present in renal sinus.

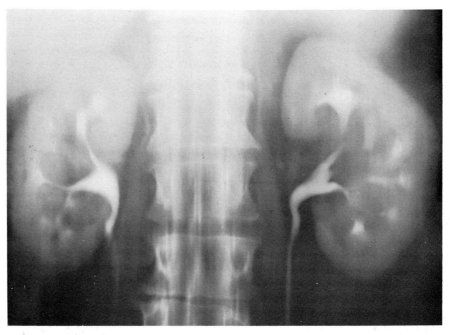

Figure 4–89. *Nephrotomogram.* **Renal sinus lipomatosis.** There is considerable flaring of calyces of both kidneys suggesting presence of multiple peripelvic cysts.

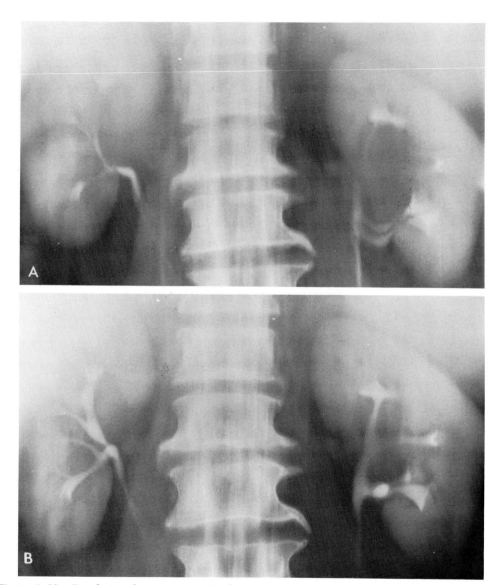

Figure 4–90. Renal sinus lipomatosis. **A,** *Nephrotomogram.* Adipose tissue, simulating peripelvic cysts, involving renal sinus of both kidneys of man 5′ 7½″ tall, weighing 226 lb. **B,** *Nephrotomogram,* 4 months later, after loss of 30 lb. Masses have disappeared, and pelvis and calyces have returned to normal.

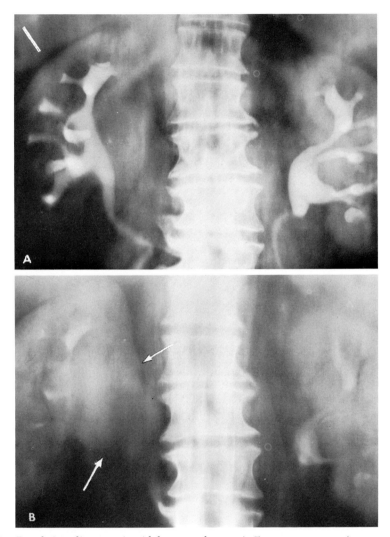

Figure 4–91. Renal sinus lipomatosis with hypernephroma. A, *Excretory urogram (tomogram)*. Extrarenal pelvis and flaring of calyces bilaterally. There is suggestion of mass on medial aspect of right kidney. **B,** *Nephrotomogram, nephrographic phase.* **Hypernephroma in hilum of right kidney** (*arrows*) **with bilateral renal sinus lipomatosis.**

FACTORS IN INTERPRETATION OF PYELOGRAMS AND UROGRAMS

Tendency to Symmetry of Renal Pelves in Same Individual

No matter how experienced one becomes in urographic interpretation, there will be times when he is confronted with an unusual pyelographic outline of a kidney in which it is almost impossible to decide whether the condition is pathologic or only an atypical variety of normal. Such questions often can be settled if a urogram is made of the opposite kidney. There is a distinct tendency toward symmetry in configuration of the kidneys in each individual (see Fig. 4–6). If a urogram of the opposite kidney is much the same in appearance as that of the kidney in question, a pathologic lesion usually can be excluded.

Unusual, Bizarre Pyelograms of Normal Kidneys

As can be surmised from the foregoing discussion, it is as difficult to describe a normal pyelogram as it is to describe a normal face; there are scarcely two alike. The following group of unusual pyelograms would no doubt raise suspicion in the minds of many urologists and radiologists, both experienced and inexperienced. After careful consideration of clinical data and review with several experienced physicians, they are presented here as variations of normal (Figs. 4–92 through 4–98).

Influence of Pelvic and Ureteral Peristalsis on the Urogram

Physiologists have shown that urine is propelled to the bladder from the kidneys by the peristaltic activity of the muscles in the wall of the pelvis and ureter. Jarre and Cumming (1930; 1934), by means of roentgenoscopy and serial pyelography, have demonstrated this action and Campbell (1966) as well as Becker and Pollack have studied it with cinefluorography. It has been observed that in the normal individual, peristaltic activity begins in the periphery of the pelvis and proceeds toward the ureteropelvic junction and thence down the ureter. In Campbell's (1966) cases studied by cinefluorography, the first detectable movement occurred at the ureteropelvic junction in 76% and in the renal pelvis or infundibulum or both in 24%. This movement was promptly followed by constriction of the ureteropelvic junction and ureteral peristalsis. A somewhat different situation has been noted in the presence of a bifid-type renal pelvis or partial duplication. In these cases the peristaltic activity is usually initiated at a pacemaker or nodal point in either the upper or the lower segment. Becker and Pollack and Campbell (1967) have found that the peristalsis originates in the infundibulum of the upper segment in most of these cases. The peristaltic contraction proceeds normally downward from its nodal point in these cases but in passing the point of bifurcation of the ureter it commonly initiates a retrograde peristaltic contraction which travels upward in the bifid or duplicated segment. (See also Figs. 12-136 and 12-148.) At times this may distend this segment of the renal collecting system (Fig. 4–99). Campbell (1967) observed retrograde peristalsis of this type in 84% of his cases and speculated that it probably occurs throughout the patient's lifetime and is of no clinical significance except in the event of pathogenic infection when serious and chronic infection or even septicemia may result. In our own experience we have found retrograde peristalsis to be very common in this type of anomaly and have noted that patients with atrophy of one (usually the lower) segment due to pyelonephritis have retrograde peristalsis in the diseased segment in most instances. The urograms of Jarre and Cumming, though rather difficult to reproduce on paper, show different contours of the pelvis when in "systole" and "diastole" and explain many of the variations seen in ordinary urograms. For instance, there is no doubt that many of the urograms in which the outline of the pelvis and calyces is rather "skeletal" in appearance are the result of the exposure being made at the time when the pelvis was in a state of systole (Fig. 4–100A and B). It is this physiologic activity that is responsible for most of the so-called strictures at or below the ureteropelvic junction which in reality are only the result of peristaltic contraction (Fig. 4–101).

While peristaltic activity in the calyces cannot be identified fluoroscopically or on cineroentgenography, some degree of activity must be present. Narath, by histologic section, demonstrated the presence of muscular tissue in the walls of the minor calyces (both fornix and calyx proper) and major calyces. In Figure 4–102A and B is demonstrated his hypothesis of the muscular activity in the alternate filling and emptying of the calyx. He has substantiated his hypothesis, to his satisfaction, by means of urograms which he interpreted as demonstrating the minor calyces in the various stages of filling and emptying. He holds that the collecting phase is brought about by relaxation of the musculus levator fornicis and sphincter fornicis, assisted by the contraction of the upper part of the musculus longitudinalis calycis, which helps the sphincter fornicis to relax. After filling has been completed, the emptying phase is ushered in by relaxation of the musculus sphincter calycis and contraction of the lower part of the musculus longitudinalis calycis; after this the sphincter fornicis closes, helped by relaxation of the upper part of the musculus longitudinalis calycis, and the levator fornicis contracts to pull the mucous membrane of the fornix over the papilla and prevent regurgitation of the urine from the pelvis into the papil-

lary ducts. If this hypothesis is correct (and Narath's evidence is quite convincing) one can easily explain the many variations seen in the appearance of the same calyces.

Difference in Appearance of Excretory Urogram and Retrograde Urogram

When one considers the peristaltic activity of the pelvis, calyces, and ureter as described in the preceding paragraphs, it is not difficult to understand why a urogram made in the retrograde manner may be considerably different in appearance from one made by the excretory method, especially when the patient is dehydrated, a small dose of contrast medium is injected, and no ureteral compression is used. In the excretory urogram the peristaltic activity is not interfered with and is constantly in progress, so that unless definite obstruction is present, there will be a tendency to incomplete filling, which is the antithesis of overdistention. For this reason the pelvis and calyces are likely to appear somewhat small and narrow, all of the calyces are likely to be incompletely filled with medium, and seldom will a ureter be entirely filled. Offsetting these shortcomings of the excretory urogram, however, are the inherent faults of the retrograde urogram, among which are distortion of the pelvis because of a coiled catheter; spasm of the ureter or ureteropelvic junction, simulating stricture but due to irritation by the catheter (Fig. 4–103); overdistention of the pelvis and calyces (Fig. 4–104); and rupture of a calyx, or pyelorenal backflow (Fig. 4–105). There is no doubt that if reasonably complete visualization can be obtained by excretory urography, it gives a more accurate picture of the urinary tract from both an anatomic and a physiologic point of view than does retrograde urography.

(Text continued on page 323.)

Fig. 4–92

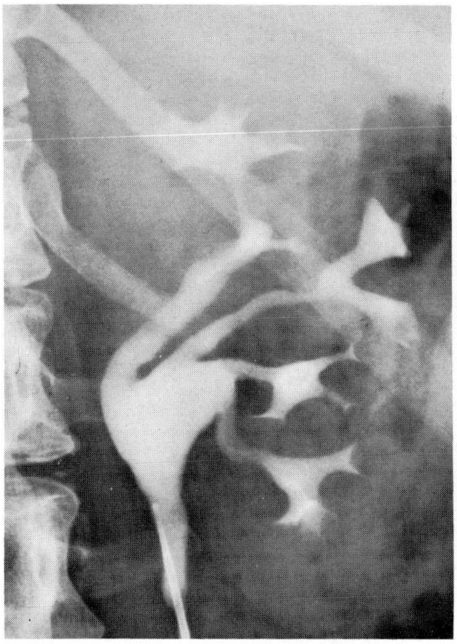

Fig. 4–93

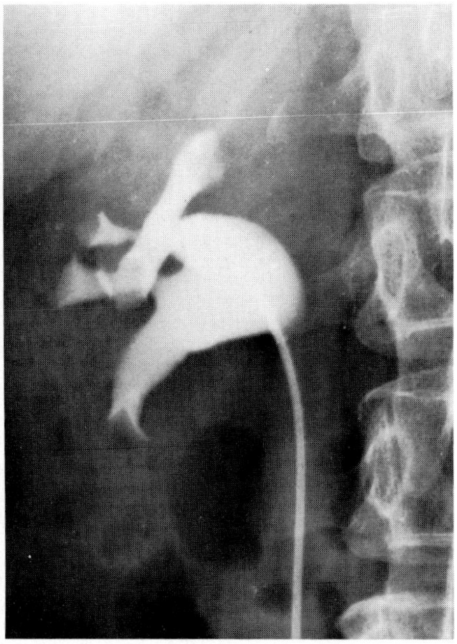

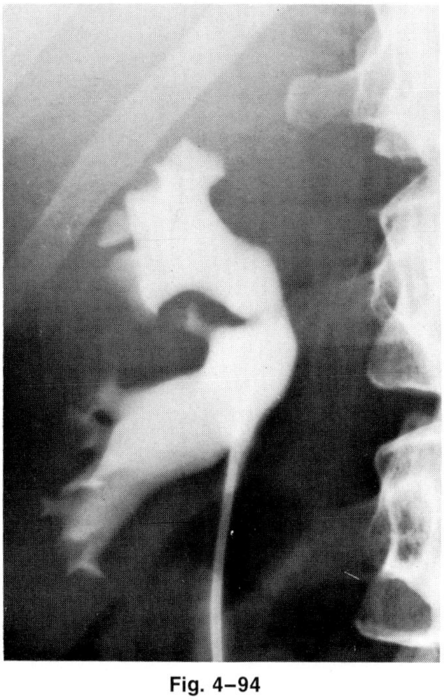

Fig. 4–94

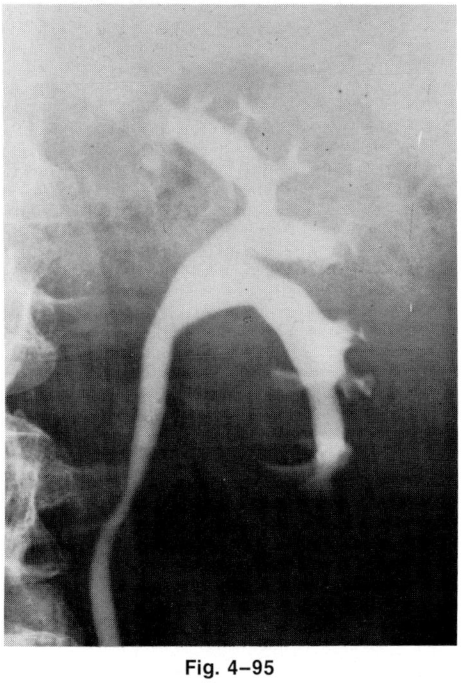

Fig. 4–95

Figures 4–92, 4–93, 4–94, and 4–95. *Pyelograms.* Variations of normal.

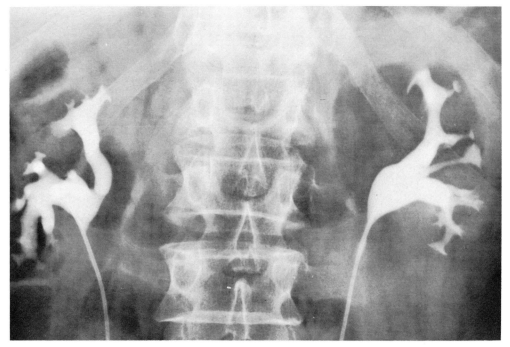

Figure 4–96. *Pyelogram.* Normal.

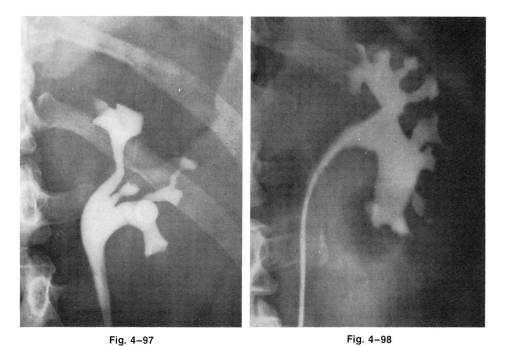

| **Fig. 4–97** | **Fig. 4–98** |

Figure 4–97. *Pyelogram.* Normal.
Figure 4–98. *Left retrograde pyelogram.* **Normal.** Minor calyces project in different planes, so that not all are seen in profile. Some calyces are seen "head-on" and overlapping other calyces.

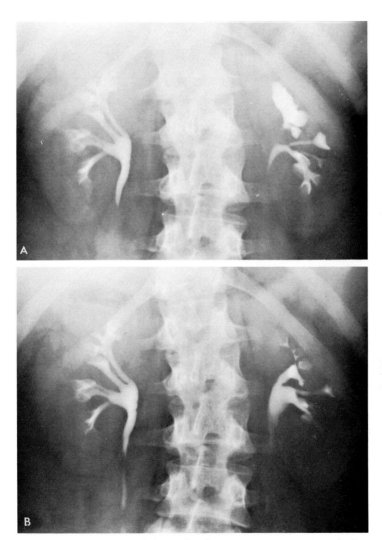

Figure 4–99. Peristaltic contraction of left renal pelvis. *Excretory urograms.* **A,** During systole. Note unusual dilatation of left upper-pole calyx (retrograde peristalsis?). **B,** During diastole. (Courtesy of Dr. M. M. Labardini and Dr. R. M. Nesbit.)

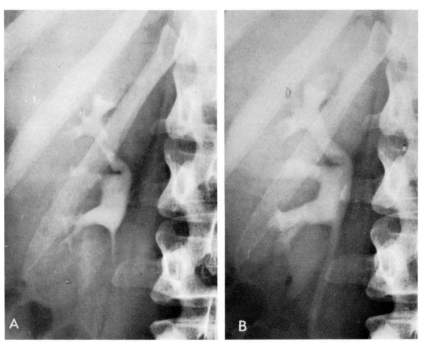

Figure 4–100.   Differences in contour of pelviocalyceal system as result of systole and diastole. *Excretory urograms.* **A,** Five-minute film. **B,** Twenty-minute film.

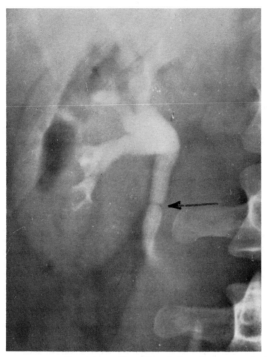

Figure 4–101. *Excretory urogram.* **Transient ring-like defect in ureter** below ureteropelvic junction (*arrow*). Not to be confused with peristaltic wave.

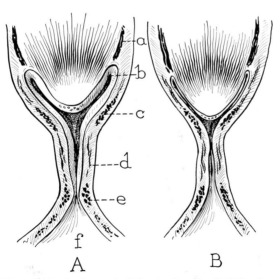

Figure 4–102. **Peristaltic activity of calyces. A,** Calyx in diastole. **B,** Calyx in systole. *a,* Musculus levator fornicis; *b,* fornix; *c,* musculus sphincter fornicis; *d,* musculus longitudinalis calycis; *e,* musculus sphincter calycis; *f,* true renal pelvis. (From Narath, P. A.)

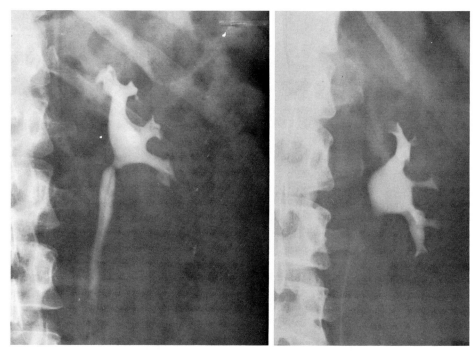

Fig. 4–103   **Fig. 4–104**

Figure 4–103. *Left retrograde pyelogram.* **Normal.** Constriction of ureteropelvic junction due to spasm resulting from irritation produced by ureteral catheter.

Figure 4–104. *Left retrograde pyelogram.* **Normal.** Overdistention of normal renal pelvis.

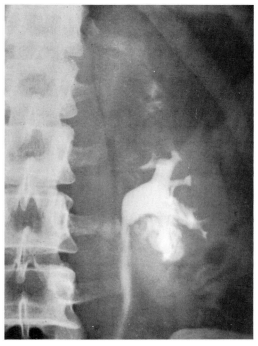

Figure 4–105. *Left retrograde pyelogram.* **Duplication of renal pelvis.** Lower half of duplicated renal pelvis shows rupture and extravasation of medium in lower calyx. (Note residual medium in upper pelvis from previous pyelogram.)

Urographic Visualization of Collecting Tubules, So-called Tubular Ectasia

The typical "brush-like" shadows projecting peripherally from minor calyces in a retrograde pyelogram have long been considered evidence of pyelotubular backflow caused by an increase in pressure in the renal pelvis that forces the contrast medium into the collecting tubules. The observation that similar shadows occur with almost equal frequency in excretory urograms has stimulated a reevaluation of this phenomenon. Vermooten in 1951 studied this problem and found outlining of the collecting tubules in approximately 5% of all excretory urograms when the films were studied carefully. In about a third of the urograms he described a "thin veiled filling of a minor calyx with a soft brush-like end" which was often difficult to distinguish from a minor calyx except on close scrutiny. In the remainder, the typical brush-like appearance was apparent in various degrees, at least half of which would be apparent to even the most casual observer (Figs. 4–106*A* and *B* and 4–107). Most authorities (Palubinskas) now consider this appearance to be one manifestation of congenital dilatation (ectasia) of renal tubules, a part of the spectrum of tubular dilatation and cystic change seen in medullary sponge kidney (see discussion of medullary sponge kidney in Chapter 9).

Pyelorenal Backflow (Calycorenal Backflow)

Pyelorenal backflow is a general term applied to the condition which results when urographic medium passes beyond the confines of the renal pelvis and calyces. It is encountered principally in retrograde pyelography, although Narath has shown that it may also occur in excretory urography. For a detailed discussion of this interesting problem, the reader is referred to the original studies of Hinman, Lee-Brown and Laidley, Narath, Abeshouse, Stapor, and Jarre and Cumming (1930).

Generally speaking, two basic types of backflow are recognized: (1) backflow from the dome of the calyces and (2) tubular backflow. Group 1 includes *pyelovenous, pyelointerstitial,* and *pyelolymphatic backflow* and *pyelosinous transflow* (Narath). Group 2 includes only *pyelotubular backflow.** Stapor has recently restudied the questions of backflow and points out that all known types occur in the parapapillary part of the calyx and in the renal papilla. He suggests, therefore, that the term *calycorenal backflow* is more appropriate than the term *pyelorenal.* It seems, however, that because of long usage the older terms will probably prevail.

Pyelotubular Backflow. In this condition the collecting tubules are outlined as brush-like lines extending from the tips of the calyces. Formerly this appearance was considered to be the result of excessive pressure of contrast medium injected in the retrograde manner that forced the medium into the tubules (Figs. 4–108 through 4–111). Its relatively common occurrence in excretory urograms plus the findings of Vermooten, however, has introduced a new concept of this phenomenon.*

Pyelovenous Backflow. The conditions spoken of as *pyelovenous, pyelosinous,* and *pyelointerstitial backflow* incite a good deal of controversy. Most authors (Hinman; Hinman and Lee-Brown; Jarre and Cumming, 1930; and Lee-Brown and Laidley) have expressed the belief that each of these represents a rupture of a minor calyx with coincidental rupture of the small arcuate or interlobular veins which are in close apposition to the minor calyces, or extravasation into the interstitial renal tissue. Narath, on the other hand, has taken a different view, which seems to be well supported by his observa-

---

*See discussion of tubular ectasia, above, and that of medullary sponge kidney in Chapter 9.

tions and demonstration. In his opinion most of the conditions loosely called *pyelovenous backflow* result from a physiologic mechanism which he terms *pyelosinous transflow*. He has expressed the belief that the mucosa of the fornix of a minor calyx has the ability to absorb fluid in case of excess pressure, thus acting as a safety valve. He has shown that excess pressure may result not only from retrograde pyelography but also from the peristaltic activity of the pelvis and calyces, with or without a secondary obstruction such as a ureteral stone. The fluid thus absorbed passes into the closed renal sinus, around the calyces and pelvis, and accounts for the urographic appearance which is most often spoken of as *pyelovenous backflow*. He prefers to call this phenomenon *pyelosinous transflow* and describes various conformations seen, such as *horn-shaped, multiform, plane-like,* and *ribbon-like* (Figs. 4–112 through 4–117).

According to Narath, this "extravasated" medium is in most cases absorbed by the capillaries or lymphatics, but in some cases in which there has actually been a traumatic rupture of a minor calyx, arcuate or interlobular veins might also be torn and allow true *pyelovenous backflow* or, as he calls it, *sino-venous ingression* to occur. In such cases the arcuate and interlobular veins may be visualized, the most characteristic appearance of which is the typical arch formation above the calyx (Figs. 4–118, 4–119, and 4–120). Often these arches are not completely filled but nevertheless can be recognized if the pyelogram is carefully studied.

If this view be accepted, one must then limit the term *pyelointerstitial backflow* to those cases in which there seems to be a *gross extravasation* of medium into the interstitial tissue of the kidney. This is characterized by the complete lack of any form or contour characteristic of the other types described previously. It consists of irregular collections of extravasated medium varying from small single or mul-

tiple areas to cases in which the medium actually has penetrated to the periphery of the kidney and collected in pools under the true renal capsule (Figs. 4–121 through 4–127).

Pyelolymphatic Backflow. Pyelolymphatic backflow is a rather unusual condition which may be seen with both retrograde pyelography and excretory urography. In this condition, one or more lymphatic channels are visualized as they pass from the hilus of the kidney medialward to the periaortic lymph nodes. They appear as multiple thread-like lines of increased density, not more than 1 or 2 mm wide, which follow an irregular course (Figs. 4–128 through 4–132). The mechanism of the pyelographic visualization of these lymphatics is not entirely clear, although in normal cases it may represent lymphatic absorption of extravasated medium in the sinus renalis or as Stapor, Narath, and others have suggested, it may result from rapid reabsorption of medium through the intact mucosa of the fornix of the calyx. This condition may also be seen in patients suffering from *chyluria,* and in such a pathologic state the phenomenon is more easily explained. It is believed that in such cases the thoracic duct is obstructed from parasitic or nonparasitic causes. This results in a secondary dilatation of the lymphatics and the establishment of a collateral circulation. Rupture of one or more of these lymphatic vessels into the pelviocalyceal system can result in chyluria and accounts for the pyelolymphatic backflow seen urographically. (See discussion of chyluria, Chapter 17.)

Variations in Contour of Renal Parenchyma

Occasionally the *lateral margin of the kidney will appear to "bulge,"* and the urologist may suspect a tumor or cyst. Frimann-Dahl in 1961, in an excellent study of this phenomenon, noted that this occurs almost exclusively in the *left kidney* and is present in approximately 10% of urograms. It is best shown with nephrotomograms, which provide excellent outlines of the renal parenchyma (Figs. 4–133A and B and 4–134A and B). By means of aortograms and pyelograms, he concluded that the condition is most likely a developmental variation of normal, which he ascribed to the presence of an overriding spleen; the calyces and vascular pattern adapt to the renal contour. Moëll stated that the left kidney is always larger than the right.

A *lobulated lateral margin of the kidney* is considered to be the remains of fetal lobulation. It is particularly well shown in the nephrotomogram (Fig. 4–135). In addition, in rare cases, bizarre renal shapes are found which have no explanation other than that of congenital anomaly. These ordinarily can be distinguished from kidneys distorted by disease by the normal thickness of the renal cortex over each calyx and by the normal or near-normal calyx supplying each part of the anomalous kidney (Fig. 4–136).

(Text continued on page 338.)

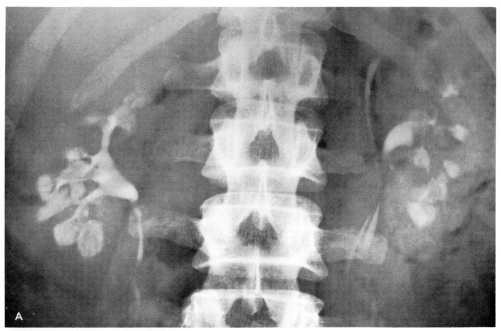

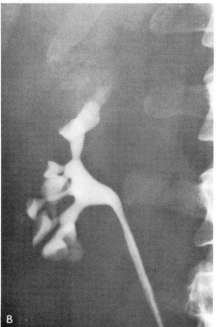

Figure 4–106. Visualization of collecting tubules.
A, *Excretory urogram.* Collecting tubules serving all
calyces of both kidneys are visible. (**Tubular ectasia,**
most marked on right. **Duplication of kidney on left.**)
B, *Retrograde pyelogram,* right kidney. Collecting
tubules of only upper and middle calyces are visualized as brush-like projections from tips of calyces.

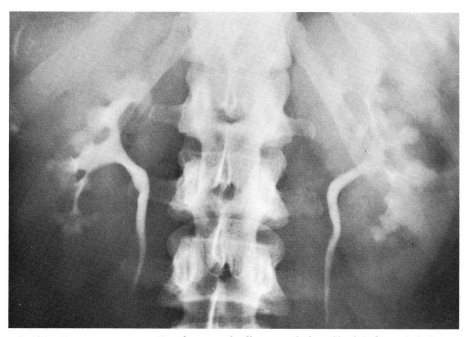

Figure 4–107. *Excretory urogram.* Visualization of collecting tubules of both kidneys (**tubular ectasia**).

Fig. 4–108

Fig. 4–109

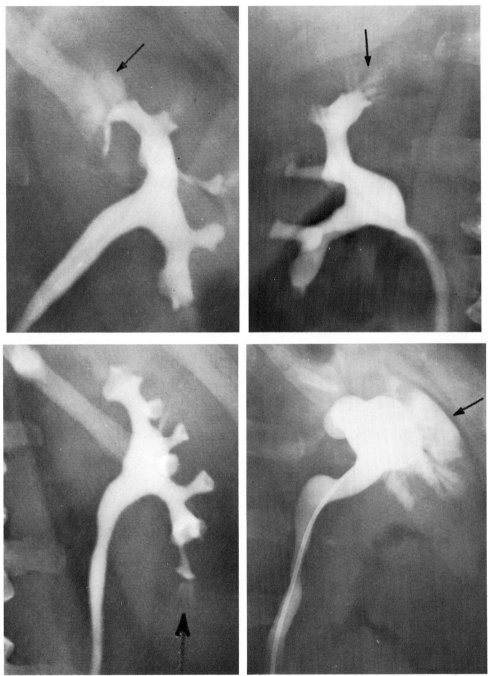

Fig. 4–110

Fig. 4–111

Figure 4–108. *Left retrograde pyelogram.* **Pyelotubular backflow** with typical tuft or brush-like appearance of medium radiating from tips of minor calyces. (See text.)

Figure 4–109. *Right retrograde pyelogram.* **Pyelotubular backflow.** (See text.)

Figure 4–110. *Left retrograde pyelogram.* **Pyelotubular backflow.** (See text.)

Figure 4–111. *Left retrograde pyelogram.* **Pyelotubular backflow in anomalous type of kidney.** (See text.)

Fig. 4–112

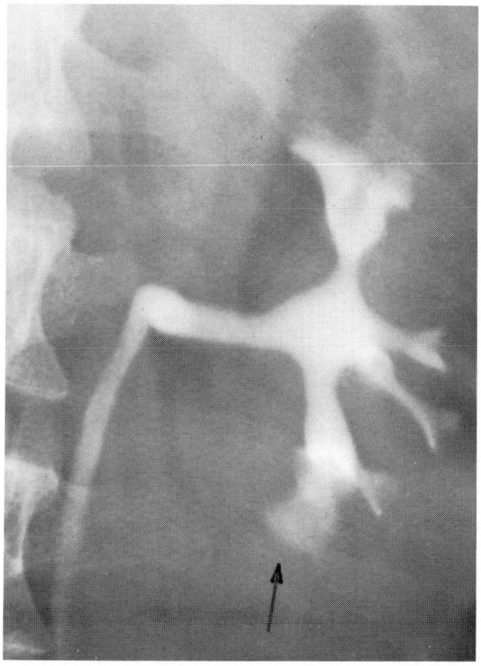

Fig. 4–113

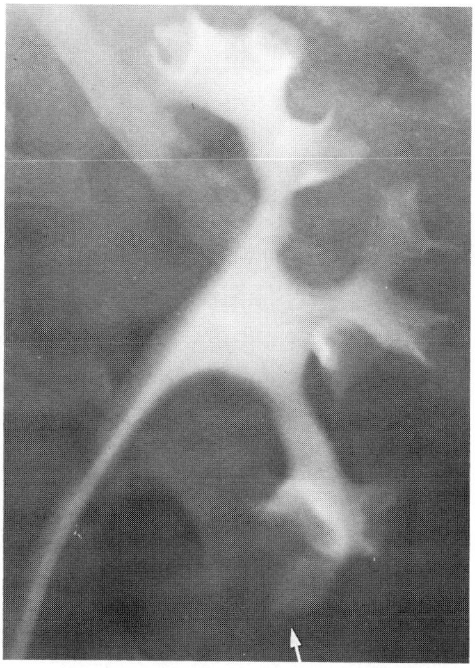

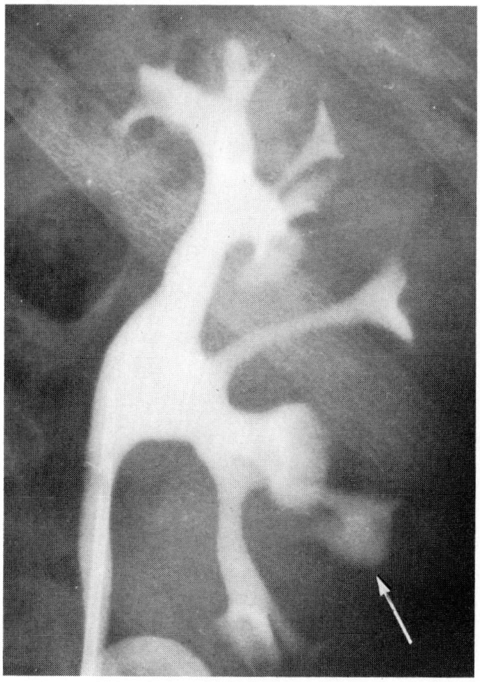

Fig. 4–114

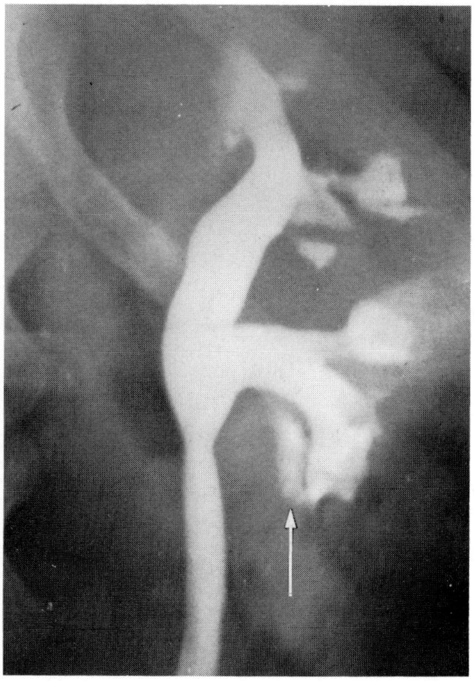

Fig. 4–115

Figures 4–112, 4–113, 4–114, and 4–115. *Left retrograde pyelograms.* Pyelosinous transflow. (See text.)

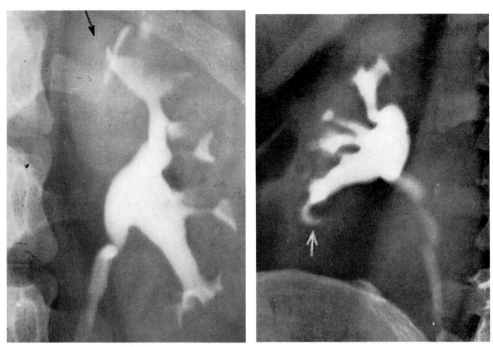

Fig. 4–116   Fig. 4–117

Figure 4–116. *Left retrograde pyelogram.* Pyelosinous transflow. (See text.)
Figure 4–117. *Right retrograde pyelogram.* Pyelosinous transflow. (See text.)

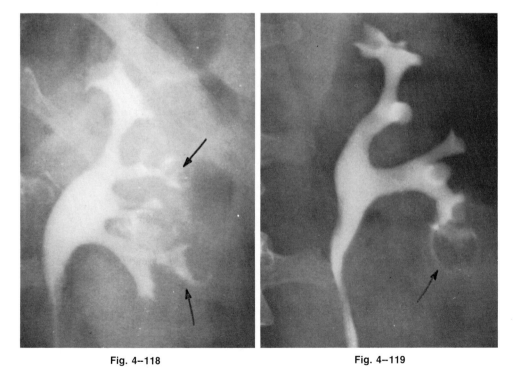

Fig. 4–118   Fig. 4–119

Figure 4–118. *Left retrograde pyelogram.* Pyelovenous backflow. (See text.)
Figure 4–119. *Left retrograde pyelogram.* Pyelovenous backflow. Excellent visualization of arcuate vessels. (See text.)

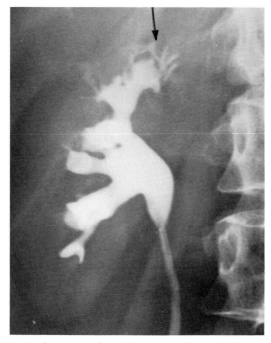

Figure 4–120. *Right retrograde pyelogram.* **Pyelovenous backflow.** (See text.)

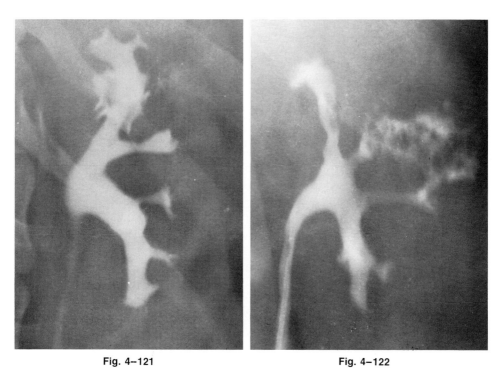

Fig. 4–121   Fig. 4–122

Figures 4–121 and 4–122. *Left retrograde pyelograms.* Extravasation of medium from calyces (pyelointerstitial backflow). (See text.)

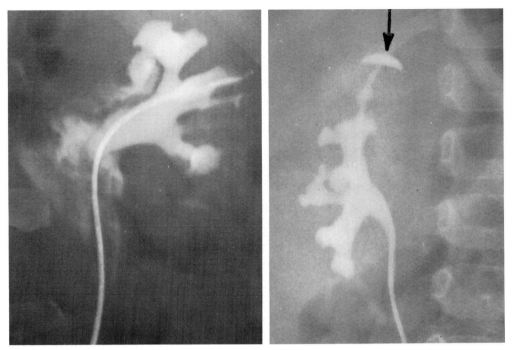

Fig. 4–123   Fig. 4–124

Figure 4–123. *Left retrograde pyelogram.* Extravasation of medium (pyelointerstitial backflow). (See text.)

Figure 4–124. *Right retrograde pyelogram.* Extravasation of medium from calyx (pyelointerstitial back-flow). Medium has collected in pool under renal capsule. (See text.)

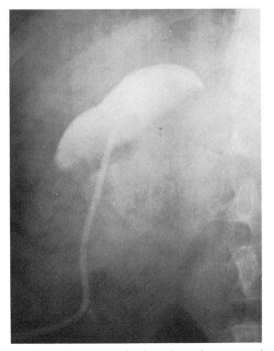

Figure 4–125. *Right retrograde pyelogram,* made through nephrostomy tube. Catheter has perforated calyx and there is extravasation of medium under renal capsule. **Pyelointerstitial backflow.**

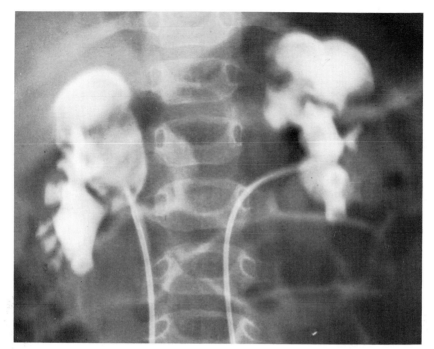

Figure 4–126. *Bilateral pyelogram.* Extravasation of medium which is collected under capsules of kidneys. Pyelointerstitial backflow. (See text.)

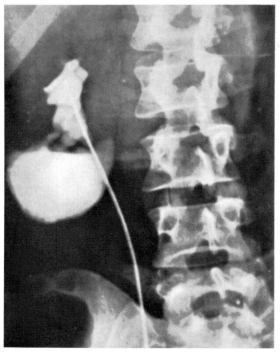

Figure 4–127. *Right retrograde pyelogram.* Extravasation of medium which is collecting under renal capsule (**pyelointerstitial backflow**). (From Williams, E. R.: Subcapsular Rupture of the Kidney—Case Report. Brit. J. Radiol. *14*:248 [July] 1941.) (See text.)

Fig. 4–128

Fig. 4–129

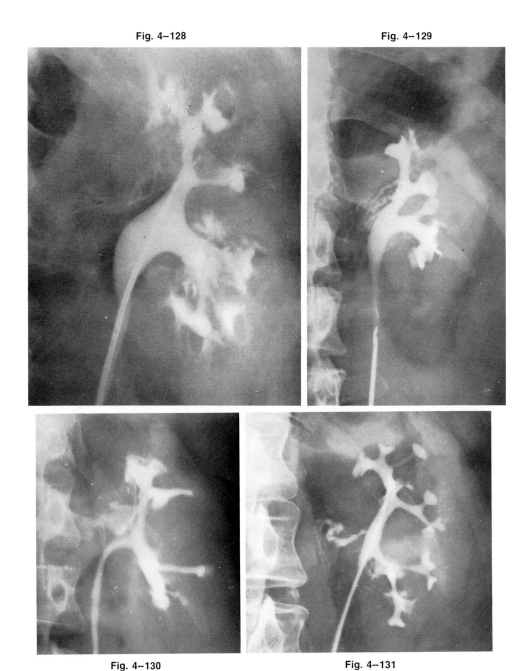

Fig. 4–130

Fig. 4–131

Figure 4–128. *Left retrograde pyelogram.* Extravasation of medium with **pyelolymphatic backflow.** Typical thread-like lines of medium which follow irregular course toward periaortic lymph nodes. (See text.)
Figures 4–129, 4–130, and 4–131. *Left retrograde pyelograms.* **Pyelolymphatic backflow.** (See text.)

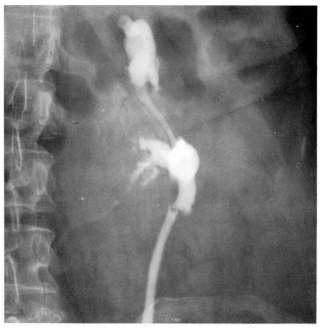

Figure 4–132. *Left retrograde pyelogram.* Unusual type of **duplication with malrotation.** Upper segment appears as composite, elongated upper calyx. **Pyelolymphatic backflow from lower calyces.** (See text.)

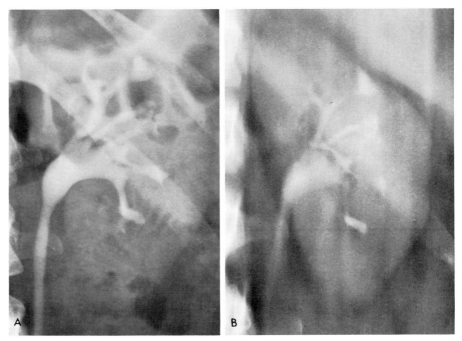

Figure 4–133.   Bulge on lateral margin of left kidney. There is small cortical scar with some blunting of underlying calyx on upper lateral aspect. **A**, *Excretory urogram*. **B**, *Nephrotomogram*. Renal outline more distinct. Lower margin of spleen well-delineated.

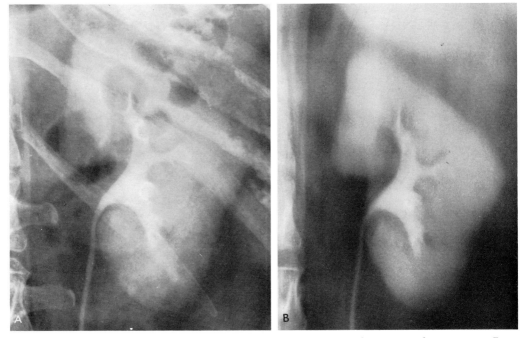

Figure 4–134.   A, *Excretory urogram*. **Bulge on lateral margin of left kidney. B**, *Nephrotomogram*. Parenchyma well-outlined. Normal calyces. **Variation of normal.** Note delineation of renal sinus with negative shadow of peripelvic fat.

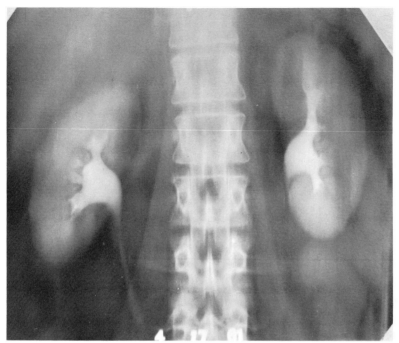

Figure 4–135. *Nephrotomogram.* **Irregular lateral margins of each kidney,** most likely remains of fetal lobulation.

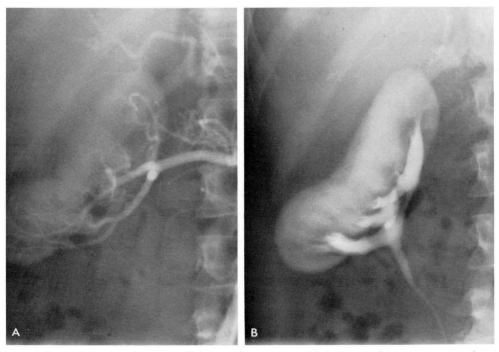

Figure 4–136. **Anomalous kidney. A,** *Renal arteriogram, arterial phase.* Renal arteries are normal. **B,** *Excretory urogram* with *arteriogram, late nephrographic phase.* **Renal parenchyma is anomalous in shape but** of normal thickness over entire kidney. **Extrarenal pelvis** with bizarre shape but otherwise normal calyces.

THE URETERS

Variations in Caliber

Because of inaccurate interpretation of urograms, the normal ureter has been too often the subject of injudicious surgical and manipulative treatment. It is highly important, therefore, that the roentgenologist and the urologist be familiar with the normal ureter in all of its urographic forms.

As has been described elsewhere, there are three main points of narrowing in the ureter, which are (1) the ureteropelvic junction, (2) where the ureter crosses the brim of the pelvis, and (3) the ureterovesical juncture. It is impossible to assert just what is the exact diameter of the normal ureter because of its wide limits of variation. It is important, therefore, that any urographic appearance of narrowing or dilatation be of a fairly marked degree before it is interpreted as being abnormal. It must also be remembered that the various parts of the ureter are not uniform in diameter. The beginning of the ureter at the ureteropelvic junction may present several varied forms. For instance, although a sphincter muscle at the ureteropelvic junction has not been demonstrated anatomically, from a urographic point of view contraction at this point from natural peristaltic activity or from irritation by a ureteral cathether is commonly seen (Fig. 4-137). This appearance may be contrasted with the long type of pelvis which merges so gradually with the ureter that one is unable to say where the pelvis ends and the ureter begins (see Fig. 4-37). At times this type of junction may give the impression of being a dilatation of the upper third of the ureter.

Another irregularity which at times results in erroneous urographic interpretation is the physiologic dilatation of the middle portion of the ureter, which is spoken of as the *spindle* (Fig. 4-138). The cause of this phenomenon is not definitely known, but it has been suggested that

it may be the result of a mild, incomplete obstruction at the brim of the pelvis where the ureter is narrowed and crosses the iliac vessels. At times this condition may be sufficiently marked to suggest pathologic ureterectasis.*

Position of Normal Ureter

Inasmuch as the position of the normal kidney is so inconstant, the course of the normal ureter is likewise difficult to define. The accepted anatomic description of the ureter has been given previously in this chapter and it applies to the majority of normal ureters seen urographically. It must be recognized, however, that great variations in the course of the normal ureter are encountered (Figs. 4-139 and 4-140), which must not be confused with pathologic conditions.

Diagnostic Errors From Incomplete Filling of Ureters

It is usually difficult to fill a ureter completely with contrast medium by either the retrograde or the excretory method. (See discussion of primary ureteral tumors, Chapter 10.) As a result incomplete filling is common in urography, and mistakes are likely to be made if this is not recognized. Apparent narrowings of the ureter (Fig. 4-141), filling defects, and ribbon-like areas of broadening and twisting (Figs. 4-142 and 4-143A, B, and C) are often seen as a result of incomplete filling. On the other hand, a ureter with definite pathologic dilatation may appear to be entirely normal if it is incompletely filled. When *air bubbles* are injected into the ureter with the contrast medium, they present a characteristic appearance which must not be confused with filling defects from clots of blood or tumor (Fig. 4-144).

When it is important that a ureter be well filled, the best method is to insert a

---

*See discussion of the right ovarian vein syndrome as a cause of ureteropyelectasis after pregnancy, Chapter 18.

snug bulb or acorn-tipped catheter just inside the ureteral orifice and inject contrast medium into the ureter from below upward (Fig. 4-145).

Ureteral Kinks and Strictures

Of all the variations of the normal ureter which have been misinterpreted and erroneously diagnosed as pathologic conditions, *kinks* and *strictures* probably hold the first place. As has been previously described, all kidneys possess a certain amount of mobility. If the excursion of the kidney is rather marked, as the kidney descends, the slack in the ureter must be taken up in some manner. This is usually done by the ureter bending on itself, forming a kink or becoming tortuous (Figs. 4-146, 4-147, and 4-148). Such deformities may be produced by descent of the kidney during deep inspiration or when the patient is in the erect position. In most cases if the patient is placed in the Trendelenburg position and instructed to exhale before the film is exposed, the kinks and curves in the ureter will disappear. If there is no pathologic dilatation of the renal pelvis above such kinks, certainly one is not justified in considering any symptoms to be the result of their presence.

Most *ureteral strictures* are diagnosed as such because the cystoscopist encounters difficulty on introducing or withdrawing a ureteral catheter or because of an evident area of narrowing in the ureterogram (Figs. 4-149 and 4-150). In most cases both findings are the result of *spasm of the ureter,* which was produced by irritation due to the passage of the ureteral catheter, or are the result of incomplete filling of the ureter. When the patient is under local anesthesia only, many ureters are extremely sensitive. Every cystoscopist knows that if a ureteral orifice is only slightly traumatized while a catheter is being introduced, it may become so spastic as to defeat all attempts to pass the catheter. If a catheter is pointed, rough, or of too large caliber, it may produce enough irritation during its passage to initiate, in any portion of the ureter, a contraction that will grasp the catheter tightly. *For this reason the diagnosis of ureteral stricture should never be made unless one can demonstrate dilatation of the ureter or pelvis above the point of narrowing.* This subject will be discussed more fully under the subject of ureteral stricture.

Nephroptosis

The subject of nephroptosis has been included in this chapter for a definite reason and with an ulterior motive in mind. We should like to impress on the student of urography the idea that ptosis should be considered a relatively normal condition, or at least only rarely a definite pathologic condition that warrants treatment. Although these statements are not scientifically accurate, yet so many unnecessary surgical operations have been done on ptosed kidneys that it is necessary to overstate the case somewhat for emphasis. Under the subject of the normal urogram, the location of the normal kidney was discussed. It was pointed out that no definite anatomic limitation can be given because the position of the normal kidney is subject to considerable variation. Arbitrarily it was stated that the normal position of the right renal pelvis is at the level of the interspace between the first and second lumbar vertebrae. The left kidney usually is situated about 2 cm higher than this. It was also stated that it is generally agreed that when the patient's position is changed from supine to erect, an excursion of the kidneys the distance of the length of one lumbar vertebra is considered within normal limits. The condition in which the kidney descends to a level lower than this is usually spoken of as *nephroptosis.*

The downward displacement of a kidney from pathologic lesions such as an enlarged liver or spleen, retroperitoneal and intra-abdominal tumors, and inflammatory processes will be considered elsewhere in this volume. All that concerns us here is the condition of simple ptosis which results from such conditions as general visceroptosis, lack of tonicity of abdominal muscles, lack of sufficient perirenal fat, and relaxed fascial support of the kidney. Nephroptosis may be either unilateral or bilateral (Figs. 4-151A and B and 4-152A and B). One may require a urogram in the erect position to demonstrate the nephroptosis or the condition may be so marked as to be apparent in the supine position (Fig. 4-153A and B). In the latter case, the kidney does not return to its normal position unless the patient is placed in the extreme Trendelenburg position or the kidney is replaced by manual manipulation against the abdominal wall. In bilateral ptosis one kidney may be considerably more ptosed than the other, so that one kidney may appear ptosed in the supine position while the other does not descend appreciably until the patient is placed erect.

In cases of marked ptosis the problem may arise as to whether the kidney is ectopic. If the kidney does not return to a more or less normal position when the patient is put in the Trendelenburg position, or if the *ureter is shortened,* suggesting that the kidney has always been in the observed position, the case for ectopia is strengthened (Fig. 4-154). There is no arbitrary level which divides a ptosed from an ectopic kidney, but most experts in urographic interpretation would no doubt insist that the kidney be fixed fairly well below the crest of the ilium before calling it ectopic. (See Chapter 12 for discussion of the various types of renal ectopy.)

The degree of descent of the kidneys varies considerably. Attempts have been made to classify this variation into various degrees of renal ptosis, but it has been found that such a classification is of little clinical value unless the renal displacement is extreme. A review of a large series of cases with renal ptosis revealed no correlation between the degree of ptosis and the patient's symptoms or urographic evidence of renal stasis. The fact that the kidney is situated below the crest of the ilium or is freely movable in the abdomen offers no evidence as to the advisability of nephropexy.

When the attachments of a kidney are so relaxed and stretched as to allow extreme freedom of renal movement, it is to be expected that the kidney may move in other planes. One of the most common changes in position during descent is *rotation around the anteroposterior axis* of the kidney so that the upper pole moves through an arc laterally and downward (Fig. 4-152). This type of motion increases the acuteness of the ureteropelvic angle and may give the appearance of an obstructive type of pelvic outlet. The kidney may also *rotate around its vertical axis* so that it may change from a normal position with the patient supine to one in which the pelvis is anterior (Figs. 4-155A and B and 4-156A and B) or even lateral when the patient is in the erect position. At times such a ptotic kidney may shift its position either medially or laterally during its descent.

It is to be expected that if a kidney is subject to a substantial amount of excursion, the form of the ureter must change as the distance from the renal pelvis to the bladder becomes shortened. The kinks, loops, and tortuosity of the ureters resulting from this condition have been discussed previously.

It is hardly within the province of this chapter to discuss the indications for treatment of this condition. Opinions differ widely as to when one can say that a ptosed kidney is the cause of pain and discomfort. Our experience has left us with the impression that the condition of nephroptosis is not commonly responsible for a patient's symptoms of pain in the loin or abdomen, unless definite signs of urinary obstruction or stasis can be demonstrated. Obstruction is evidenced by dilatation of the ureter, pelvis, and calyces or definite evidence of retention in a delayed urogram. One should be rather liberal in the interpretation of roentgenograms in which renal ptosis is present, or he is likely to make a diagnosis of pyelectasis or calycectasis more often than it is actually present. Owing to the marked mobility and tendency to rotation in such kidneys, the pelvis and calyces may be projected in unusual positions and may appear dilated when in reality they are not. The urologist is wise who remembers that renal ptosis is a common condition in normal persons who never complain of symptoms referable to the urinary tract. Therefore, it should require a very careful examination and a long period of study before even the most expert urologist should advise nephropexy. This is especially true in the absence of signs of a substantial amount of urinary obstruction or stasis.

(Text continued on page 350.)

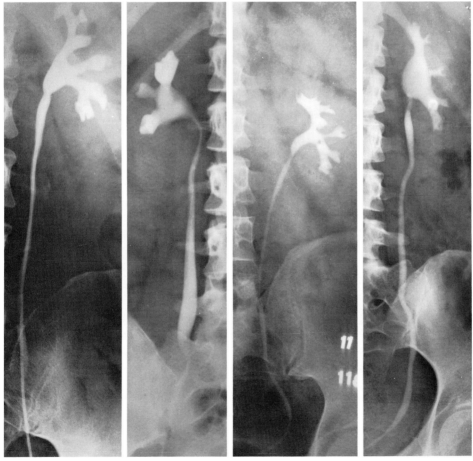

Fig. 4–137   Fig. 4–138   Fig. 4–139   Fig. 4–140

Figure 4–137. *Left retrograde pyelogram.* **Spasm at ureteropelvic junction** caused by irritation from ureteral catheter.

Figure 4–138. *Right retrograde pyelogram.* **Normal.** Physiologic dilatation of midportion of ureter known as *spindle* of ureter.

Figures 4–139 and 4–140. *Left retrograde pyelogram.* **Normal.** Variations in course of normal ureter.

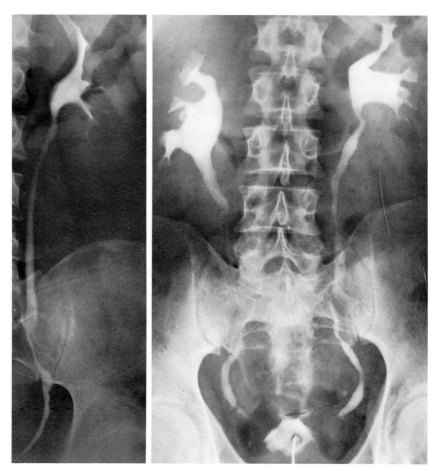

Fig. 4–141   Fig. 4–142

Figure 4–141. *Left retrograde pyelogram.* **Normal.** Apparent narrowing of ureter due to incomplete filling.

Figure 4–142. *Bilateral retrograde pyelogram.* **Normal.** Twisting, "ribbon" type of ureters, due to incomplete filling.

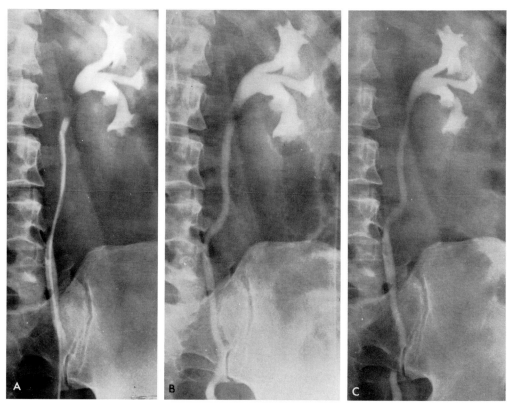

Figure 4–143. Diagnostic error which may occur with incomplete filling of normal ureter. A and B, *Left retrograde pyelograms* suggest filling defect just below ureteropelvic juncture. In **C**, with ureter filled, no filling defect is present. In **C** there is suggestion of filling defect in lower third of ureter overlying brim of pelvis. In **B**, ureter in this area is filled and is normal.

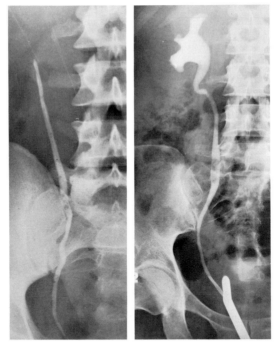

Fig. 4–144   Fig. 4–145

Figure 4–144. *Right retrograde ureterogram.* (Previous nephrectomy on right.) Multiple "filling defects" in ureter caused by air bubbles in medium.

Figure 4–145. *Retrograde ureterogram* made with bulb catheter inserted just within ureteral orifice. Note typical *spindle* of midureter. Intestinal gas shadows over spindle could be misinterpreted as negative filling defects.

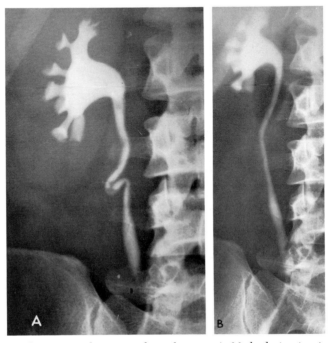

Figure 4–146. Normal ureter. *Right retrograde pyelograms.* **A,** Made during inspiration. Kink in ureter. **B,** Made during expiration. Kink in ureter has disappeared.

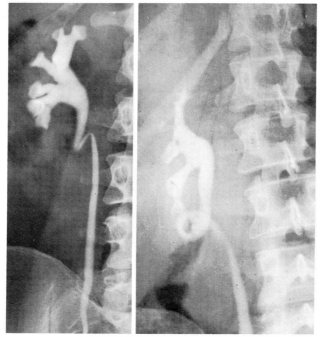

Fig. 4–147   Fig. 4–148

Figure 4–147. *Right retrograde pyelogram.* **Normal.** Kinks in ureter.
Figure 4–148. *Right retrograde pyelogram.* **Normal.** Complete loop in ureter.

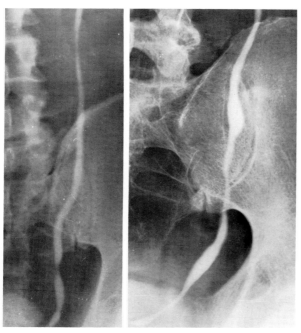

Fig. 4–149   Fig. 4–150

Figure 4–149. *Left retrograde pyelogram.* **Normal.** Areas of incomplete filling in lower part of ureter, such as are occasionally interpreted erroneously as ureteral strictures.
Figure 4–150. *Left ureterogram.* **Normal.** Areas of incomplete filling in lower part of ureter which might be erroneously interpreted as stricture.

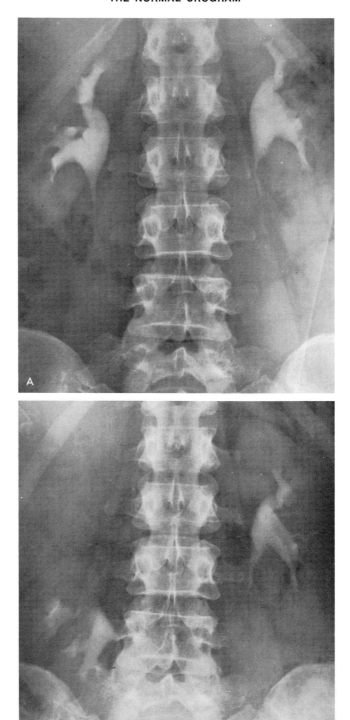

Figure 4–151. Bilateral nephroptosis. *Excretory urograms.* **A,** In supine position. Kidneys are at normal level. **B,** In upright position. There is marked descent of right kidney, with rotation around its anteroposterior axis. Slight descent of left kidney.

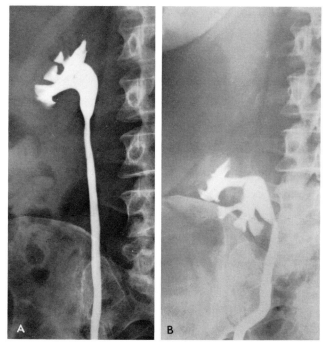

Figure 4–152. Right renal ptosis. *Right retrograde pyelograms.* **A,** In supine position. **B,** In upright position. Kidney rotates around anteroposterior axis.

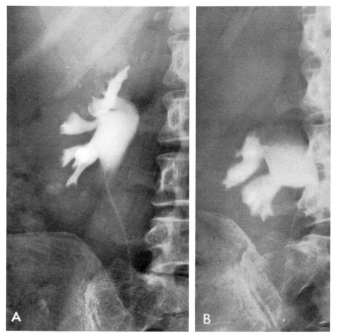

Figure 4–153. Nephroptosis. *Right retrograde pyelograms.* **A,** In supine position. Renal pelvis is opposite third lumbar interspace. **B,** Upright. Pelvis descends to fourth lumbar interspace.

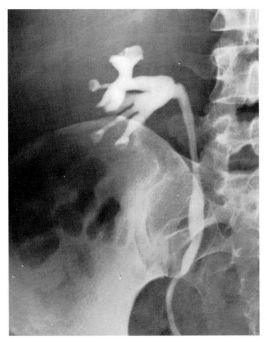

Figure 4–154. *Right retrograde pyelogram.* **Right renal ptosis versus ectopia.** Pyelogram made with patient in supine position. Short ureter suggests that this may be normal position of kidney. Hardly sufficient displacement to class as congenital ectopic kidney.

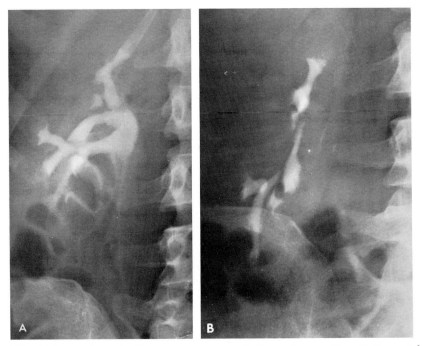

Figure 4–155. Right renal ptosis. *Excretory urograms.* **A,** In supine position. **B,** In upright position. Kidney has rotated around vertical axis during descent, so that calyces are projected in anteroposterior position.

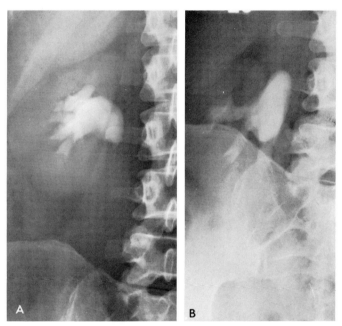

Figure 4–156. Renal ptosis. *Excretory urograms.* **A,** In supine position. **B,** In upright position. Kidney has rotated around anteroposterior axis and vertical axis, so that calyces point downward and anteroposteriorly. Mild pyelectasis.

THE BLADDER AND URETHRA

Excretory and Retrograde Cystograms

Roentgenographic visualization of the bladder with contrast medium (excretory or retrograde cystography) is of less importance than urographic visualization of the kidneys and ureters, because it is possible in most cases to view the interior of the bladder satisfactorily by means of cystoscopy. The best cystogram is made by the retrograde method, either opaque medium, air, or a combination of the two being used. However, the excretory cystogram, even though often poor owing to incomplete filling, may suggest the etiologic factor involved in lesions of the ureters and kidneys, or call attention to coincident lesions of the bladder which otherwise might be overlooked. In selected cases a cystogram of the well-filled bladder may be necessary for diagnosis. In such cases a catheter is inserted into the bladder, the urine is evacuated, and approximately 150 ml of contrast medium or air is injected. The technique is described in Chapter 1.

Hansen stated that the normal, inactive, filled bladder in the normal adult is either transverse, oval, or roundish. It is never longitudinally oval (Figs. 4-157 through 4-161). In children, however, it may be either longitudinally or transversely oval (Fig. 4-162A and B).

Distortion of the Cystogram in the Female by Pressure of the Uterus on the Bladder

Characteristic alterations in the outline of the bladder in the female are produced by the uterus which, if enlarged, may encroach on the base and posterior wall of the bladder, producing the typical "saddle deformity" seen in so many cystograms. Depending on the position and size of the uterus, the compression may be either in the midline or to either side.

If in the midline, the characteristic saddle contour results. If to the side, the vesical outline appears asymmetrical or lopsided (Figs. 4-163 through 4-167). If fibroid tumors are present in the uterus, they may poke into the bladder wall and produce a filling defect that might be mistaken for an intrinsic lesion such as a vesical tumor (Fig. 4-168).

Visualization of Trigone and Interureteric Ridge

Often a routine excretory cystogram is seen in which the trigone and interureteric ridge are outlined (Fig. 4-169). This usually occurs in male patients in whom the trigone and interureteric ridge are well developed, but may be seen in the female as well. To secure such a film the central beam of the x-ray apparatus must be directed to give a tangential view of the trigone and base of the bladder. Edling (1948) pointed out that with the patient supine the anteroposterior axis of the bladder is inclined several degrees in the caudocranial direction. If the x-ray beam is tilted in this direction, the interureteric ridge may be visualized as having a crescentic contour with the concave border looking cranially. The increased density of contrast medium immediately cranial to the crescentic border is due to the anteroposterior depth of the bladder being greatest in this area. Edling also called attention to the fact that the intramural portions of the ureters course laterally and caudally to this crescentic contour in a symmetrical manner, being separated from the contour by 2 to 3 mm (Figs. 4-170, 4-171, and 4-172; see also Figs. 6-164, 6-165, and 6-166). He made use of this observation in difficult diagnostic problems, such as nonopaque stones or tumors in the intramural part of a ureter. Edema of this portion of the ureter will result in asymmetry and an increase in distance between the ureter and the crescentic contour of the interureteric ridge.

Visualization of Jet of Urine From Ureteral Orifice

A rather unusual urographic phenomenon which may be difficult to explain at times is the apparent projection of one ureter across the midline to the opposite side of the interureteric ridge. This observation is simply the result of exposure at the instant a jet or bolus of urine containing a good concentration of contrast medium is ejected by the ureter (Fig. 4–173). It has no pathologic significance in either children or adults.

Common Errors in Interpreting Cystograms

If the greatest diameter of the bladder is its anteroposterior dimension, a double shadow may be cast which might be mistaken for a diverticulum (Fig. 4–174). This situation is most commonly encountered in the male bladder. Poor visualization or incomplete filling may produce unusual contours suggestive of pathologic conditions that are not present (Figs. 4–175 through 4–179). The physician must be careful not to rely too much on cystograms of incompletely filled bladders, since they may be the source of diagnostic error. Gas in the rectum overlying the bladder can easily be mistaken for a filling defect in the bladder if the film is not carefully studied (Fig. 4–180).

(Text continued on page 358.)

Fig. 4–157   Fig. 4–158

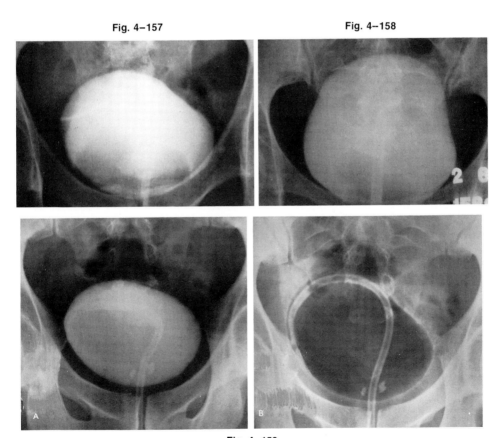

Fig. 4–159

Figure 4–157. *Retrograde cystogram.* Normal round bladder in male.
Figure 4–158. *Retrograde cystogram.* Normal oblong bladder in female.
Figure 4–159. Normal oval bladder in male. **A,** *Retrograde cystogram* made with contrast medium. **B,** *Retrograde cystogram* made with air.

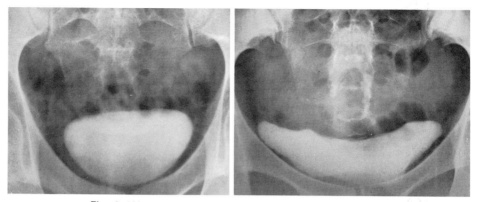

Fig. 4–160   Fig. 4–161

Figures 4–160 and 4–161. *Excretory cystograms.* **Normal bladder in female.** Greatest diameter in transverse axis.

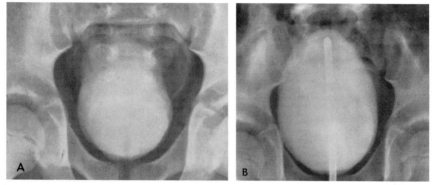

Figure 4–162. **Normal bladder** of boy 7 years of age. Greatest diameter in anteroposterior axis. **A,** *Excretory cystogram.* **B,** *Retrograde cystogram.*

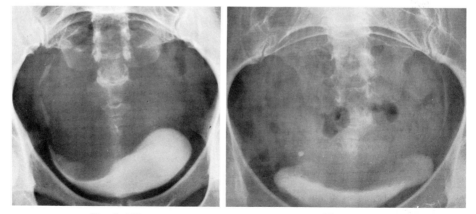

Fig. 4–163   Fig. 4–164

Figures 4–163 and 4–164. *Excretory cystograms.* **Normal bladder in female.** Typical deformity from extravesical pressure of uterus.

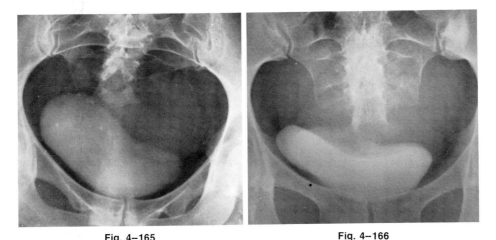

Fig. 4–165   Fig. 4–166

Figures 4–165 and 4–166. *Excretory cystograms.* **Normal bladder in female.** Typical deformity from extravesical pressure of uterus.

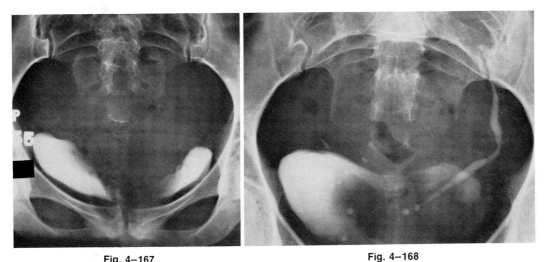

Fig. 4–167   Fig. 4–168

Figure 4–167. *Excretory urogram.* **Bladder incompletely filled.** Saddle-shaped deformity from pressure of uterus.

Figure 4–168. *Excretory urogram.* **Incomplete filling of bladder.** Filling defect in bladder caused by extravesical pressure from pedunculated fibroid tumor of uterus "poking" wall of bladder.

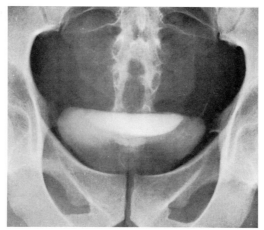

Figure 4--169. *Excretory cystogram.* Normal bladder in male. Delineates position of interureteric bar.

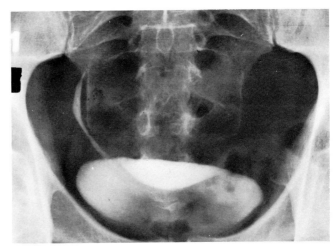

Figure 4–170. *Retrograde right pyelogram.* Medium has run back into bladder, forming cystogram. **Trigone and interureteric ridge sharply outlined.** Terminal right ureter can be seen coursing lateral and caudal to ridge and separated from it by about 3 mm.

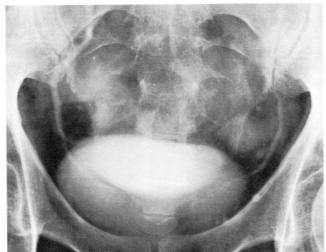

Figure 4–171. *Excretory cystogram.* Crescentic outline of **interureteric ridge, which outlines trigone. Intramural ureters** course just lateral and caudal to interureteric ridge, being separated from ridge by 2 to 3 mm.

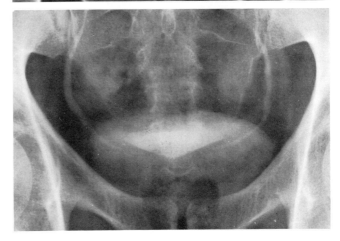

Figure 4–172. *Excretory cystogram.* Crescentic **outline of interureteric ridge,** which outlines trigone. Intramural ureters course just lateral and caudal to it, being separated from ridge by 2 to 3 mm.

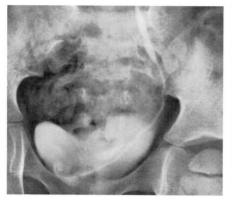
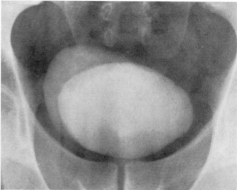

Fig. 4–173   **Fig. 4–174**

Figure 4–173. *Excretory urogram.* Jet of urine being ejected from left ureter crosses midline and curls around right side of bladder. (Courtesy of Dr. Donald D. Albers.)

Figure 4–174. *Excretory cystogram.* **Normal bladder** of male. Greatest diameter of bladder is in antero-posterior axis. Bladder casts superimposed shadow suggesting diverticulum, which is not present. Results of cystoscopy were negative.

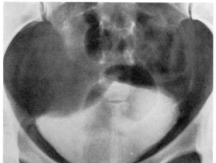
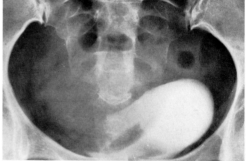

Fig. 4–175   **Fig. 4–176**

Figure 4–175. *Excretory cystogram* of female. **Incomplete filling.** Suggests filling defects, which are not present. Illustrates danger of attempting diagnosis on basis of cystogram of incompletely filled bladder.

Figure 4–176. *Excretory cystogram* of female. Typical **asymmetric deformity** from extravesical pressure of uterus.

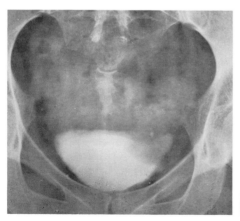
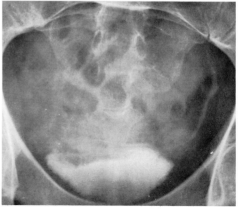

Fig. 4–177   **Fig. 4–178**

Figure 4–177. *Excretory cystogram.* **Normal bladder** of female. Incomplete filling, suggesting filling defect in left side of bladder, which was not present.

Figure 4–178. *Excretory cystogram* of male. **Normal.** Incomplete filling, suggesting filling defect, which is not present.

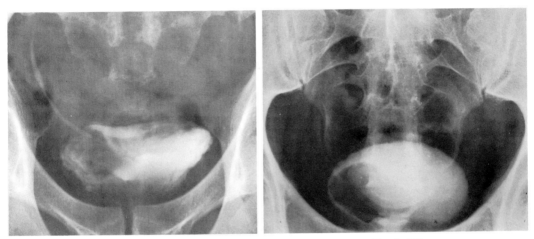

Fig. 4–179   Fig. 4–180

Figure 4–179. *Excretory cystogram* of man. Incomplete filling of bladder suggests filling defect on right. Cystoscopic examination negative.

Figure 4–180. *Excretory urogram.* Gas in rectum overlying bladder. This could be misinterpreted as filling defect in bladder from possible vesical neoplasm.

Cystourethrograms

THE NORMAL CYSTOURETHROGRAM IN THE ADULT MALE

Anatomic Considerations

Anatomically the male urethra has always been considered to be divided into two parts: (1) the posterior urethra, which includes the prostatic and membranous portion, and (2) the anterior urethra, which extends from the urogenital diaphragm to the urethral meatus. The membranous urethra is the section surrounded by the external sphincter muscle; it begins immediately distal to the apex of the prostate gland (and verumontanum) and lies between the two layers of the triangular ligament (urogenital diaphragm) (Fig. 4–181). Clinically, however, the "bulbomembranous urethra" is often spoken of as the *posterior urethra;* the anterior urethra is regarded as the pendulous urethra (including the fossa navicularis) and the region of the penoscrotal junction. The caliber of the urethra varies in its various parts. On study of micturition cystourethrograms in the adult male, Hansen stated that the prostatic urethra is usually about 1 cm in diameter at the vesical neck, narrowing to about 0.5 cm at the level of the verumontanum. The bulbous urethra measures about 1.5 cm, and the pendulous urethra about 1 cm "whereafter it narrows off." He pointed out, however, that these measurements vary with voiding pressure. Also, in the retrograde urethrogram the anterior urethra may be much more distended.

Urographic Considerations

Since both normal landmarks and pathologic lesions of the urethra are best shown on urethrograms taken in either the *right or left semilateral (oblique) positions* (Waterhouse) (see Fig. 1–39), the normal urethrogram will be described in this projection (Figs. 4–182 through 4–185). The caliber of the various parts of the urethra appears exaggerated (larger than actual calibration would suggest) because, as in all roentgenograms, there is some enlargement of the part because of the distance between the object and films. Also, the anterior urethra (including the bulb) appears of much larger caliber in the *retrograde cystourethrogram* due to greater distention of the urethra during injection of contrast medium against the resistant external urethral sphincter. *In the retrograde urethrogram made with viscous medium,* the vesical neck (internal urethral orifice or internal urethral sphincter) appears as a wide-caliber constriction of the prostatic urethra. Recognition of this landmark is important because occasionally the lumen may appear to be widened proximal to this constricted area, and this may seem to be a widening of the prostatic urethra itself, whereas in reality the image is not made by the prostatic urethra but by an overflow of the viscous medium into the lowermost portion of the bladder. This overflow may occur because the internal orifice is not always in the lowest (most distal) portion of the bladder. When it is not at the lowest point in the bladder, some of the medium may flow into the bladder and collect at the lowest portion immediately distal to the internal orifice.

Effect of Micturition on Fundus of Bladder, Vesical Neck, and Prostatic Urethra. At the beginning of micturition the fundus* lowers and the vesical neck widens. As a result the vesical neck and prostatic urethra becomes funnel-shaped, and this may give an impression of shortening of the prostatic urethra. The widening or dilatation of the prostatic urethra may vary with such factors as tonicity (or relaxation) of the external sphincter and whether the patient is voiding freely or

---

*The term *fundus* is used to denote the part of the bladder in the area of the vesical neck. Other terms are *floor* and *base* of bladder.

voiding against resistance. The resistance is provided either (1) by partial occlusion of the meatus with a penile clamp or (2) by having the patient void against the plunger of a syringe which is held tightly against the meatus. Edling (1945), in his excellent thesis on cystourethrography in the male, carefully compared films made by these two methods (Figs. 4–186*A, B,* and *C* and 4–187*A* and *B*).

The Prostatic Urethra. In the oblique projection the prostatic urethra appears as a gently curved section with its concavity directed ventrally (anteriorly). As mentioned previously, its diameter on the urethrogram depends on the technique used. For example, *in voiding cystourethrograms* it is well distended owing to the resistance of the external sphincter, whereas *in retrograde urethrograms* it is usually distended very little. (If viscous medium is used, distention will be a little better than with the use of liquid medium.) The length of the prostatic urethra is normally 3 to 4 cm. In the midportion of its posterior wall, an oval-shaped negative shadow or filling defect (to 1 cm in length) is often noted which represents the *verumontanum* (*colliculus seminalis*). Occasionally small folds may be seen as linear filling defects arising from the verumontanum, running distally and laterally and terminating in the wall of the membranous urethra. These folds represent the finger-like projections or small ridges seen on cystoscopy which appear to originate from the base of the verumontanum. These ridges (congenital urethral valves) are more predominant in the newborn infant and can be the cause of urinary obstruction if they fail to obliterate in due time (see Figs. 5–203 through 5–219).

The Membranous Urethra. The membranous urethra is seen as a narrowing of the lumen distal to the verumontanum. Usually this portion is less adequately filled with contrast medium than the prostatic urethra and is identified either as an area containing no contrast medium or as a thin line of contrast medium which tapers at both ends but which enlarges distally into the bulbous urethra and proximally into the prostatic urethra. The diameter of the membranous urethra depends on the relative state of tonicity of the external urethral sphincter; it usually appears wider in the voiding than in the retrograde urethrogram.

The Anterior Urethra. The anterior urethra appears as a wide channel on the urethrogram, in fact, appreciably wider than would have been thought. The bulbous urethra appears as a wide tube forming a gentle curve between the prostatic urethra and the penoscrotal juncture where the pendulous (penile) urethra begins. The caliber (degree of distention) appears greatest in the retrograde cystourethrogram, next in the voiding cystourethrogram (voiding against resistance), and least in the free voiding films.

THE NORMAL CYSTOURETHROGRAM IN MALE INFANTS AND CHILDREN

The *cystourethrogram* in the male child does not differ greatly from that in the adult, except in caliber and length (Figs. 4–188 through 4–191), and except that the fundus of the bladder usually lies on a higher level than in the adult. Some *voiding cystourethrograms,* however, have given rise to considerable controversy which has been chiefly concerned with the region of the vesical neck and prostatic urethra. Some workers including Kjellberg, Ericsson, and Rudhe have pointed out urographic contours which to them suggested abnormalities such as failure of relaxation of the vesical neck (internal sphincter). They called this a *fundus ring* and considered it an indication of pathologic obstruction. More recently Griesbach, Waterhouse, and Mellins; Shopfner (1967a and b); Shopfner and Hutch (1967; 1968); and others have disputed this view and have demonstrated that most if not all of these are only "physiologic variations" in contractions of the trigonal region and the sphincteric mechanisms, which are apparent only on "instantaneous roentgenograms." Griesbach, Waterhouse, and Mellins suggested that films taken moments later may not show these "deformities" (Figs. 4–192*A* and *B* and 4–193) and, therefore, warned against making too definite conclusions from individual films. They stated that "micturition produces dynamic changes in the appearance of the bladder neck and posterior urethra. Thorough familiarity with these variations is necessary to differentiate them from pathologic changes." Shopfner (1967a and b) in a recent discussion said that the roentgen features of bladder neck narrowing, contracture, anterior defect, and posterior defect are not valid criteria in diagnosis of bladder neck obstruction. He pointed out that these features are seen in the case of normal persons as frequently as in the case of symptomatic patients and do not correlate well with diagnoses of bladder neck obstruction made by other means (see discussion and Figs. 5–201 and 5–202 in Chapter 5).

CYSTOURETHROGRAM IN THE FEMALE

Because of the shortness of the urethra and the difficulty of obtaining films of the filled urethra during micturition, the older techniques of cystourethrography in the female, which depend on single or at best a very few blindly exposed films to demonstrate vesical and urethral anatomy, have been of limited value. They have been used rather unsuccessfully (Nilsen) to study vesical function and cases of urethral incontinence. However, the retrograde urethrogram made with a special technique, under pressure, has been of definite value in demonstrating urethral diverticula (see Figs. 1–37 and 1–38). Since development and popularization of the fluoroscopic technique of voiding cystourethrography with cine or multiple spot filming, cystourethrography has become a commonplace study for female patients, especially for girls in the pediatric age group. For female patients with repeated urinary-tract infection enuresis, and a variety of other urinary complaints, this technique has proved to be as effective a method for demonstrating vesicoureteral reflux and abnormalities of the bladder and urethra as it has for male patients (Fig. 4–194) (see Chapter 5).

(References begin on page 367.)

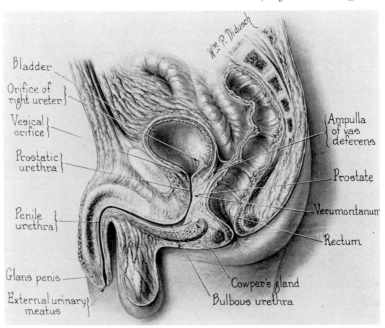

Figure 4–181. *Saggital section.* Normal male anatomy. (See text.) (Courtesy of Mr. William P. Didusch.)

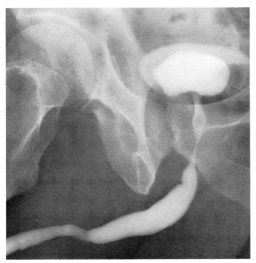 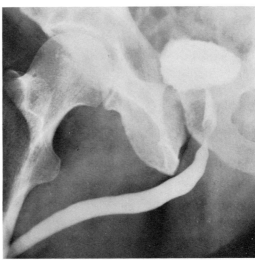

Fig. 4–182   **Fig. 4–183**

Figures 4–182 and 4–183. *Retrograde urethrograms.* Normal urethra of adult male.

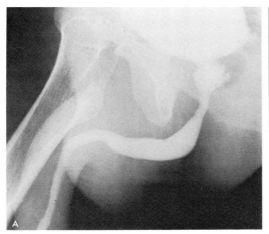 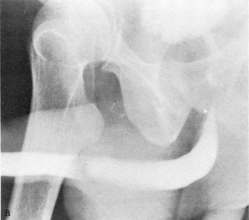

Figure 4–184.   Comparison of retrograde and voiding cystourethrograms. **A,** *Voiding cystourethrogram* of man, 47 years of age, with prostatitis and dilated prostatic duct abscesses. Note good distention and filling of prostatic urethra and lowering of floor of bladder and widening of vesical neck. **B,** *Retrograde urethrogram* in same case. Greater distention of anterior urethra but typical poor delineation and filling of prostatic urethra. (Courtesy of Dr. H. W. ten Cate.)

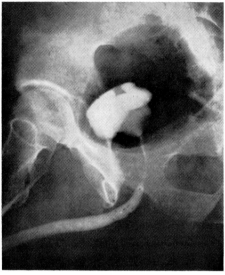

Figure 4–185. *Retrograde cystourethrogram* with semisolid medium, right oblique position. **Normal bladder and urethra.** Note width of anterior urethra of normal patient. (See text.) (Courtesy of Dr. R. H. Flocks.)

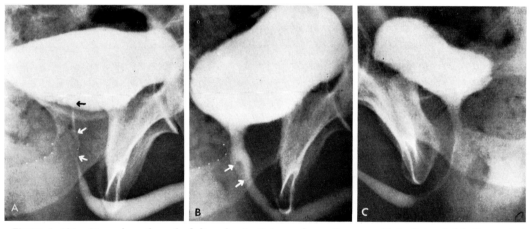

Figure 4–186. Normal urethra of adult male. **A,** *Retrograde urethrogram.* Note distended bulb, conical membranous urethra, and contracted prostatic urethra. **B,** Same case. *Voiding urethrogram (against resistance).* Note lowering of fundus, funnel shape of vesical neck, widening of lumen of prostatic urethra, better outline of verumontanum, and less distention of bulbomembranous urethra. **C,** Same case. *Voiding urethrogram (free voiding).* Opposite oblique view. Entire urethral lumen is less distended although funnel shape of vesical neck and prostatic urethra still are well seen. (From Edling, N. P. G., 1945.)

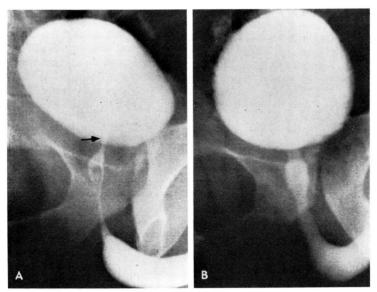

Figure 4–187.   Normal urethra of adult male. **A,** *Retrograde urethrogram.* **B,** *Voiding urethrogram (against resistance).* (From Edling, N. P. G., 1945.)

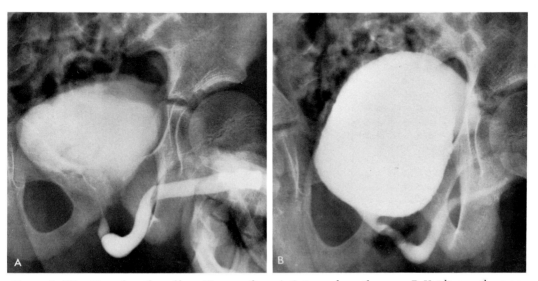

Figure 4–188.   Normal urethra of boy, 10 years of age. **A,** *Retrograde urethrogram.* **B,** *Voiding urethrogram.*

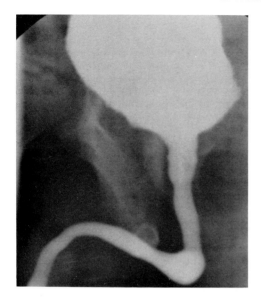

Figure 4–189. *Voiding urethrogram.* Normal male, age 7.

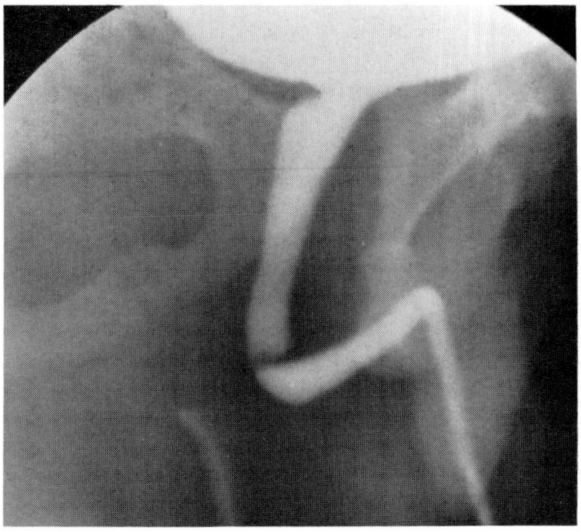

Figure 4–190. *Voiding urethrogram.* Normal male, age 6.

Figure 4–191. *Voiding urethrogram.* Normal male, age 4.

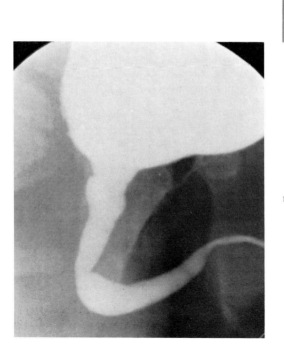

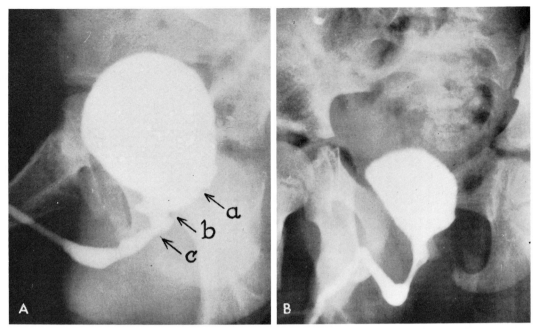

Figure 4–192. Normal. *Voiding cystourethrograms.* A, Note interureteric ridge (a), contracted trigonal area (b), called by Kjellberg and associates *fundus ring*, and internal sphincter (c). B, Same case few moments later. (From Griesbach, W. A., Waterhouse, R. K., and Mellins, H. Z.)

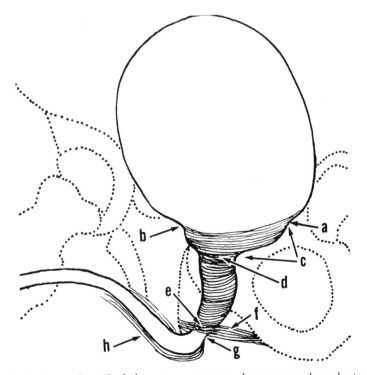

Figure 4–193. Posterior urethra. Shaded portions represent detrusor muscle, voluntary muscle of the urethra, and deep transverse muscle fibers from urogenital diaphragm: a, indicates interureteric ridge; b, fundus ring; c, trigone; d, internal sphincter; e, external sphincter; f, urogenital diaphragm (deep transverse muscle); g, pars nuda (membranous urethra); and h, bulbocavernosus muscle. (From Griesbach, W. A., Waterhouse, R. K., and Mellins, H. Z.)

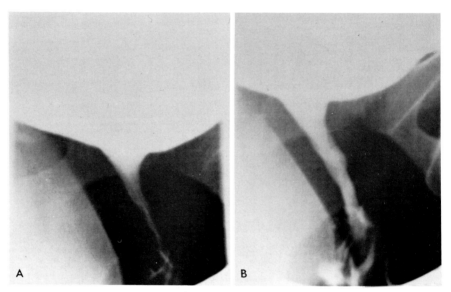

Figure 4–194.   Normal urethra of girl age 8. *Voiding cystourethrogram.* **A,** Early voiding. Urethra incompletely distended. **B,** Later stage. Urethra distended by good urine flow showing appearance of normal urethra.

REFERENCES

Abeshouse, B. S.: Pyelographic Injection of the Perirenal Lymphatics: Report of 2 Cases and Review of the Literature; a Consideration of the Relation of Pyelolymphatic Backflow to Chyluria, the Anatomy of the Lymphatics of Kidney and Mechanism of Backflow From the Renal Parenchyma and Pelvis. Am. J. Surg. 25:427-450 (Sept.) 1934.

Baum, S., and Gillenwater, J. Y.: Renal Artery Impressions on the Renal Pelvis. J. Urol. 95:139-145 (Feb.) 1966.

Becker, J. A., and Pollack, H.: Cinefluorographic Studies of the Normal Upper Urinary Tract. Radiology 84:886-893 (May) 1965.

Campbell, J. E.: A Cinefluorographic Analysis of Normal Pyelo-ureteral Dynamics. Invest. Radiol. 1:198-204 (May-June) 1966.

Campbell, J. E.: Ureteral Peristalsis in Duplex Renal Collecting Systems. Am. J. Roentgenol. 99:577-584 (Mar.) 1967.

Crenshaw, J. L.: Personal communication to the author.

Cunningham, D. J.: Cunningham's Text-Book of Anatomy. Ed. 7, New York, Oxford University Press, 1937, pp. 1422-1423.

Dell, J. M., Jr., and Barnwell, C. H.: The Normal Lateral Retrograde Pyelogram. Radiology 47:163-165 (Aug.) 1946.

Edling, N. P. G.: Urethrocystography in the Male With Special Regard to Micturition. Acta radiol. Suppl. 58, 1945, pp 1-144.

Edling, N. P. G.: Further Studies of the Interureteric Ridge of the Bladder. Acta radiol. 30:69-75, 1948.

Faegenburg, D., Bosniak, M., and Evans, J. A.: Renal Sinus Lipomatosis: Its Demonstration by Nephrotomography. Radiology 83:987-997 (Dec.) 1964.

Fisher, O. D., and Forsythe, W. I.: Micturating Cystourethrography in the Investigation of Enuresis. Arch. Dis. Childhood 29:460-471 (Oct.) 1954.

Flocks, R. H.: The Roentgen Visualization of the Posterior Urethra. J. Urol. 30:711-736 (Dec.) 1933.

Fraley, E. E.: Vascular Obstruction of Superior Infundibulum Causing Nephralgia: A New Syndrome. New England J. Med. 275:1403-1409 (Dec. 22) 1966.

Fraley, E. E.: Dismembered Infundibulopyelostomy: Improved Technique for Correcting Vascular Obstruction of the Superior Infundibulum. J. Urol. 101:144-148 (Feb.) 1969.

Frimann-Dahl, J.: Normal Variations of the Left Kidney: An Anatomical and Radiologic Study. Acta radiol. 55:207-216 (Mar.) 1961.

Griesbach, W. A., Waterhouse, R. K., and Mellins, H. Z.: Voiding Cystourethrography in the Diagnosis of Congenital Posterior Urethral Valves. Am. J. Roentgenol. 82:521-529 (Sept.) 1959.

Hansen, L. K.: Micturition Cystourethrography With Automatic Serial Exposures: An Opinion on the Value of the Method. Acta radiol. Suppl. 207, 1961, pp. 1-139.

Hinman, F.: The Principles and Practice of Urology. Philadelphia, W. B. Saunders Company, 1935, p. 75.

Hinman, F., and Lee-Brown, R. K.: Pyelovenous Back Flow: Its Relation to Pelvis Reabsorption, to Hydronephrosis and to Accidents of Pyelography. J.A.M.A. 82:607-612 (Feb. 23) 1924.

Jarre, H. A., and Cumming, R. E.: Cinex-Camera Studies on the Urinary Tract: A New Method of Functional Investigation. J. Urol. 24:423-431 (Oct.) 1930.

Jarre, H. A., and Cumming, R. E.: Pyelo-peristalsis Characteristically Altered by Infection, With Notes on Functional Behavior of Other Hollow Viscera. Radiology 23:299-314 (Sept.) 1934.

Kjellberg, S. R., Ericsson, N. O., and Rudhe, U.: The Lower Urinary Tract in Childhood: Some Correlated Clinical and Roentgenologic Observations. Chicago, Year Book Publishers, 1957, 298 pp.

Knutsson, F.: On the Technique of Urethrography. Acta radiol. 10:437-440, 1929.

Knutsson, F.: Urethrography: Röntgen Examination of the Male Urethra and Prostate After Injection of Contrast Material Into the Urethra; Experience Gained From the Examination of 154 Patients in Maria Hospital, Stockholm. Acta radiol. Suppl. 28, 1935, pp. 1-150.

Kreel, L., and Pyle, R.: Arterial Impressions on the Renal Pelvis. Brit. J. Radiol. 35:609-614 (Sept.) 1962.

Lee-Brown, R. K., and Laidley, J. W. S.: Pyelovenous Backflow. J.A.M.A. 89:2094-2098 (Dec. 17) 1927.

Meng, C.-H., and Elkin, M.: Venous Impression on the Calyceal System. Radiology 87:878-882 (Nov.) 1966.

Mertz, H. O.: The Lateral Pyelogram (a Neglected Procedure in the Diagnosis of Various Abdominal Conditions). J. Indiana M. A. 24:537-540 (Oct.) 1931.

Mertz, H. O., and Hamer, H. G.: The Lateral Pyelogram: An Investigation of Its Value in Urologic Diagnosis. J. Urol. 31:23-55 (Jan.) 1934.

Moëll, H.: Size of Normal Kidneys. Acta radiol. 46:640-645 (Nov.) 1956.

Morales, O., and Romanus, R.: Urethrography in the Male: Delimitation of the Anterior and Posterior Urethra, the Pars Diaphragmatica, the Pars Nuda Urethrae and the Presence of a Musculus Compressor Nudae. Acta radiol. 39:453-476, 1953.

Narath, P. A.: The Hydromechanics of the Calyx Renalis. J. Urol. 43:145-176 (Jan.) 1940.

Nilsen, P. A.: Cystourethrography in Stress Incontinence. Acta obst. et gynec. scandinav. 37:269-285, 1958.

Olsson, O., and Weiland, P.-O.: Renal Fibrolipomatosis. Acta radiol. [Diagn.] N.S. 1:1061-1070 (Sept.) 1963.

Palubinskas, A. J.: Medullary Sponge Kidney. Radiology 76:911-918 (June) 1961.

Shopfner, C. E.: Roentgen Evaluation of Distal Urethral Obstruction. Radiology 88:222-231 (Feb.) 1967a.

Shopfner, C. E.: Roentgenological Evaluation of Bladder Neck Obstruction. Am. J. Roentgenol. 100:162-176 (May) 1967b.

Shopfner, C. E., and Hutch, J. A.: The Trigonal Canal. Radiology 88:209-221 (Feb.) 1967.

Shopfner, C. E., and Hutch, J. A.: The Normal Urethrogram. R. Clin. North America 6:165-189 (Aug.) 1968.

Simril, W. A., and Rose, D. K.: Replacement Lipomatosis·and Its Simulation of Renal Tumors: Report of Two Cases. J. Urol. 63:588-592 (Apr.) 1950.

Stapor, K.: Calycorenal Backflow. Brit. J. Urol. 39:753-758 (Dec.) 1967.

Vermooten, V.: Congenital Cystic Dilatation of the Renal Collecting Tubules: New Disease Entity. Yale J. Biol. & Med. 23:450-453 (June) 1951.

Waterhouse, K.: Voiding Cystourethrography: A Simple Technique. J. Urol. 85:103-104 (Jan.) 1961.

CHAPTER 5

Urinary Stasis: The Obstructive Uropathies, Atony, Vesicoureteral Reflux, and Neuromuscular Dysfunction of the Urinary Tract

TERMINOLOGY

Nomenclature has been a source of much confusion in this subject. The terms *hydronephrosis* and *hydro-ureter* have been widely used to denote dilatation of the renal pelvis (and calyces) and ureter, respectively. Obviously, however, they are inaccurate terms. More accurate terms are *calycectasis, pyelectasis,* and *ureterectasis.* Combinations of these terms, such as *ureteropyelocaliectasis, ureteropyelectasis,* and *pyelocaliectasis,* have been used. Because dilatations of the calyces and pelvis are so often associated, many urologists use the term *pyelectasis* to mean dilatation of both pelvis and calyces. However, the terms *hydronephrosis* and *hydro-ureter,* like the term *hypernephroma,* have become so well entrenched in medical writing that undoubtedly they will continue to be used.

CLASSIFICATION OF STASIS

Obstructive Versus Nonobstructive (Obscure) Varieties of Stasis

Dilatation in the urinary tract usually is the result of obstruction. However, it also may be present in the absence of demonstrable obstruction. The cause of urinary stasis in cases of the latter type is poorly understood. Although the problem of etiology cannot be adequately treated in a book of this kind, a brief *etiologic classification* may be suggested. Two groups of lesions usually are recognized; namely, (1) *obstructive* and (2) *nonobstructive* (or *obscure*). The second group includes conditions which have been referred to as *inflammatory, atonic, neurogenic,* and *congenital.* This group might be referred to as the *wastebasket* for types of dilatation which are not well understood.

369

PYELECTASIS (HYDRONEPHROSIS)

Physiopathologic Changes in the Kidney

The primary effect of the back pressure of urine in hydronephrosis is parenchymal atrophy (so-called back-pressure atrophy). This results from (1) ischemic atrophy from impairment of renal blood flow secondary to compression of the interlobar and arcuate arteries (Figs. 5–1 and 5–1$_a$)* (Hinman; Widén) and (2) direct parenchymal damage from pressure. Some protection is provided the kidney by the reverse flow of urine from the renal pelvis, and calyces (pyelosinous back-flow)† back into the circulation. Whereas previously emphasis has been on the degree of pyelocaliectasis, it has now shifted to the degree of atrophy of the renal cortex (Hodson and Craven).

Roentgenographic Changes

As has been mentioned previously (see Chapter 4 – "The Normal Urogram"), it is difficult or impossible to stipulate arbitrarily a dividing line between a large normal pelvis and early pyelectasis. Comparison with the opposite (normal) kidney may supply a reasonable answer because of the tendency to symmetry of the two kidneys (Figs. 5–2, 5–3, and 5–4). In the absence of a normal contralateral kidney, one may require comparison with previous films if they are available.

Changes in the Calyces, Renal Papillae, and Renal Pyramids

The first observable radiologic signs of obstructive back pressure occur in the calyces. To appraise early changes accurate-

ly, it is important that the variations in appearance of normal calyces be understood (see Chapter 4, pages 296–297). The shape of a calyx depends on the contour of the renal papillae. A narrow pointed papilla presents a narrow deep conical calyx; a large broad fleshy papilla presents a widely "cupped" calyx; other papillae may present a sessile, almost flat, contour. In general, however, as Hodson and Craven indicated, the general configuration of the normal calyx is that of a "Y." Progressive papillary atrophy and flattening allow more contrast medium to collect at the base of the papilla, finally resulting in a definite "clubbing" of the calyx. As the process continues, the papilla no longer projects into the calyx, but it becomes flat and, later, concave; also, the walls of the calyx separate and become widened (Figs. 5–5, 5–6, and 5–7). In the majority of cases, this latter state represents essentially complete atrophy of the renal papilla. Urographically, this lesion simulates renal papillary necrosis after the papilla has separated and been passed. The differential point is that in the case of obstruction all calyces are more or less evenly involved, whereas in papillary necrosis the changes are spotty and uneven with some calyces being involved and others not.

It has been pointed out (Hodson and Craven) that occasional diagnostic errors are possible if one assumes that a papilla is atrophied just because the calyx is clubbed and dilated. This situation may arise in the case of a rather markedly dilated calyx filled with dense contrast medium that has completely obscured the papilla. Careful radiologic technique with meticulous search for evidence of a papilla in the early film before the contrast medium has become too dense may keep such errors to a minimum (Fig. 5–8A and B).

The process of atrophy is not limited to the renal papilla, rather it proceeds throughout the entire renal substance. Although the obstructed kidney may appear either enlarged, unchanged, or reduced in size, the end result is nearly

---

*Reduction in the caliber of the renal arteries is considered to be a sign of parenchymal atrophy.

†See Chapter 4.

always some reduction in size and dimensions of the renal cortex (hydronephrotic atrophy) (Fig. 5-9A, B, and C). It has been shown by Hodson and Craven that similar parenchymal atrophy also may occur as a result of short intervals of obstruction such as are produced by obstruction from a ureteral stone. In some of these cases, for some unexplained reason, the papilla apparently returns to normal contour despite some degree of definite generalized parenchymal atrophy with decrease in renal size. It seems logical that, in some cases, unexplained renal atrophy which in the past has been attributed to "congenital hypoplasia" may be the end result of forgotten or asymptomatic previous episodes of temporary obstruction. It is usually possible to distinguish obstructive parenchymal atrophy from the inflammatory variety (pyelonephritis), because the former tends to be even and symmetrical while the latter tends to be focal and spotty (see discussion in Chapter 7, pages 751–752). When estimating the degree of renal atrophy, the basis of comparison is usually the "normal" contralateral kidney. This may provide a possible source of error, however; for instance, if renal damage is of long standing and the kidney has relatively poor function, compensatory hypertrophy of the "normal" contralateral kidney may have increased its size.

Changes in the Renal Pelvis

The problem of distinguishing between a large normal renal pelvis and an early pyelectasis has already been discussed (see Figs. 5-2, 5-3, and 5-4). Usually dilatation of the pelvis and calyces proceeds at a fairly uniform rate. In some cases, however, this progression is unequal, and it is not uncommon to see substantial degrees of pyelectasis with entirely normal calyces (Figs. 5-10, 5-11, and 5-12) or significant calycectasis with little or no pyelectasis (Figs. 5-13, 5-14, and 5-15). It has been opined that obstruction near the renal pelvis predisposes to dilatation of the pelvis whereas more distal obstruction produces more dilatation of the calyces than pelves. The value of this observation, however, is open to question (Figs. 5-16 and 5-17). It is also apparent that an extrarenal type of pelvis dilates more easily than does the intrarenal variety which is supported and contained within a more rigid and confined space (see Figs. 5-10, 5-11, and 5-12). Hodson and Craven wondered if pyelectasis in the presence of normal calyces might represent some local neuromuscular disturbance rather than obstruction with back pressure and theorized that (in the absence of infected urine) such a situation may be of no danger to renal integrity. One must keep in mind, however, that stasis of urine in a dilated pelvis can conceivably predispose to urinary infection and ascending pyelonephritis.

ADVANCED DEGREES OF PYELOCALIECTASIS

In advanced cases of pyelocaliectasis, dramatic urograms may be obtained. Huge, round, dilated calyces may be all that are visualized in an excretory urogram, because there may not be sufficient function to enable one to visualize the large hydronephrotic pelvis (Fig. 5-18). In such a case, the pelvis may be visualized if a 2- to 6-hour delayed film is taken.

The pelvis may become so large that by its own weight the kidney descends and rotates on the anteroposterior axis, thereby decreasing the angle at the ureteropelvic junction and increasing the degree of obstruction. In far-advanced cases a huge dilated sac may be all that remains of the kidney and pelvis. Occasionally the wall of a hydronephrotic sac is calcified or the interior surface of the sac is covered with an exudate that contains sufficient calcium to cast a shadow (Figs. 5-19 and 5-20). Crescentic collections of contrast material in the renal parenchyma overlying nonopacified dilated calyces are occasionally observed in cases of severe hydronephrosis (Fig. 5–21). This abnormality, which is termed the *crescent sign of hydronephrosis*, is detectable during the early phases of excretory urography and then gradually disappears as the calyces and pelvis are opacified. It is attributed to the accumulation of contrast material in collecting tubules that have been flattened and displaced by the hydronephrotic calyces so that they lie parallel to the renal convexity and close to its surface (LeVine and associates).

In advanced hydronephrosis, in which little or no function remains, diagnosis by excretory urography may be impossible even with the use of infusion type excretory urography and delayed films. If pressure or angulation from the greatly dilated pelvis has occluded the ureter and a catheter cannot be passed, it may be impossible to make a retrograde pyelogram. In such cases the lesion may easily be confused with tumor (Figs. 5–22 through 5–27).

Blood Clots and Fluid Level

Unusual and bizarre urograms occasionally are encountered in cases of hydronephrosis. Evidence of a fluid level in a large hydronephrotic kidney indicates that air or gas is present (Fig. 5–28). Bleeding is not uncommon in hydronephrosis, and coincident blood clots may be the cause of unusual urograms (Fig. 5–29). Pyelectasis may result from renal tumors, especially epithelial tumors of the calyces or pelvis (see Chapter 10, "Tumors").

(*Text continued on page 388.*)

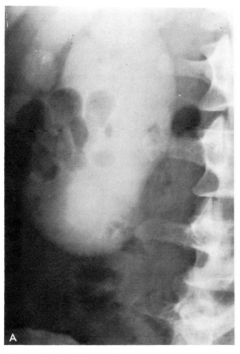
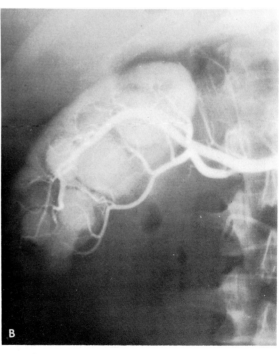

Figure 5–1. Obstruction at ureteropelvic junction and marked pyelectasis. **A,** *Excretory urogram.* Large distended renal pelvis. Some circular dilated calyces may be seen overlying lateral margin of pelvis near upper pole. **B,** *Selective renal arteriogram.* Marked displacement of branches of renal arteries around dilated calyces. Thinning of renal cortex.

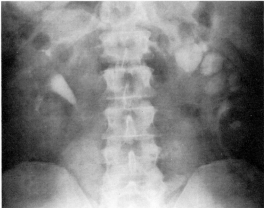

A

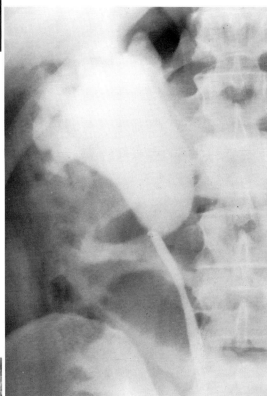

B

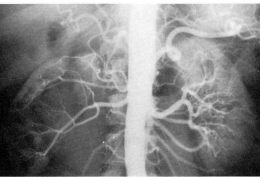

C

Figure 5–1ₐ. Arteriographic demonstration of **displacement and compression of interlobar vessels in hydronephrosis** (ureteropelvic junction obstruction). **A,** *Excretory urogram. Right*—dilatation of calyces; pelvis is not visualized. *Left*—**normal. B,** *Right retrograde pyelogram.* **Marked dilatation of pelvis and calyces.** (At operation marked narrowing of short segment of ureter adjacent to ureteropelvic junction found to be cause of obstruction.) **C,** *Midstream arteriogram.* **Two arteries serve right kidney.** Note displacement and reduction in number of arterial branches stretched around dilated calyces and the nephrographic demonstration of thinning of the renal parenchyma. Compare with appearance of normal left kidney.

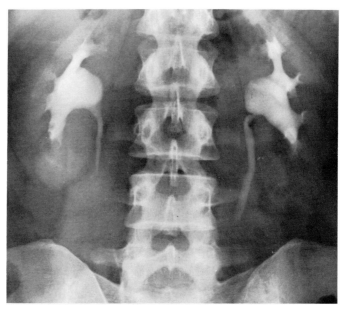

Figure 5–2. *Excretory urogram.* **Minimal bilateral pyelectasis.** Calyces are normal. Difficult to be sure if ureteropelvic junctions are pathologic or variations of normal, but left is not funnel shaped, as is right. Both give impression that retrograde pyelograms might demonstrate greater degree of pyelectasis.

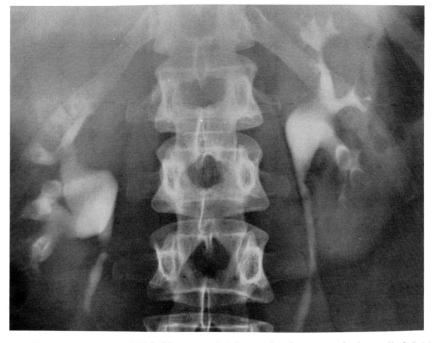

Figure 5–3. *Excretory urogram.* **Mild dilatation of right renal pelvis,** typical of so-called flabby type of pelvis. Ureter not inserted in most dependent position. Compare with left kidney, which is normal.

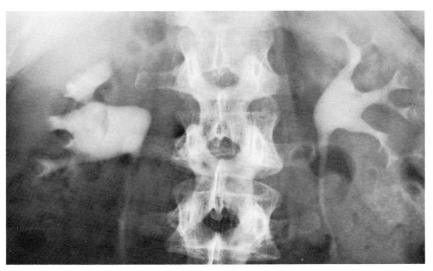

Figure 5–4. *Excretory urogram.* **Minimal pyelectasis on right.** Comparison with left kidney suggests pathologic rather than large normal pelvis.

Renal Papillae

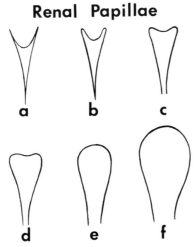

Figure 5–5. Papillary and calyceal changes in obstructive atrophy from normal (*a*) to clubbed (*f*). See text for explanation. (From Hodson, C. J., and Craven, J. D.)

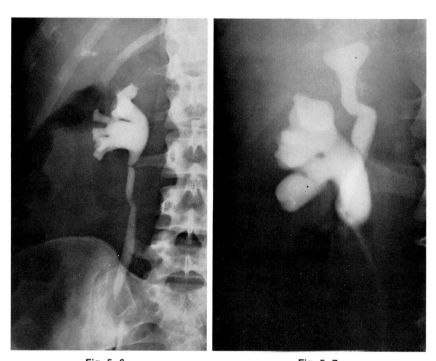

Fig. 5–6   Fig. 5–7

Figure 5–6. *Right retrograde pyelogram.* Clubbing of all calyces with associated mild pyelectasis graded 1. Difficult to say whether pathologic or only result of overdistention.

Figure 5–7. *Right retrograde pyelogram.* More advanced clubbing of minor calyces, with broadening of major calyces, in bifid type of pelvis. Dilatation of pelvis graded 1.

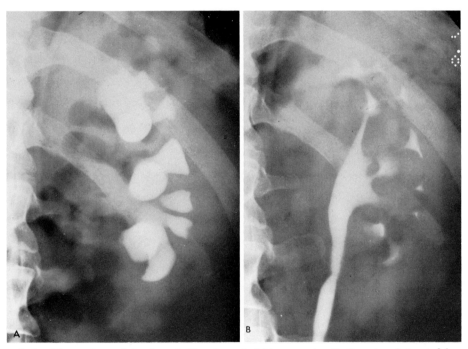

Figure 5–8. Obstructive pelviocalyceal dilatation mimicking atrophy. (Left ureter obstructed from retroperitoneal fibrosis.) **A,** *Preoperative excretory urogram.* Calyceal dilatation and apparent papillary atrophy. **B,** *Excretory urogram* after surgical relief of obstruction. Papillae appear nearly normal once calyceal dilatation has subsided. (From Hodson, C. J., and Craven, J. D.)

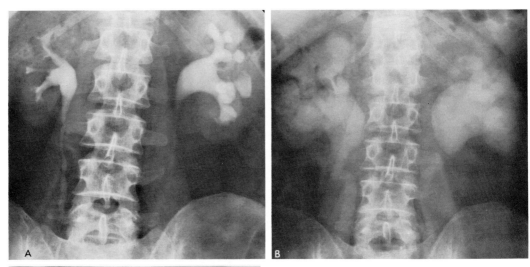

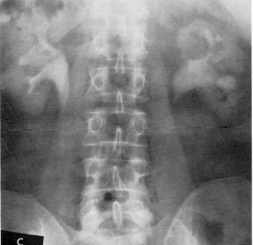

Figure 5–9. Hydronephrotic atrophy of kidney secondary to long-standing urethral stricture with recurring periods of obstruction and vesical distention. **A,** *Excretory urogram,* 1957. **Moderate left pyelocaliectasis,** but left kidney is as large as or larger than right. **B,** *Excretory urogram,* August 1966. Bladder had been distended (6,200 ml residual) for several months because stricture had been neglected. **Advanced bilateral hydronephrosis and hydroureter.** (Stricture dilated and retention relieved.) **C,** *Excretory urogram,* 3 months later. **Minimal left pyelocaliectasis** persists, but there has been reduction in size of kidney—**parenchymal atrophy.**

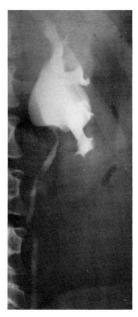

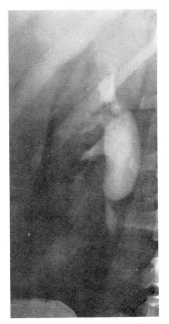

Fig. 5-10   Fig. 5-11

Figure 5–10. *Left retrograde pyelogram.* **Pyelectasis with almost no dilatation of calyces.** Abnormal ureteropelvic junction. Ureter is not inserted in most dependent position. (Anomalous vessels found at operation, one in upper and one in lower pole, and angulation of ureter at ureteropelvic junction.)

Figure 5–11. *Excretory urogram.* **Extrarenal, elongated type of pelvis, with pyelectasis.** Abnormal ureteropelvic junction.

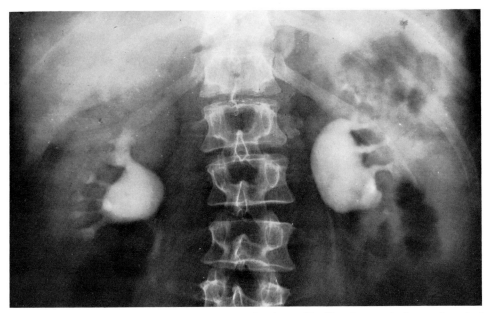

Figure 5–12. *Excretory urogram.* **Bilateral extrarenal pelves with dilatation, grade 2; no calycectasis.** No surgical exploration.

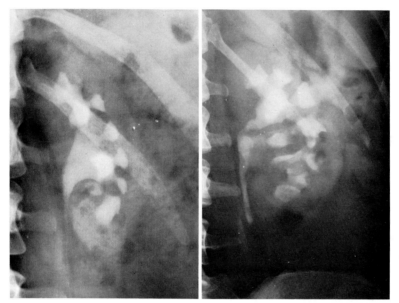

Fig. 5–13   Fig. 5–14

Figure 5–13. *Excretory urogram.* Calyces dilated, grade 1; no pyelectasis.

Figure 5–14. *Excretory urogram.* Moderate calycectasis with minimal pyelectasis. Note marked cortical damage with irregular scarring and thinning of renal parenchyma, resulting from infection or obstruction or both.

Figure 5–15. *Excretory urogram.* Stricture of terminal portion of left ureter, producing calycectasis and ureterectasis, but minimal pyelectasis.

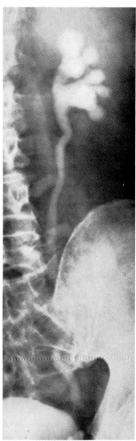

Fig. 5–15

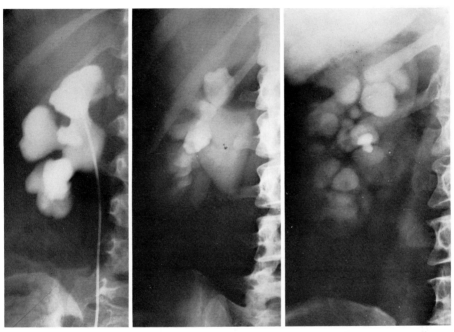

Fig. 5–16   **Fig. 5–17**   **Fig. 5–18**

Figure 5–16. *Right retrograde pyelogram.* Calycectasis, grade 3, and little if any pyelectasis. At operation ureter was found to be inserted about halfway up pelvis, not giving dependent drainage. Y type of plastic operation was done.

Figure 5–17. *Excretory urogram.* Calycectasis, grade 2, with minimal pyelectasis. At operation congenital stricture of upper third of ureter was found.

Figure 5–18. *Excretory urogram.* Right hydronephrosis with advanced dilatation of calyces. Not enough medium was excreted to outline pelvis adequately. At operation anomalous vessels obstructing ureteropelvic junction were found.

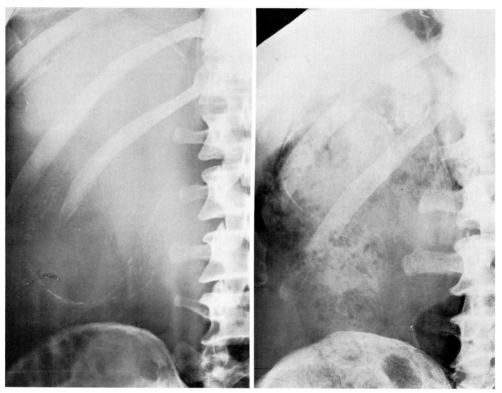

Fig. 5–19   Fig. 5–20

Figure 5–19. *Excretory urogram.* **Advanced pyelectasis on right with no renal function.** Hydronephrotic sac outlined with thin curvilinear shadow of calcium. (Nephrectomy. Pathologic study showed the pelvis extensively involved with **leukoplakia, containing many focal areas of calcification.**)

Figure 5–20. *Excretory urogram.* **Huge nonfunctioning hydronephrotic right kidney.** Hydronephrotic sac lined with inflammatory exudate, with calcification.

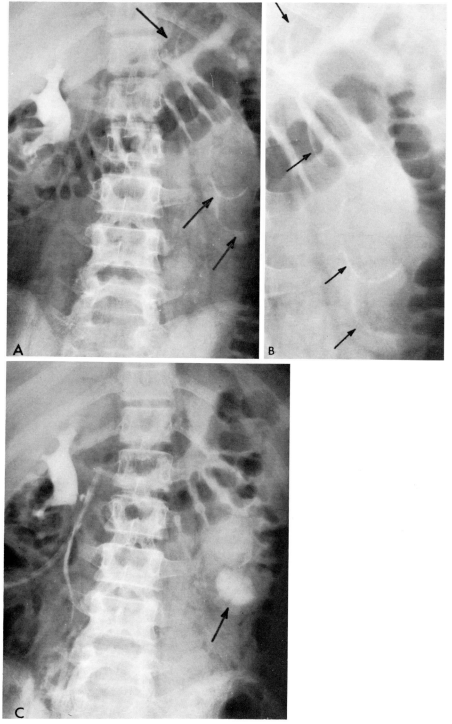

Figure 5–21. Appearance and disappearance of crescent sign of hydronephrosis. **A,** *Excretory urogram, 5-minute film.* There is good opacification of right renal pelvis and calyces. Pelvis and calyces of left kidney are not opacified, but crescentic collections of medium (crescent sign) are seen in renal parenchyma overlying dilated calyces (*arrows*). **B,** Enlargement of part of film shown in **A.** Crescent sign of hydronephrosis is exaggerated (*arrows*). **C,** *Excretory urogram, 60-minute delayed film.* Some medium has collected in dilated calyces (*arrow*). Crescent sign has almost completely disappeared.

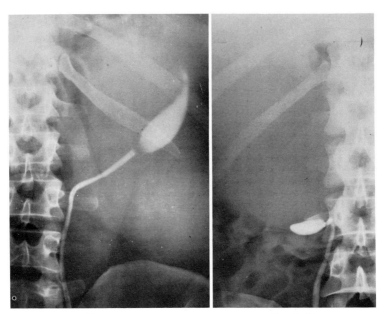

Fig. 5–22   Fig. 5–23

Figure 5–22. *Left retrograde pyelogram.* **Huge hydronephrosis** producing so much pressure at uretero-pelvic junction that only periphery of pelvis and adjacent portion of ureter can be filled. (At operation **anomalous vessels** were found crossing kidney at ureteropelvic junction.)

Figure 5–23. *Right retrograde pyelogram.* **Huge hydronephrosis** (pelvis not visualized, as contrast medium will not enter pelvis). Point of obstruction at angulation of ureter in region of ureteropelvic junction. (At operation huge hydronephrosis found, with **small caliber ureter.**)

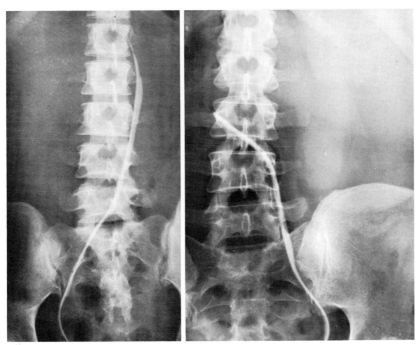

Fig. 5–24 **Fig. 5–25**

Figure 5–24. *Attempted right retrograde pyelogram.* **Huge hydronephrosis** (pelvis not visualized), **completely displacing right ureter across midline.** Unable to introduce contrast medium into pelvis because of obstruction. Condition could be easily confused with renal tumor. (At operation huge hydronephrotic kidney was found, filling right side of abdomen.)

Figure 5–25. *Left retrograde pyelogram.* **Huge hydronephrosis, which displaces ureter to right of midline,** obstructing ureter so that contrast medium does not enter pelvis. Could be confused with renal tumor or crossed renal ectopia. (At operation elsewhere, huge hydronephrotic left kidney was found, pelvis extending across vertebral column.)

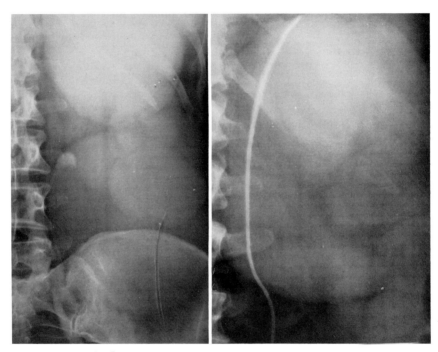

Fig. 5–26   Fig. 5–27

Figure 5–26. *Excretory urogram.* **Huge hydronephrosis** which on exploration was found to be size of football. **Marked angulation and obstruction at ureteropelvic junction.** Dilatation of ureter unexplained.

Figure 5–27. *Left retrograde pyelogram.* **Huge hydronephrosis** which was not visible on excretory urogram. Contrast medium injected shows faint outline of huge hydronephrotic sac. Obstruction of undetermined origin at ureteropelvic juncture. In this type of case all other means of diagnosis should be exhausted before retrograde pyelography is attempted. Even then, it should be done with caution.

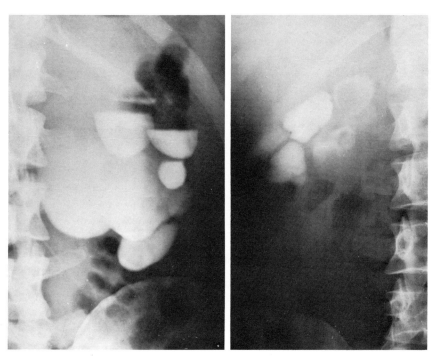

Fig. 5–28   Fig. 5–29

Figure 5–28. *Left retrograde pyelogram.* **Advanced hydronephrosis with fluid level,** indicating that air is present. (At operation several **anomalous vessels** were found; one large vein crossed upper end of ureter and bound it against pelvis.)

Figure 5–29. *Right retrograde pyelogram.* **Hydronephrosis with dilated calyces.** Two of calyces show **filling defects due to blood clots.** (At operation obstruction was found at ureteropelvic junction. Right nephrectomy was done.)

*INTERPRETATION OF UROGRAMS; VALUE OF
SPECIAL TECHNIQUES*

Inconsistencies Between Excretory and Retrograde Urograms

A finding that is often misunderstood is the occasional great difference in appearance between a routine excretory urogram in which considerable abdominal pressure is used to partially obstruct the ureters and a retrograde pyelogram. All experienced urologists have encountered cases in which the kidneys and ureters looked normal in excretory urograms, yet the retrograde pyelograms demonstrated marked pyelectasis or pyeloureterectasis, or a case in which the excretory urogram without abdominal pressure appeared normal, but a urogram made with abdominal pressure showed marked pyeloureterectasis. Overdistention of the normal pelvis or ureter or both is occasionally seen in retrograde pyelography (see Chapter 4, page 277) and usually presents no problem. Marked pyeloureterectasis on the other hand is a distinctly different problem. At the present writing knowledgeable authors think this results from previous damage to the urinary tract from obstruction or infection or both (Figs. 5–30, 5–31, and 5–32). (See also discussion in Chapter 7, page 779.)

Value of Delayed Retrograde Pyelogram

One procedure which may be helpful in distinguishing a large normal pelvis from pathologic dilatation is the delayed retrograde pyelogram which is made as follows: After the contrast medium has been injected through the catheter and the initial pyelogram has been made, the catheter is withdrawn and the patient is allowed to be up on his feet. Subsequent pyelograms are then made at intervals of 10, 20, and 30 minutes. The degree of obstruction may be surmised from the elapsed time and the amount of medium which is retained in the pelvis. Although helpful, this diagnostic procedure is not infallible and the result must be interpreted with caution, since it is possible with the passage of the catheter to irritate the ureteropelvic junction, ureter, or ureteral orifice enough to produce spasm which could account for delayed emptying time of the medium (Figs. 5–33, 5–34, and 5–35).

Value of Re-injection and Infusion Types of Excretory Urography

In advanced cases of hydronephrosis, function may be so reduced that in the routine series of excretory urograms the usual 20- and 45-minute films show nothing. In such cases the use of re-injection or infusion type excretory urography plus delayed films of several hours may result in visualization sufficient for diagnosis (Figs. 5–36 and 5–37A and B; see also Fig. 12–177). As a matter of fact, in occasional cases urograms made 24 hours after injection of contrast medium may finally visualize conditions enough for diagnosis (Fig. 5–38).

(Text continued on page 394.)

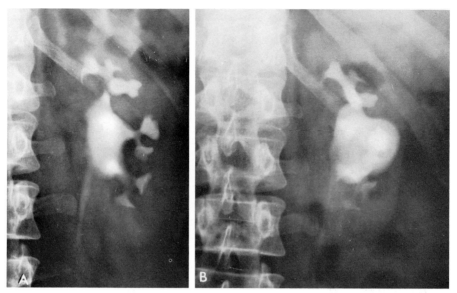

Figure 5–30. *Excretory urograms.* **A,** *Twenty-minute film.* **Apparently mild pyelectasis** of left kidney. **B,** *Sixty-minute film,* with more complete filling. **Pyelectasis of much greater degree** than one would suspect from 20-minute film. (At operation anomalous vessels at ureteropelvic junction were found and sectioned.)

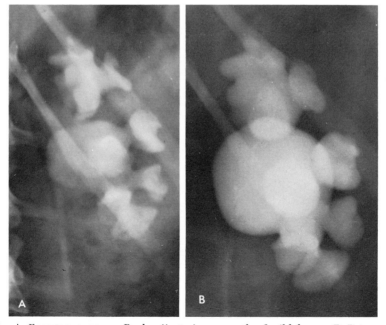

Figure 5–31. **A,** *Excretory urogram.* **Pyelocaliectasis apparently of mild degree. B,** *Retrograde pyelogram.* More complete filling shows that **degree of pyelocaliectasis is much greater than suspected** from excretory urogram.

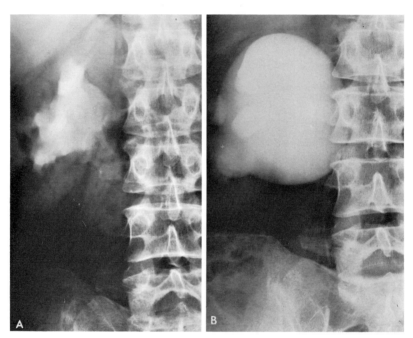

Figure 5–32.   Possible diagnostic errors from incomplete filling of pelvis with contrast medium. **A,** *Excretory urogram, 20-minute film.* Moderately severe hydronephrosis on right. It was minimal on left (not shown). **B,** *Right retrograde pyelogram.* Complete filling shows pyelectasis to be of much greater degree.

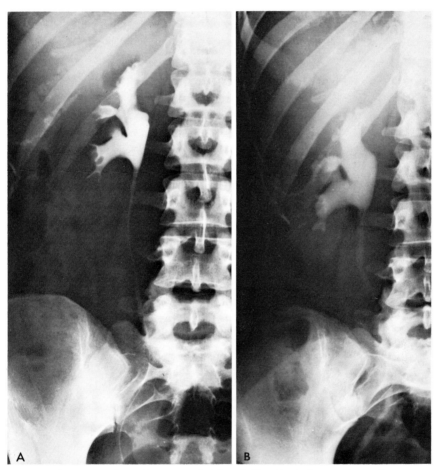

Figure 5–33. *Right retrograde pyelogram and delayed film.* **A,** *Pyelogram.* **Normal. B,** *Twenty-minute delayed pyelogram.* **Pelvis and ureter dilated, grade 1.** Ureter is entirely filled with medium down to bladder because of irritation of ureter during catheterization. (No surgical exploration.)

Fig. 5–34

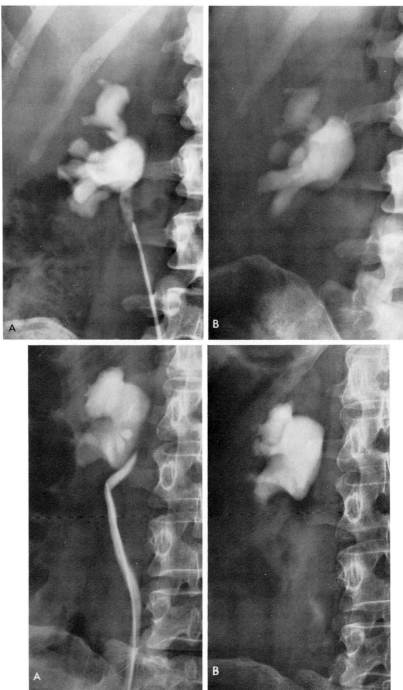

Fig. 5–35

Figure 5–34. *Right retrograde pyelogram with delayed film.* **A,** *Pyelogram.* **Pyelectasis from obstruction of ureteropelvic junction.** Pelvis is of globular type; it and calyces are dilated, grade 1. **B,** *Twenty-minute delayed pyelogram.* Medium retained in pelvis, none in ureter, indicating obstruction at ureteropelvic junction. (Anomalous vessel was found at operation and plastic operation done on ureteropelvic junction.)

Figure 5–35. *Right retrograde pyelogram with delayed film.* **A,** *Pyelogram.* **Pyelocaliectasis with high lying ureteropelvic junction.** Ureter is not inserted at most dependent portion of pelvis. **B,** *Twenty-minute delayed pyelogram.* Medium is retained in pelvis and calyces; very slight amount in right ureter, indicating obstruction at ureteropelvic junction.

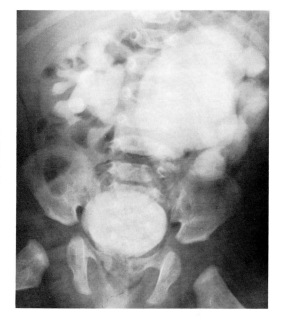

Figure 5–36. *Excretory urogram* of boy, aged 4 months. **Bilateral obstruction at ureteropelvic junctures with pyelectasis,** grade 4 on left and grade 2 on right. This film, made 2½ hours after injection of contrast medium, indicates value of late films.

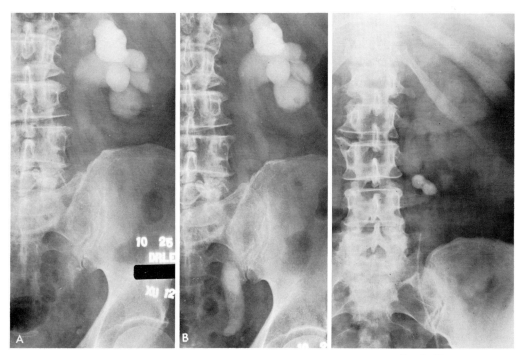

Fig. 5–37   Fig. 5–38

Figure 5–37. Value of delayed or late excretory urogram. (There had been **recently attempted manipulation of left ureteral stone;** and *20-minute excretory urogram* showed suggestion of dilated calyces, but pelvis and ureter were not outlined.) **A,** *Excretory urogram, 2-hour film.* **Pyelocaliectasis with dilatation of upper part of ureter.** Lower part of ureter not outlined. **B,** *Three-hour film.* Entire ureter filled. Obstruction at intramural portion of ureter.

Figure 5–38. Value of delayed or late excretory urogram. *Plain film* with lead catheter in left ureter. (Excretory urogram made 24 hours previously had shown no function.) There is now contrast medium present in kidney. **Hydronephrosis secondary to obstruction at ureteropelvic juncture and calculous obstruction.** (No medium was injected through catheter.)

LOCALIZED DILATATION OF CALYX (HYDROCALYX, CALYCEAL DIVERTICULUM, AND PYELOGENIC CYST); HYDROCALYCOSIS

Localized dilatation of an entire calyx or a portion of a calyx, a fairly common condition, has caused a good deal of confusion in the literature especially from the standpoint of terminology and etiology. Bona fide obstruction of a calyx may result from stricture of the infundibulum (Figs. 5–39 and 5–40), stone, tumor, peripelvic cyst (Fig. 5–41), or an overlying blood vessel.

When obstruction is not apparent and the etiology is obscure, the condition has been described by such terms as *pyelogenic cyst* (Holm), *calyceal diverticulum* (Prather), and *hydrocalyx* (Figs. 5–42 through 5–55). It has also been suggested that these lesions may represent simple parenchymal cysts or cortical abscesses which have ruptured and drained into a calyx. Holm thinks pyelogenic cysts arise from the Wolffian ducts in contradistinction to simple renal cysts which arise from metanephrogenic tissue. A pyelogenic cyst, therefore, in his opinion must be lined by typical uroepithelium (transitional epithelium). This would distinguish it from a simple cyst or cortical abscess which had ruptured into a calyx. Vermooten suggested that tubular dilatation (as seen in sponge kidney) is a possible etiologic agent. In all cases, a communication between the cavity and the pelviocalyceal system can be demonstrated either urographically or at operation.

The term *hydrocalyx* should be used to indicate that the **entire** calyx is involved and that the communication is directly into the pelvis rather than into another part of the calyx (either minor or major calyx). The terms *calyceal diverticulum* and *pyelogenic cyst* indicate that there is a communication between the cavity and a calyx. Abeshouse tried to distinguish

these two entities on the basis of the length of the narrow communicating channel. In his opinion, a long narrow channel indicated a calyceal diverticulum whereas a short one suggested a pyelogenic cyst. Calyceal diverticula and pyelogenic cysts are usually small or of only moderate size in contrast to a hydrocalyx, which may be large, or to hydrocalycosis, in which the cyst may reach extreme proportions. It should be appreciated that accurate distinction may be impossible even at operation or at the time of gross and microscopic examination of a kidney which has been removed. In most cases, especially if the lesion is of small or only moderate size, calyceal cysts are of no clinical importance; diagnosis is made accidentally when an excretory urogram is made for some unrelated problem. In some cases, however, infection or stones may complicate the situation and require surgical excision.

Hydrocalycosis

An extreme degree of hydrocalyx in which the calyx becomes so large that it may present as a palpable abdominal tumor has been described as a distinct clinical entity and given the name *hydrocalycosis*. Williams and Mininberg reported three cases in children, which they state comprised the third, fourth, and fifth pediatric cases reported in the literature. They found 12 "well documented" cases in adults in the literature. They define this condition as a cystic dilatation of a major calyx with no obvious obstructive etiology; there must be a demonstrable connection with the renal pelvis and the cyst wall must be lined with uroepithelium. Urographic diagnosis may be difficult as findings are not pathognomonic. In their three pediatric cases, the problem was essentially that of a mass in the upper pole of the kidney with absent or very poor visualization of the involved calyx on excretory urography and little or no filling during retrograde pyelography. Two of their cases also had posterior urethral valves. Theoretical considerations of the etiology of this condition (Moore; Watkins, 1939) suggest the possibility of a ring of muscle at the juncture of the calyceal infundibulum and renal pelvis.

(Text continued on page 405.)

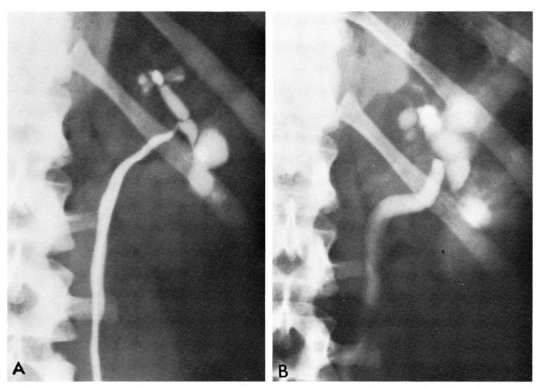

Figure 5–39. Congenital solitary kidney with stricture at juncture of ureter and calyces. (At surgical exploration there seemed to be no true pelvis.) **A,** *Retrograde pyelogram,* in 1955. **B,** *Retrograde pyelogram,* 1958. **Progression of pyelectasis.** (At operation, cause of stricture was not apparent. Ureterolysis was done.) (Courtesy of Dr. C. D. Creevy.)

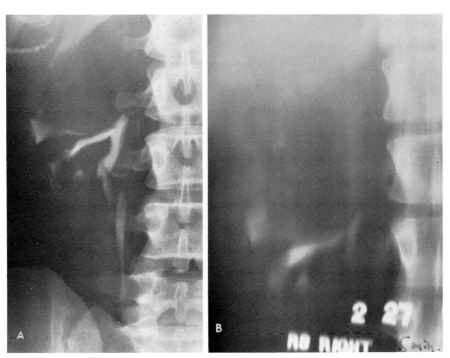

Figure 5–40. Stricture of infundibulum of upper calyx of right kidney, producing huge hydrocalyx suggesting tumor. **A,** *Excretory urogram.* Middle calyx displaced downward by "mass" in upper pole. **B,** *Nephrotomogram.* "Mass" is large negative shadow from dilated calyx. (Nephrectomy done.)

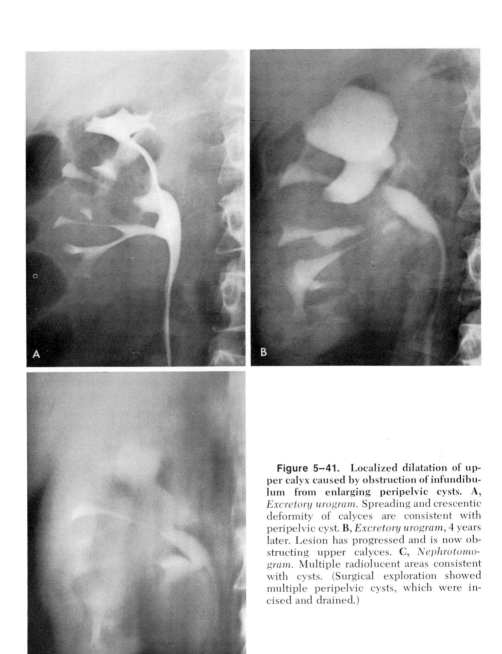

Figure 5–41. Localized dilatation of upper calyx caused by obstruction of infundibulum from enlarging peripelvic cysts. **A,** *Excretory urogram.* Spreading and crescentic deformity of calyces are consistent with peripelvic cyst. **B,** *Excretory urogram,* 4 years later. Lesion has progressed and is now obstructing upper calyces. **C,** *Nephrotomogram.* Multiple radiolucent areas consistent with cysts. (Surgical exploration showed multiple peripelvic cysts, which were incised and drained.)

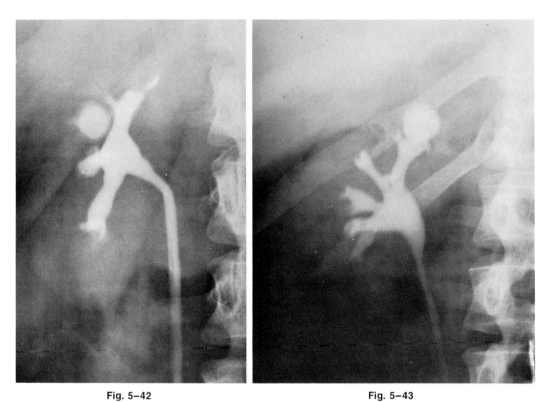

Fig. 5–42   Fig. 5–43

Figures 5–42 and **5–43.**   *Retrograde pyelograms.* Calyceal diverticula or pyelogenic cysts communicating with branches of upper calyces.

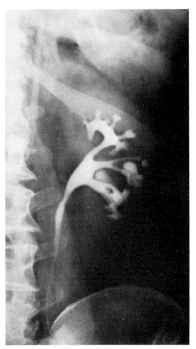

Figure 5–44. *Left retrograde pyelogram.* **Small calyceal diverticulum or pyelogenic cyst** which communicates with branch of middle calyx.

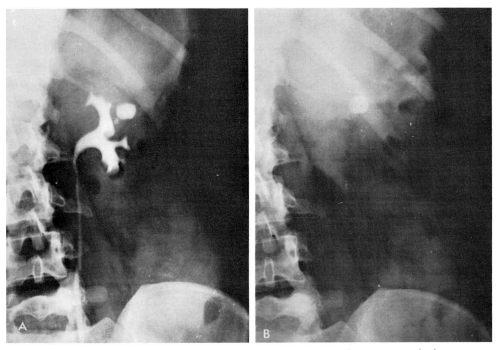

Figure 5–45. **A,** *Retrograde pyelogram.* **Calyceal diverticulum or pyelogenic cyst** which communicates with branch of upper calyx. **B,** *Delayed film.* Contrast medium is retained in cyst.

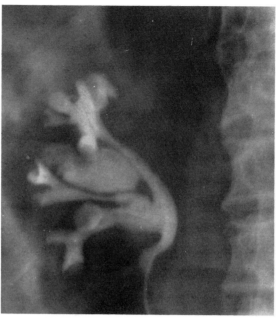

Figure 5–46. *Retrograde pyelogram.* **Rather large pyelogenic cyst or calyceal diverticulum** which communicates with infundibulum of upper calyx. (Courtesy of Dr. Hugh Rives.)

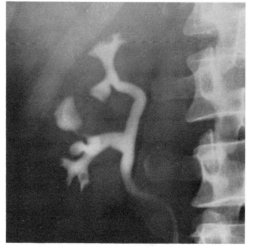

Figure 5–47. *Right retrograde pyelogram.* **Calyceal diverticulum or pyelogenic cyst** communicating with branch of lower calyx. (According to Abeshouse, this should be considered diverticulum because of long communicating channel.)

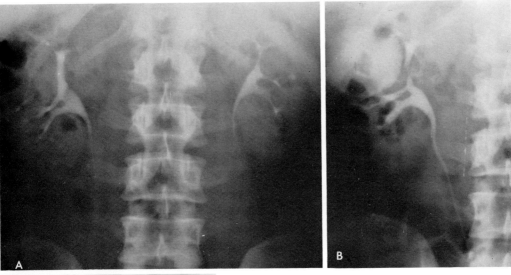

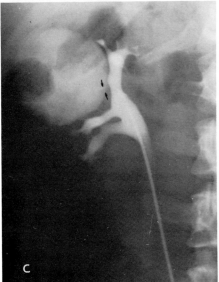

Figure 5–48. Large calyceal diverticulum of right kidney of 35-year-old woman. **A,** *Excretory urogram, 5-minute film.* Spreading of middle and upper calyces, but no contrast medium is visible in diverticulum. **B,** *Excretory urogram, 15-minute film.* Large diverticulum is now fairly well filled. **C,** *Retrograde pyelogram.* Diverticulum is better filled. Narrow communication (*arrows*) can be seen between upper calyx and diverticulum. (Courtesy of Dr. H. W. Calhoon.)

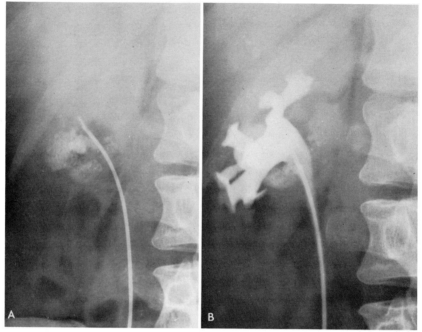

Figure 5–49. Pyelogenic cyst or calyceal diverticulum filled with many small calculi. **A,** *Plain film.* Calculi overlie midrenal area. **B,** *Retrograde pyelogram.* Diverticulum filled with stones is overlying normal appearing pelvis and calyces. (Surgical exploration showed that diverticulum communicated with branch of middle calyx in anteroposterior plane, so it is not shown in this projection.)

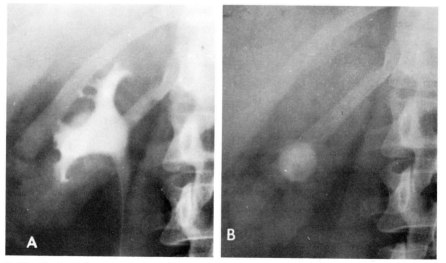

Figure 5–50. Pyelogenic cyst or calyceal diverticulum with retained medium. **A,** *Right retrograde pyelogram.* Cyst communicates with lower major calyx of right kidney and is partially obscured by this calyx. **B,** *Delayed film.* Residual contrast medium remains in cyst.

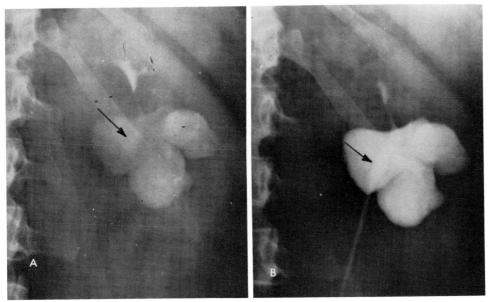

Figure 5–51. Large pyelogenic cyst, calyceal diverticulum, or hydrocalyx. **A,** *Excretory urogram.* Large irregular collection of contrast medium overlies and partially obscures pelvis and middle and lower calyces of left kidney. Pelvis, however, can be seen through the medium (*arrow*). **B,** *Left retrograde pyelogram.* Better visualization of large pyelogenic cyst. Outline of normal pelvis can be seen through medium. (On exploration, large pyelogenic cyst was found, which apparently arose from middle calyx. Calyx was obliterated and midportion of kidney was almost destroyed. This might be more accurately described as hydrocalyx.) (Courtesy of Dr. David Cristol.)

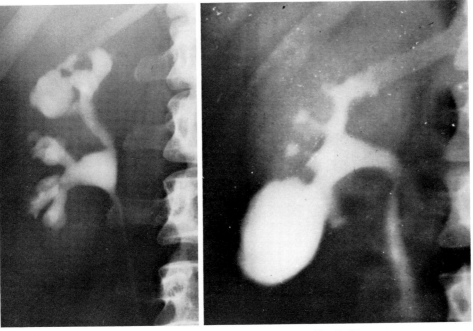

Fig. 5–52   Fig. 5–53

Figure 5–52. *Right retrograde pyelogram.* Calyceal diverticulum or pyelogenic cyst communicates with branch of upper calyx of right kidney.

Figure 5–53. *Retrograde pyelogram.* Large calyceal diverticulum or hydrocalyx communicating with lower calyces. (Not explored.)

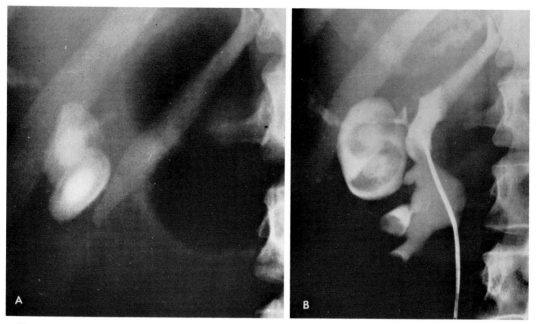

Figure 5–54. Calculi in calyceal diverticulum. A, *Plain film.* Laminated stones overlying right kidney. B, *Right retrograde pyelogram.* Stones are seen to be included in diverticulum which apparently communicates with branch of upper calyx. (Courtesy of Dr. Edwin Davis.)

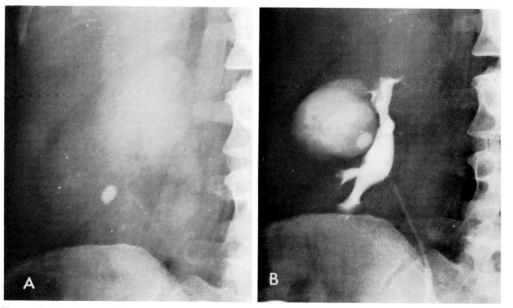

Figure 5–55. Stone in large calyceal diverticulum, pyelogenic cyst, or simple cyst which had ruptured into renal pelvis. A, *Plain film.* Multiple shadows over midportion of right kidney. B, *Right retrograde pyelogram.* Large pyelogenic cyst which apparently communicates with middle calyx and extends to periphery of kidney. Calculi included in cyst. (At operation, there appeared to be large simple cortical cyst which had ruptured into pelvis, but it could not be differentiated from pyelogenic cyst.)

Vascular Obstruction of the Infundibulum of the Upper Calyx

by

Elwin E. Fraley

That renal vessels can impinge on the proximal collecting system and cause persistent radiographic filling defects has been recognized by radiologists for a long time. Baum and Gillenwater, Kreel and Pyle, and Tille showed that vascular impressions can produce filling defects similar to those caused by tumors and stones. Not until recently, however, was the possible physiologic significance of vessels crossing the infundibulum recognized. A syndrome consisting of nephralgia and vascular obstruction of the superior infundibulum was first described in 1966 (Fraley). Subsequently, the clinical and radiographic findings associated with functionally significant *intrarenal vascular obstruction* were documented further (Fraley, 1967; Nebesar, Pollard, and Fraley).

In cases of vascular obstruction of the superior infundibulum, a persistent, well-marginated, transversely oriented filling defect of the infundibulum is evident on the intravenous pyelogram. Usually, of course, the remaining calyces of the obstructed kidney and the collecting system

of the contralateral kidney are normal. Proximal to the filling defect there is marked calycectasis (Fig. 5–56A). The delayed drainage radiographs of the retrograde pyelogram show selective entrapment of dye in the superior calyx (Fig. 5–56B), and selective angiography usually demonstrates a vessel, artery or vein, crossing the infundibulum in the region of the filling defect (Fig. 5–56C).

If wires are placed in the offending vessels through the angiogram catheters, the precise anatomic relations between the vessels and the infundibulum can be studied by radiographs taken in multiple projections (Doppman and Fraley) (Fig. 5–57A through D). Angiograms are also useful in these cases to rule out mass lesions of the kidney which either can compress the infundibulum extrinsically or, as with renal tumors, produce infundibular obstruction by direct invasion.

Vascular obstruction of the superior infundibulum is sometimes difficult to differentiate from infundibular obstruction produced by strictures such as are often seen late in tuberculosis or from other intrinsic lesions such as stones and tumors. However, the characteristic radiographic findings and routine clinical studies usually serve to clarify the differential diagnosis.

(Text continued on page 408.)

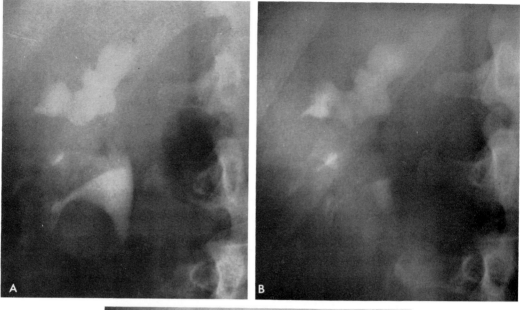

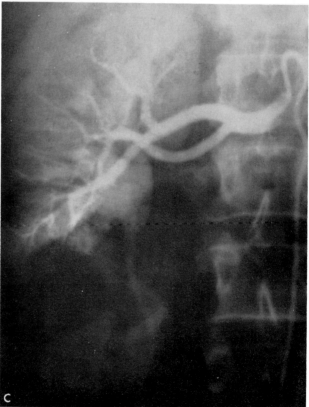

Figure 5–56. Vascular obstruction of superior infundibulum. A, *Excretory urogram.* Persistent filling defect in infundibulum and marked superior calycectasis. B, *Retrograde pyelogram, delayed film.* Selective entrapment of dye proximal to point of infundibular obstruction. C, *Selective renal angiogram.* Large artery crosses infundibulum in area of filling defect seen on excretory urogram (A). Dilated calyx can be seen in background.

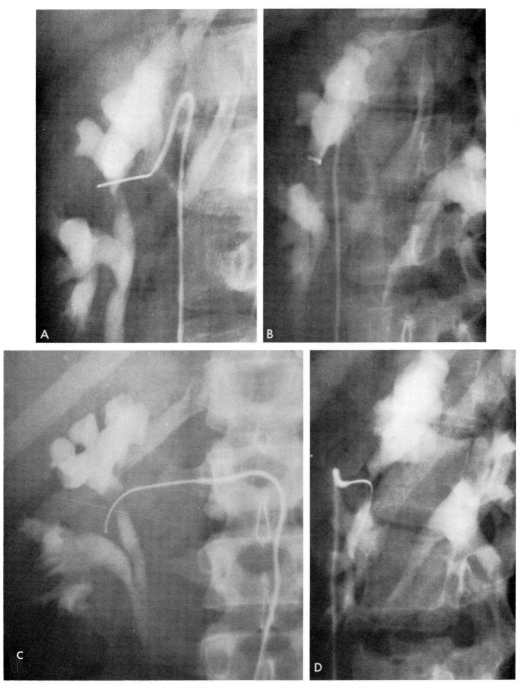

Figure 5–57. Obstruction of infundibulum by vascular vise consisting of two arteries. *Excretory urograms.*
A, *Anteroposterior view.* Guide wire in what appeared to be obstructing artery on selective angiogram.
B, *Oblique view.* Artery supplying middle vascular segment can be seen to pass ventral to infundibulum.
C, *Anteroposterior view.* Wire now positioned in vessel to posterior vascular segment. **D,** *Oblique view.* This
vessel is dorsal to infundibulum; thus it forms obstructive vascular vise with artery to middle segment.

"OBSTRUCTION" AT THE URETEROPELVIC JUNCTION

Ureteropelvic obstruction with pyelectasis is by far the commonest congenital anomaly of the urinary tract and is one of the commonest urologic problems in infants and children.* Excretory urography finds one of its greatest fields of usefulness in this condition. Severe degrees of "obstruction" at the ureteropelvic junction usually give rise to symptoms and findings early in life, whereas milder degrees may not become clinically apparent until adult life.

Tendency to Bilaterality

There is a distinct tendency to bilateral obstruction of the ureteropelvic junction. Fortunately, however, in most cases the dilatation is less on one side than on the other (Figs. 5–58, 5–59, and 5–60), so that surgical intervention on one side may be all that is required. It is usually wise to examine the nonoperated kidney periodically by means of excretory urography for a period of years to determine whether the pyelectasis is progressing.

Occurrence in Infants and Children

The commonest cause of an upper abdominal mass in a child is *not* a renal tumor (Wilms' tumor or neuroblastoma; see Chapter 10) but rather a hydronephrotic kidney from obstruction of the ureteropelvic junction. This is true even though the mass may feel firm and solid. An important axiom, which should be repeated, is that *an abdominal mass in a child should be considered hydronephrosis until proved otherwise.* Exploratory operation should not be carried out for a suspected renal tumor on an infant or child until an excretory urogram (plus a retrograde pyelogram if necessary) has been made to exclude hydronephrosis.

As has been mentioned previously, the degree of obstruction of the ureteropelvic junction varies greatly. In cases of minimal obstruction, it may be necessary to compare the involved kidney with the contralateral kidney to determine if pyelectasis is really present. Such minimal degrees of pyelectasis may be of clinical importance in recurring urinary infection. Examples of various degrees of obstruction at the ureteropelvic junction in infants and children are shown in Figures 5–61 through 5–67.

Etiology and Pathogenesis

Concept of Mechanical Obstruction

Opinions expressed in the literature have differed greatly concerning the various types and causes of obstruction of the ureteropelvic junction. For instance, some workers have ascribed the primary causative role to *anomalous vessels* which cross the ureteropelvic junction (Figs. 5–68 through 5–73). To others these vessels are of secondary or no importance and become apparent only because pyelectasis has resulted either from positional malrelationship or some *intrinsic or extrinsic obstructive lesions such as stenoses, strictures, bands, or adhesions.* Some workers think the term *high insertion of the ureter into the renal pelvis* is a misnomer representing an erroneous concept which falls into the same category as obstruction from anomalous vessels. In other words it is a secondary not a primary situation. They think that the pelvis, because of its anatomic relationships, can enlarge only anteriorly and caudally, bulging over blood vessels or any "fibrous bands" that may be in the vicinity.* This results in the appearance of the so-called pyelectasis with "high insertion of the ureter." Currently, however, the majority of urologists seem

---

*Shopfner (1965; 1966a; 1966b) has challenged this concept. He thinks most cases of pyelectasis result from infection rather than obstruction. (See discussion of "concept of nonobstructive dilatation," page 409.)

*Because of this anterior sagging of the renal pelvis, films made with the patient in the prone position often will reveal the dilated pelvis better than will those made with the patient in the ordinary supine position.

to think that the contour of the ureteropelvic junction, its caliber, and the caliber of the adjacent ureter are important. Serious diagnostic effort is expended before operation to determine these factors urographically (Figs. 5–74 through 5–79).

Concept of "Nonobstructive Dilatation"; Flow Rate Versus Capacity

The profession has been more or less startled by recent publications of Shopfner (1965; 1966a; 1966b), in which he asserts that mechanical obstruction of the ureteropelvic junction is extremely rare, and that most cases of pyelectasis are nonobstructive and the result of primary infection. As proof of this contention he cites statistics from the Children's Mercy Hospital in Kansas City where he is director of the Department of Radiology. He points out that in 1953 in that hospital the diagnosis of obstruction of the ureteropelvic junction was made in 63 cases and that plastic operations were performed on the ureteropelvic junction in 44 cases. In contrast, during 1963 the diagnosis was made in only five cases. He concludes that the problem is chiefly medical rather than surgical, most cases being "nonobstructive." The rare obstructive type case he maintains is seen only in the very young infant and is congenital in origin.

Further explanation of Shopfner's (1965; 1966a; 1966b) position follows: Primary infection (pyelonephritis, cystitis, and so on) results in ileus of the collecting system (calyces, pelvis, and ureter), which predisposes to vesicoureteral reflux. The reflux further aids and abets the ileus. *If the flow rate of urine from the kidneys is greater than the emptying rate of the sluggish pelvis and ureter, these structures tend to dilate.*＊

＊Flow rate versus capacity is receiving more and more attention as an etiologic factor in pyelectasis. (See discussion of intermittent hydronephrosis below.)

Hutch and Tanagho have further elaborated this concept by showing that vesicoureteral reflux can increase flow rates beyond the emptying capacity of the structures. They state that "any tube will become obstructive if the flow rate through it exceeds its emptying capacity." In the human ureter, the points of lowest emptying capacity are the ureteropelvic and ureterovesical junctions; therefore, nonobstructive dilatation begins above these points.

Conditions which can result in abnormally large flow rates include forcing of fluids (such as excessive beer drinking), diabetes insipidus, increased output of one kidney after removal of the other, and vesicoureteral reflux.

Shopfner further pointed out that minimal degrees of pyeloureterectasis, which were formerly regarded as variations of normal, may be pathologic; this also holds for the ureter, where minimal degrees of segmental dilatation (such as the "spindle") are manifestations of impaired peristalsis. As the condition progresses, generalized dilatation of the collecting system results, the ureters become tortuous and elongated, and reversed ureteral peristalsis occurs—the consequent back-and-forth movement of urine contributing to the persistence of infection.

As the ureter dilates, elongates, and becomes tortuous, "kinking" appears. This occurs first at the points of junction of the mobile and fixed portions of the ureter (the ureteropelvic junction—brim of the pelvis—and the ureterovesical junction). Periureteritis with exudation and necrosis results in stenosis and adhesions between adjacent and parallel segments of the tortuous ureter. Ureteral dilatation below the "point of obstruction" and vesicoureteral reflex are considered specific signs that the stasis and dilatation are acquired, that is, secondary to infection. Treatment should be directed toward eradication of the infection rather than toward the selection of surgical procedures to eliminate "obstruction."

Although this concept appears to be rather radical and revolutionary, the reader is urged to give it thoughtful and serious consideration before completely discarding it. It is common knowledge that the results of plastic surgical procedures on the ureteropelvic junction have not been consistently brilliant; the multiplicity of operations advocated provides elo-quent proof of this statement. Also, knowledgeable workers in this field (Hodson, 1967; Hope) are more and more expressing opinions that infection and reflux are high on the list of etiologic factors in the so-called obstructive uropathies. Certainly it behooves the urologist to carefully exclude vesicoureteral reflux and ureterectasis before making an unqualified diagnosis of mechanical obstruction of the ureteropelvic junction.

(Text continued on page 420.)

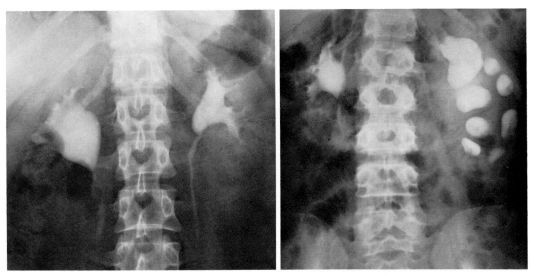

Fig. 5–58   **Fig. 5–59**

Figure 5–58. *Excretory urogram.* Obstruction of both ureteropelvic junctions, greater on right than left.
Figure 5–59. *Excretory urogram.* Obstruction of both ureteropelvic junctions of boy age 12 years, greater on left than right. (Left nephrectomy.)

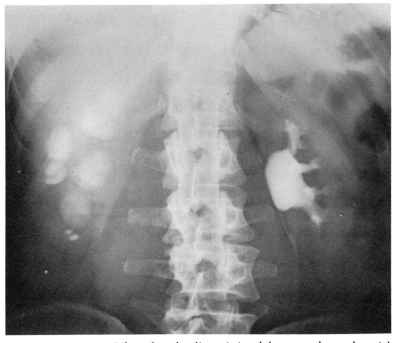

Figure 5–60. *Excretory urogram.* Bilateral pyelocaliectasis in adult; more advanced on right than on left. (At operation **anomalous vessels** were found running into lower pole. **Two stones** measured 3 mm in diameter.)

Fig. 5–61

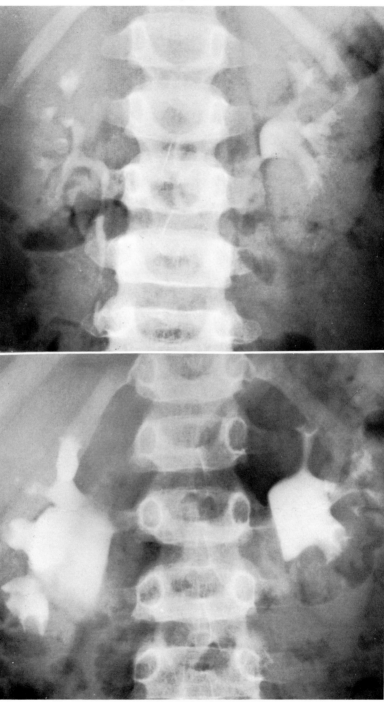

Fig. 5–62

Figure 5–61. *Excretory urogram* of 6-year-old girl. **Minimal obstruction of ureteropelvic junction** on left. Normal pelvis on right.

Figure 5–62. *Excretory urogram* of 4-year-old boy. **Obstruction of both ureteropelvic junctions.** Obstruction greater on right than on left. (Y-plasty operation done on right.)

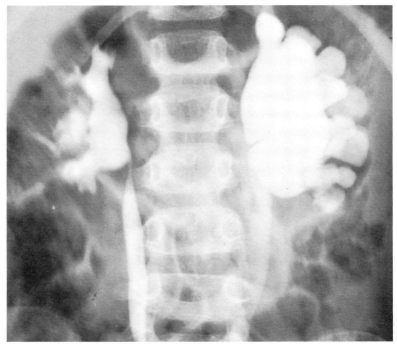

Figure 5–63. *Retrograde pyelogram.* **Obstruction of both ureteropelvic junctions** of girl, 4 years of age. **Right pyelectasis, grade 1; left, grade 3.** (Y-plasty operation was done on left.)

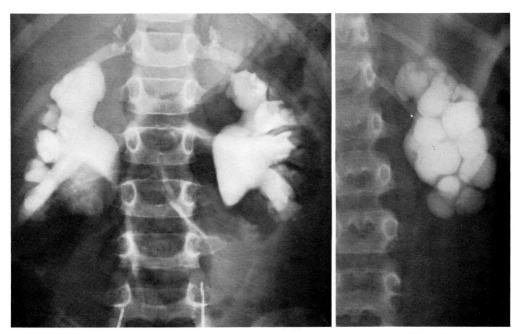

Fig. 5–64   Fig. 5–65

Figure 5–64. *Retrograde pyelogram.* **Obstruction of both ureteropelvic junctions** of boy, 6 years of age. **Bilateral pyelectasis, grade 2.** (Spiral-flap operation done on right.)

Figure 5–65. *Left retrograde pyelogram.* **Obstruction at ureteropelvic juncture with pyelocaliectasis, grade 4,** in boy, 9 years of age. (Almost all of kidney was destroyed, so nephrectomy was performed. Preoperative excretory urogram showed right pyelectasis, grade 1.)

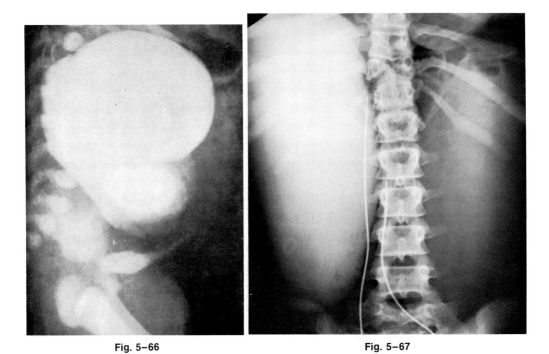

Fig. 5–66   Fig. 5–67

Figure 5–66. *Contrast medium injected with needle introduced through lumbar region.* **Huge left hydronephrosis and hydroureter** in newborn male infant. Right kidney was normal on excretory urogram, but left kidney showed no function. (Courtesy of Dr. S. A. Vest.)

Figure 5–67. *Retrograde pyelogram.* **Bilateral pyelectasis, grade 4,** in girl, 13 years of age, from **obstruction of ureteropelvic junctures.** No visualization on excretory urogram. (Y-plasty was done on right, nephrectomy on left.)

Fig. 5–68

Fig. 5–69

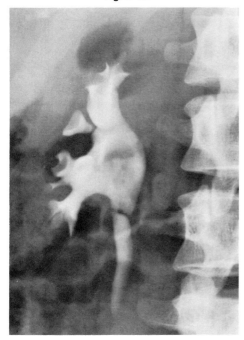

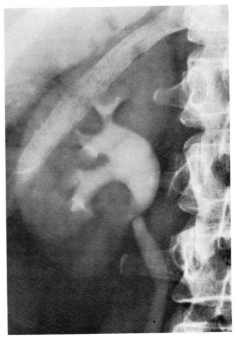

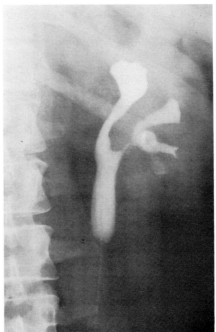

Fig. 5–70

Figure 5–68. *Retrograde pyelogram, right.* Filling defect apparently from anomalous vessel crossing ureteropelvic juncture. **Pyelectasis, grade 1.**

Figure 5–69. *Excretory urogram.* Filling defect from vessel crossing ureteropelvic juncture of right kidney. **Pyelectasis, grade 1.**

Figure 5–70. *Retrograde pyelogram.* **Partial obstruction of ureter** 4 cm below ureteropelvic juncture. **Stone** 1 cm in diameter in anterior projection of middle calyx. (At operation, obstruction was found to be caused by plexus of veins which crossed ureter at point of obstruction. They were excised, and stone was removed.)

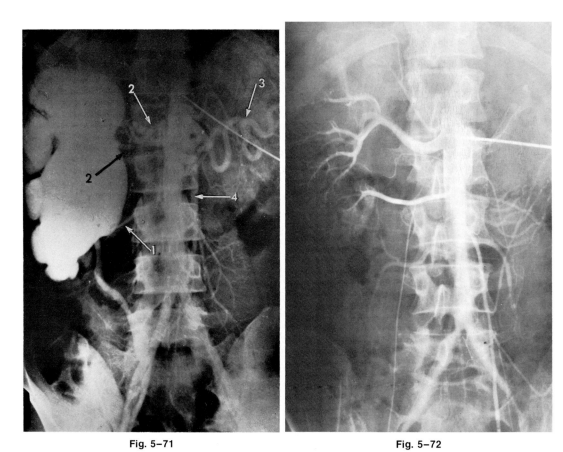

Fig. 5–71   **Fig. 5–72**

Figure 5–71. *Right retrograde pyelogram* of 27-year-old man, *with aortogram superimposed.* **Marked pyelectasis with aberrant artery (*1*) seen to be obstructing ureteropelvic junction.** Right renal artery (*2*), splenic artery (*3*), and superior mesenteric artery (*4*) are well-outlined. (Courtesy of Dr. A. K. Doss.)

Figure 5–72. *Aortogram.* **Aberrant artery** of type often found crossing ureteropelvic junction serves lower pole of right kidney. (Courtesy of Dr. C. K. Pearlman.)

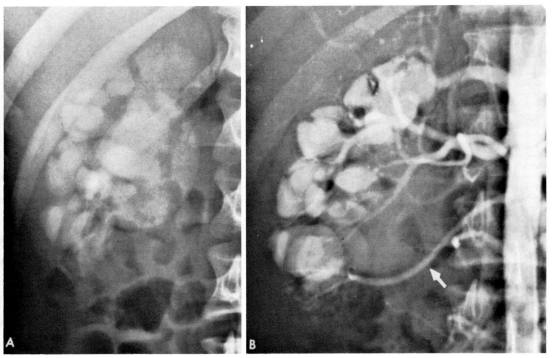

Figure 5–73. Hydronephrosis with accessory renal artery crossing right ureteropelvic junction. A, *Excretory urogram.* B, *Arteriogram.* Accessory renal artery to lower pole of kidney passes across ureteropelvic junction (*arrow*). (From Siegelman, S. S., and Bosniak, M. A.)

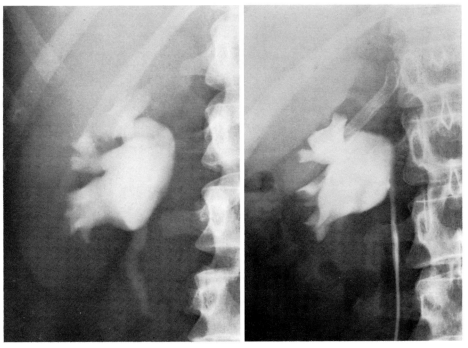

Fig. 5–74   Fig. 5–75

Figure 5–74. *Excretory urogram.* Obstruction of right ureteropelvic juncture from high insertion of ureter.
Figure 5–75. *Retrograde pyelogram,* right. Obstruction of ureteropelvic juncture from high insertion of ureter.

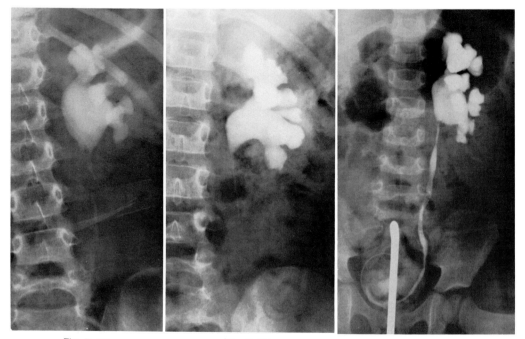

Fig. 5–76   Fig. 5–77   Fig. 5–78

Figure 5–76. *Retrograde pyelogram, left.* Stricture of upper part of left ureter causing moderate pyelo-caliectasis in girl, 5 years of age. (At operation, stricture was found to be about 2.5 cm long and was situated immediately below ureteropelvic juncture. It was treated as obstruction of ureteropelvic juncture. Flap turned down to replace entire area of narrowing.)

Figure 5–77. *Excretory urogram.* Unilateral (left) pyelectasis in boy, 5 years of age, secondary to obstruction of ureteropelvic juncture. Ureteropelvic juncture is in normal dependent position, but it and adjacent ureter are narrowed.

Figure 5–78. Obstruction of ureteropelvic junction of child, age 5 years. Note long segment of narrow ureter adjacent to dilated renal pelvis. (Culp-Scardino spiral-flap pyeloplasty was performed.) (Courtesy of Dr. Jerry D. Giesy.)

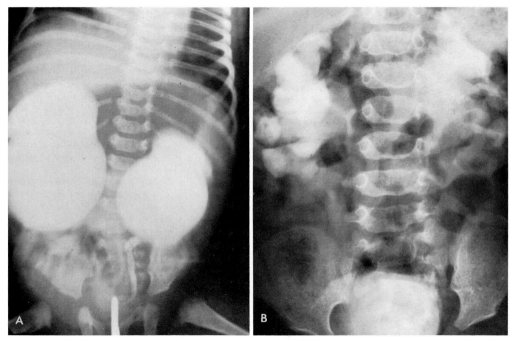

Figure 5–79. Infant with advanced bilateral hydronephrosis. **A,** *Retrograde pyelograms,* at 8 weeks of age. Previous excretory urogram had shown function on right in 5-hour film and slight function on left. (Surgical exploration revealed narrowing of both ureters just below ureteropelvic juncture. Bilateral spiral-flap operation was performed.) **B,** *Excretory urogram,* 8 months after operation.

INTERMITTENT HYDRONEPHROSIS

The syndrome of intermittent hydronephrosis has added considerably to our knowledge of the problem of obstruction of the ureteropelvic junction. This was first brought to the attention of the profession in 1956 by Nesbit who described patients with intermittent attacks of flank pain. Excretory urograms made between attacks of pain were normal; during an attack, pyelectasis was demonstrated on the painful side. Bourne; Falk; and Ansell and Paterson have confirmed this syndrome and added cases to the literature.

Hanley in 1959 and 1960 studied the problem and made the observation that the bifid "funnel type" pelvis (Fig. 5–80A) was almost never involved in this condition; it was the "closed type" or "ampullary" pelvis (Fig. 5–80B) that was the offender. This type of pelvis tends to be full and extrarenal and to have short infundibula of the calyces. His cinepyelographic studies with *overhydration* showed the bifid funnel type of pelvis to handle the increased fluid load easily without pelvic dilatation whereas the ampullary type of pelvis appeared to have difficulty handling the increased flow of urine. The "hold up," which appeared to be at the ureteropelvic junction, resulted in temporary pyelectasis until the urine flow dropped to a more normal level. Hanley further observed that clinically at least 90% of all ureteropelvic obstructions occur in the ampullary type of pelvis. Murnaghan studied the problem of the ureteropelvic junction in "congenital ureteropelvic obstruction" and came to the conclusion that the obstruction is due to replacement of normal muscular spirals of the pelvis by longitudinal fibers. Increased distention of the pelvis caused elongation of the longitudinal muscle fibers without increasing their girth, resulting in narrowing rather than distention of the ureteropelvic lumen. The cinefluorographic studies of Becker and Pollack tend to confirm the work of both Hanley (1959; 1960) and Murnaghan.

Kendall and Karafin recently reported two typical cases. The first was of a woman, aged 22 years, who had had intermittent right flank pain since puberty. She had noticed that excessive fluid intake seemed to bring on pain, and had learned to keep fluid intake to a minimum (even 2 cups of coffee for breakfast would precipitate the pain). The pain could often be relieved by strenuously arching her back. An excretory urogram revealed minimal right pyelectasis with normal calyces (Fig. 5–81A). The pelvis was of the ampullary type. A repeat excretory urogram was made during overhydration.[*] The right flank pain was reproduced and the urogram revealed a marked right hydronephrosis (Fig. 5–81B). The patient then proceeded to hyperextend her spine, change position, and so on until the pain eventually disappeared. A film taken after the pain disappeared is shown in Figure 5–81C which shows the pelvis to have returned to its previous size. Surgical exploration was carried out and a right pyeloplasty was done for "ureteropelvic stricture." The patient's symptoms have been relieved.

Their second case is illustrated in Figure 5–82A and B. A 28-year-old woman had recurring episodes of severe left flank pain. An excretory urogram showed mild left pyelectasis but essentially normal calyces. During overhydration, minimal flank pain recurred and a repeat excretory urogram showed moderate left hydronephrosis (Fig. 5–82B). Operation disclosed a "ureteropelvic obstruction secondary to a ureteral stricture with an overlying aberrant vessel." The patient has been asymptomatic since a pyeloplasty.

---

[*]Hydration pyelography is accomplished by administering (about 1 hour before injection of the excretory urographic medium) either 1,000 ml of fluid orally or 1,000 ml of 5% dextrose intravenously. Probably an even better method is the intravenous injection of 500 ml of 10% mannitol.

Ten Cate's case (Fig. 5–83) was also associated with ureteropelvic junction obstruction.

Bourne reported two cases of intermittent hydronephrosis. In both cases, the hydronephrosis resulted from overhydration associated with beer drinking (Fig. 5–84).

(Text continued on page 426.)

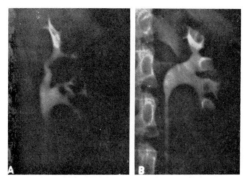

Figure 5–80. A, Funnel or bifid type of pelvis. B, Ampullary or closed type of pelvis. (From Kendall, A. R., and Karafin, L.)

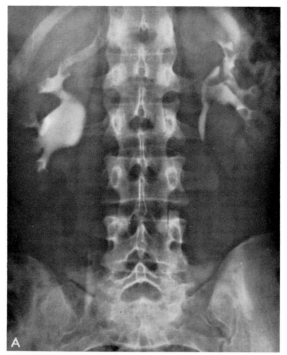

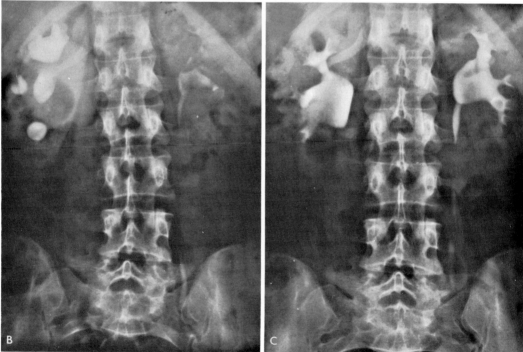

Figure 5–81. Intermittent right hydronephrosis of 22-year-old woman. **A**, *Excretory urogram* during asymptomatic period. **Mild right pyelectasis** but normal calyces. **B**, *Excretory urogram*. Film made during flank pain induced by hydration. **Moderate hydronephrosis**. **C**, Film made after pain had subsided. Pelvis has returned to original size. (From Kendall, A. R., and Karafin, L.)

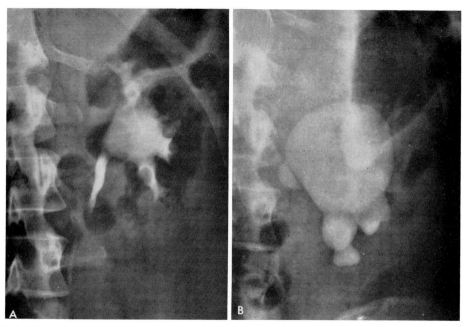

Figure 5–82. Intermittent left hydronephrosis. **A,** *Excretory urogram* during asymptomatic period. Mild pyelectasis but normal calyces. **B,** *Hydration excretory urogram* (patient having mild flank pain). Moderate hydronephrosis. (From Kendall, A. R., and Karafin, L.)

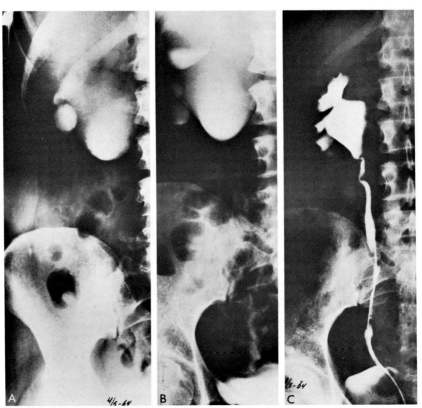

Figure 5–83.   Intermittent hydronephrosis due to obstruction at ureteropelvic junction. A and B, *Excretory urograms* during attack of right flank pain. C, *Retrograde pyelogram* only 4 days later, during absence of pain, showing almost complete reduction of hydronephrosis and well-delineated area of obstruction in ureteropelvic junction. (Courtesy of Dr. H. W. ten Cate.)

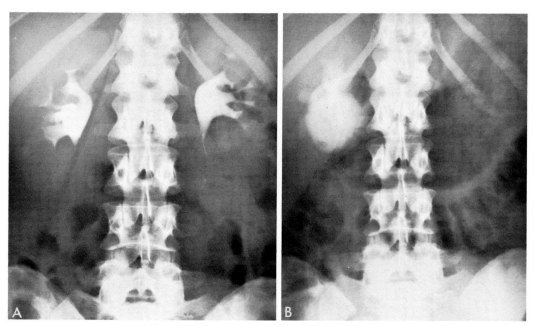

Figure 5–84. Intermittent **hydronephrosis** in woman aged 33. **A,** *Excretory urogram* when patient was free of pain. Normal. **B,** *Excretory urogram* during acute pain after drinking three glasses of beer. Note definite right hydronephrosis. (Medium has been almost entirely evacuated from left kidney.) (From Bourne, R. B.)

The Clinical Problem—Surgical Considerations

A few brief statements concerning surgical therapy accompanied by illustrative drawings may help the reader to understand the diagnostic problem of obstruction at the ureteropelvic junction.

In general, mild degrees of ureteropelvic obstruction with pyelectasis and little or no calycectasis are best left alone. Indications for surgical intervention include pain, calculi, infection, and destruction of renal substance. In borderline situations it is usually wise to lean toward conservatism and follow the patient with yearly excretory urograms to determine whether the condition is progressing. Whenever a kidney is operated on for stone, the surgeon should consider the possibility of associated obstruction of the ureteropelvic junction as an etiologic factor in the calculous formation. If such obstruction is present, it should be corrected at the time of operation. The choice between nephrectomy and conservative operation in cases of advanced pyelectasis is often difficult. The age of the patient and the condition of the opposite kidney will influence the decision, which is usually made when the kidney is exposed surgically.

So many types of surgical procedures have been described to correct obstruction at the ureteropelvic junction that it is impractical to consider them here. Figures 5–85 through 5–90 show the principal types of obstruction encountered at the ureteropelvic junction and the methods of operation presently employed at the Mayo Clinic to correct them. These drawings have been taken from articles by Culp (1955; 1961) and by Culp and De-Weerd. The interested reader should consult these articles for more detailed information.

Success of operation on the ureteropelvic junction is evaluated on the basis of (1) clinical and (2) urographic results. A patient may be relieved of pain, infection, and recurring formation of stones, and yet the postoperative urograms may show little or no change. In other cases postoperative urograms show the pelvis and calyces to have returned almost to normal size. In the majority of cases conditions vary between these two extremes (Figs. 5–91 through 5–94).

(*Text continued on page 432.*)

Figure 5–85. High insertion of ureter on renal pelvis. (From Culp, O. S., 1955.)

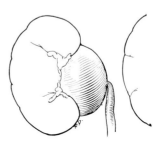

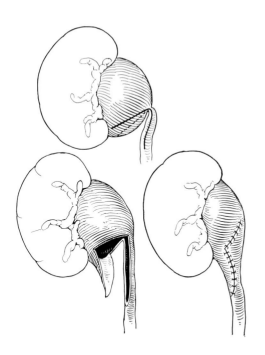

Figure 5–86. Technique of Y-plasty in cases of high insertion of ureter. Incisions are made on anterior and posterior surfaces of dilated pelvis and along medial aspect of ureter, thereby creating flap of pelvic tissue which is sutured to incised ureter in form of **V**. (From Culp, O. S., 1961.)

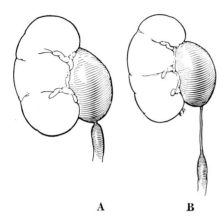

A   B

Figure 5–87. Obstructed ureteropelvic juncture that already has dependent position. Constriction may be located as shown in **A**, or it may be much longer as in **B**. (From Culp, O. S., and DeWeerd, J. H.)

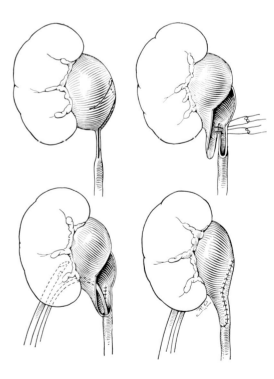

Figure 5–88. Technique of spiral-flap operation in cases in which ureteropelvic juncture is already in dependent position. Converging incisions from broad, slightly oblique base adjacent to original juncture are joined after following spherical contour of dilated renal pelvis for sufficient distance to assure flap longer than constricted segment of the ureter. This flap is interposed between edges of split ureter, and defect in pelvis is closed. (From Culp, O. S., and DeWeerd, J. H.)

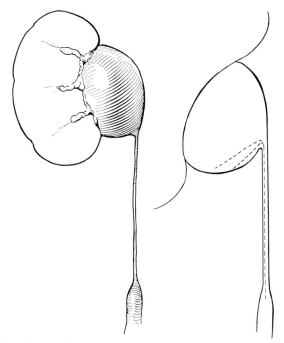

Figure 5–89. Unusually long constriction of ureter. (From Culp, O. S. 1955.)

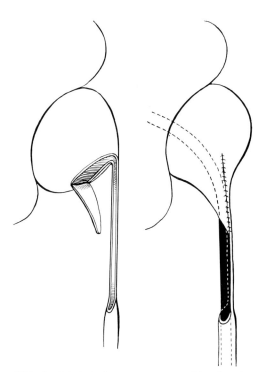

Figure 5–90. Technique of Davis, intubated ureterotomy combined with Y-plasty, used in cases which have long segment of ureteral constriction. (From Culp, O. S., 1955.)

Fig. 5–91

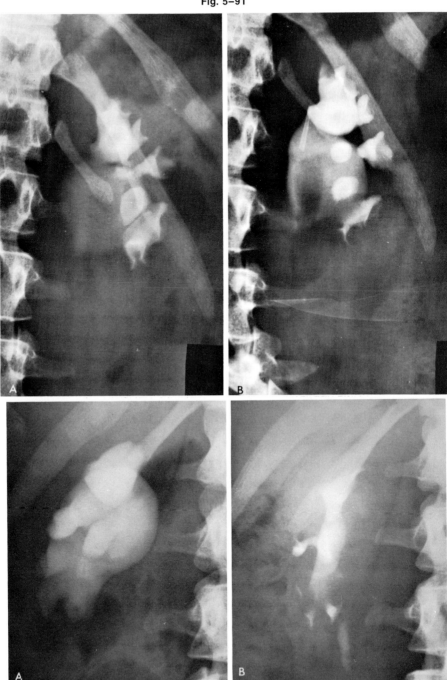

Fig. 5–92

Figure 5–91.   Fair to poor result of operation for obstruction. **A,** *Preoperative excretory urogram.* Pyelectasis, grade 2. **B,** *Postoperative film,* almost 6 months after severing anomalous vessels and performing Y-plasty on ureteropelvic juncture. Urographic change is not spectacular. **Moderate pyelectasis persists.**

Figure 5–92.   Good result of operation for obstruction. **A,** *Retrograde pyelogram, 25-minute delayed exposure.* **Grade 2 pyelectasis and calycectasis.** Marked retention of medium due to obstruction at ureteropelvic juncture. **B,** *Excretory urogram,* after plastic operation on ureteropelvic juncture. **Anomalous artery and vein at lower pole** cross ureter and produce partial obstruction. Pelvis and calyces have returned almost to normal. Some malrotation of kidney.

Fig. 5–93

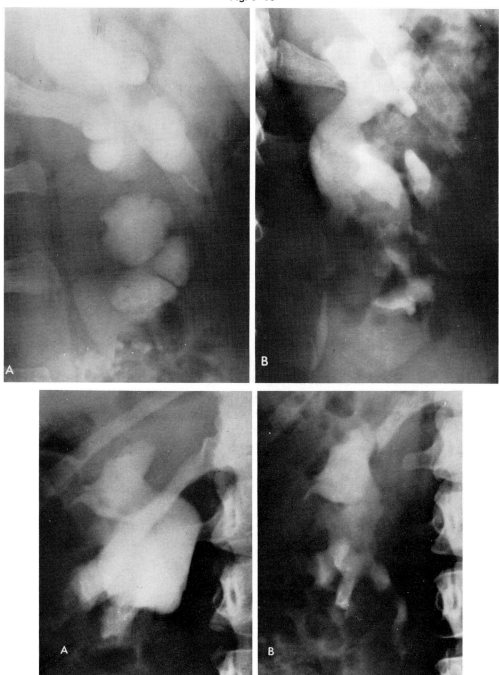

Fig. 5–94

Figure 5–93.   Good result of plastic operation on renal pelvis for hydronephrosis. A, *Preoperative excretory urogram.* **Marked left hydronephrosis,** showing huge dilated calyces. Pelvis not filled. Reduced function of kidney. (Left retrograde pyelogram showed **obstruction at ureteropelvic juncture** from pressure of large dilated renal pelvis. Contrast medium would not enter pelvis.) **B,** *Excretory urogram,* 13 months after operation. Improvement in function of kidney. Reduction in dilatation of pelvis and calyces.

Figure 5–94.   Good result of operation for obstruction. A, *Preoperative excretory urogram.* **Moderate right pyelectasis caused by obstruction at ureteropelvic juncture.** B, *Postoperative excretory urogram.* **Marked reduction in degree of dilatation of pelvis and calyces** after plastic operation on ureteropelvic juncture. Ureteropelvic juncture now patent, and medium freely enters ureter.

URETERECTASIS AND URETEROPYELECTASIS

GENERAL PRINCIPLES AND CONSIDERATIONS

It may be difficult to distinguish minimal degrees of ureterectasis from the normal because of the considerable variation in the size of "normal" ureters and the completeness with which the ureter is filled with contrast medium. *Unless ureterectasis is definite, it should be considered of doubtful clinical significance.*

Widening of the ureter is the first sign of dilatation (Fig. 5–95). As the process continues, the ureter also may lengthen and become tortuous (Figs. 5–96 and 5–97). If ureterectasis results from obstruction, the dilatation usually is confined to the part of the ureter above the point of the obstruction (Fig. 5–98). If infection is present, however, there also may be dilatation below. Dilatation of the lower third of each ureter is a fairly common result of urinary infection, especially of recurring cystitis (Fig. 5–99). It also may be the first manifestation of obstruction of the vesical neck or urethra.

Diagnostic Errors From Incomplete Filling

As mentioned previously, serious diagnostic errors may occur with either the excretory urogram or retrograde pyelogram if complete filling of the pelvis and ureter is not obtained. Examples of such possibilities are seen in Figures 5–100, 5–101, and 5–102. Attention has already been called to the propensity of pelves and ureters which have been previously infected and dilated (or are involved with vesicoureteral reflux) to dilate readily from retrograde injection of contrast medium or from ureteral compression during excretory urography.

Segmental Ureterectasis

Dilatation of isolated segments of the ureter provides interesting urograms. Usually, the explanation of the dilatation is not clear. It is most likely the result of some congenital error in development.* The most common site is the lower third of the ureter (Figs. 5–103, 5–104, and 5–105), although other parts of the ureter may be involved (Figs. 5–106 and 5–107). Abnormalities of the intramural ureter (both physiologic and pathologic) as causes of dilatation of the terminal ureter will be discussed further on in this chapter.

---

*See discussion of reflux and infection as causes of segmental ureterectasis (page 409).

(Text continued on page 440.)

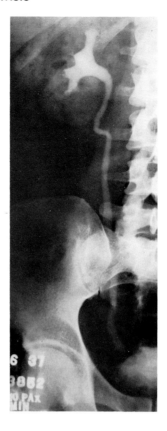

Figure 5–95. *Excretory urogram.* Right ureteropyelectasis, grade 1, with filling defect in region of ureterovesical juncture due to edema secondary to recently passed stone.

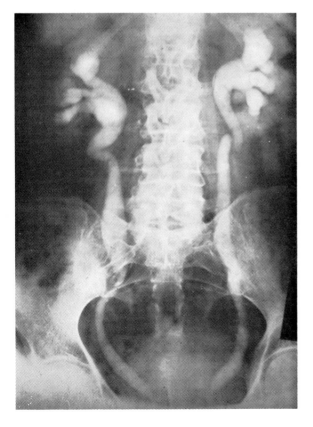

Figure 5–96. *Excretory urogram.* Bilateral ureteropyelectasis caused by obstruction from carcinoma of cervix.

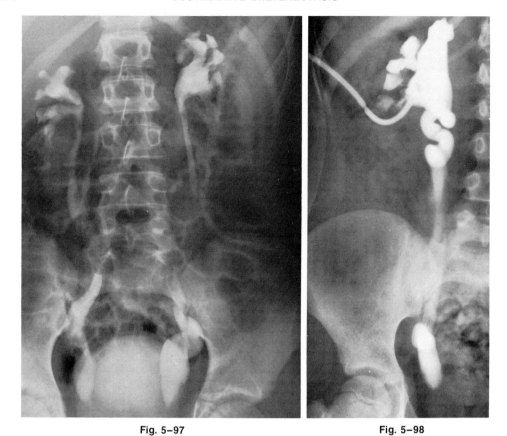

Fig. 5–97   Fig. 5–98

Figure 5–97. *Excretory urogram.* **Marked dilatation of lower third of each ureter, with lesser degree of ureterectasis above.** Cicatricial and inflammatory changes in both pelves and calyces from long-standing infection. Patient had **urinary obstruction due to stenosis of urethral meatus.** Cystogram in this case showed reflux up both ureters. Cystoscopy showed bladder trabeculation, grade 1.

Figure 5–98. *Pyelogram made through nephrostomy tube.* Boy, aged 12 years, had **long-standing congenital obstruction of vesical neck. There are marked tortuosity and dilatation of ureter, with associated pyelocaliectasis.**

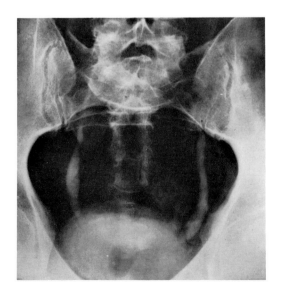

Figure 5–99. *Excretory urogram.* **Dilatation of lower third of each ureter.** Apparently result of ascending infection. (No surgical exploration.)

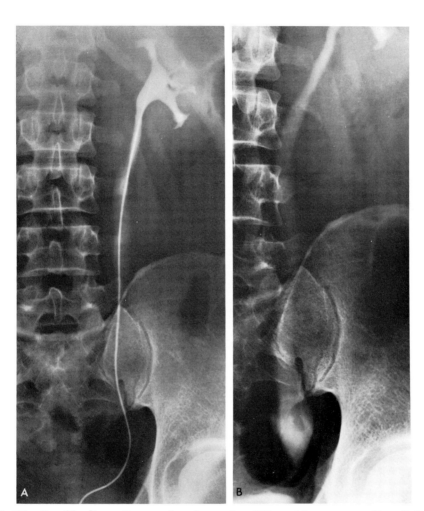

Figure 5–100.   Possible diagnostic error from incomplete filling with contrast medium. *Left retrograde pyelograms.* **A,** *First pyelogram, made with only upper half of ureter filled.* Pelvis and calyces normal. Suggestion of **mild ureterectasis in middle third.** **B,** *Second pyelogram, made with ureter completely filled.* **Marked dilatation in lower third of left ureter,** which could be missed because of incomplete filling in first pyelogram. Note that ureter narrows to normal size at its intramural site. No reflux.

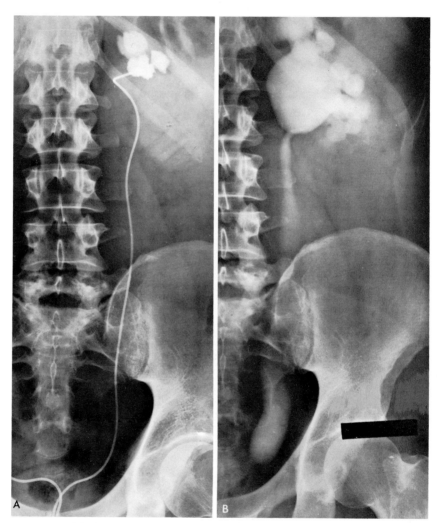

Figure 5–101. Possible diagnostic error from incomplete filling with contrast medium. *Left retrograde pyelograms.* **A,** Only group of calyces in upper half of left kidney outlined. Calyces irregularly dilated, suggesting possibility of renal tuberculosis. **B,** *Pelvis and ureter completely filled.* Lesion shown to be marked hydronephrosis and hydro-ureter, with marked dilatation of lower third of left ureter. Note that ureter narrows to normal size at its intramural site. No reflux. (At operation no evidence of obstruction to ureter was found.)

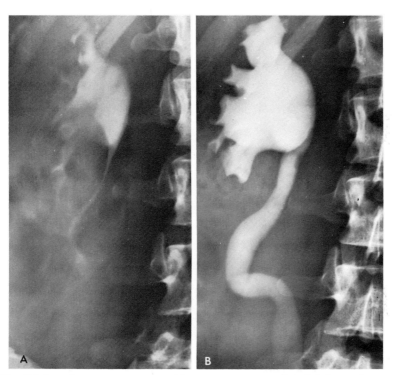

Figure 5–102. Pelvis and ureter appear normal in excretory urogram but definite pyeloureterectasis demonstrated in retrograde pyelogram. **A,** *Excretory urogram.* **Pyelectasis, grade 1. B.** *Right retrograde pyelogram* few days later. Pelvis and ureter completely filled and dilated—**pyeloureterectasis, grade 2.** (No surgical exploration.)

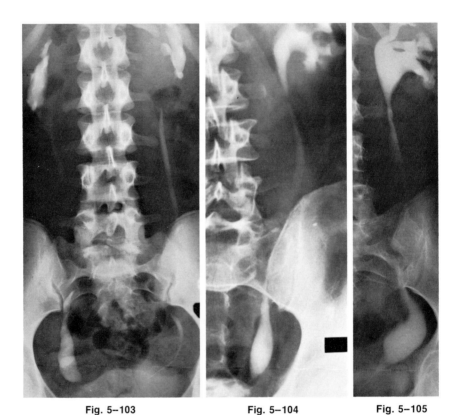

Fig. 5–103   Fig. 5–104   Fig. 5–105

Figure 5–103. *Excretory urogram.* Localized dilatation of lower third of right ureter with apparently normal intramural ureter. Bilateral malrotation of kidneys.

Figures 5–104 and 5–105. *Left retrograde pyelogram.* Localized, apparently congenital, dilatation of lower third of left ureter with little or no dilatation above. Ureter narrows to normal size before entering bladder. No reflux.

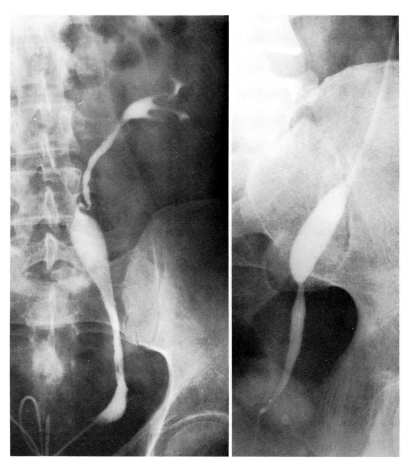

Fig. 5–106   Fig. 5–107

Figure 5–106. *Left retrograde pyelogram.* **Dilatation of lower two thirds of ureter** with no dilatation above. Marked angulation at junction of normal upper third and dilated lower two thirds of ureter. (No surgical exploration.)

Figure 5–107. *Left retrograde pyelogram.* **Unusually localized dilatation of ureter over promontory of sacrum.** Could be regarded as exaggerated spindle. (No surgical exploration.)

Obstructive Ureterectasis: Obstruction at or Above the Ureterovesical Junction

INTRINSIC OBSTRUCTION

Obstructive ureterectasis may result from obstruction within or without the urinary tract. The common causes of obstruction within the ureter itself are *stone, tumor, stricture, stenosis of the ureteral meatus,* and *ureterocele.* Ureterectasis caused by stone will be discussed in Chapter 6; by tumor, in Chapter 10; and by ureterocele, in Chapter 12.

Stricture of the Ureter

Strictures may be of inflammatory, traumatic, or congenital origin. *Stricture of inflammatory origin* may result from infection within the urinary tract or from infection of nearby structures (such as an appendiceal abscess) which infect the ureter from without (see Chapter 7). *Congenital stricture* is seen most frequently in the upper third of the ureter and usually is considered with the subject of obstruction of the ureteropelvic junction (see pages 408, 409, and 426; see also Figs. 5–76 through 5–78 and Figs. 5–87 through 5–90). The next most common site is the ureteral meatus or intramural portion of the ureter or both. The accuracy of the diagnosis of many reported cases of so-called congenital stenosis of the ureteral orifice, however, may be questioned, because they represent the poorly understood problem of the abnormal ureterovesical junction. If a size 5-F catheter will pass unobstructed through the meatus and intramural portion of the ureter, the diagnosis is certainly open to question. This subject will be discussed more fully later in this chapter under the subject of "nonobstructive" or "obscure" ureterectasis.

Iatrogenic Stricture of Ureteral Meatus and of Intramural Ureter. Postoperative stricture of the ureteral meatus and intramural portion of the ureter is a definite and not infrequently encountered condition. Usually it is the result of transurethral prostatic resection, although it also may result from open or transurethral resection of the bladder for tumor, open prostatectomy, or other surgical procedure on the bladder. When it occurs after transurethral prostatic resection, the operation usually has been carried a little too far cephalad so that either the ureteral orifice was damaged or the adjacent bladder was resected so near the orifice that in healing the scar tissue involved the ureteral orifice. Cystoscopically, the orifice then is seen to be pulled into the scarred vesical neck, and it may or may not be identified. This situation is a common complication of postoperative contracture of the vesical neck (see page 576). The degree of obstruction may vary from minimal to advanced or even complete occlusion (Figs. 5–108 and 5–109A and B).

A less common type of iatrogenic ureteral stricture is that resulting from implantation of radon seeds near the ureteral orifice or near the intramural ureter in cases of bladder tumor (Fig. 5–110). Ureteral stricture may also result from ureteral trauma from manipulation of ureteral calculi (Figs. 5–111 and 5–112).

EXTRINSIC (EXTRA-URETERAL) OBSTRUCTION

An endless variety of neoplastic or inflammatory intra-abdominal or retroperitoneal lesions may obstruct the ureter by pressure, constriction, or direct invasion.

Neoplastic. Among the neoplasms which may involve the ureter are *carcinoma of the colon,* especially of the rectosigmoid (Figs. 5–113, 5–114, and 5–115). All pelvic tumors in women, including carcinoma of the cervix, are potential causes of obstruction (see Chapter 18, pages 1973, 1974). *Retroperitoneal tumors* such as sarcoma, lymphoma, and carcinoma of the pancreas may obstruct the ureters (Fig. 5–116; see also Chapter 10). Of course, any malignant tumor can metastasize and compromise the ureter at some level. Extravesical extension of *carcinoma of the prostate* is a not uncommon cause of obstruction of the lower part of the ureter (Fig. 5–117*A* and *B*). Bilateral orchiectomy or estrogen therapy may relieve the obstruction in this instance. Ureteral obstruction from carcinoma of the bladder is shown in Figure 5–118.

Endometriosis is usually classified with tumors, but it will be discussed separately in Chapter 18.

Inflammatory. Probably the inflammatory lesion that most frequently causes ureteral obstruction is *pelvic inflammatory disease in women* (see Chapter 18, page 1974, Figs. 18–40 and 18–41).

Ureteral obstruction from *retroperitoneal fibrosis* will be discussed separately in Chapter 17.

Vascular. Aneurysms of the abdominal aorta not infrequently cause ureteral obstruction (see Chapter 14). Obstruction of the *ureteropelvic junction* and upper part of the ureter by anomalous blood vessels is a common well-documented occurrence (see page 408). Obstruction of the lower part of the ureter from this cause is less common. Relatively few such cases have been reported; and, in the majority of these, the primary obstruction was near the *ureterovesical junction,* and the vessel compromised the ureter only after the ureter had become dilated. In a few cases (Greene and associates, 1952), however, anomalous vessels are the primary cause of obstruction low in the ureter (Greene and associates, 1954) (see Chapter 14, Figs. 14–48 and 14–49).

Miscellaneous. *Vesical diverticula* not uncommonly cause ureteral obstruction. The ureter may be compressed and displaced as it circles around the diverticulum to enter the bladder (Fig. 5–119). (This subject is discussed in greater detail on page 553.)

Pregnancy results in ureteral obstruction and infection which is called either *pyelitis* or *pyeloureterectasis of pregnancy.* This will be discussed in Chapter 18.*

Bands and *adhesions* may occasionally be responsible for ureteral obstruction. Obstruction of the right ureter at the brim of the pelvis of a 12-year-old boy who complained of intermittent right renal pain is shown in Figure 5–120. Operation showed obstruction and angulation of the ureter, apparently from fixation by the sheath of the ureter and adjacent periureteral tissue. When the sheath and adjacent tissues were divided, the ureter became straight and the obstruction and dilatation disappeared.

---

*See also discussion of the "Right Ovarian Vein Syndrome," Chapter 18.

(Text continued on page 448.)

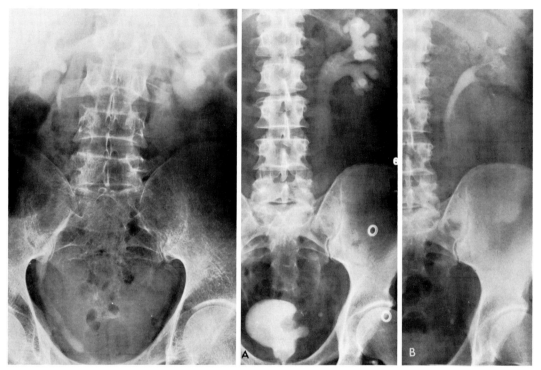

Fig. 5–108   Fig. 5–109

Figure 5–108. *Excretory urogram.* Bilateral obstruction of ureteral orifices secondary to repeated transurethral resection of bladder tumor and vesical neck. Obstruction most marked on left, with **pyelectasis, grade 3**, and ureter not filled. On right, entire ureter outlined showing mild obstruction at ureteral orifice.

Figure 5–109. **Stenosis of left ureteral orifice after transurethral resection.** No function on left. Normal kidney and ureter on right. *Excretory urograms.* **A,** Two weeks after left ureteroneocystostomy. Function has returned. **Pyeloureterectasis, grade 2.** Note negative filling defect from cuff of ureter in bladder. **B,** Fourteen months after operation. Kidney and ureter have returned almost to normal.

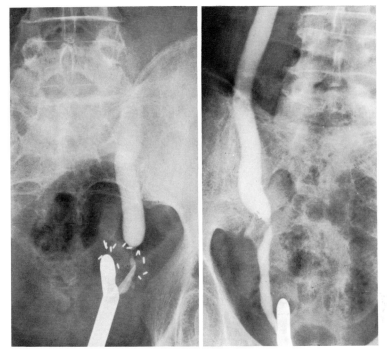

Fig. 5–110   Fig. 5–111

Figure 5–110. *Retrograde pyelogram made with bulb catheter inserted just inside ureteral meatus.* Ureteral stricture resulting from radon seeds implanted into bladder tumor. (Tumor was eradicated.) Ureter is kept open and kidney function maintained by ureteral dilatation every 4 months.

Figure 5–111. *Retrograde pyelogram.* Stricture of right ureter following transurethral manipulation of ureteral stone. (Excision and end-to-end anastomosis.)

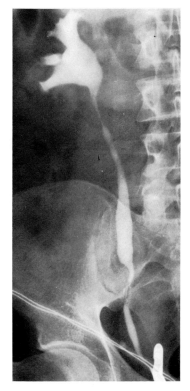

Figure 5–112. *Retrograde pyelogram.* Stricture and deformity of lower third of right ureter after traumatic manipulation of ureteral stone.

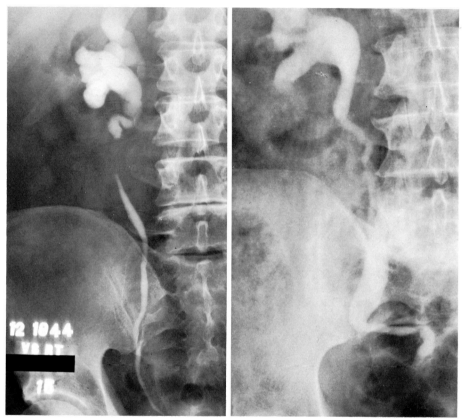

Fig. 5–113　　　　　　　　　　**Fig. 5–114**

Figure 5–113. *Right retrograde pyelogram.* Obstruction in upper third of right ureter caused by extension of carcinoma of hepatic flexure of colon.

Figure 5–114. *Retrograde pyelogram.* Postoperative recurrence of carcinoma of rectosigmoid. Obstruction of right ureter. Later, left ureter also became obstructed. (Palliative left nephrostomy was done.)

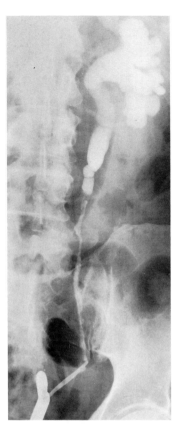

Figure 5–115. *Retrograde pyelogram.* **Ureteral obstruction from recurring carcinoma of lower part of sigmoid.** Narrowing of lower two thirds of ureter. Kidney showed no function on excretory urography.

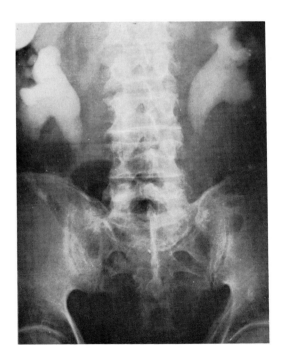

Figure 5–116. *Excretory urogram.* **Bilateral ureteral obstruction caused by carcinoma of pancreas.** (Courtesy of Dr. R. O. Pearman.)

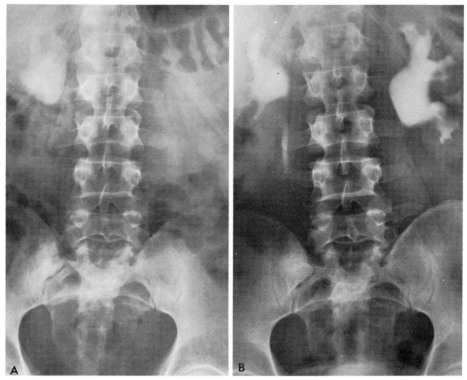

Figure 5–117. Lower ureteral obstruction from cephalad extravesical extension of carcinoma of prostate. A, *Excretory urogram.* **Nonfunctioning left kidney. Pyelectasis on right.** B, *Excretory urogram* made 14 months after bilateral orchiectomy. Regression in growth. Left kidney now functioning, although pyelectasis persists. Reduction in degree of pyelectasis on right.

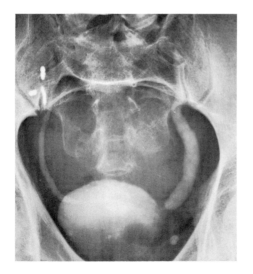

Figure 5–118. *Excretory urogram.* Obstruction of left ureter from infiltrating carcinoma of bladder.

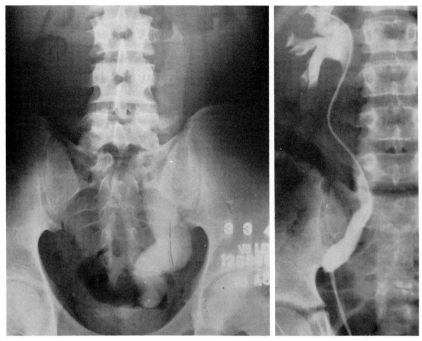

Fig. 5–119   **Fig. 5–120**

Figure 5–119. *Forty-five-minute excretory urogram.* **Huge dilatation of left ureter, resulting from obstruction by vesical diverticulum and congenital obstruction of vesical neck** in man of 19 years. Right kidney urographically normal, as was shown in 15- and 20-minute urograms. In this urogram most of medium had emptied out of right kidney.

Figure 5–120. *Retrograde pyelogram.* **Ureteral obstruction from fixation by band of periureteral tissue** (in boy, age 12). (Operation showed abrupt transition between dilated flabby portion of ureter and normal ureter below. There appeared to be angulation at this point. Sheath of ureter and adjacent tissues were divided and ureter became perfectly straight.) Subsequent excretory urogram showed that ureter had returned to normal.

Nonobstructive (Obscure) Ureterectasis

This subject constitutes one of the most obscure, controversial, and unsolved problems in urology (Williams, 1954a). It presents itself primarily as a problem in pediatric urology, because in most cases the disease is congenital and because a high percentage of patients die before they reach adult life. In some cases, however, the lesion is less severe and renal function is less impaired, so that patients may survive to a later age. Most cases of extreme ureterectasis are associated with ureteral reflux and may progress to the stage in which the bladder, ureters, and renal pelvis become one continuous, common reservoir of urine.

WITHOUT REFLUX

Fusiform Terminal Ureterectasis

Widely dilated ureters which narrow to normal caliber as they pass through the wall of the bladder and terminate with normal-appearing, competent ureteral orifices (without reflux) have been difficult to explain (Fig. 5–121). (This condition has been described on page 432; see also Figs. 5–103 through 5–107.) Associated pyelectasis may or may not be present. Creevy (1967a) has suggested the term *fusiform terminal ureterectasis*. The cause of this condition is not known and it is not clear if the primary lesion is in the nerve supply or the muscularis, for as he points out it is still not clear if ureteral peristalsis is of neurogenic or myogenic origin. In some cases this condition may be present for years, causing the patient no symptoms, no infection, and no progressive dilatation of the ureter or renal pelvis (Fig. 5–122). Creevy (1967a) states that in other cases progressive ureteropyelectasis with associated infection may demand treatment.

Surgical exposure of the ureter discloses a thick-walled bulbous dilatation of the distal pelvic ureter with an abrupt but smooth transition to an intramural segment of normal caliber. The dilatation diminishes less abruptly above at a variable level. Pinching the ureter evokes peristalsis except in its terminal portion if urine is passing down the ureter. Division of the ureter at its entrance into the bladder yields only a trickle of urine. However, as successively higher short segments are snipped off, a gush will occur, along with partial collapse of the dilated segment.

Surgical experience with four cases in which the "atonic" segment of ureter was excised and the cut end reimplanted into the bladder with "antireflux techniques" was favorable (Figs. 5–123 and 5–124).

(Text continued on page 451.)

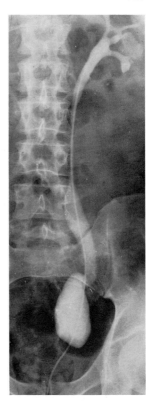

Figure 5–121. *Retrograde pyelogram.* Dilatation (congenital?) of lower half of left ureter with normal ureteral orifice and intramural ureter. No reflux. (Plastic operation performed, reducing width of ureter. Intramural ureter not disturbed.)

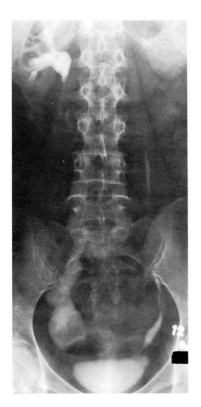

Figure 5–122. *Excretory urogram* of woman, aged 26. **Atonic distal ureteral segment (ureteral achalasia). Fusiform terminal ureterectasis** has remained static for at least 14 years. (No surgery.) (From Creevy, C. D.)

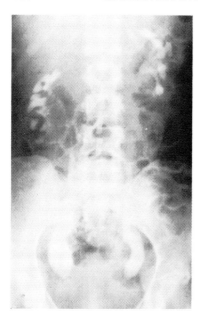

Figure 5–123. *Excretory urogram.* **Fusiform terminal ureterec-tasis** in woman, aged 26. Condition is known to have remained static for 14 years. (From Creevy, C. D.)

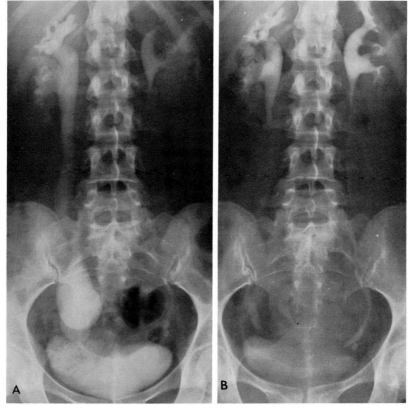

Figure 5–124. **Fusiform terminal ureterectasis with associated pyelectasis and recurring urinary infection.** **A,** *Preoperative excretory urogram* of woman, aged 22. (Excision of terminal ureteral segment with reimplantation.) **B,** *Excretory urogram* 2 years postoperatively. Ureter appears essentially normal. (From Creevy, C. D.)

Although it occurs in patients of all ages, vesicoureteral reflux of obscure etiology constitutes one of the most troublesome urologic problems affecting infants and children. It is associated with infection and ureteropyelectasis varying in degree from minimal ureterectasis to advanced disease, with enormous dilation of the ureters and renal pelves, in which the bladder, ureters, and renal pelves constitute one common reservoir of urine. Although ureteropyelectasis and infection are invariably associated, it is not yet clear which is the primary condition. Progressive renal deterioration makes the condition potentially lethal and of urgent importance. Imperfect knowledge of the physiology and mechanics of the ureterovesical junction in the past has contributed to the slow pace of therapeutic progress in this disease. Definite advances in recent years in the understanding of the complex mechanism of this disorder have greatly improved the outlook of the unfortunate patients so afflicted.

VESICOURETERAL REFLUX

Physiology of the Ureterovesical Junction

"Flap-Valve" Theory

In recent years there has been a revival of Sampson's theory that the intramural part of the ureter operates as a "flap valve" to prevent reflux; this theory postulates that the intravesical tension of urine compresses the intramural portion of the ureter against the firm vesical musculature through which it passes (Sampson). This concept was supported by Graves and Davidoff (1923; 1924; 1925) and Gruber, who showed that in animals, such as the rabbit, which have short and poorly developed intravesical ureters, the incidence of vesicoureteral reflux is great.

More recent work with human beings (McGovern, Marshall, and Paquin; Paquin; Paquin, Marshall, and McGovern) also suggests that a substantial length of intramural ureter is necessary in the prevention of reflux.

Trigonal-Muscle Theory

The results of meticulous anatomic studies of the ureterovesical junction by Tanagho and Pugh, who used a microdissection technique, have yielded fresh new concepts of the mechanism of the ureteropelvic junction. A brief summary of their work follows:[*] The muscle fibers of the terminal portion of the ureter (juxtavesical and intramural segments) are mainly longitudinal, although a few oblique and circular fibers can be identified at the ureteral orifice. The longitudinal fibers in the roof of the intramural ureter diverge and sweep around to become continuous with the fibers in the floor, which then pass distally as the superficial trigonal muscle to be firmly attached near the verumontanum. This superficial trigonal muscle acts as a type of obliquely disposed "sphincter" to provide a simple but quite efficient means of closure of the lower end of the ureter.

At the completion of micturition the superficial trigonal muscle is relaxed and the intravesical pressure is low, but the resting "tone" of the trigonal muscle apparently is still sufficient to ensure competence of the ureteral orifice. As urine accumulates in the bladder, there is a gradual (but minimal) rise in the intravesical pressure; concomitant stretching of the longitudinal fibers of the ureteric and superficial trigonal muscles approximates the roof and floor of the intramural ureter and narrows the ureteral orifice.

During micturition, both the detrusor and superficial trigonal muscles contract. Thus, in addition to closing the ureteral

---

[*]See also description of this theory by Tanagho, Hutch, Meyers, and Rambo on page 461.

orifice, the trigonal muscle assists in opening the vesical neck, as its fibers pass through the vesical neck down to their attachment near the verumontanum. (This latter action was postulated many years ago by Wesson and Fulmer.) The question still arises as to why *no* reflux occurs during the opening of the ureteral orifice to permit efflux of urine. The answer is that, normally, intraureteric pressure during efflux exceeds intravesical pressure unless the bladder is contracting for micturition.

The authors point out that their anatomic findings and theory of the mechanics of the ureterovesical junction explain numerous observations on the subject of reflux better than does Sampson's "flap-valve" theory. For instance, the inconsistent results with "delayed cystography" (Bunge; Stewart, 1953; 1955) can be explained by fatigue of the trigonal muscles and recovery after a period of rest. The theory also clarifies the "maturation theory" of Hutch (1961b), the excessively large trigones of children with reflux (McGovern, Marshall, and Paquin), and the large trigone associated with the so-called megacystis syndrome (Paquin, Marshall, and McGovern; Stewart, 1955; Williams, 1959), the explanation being that the trigonal muscle fibers are likely to be smaller than usual and to have reduced tone and contractile powers, allowing the ureteric orifices to lie farther apart than normally. The patulous orifices of patients with reflux (Garrett and Switzer) also could be due to decreased size and lack of tone of the trigonal muscle fibers. Reflux occurring *secondary* to infection (cystitis) could be explained by *inflammatory* interference with the action of the trigonal muscle, which could render it incapable of efficient sustained stretch or contraction.

There is one other area in which this theory would offer a helpful physiologic explanation of controversial observations. This concerns the role of vesical-neck obstruction (especially in infants and children) in reflux. Is such obstruction present or is it not? In most cases it is impossible to settle this quandary urographically or visually (either by cystoscopy or by suprapubic exposure of the vesical neck). Should ureterovesicoplasty be done in every case of ureteroneocystostomy for reflux? There is a wide divergence of opinion concerning the incidence of vesical-neck obstruction as an etiologic agent in reflux as follows: Stewart (1960) found 95% and Hutch (1961b), 5%. There is evidence that widening of the bladder neck (Y-V plasty or transurethral resection) has been helpful (Williams, Scott, and Turner-Warwick). If it is true that substantial assistance to opening of the bladder neck during micturition is provided by contraction of the trigonal muscle, then congenital weakness or maldevelopment of this muscle could explain this apparently paradoxical situation.

Comment

It should be pointed out, before proceeding with the discussion of reflux, that both of the described postulates emphasize the *importance of the length of the intramural ureter* in the prevention of reflux. In that respect, they complement one another rather than compete.

In the following discussion, some of the referenced dissertations by various interested workers in this field were written before the trigonal-muscle postulate of Tanagho and Pugh was published in 1963; thus, they must be evaluated with this in mind. Many of the authors now tend to support this postulate.

Specific Etiologic Considerations

ACQUIRED FACTORS WHICH CAUSE OR CONTRIBUTE TO REFLUX

Iatrogenic Factors

A common cause of reflux is surgical trauma to the ureteral orifice and intramural ureter—such as occurs incidental to meatotomy and excision of ureterocele and inadvertently during transurethral prostatic resection or transurethral or open removal of bladder tumors. Traumatic manipulation of a ureteral stone with tearing of the meatus may result in either reflux or obstruction from scarring (Figs. 5–125 through 5–130).

Infection

Infection is considered to be a potential cause of ureteral reflux, although it is difficult to be sure whether the infection or the reflux is primary. Disappearance of reflux after the infection is controlled tends to support the thesis that infection is the primary lesion.

CONGENITAL ANOMALIES WHICH CAUSE OR CONTRIBUTE TO REFLUX (URETERAL DUPLICATION; ECTOPIC URETERAL ORIFICES)

Congenital malformations of the termination of the ureter such as duplication and ectopy may contribute to reflux (Figs. 5–131, 5–132, and 5–133). In the case of complete duplication (see Chapter 12, page 1452), it is well known that reflux is more common in the lower-pole (orthotopic) ureter (cephalad and laterally located orifice) whereas obstruction is more common in the upper-pole ectopic ureter (caudally and medially located orifice). The short intramural length of the lower-pole ureter is considered to be the reason for this. However, it should not be forgotten that the lower (ectopic) orifice, located near the vesical neck, may also reflux. Moreover, approximately 20% of ectopic ureters emptying into the urethra will reflux (King and associates). Duplicated ureters that join within the intramural ureter (just inside or on the edge of a common orifice) may present unusual diagnostic and surgical problems.

NEUROGENIC DYSFUNCTION AND CONGENITAL ABSENCE OF ABDOMINAL MUSCLES

There is a high incidence of vesicoureteral reflux in neurogenic bladder (both congenital and acquired). The congenital lesions, such as *spina bifida* and *myelodysplasia*, predominate in children. Adults more commonly have acquired lesions (degenerative and traumatic). The original observations of Hutch and Bunts (which initiated the modern concepts of reflux) were made in paraplegic patients and are documented further on in this chapter (page 460).

The association of vesicoureteral reflux in cases of "prune belly" is well-known (congenital absence of the abdominal muscles). (See Chapter 12, page 1569.)

(*Text continued on page 460.*)

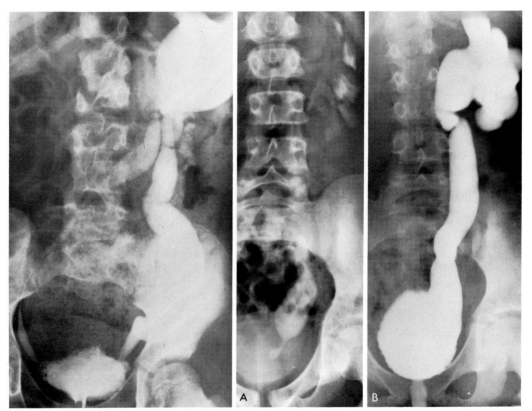

Fig. 5–125   Fig. 5–126

Figure 5–125. *Retrograde cystogram* of boy, 8 years of age, with persistent pyuria and urinary incontinence who had been operated on for imperforate anus at the age of 3 days. Vesicorectal fistula suspected. Note **bilateral reflux showing crossed renal ectopy.** (Courtesy of Dr. H. W. ten Cate.)

Figure 5–126. Reflux after transurethral meatotomy for ureterocele of girl, 8 years of age. **A,** *Excretory urogram.* Dilatation of lower third of ureter which narrows down to normal size in intramural ureter, then ends in small ureterocele. **B,** *Voiding cystourethrogram* made 8 months after transurethral meatotomy. **Vesicoureteral reflex with advanced ureteropyelectasis.**

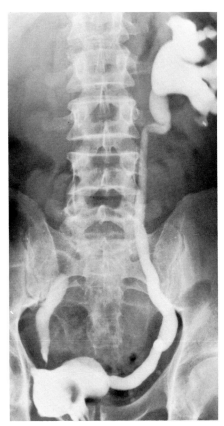 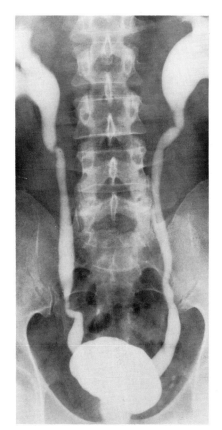

Fig. 5–127   Fig. 5–128

Figure 5–127. *Retrograde cystogram.* Bilateral ureteral reflux secondary to transurethral resection of extensive high-grade infiltrating tumor of bladder, followed by implantation of radon seeds and irradiation with cobalt-60.

Figure 5–128. *Retrograde cystogram.* Bilateral ureteropyelectasis with reflux, after repeated transurethral fulguration of extensive infiltrating transitional cell carcinoma of trigone, which also invaded prostate.

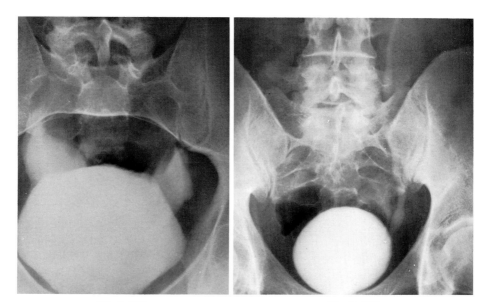

Fig. 5–129   Fig. 5–130

Figure 5–129. *Retrograde cystogram.* Reflux up hugely dilated ureters resulting from bilateral (suprapubic) ureteral meatotomy to relieve bilateral congenital hydro-ureter without reflux.

Figure 5–130. *Retrograde cystogram.* Reflux up left ureter resulting from transurethral fulguration of inflammatory lesion in vicinity of left ureteral orifice.

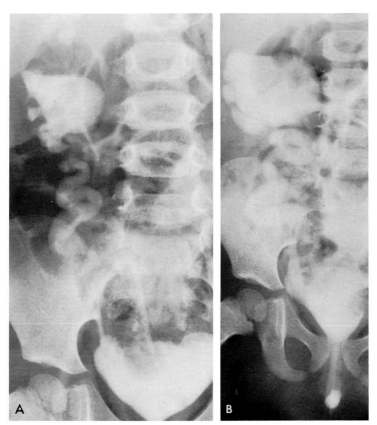

Figure 5–131. Reflux associated with ureteral duplication. **A,** *Excretory urogram.* **Duplication on right.** Upper segment normal; lower, dilated grade 2. **B,** *Retrograde cystogram.* **Reflux up ureter serving lower pelvis, which is dilated, grade 2.** (At cystoscopy upper meatus [serving lower pelvis] was dilated to about 1 cm in diameter; meatus serving upper segment was of normal size and could be seen just within edge of dilated orifice.)

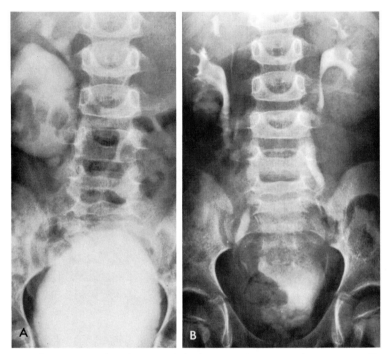

Figure 5–132. Reflux associated with ureteral duplication. **A**, *Retrograde cystogram*. Duplicated ureter on right (juncture within intramural ureter) with reflux up both limbs. Hydronephrosis of lower segment only. (At ureteroneocystostomy orifices not separated, but entire ureter brought through tunnel under vesical mucosa.) **B**, *Postoperative excretory urogram*. Normal. Note negative filling defect from "turned back" cuff of ureter projecting into bladder.

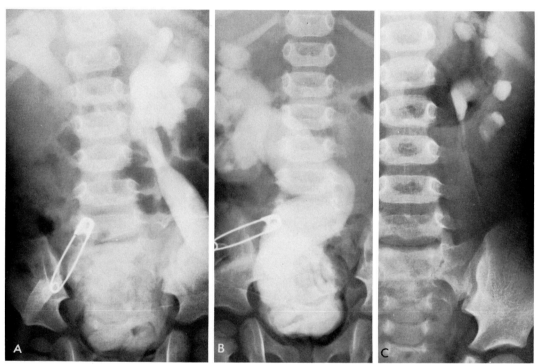

Figure 5–133. Obstruction of vesical neck in boy, 4 years of age. A, *Excretory urogram.* Duplication on right with no function in lower segment. Ureteropyelectasis of upper right segment and of left kidney and ureter. B, *Retrograde cystogram.* Reflux up huge ureter (right) serving lower pelvis. (On cystoscopy upper meatus [serving lower pelvis] was found to be greatly dilated. Meatus for upper pelvis was of normal size and could be seen on lower edge of it. Right nephrectomy [ureters could not be separated] and plastic Y-V operation on vesical neck were performed.) C, *Excretory urogram* 2 months after operation. Left kidney greatly improved. Patient voiding normally.

Modern Concepts of Reflux (Hutch Diverticulum; Maturation of Intramural Ureter; "Megacystis")

The work of Hutch (1952; 1957; 1958; 1961a; 1961b; Hutch, Ayres, and Loquvam; Hutch and Bunts) provided an attractive approach to this complex problem. Hutch and Bunts observed the frequency with which vesicoureteral reflux developed in *paraplegic patients,* even when the bladder was kept empty with either an indwelling urethral catheter or a suprapubic cystostomy tube. After careful study and observation, they concluded that the basic underlying difficulty is the formation of trabeculation and cellules or saccules in the bladder. Briefly, their explanation is as follows:[*]

Trabeculation of the bladder results from pulling of the muscle fibers of the bladder wall in bands which in turn are the result of work hypertrophy. This leaves weak areas between the muscular bands that are recognized as cellules, saccules, or diverticula. Work hypertrophy may result from obstruction at the vesical neck (with the bladder working to expel urine through it) or from a neurogenic bladder caused by transection of the spinal cord above the conus. In the latter case, repeated uncontrolled impulses from the isolated stump of the spinal cord cause frequent detrusor contractions. The point at which the ureter pierces the bladder wall is naturally a weak spot and is easily compromised by saccule formation. The saccule in this region is almost always situated lateral and cephalad to the ureteral orifice, which usually is located on the medial inferior lip of the saccule (Fig. 5–134). The ureter courses along the floor of the saccule so that it no longer has any support from the bladder musculature. In effect, then, the intramural ureter is no longer intramural; it is now extravesical, with no bladder wall to support it.

Hutch stated that the normal ureter has two muscle layers: an internal longitudinal layer and an outer circular layer. The circular layer of muscle compresses the ureter and supplies the peristaltic action which propels the urine downward into the bladder. As the ureter pierces the bladder wall to become the "intramural ureter," the circular layer blends with the middle muscular layer of the bladder wall and only the longitudinal muscle layer is left for the intramural ureter (Fig. 5–135A). If the *intramural ureter* is compromised by an adjacent saccule or by thinned-out areas between trabeculae, *it becomes extravesical* and is no longer supported by the bladder wall (Fig. 5–135B). In its extravesical state it is left without any circular muscle fibers to provide peristaltic activity. This segment, therefore, becomes a fixed tube without peristaltic activity and acts as an obstruction similar to the way the aganglionic rectum acts as an obstruction to the colon in Hirschsprung's disease. The ureter above this segment becomes dilated as a result of work hypertrophy of the circular muscle fibers. The short, fixed tube segment (former intramural ureter) does not dilate (Fig. 5–135C). In addition, there is no longer any flap-valve action, because there is no intravesical ureter with bladder wall support. With the valve action gone, reflux occurs and increases the degree of ureterectasis. The final stage is stretching and dilatation of the ureteral orifice and terminal ureter. Hutch (1958) has named this concept of ureterectasis (caused by the inert displaced intramural ureter) plus later reflux (caused by loss of the flap-valve action) "hydroflux."

Although this theory seems reasonable in cases in which trabeculation and saccule formation of the bladder are present, it is common knowledge that in a large

---

[*]For modification of Hutch's explanation of ureteral reflux in light of Tanagho and Pugh's trigonal-muscle postulate of ureterectasis the reader is urged to read (1) "Primary Reflux" by Tanagho and Hutch, J. Urol. 93:158-164 (Feb.) 1965 and (2) "Primary Vesicoureteral Reflux: Experimental Studies of Its Etiology" by Tanagho, Hutch, Meyers, and Rambo, J. Urol. 93:165-176 (Feb.) 1965.

proportion of cases there is little or no trabeculation and, in fact, the bladder appears distended and the wall thin. Hutch stated that this situation is essentially the same; namely, that the bladder wall is too thin to support the oblique passage of the ureter through it, so that in reality there is no normal intramural ureter. The ureter in such cases enters the bladder in a perpendicular rather than an oblique position, so that the segment of the ureter which would normally be the intramural ureter is now in an extravesical position, without any circular muscle fibers and without any support from the bladder musculature (Figs. 5–135D and 5–136).

Urographic demonstration of Hutch's theory is shown in Figures 5–137A and B and 5–138A, B, and C). The saccule adjacent to the ureteral orifice is usually not difficult to demonstrate. In some cases, however, Hutch was unable to demonstrate it except in the voiding cystogram when sufficient pressure caused herniation of the saccule through the region of the ureteral orifice. The clinical problem of the *ureteral orifice situated in the rim of, or within, an adjacent small vesical diverticulum with associated ureterectasis and reflux* is a common one which has long been recognized (Fig. 5–139).

Most of the above observations published in 1961 have stood the test of time for *secondary* reflux in obstructive and neurologic disease. For cases of primary reflux, Hutch has now embraced the trigonal muscle postulate of Tanagho and Pugh (see page 451). As a matter of fact, Tanagho came to this country and continued his investigation with Hutch. From this association several studies have emerged (Hutch and Tanagho; Tanagho and Hutch; Tanagho and associates).

In 1965, in an introduction to an experimental study on the etiology of primary vesicoureteral reflux, Tanagho and associates wrote as follows:

A recent study by Tanagho and Pugh of the anatomy of the human ureterovesical junction demonstrates that the ureter does not end at the ureteral orifice. It loses its lumen at this level but its musculature, without interruption, continues downward as the *superficial trigone to end at the verumontanum.* In addition, Waldeyer's sheath, which surrounds the distal end of the lower ureter, does not end at the ureteral hiatus but proceeds downward and medially under the superficial trigone to form the *deep trigone.* These two layers together *constitute the trigone of the bladder, which is embryologically, anatomically, and functionally a direct continuation of the ureter* and will be referred to as the trigonal muscle. [Emphasis added.]

Our aim is to show that a physiologic relationship exists between the trigonal muscle and the lower end of the ureter, and to test the hypothesis that the competency of the ureterovesical junction is maintained by the integrity and efficiency of the trigonal muscle.

It is apparent that the blame for ureteral reflux is gradually being shifted from the ureter to the bladder (and trigone). The new concept explains the enlarged trigone and widely separated ureteral orifices in "megacystis" (Paquin, Marshall, and McGovern; Williams, 1958). Also, it provides a more logical reason for Hutch's concept of maturation of the intravesical ureter, in which he pointed out that it often requires 10 to 12 years for the intramural ureter of the child to attain "sufficient length" to prevent reflux with associated infection. (From this observation has come the saying that little girls will "outgrow" their recurring infection and reflux at puberty.)

Techniques to Demonstrate Ureteral Reflux

UROGRAPHIC DEMONSTRATION

The Cystogram

It is generally agreed that the most important examinations for evaluating ureteral reflux and its associated ureterectasis are the *retrograde and voiding cystograms* (Waterhouse). If they are made with *cinefluoroscopy* and television control, reflux may be demonstrated in an even higher percentage of cases. It is also generally conceded that ureteral reflux does not occur in the normal urinary tract of the human being (Peters, Johnson, and Jackson). Ureteral reflux has been described as an evanescent condition, sometimes present, sometimes absent, sometimes unilateral, and at other times bilateral. Recent cinefluoroscopic studies have demonstrated that reflux may indeed be an intermittent phenomenon, its appearance and disappearance depending on detrusor activity (Fig. 5–140). This partially explains why in some cystograms reflux can be seen and in others it does not appear. Often reflux can be demonstrated only in the *voiding cystogram* exposed during micturition (Figs. 5–141*A*, *B*, and *C* and 5–142*A* and *B*). At other times the *delayed cystogram* (Bunge; Stewart, 1953; 1955) with films exposed at intervals of 15 to 45 minutes after injection of the medium will demonstrate the reflux. The amount of contrast medium introduced into the bladder, the degree of vesical filling, and the intravesical pressure are all important factors in technique. (See discussion of Tanagho and Pugh's explanation of this phenomenon, pages 451 and 461.)

In order to standardize the examination to some extent, Paquin, Marshall, and McGovern performed cystography under cystometric control. Their technique consists of first filling the bladder with opaque medium to a pressure of 15 cm of water. If the film does not show reflux, another film is exposed after additional solution has raised the intravesical pressure to 25 cm or more. They showed that the incidence of reflux increases as the intravesical pressure rises. They have assumed that reflux which occurs at low intravesical pressure is more serious than that which occurs only at high pressure and have used this information in selecting patients for surgical treatment. Some workers, however, recently have questioned the importance of these data (King and associates).

Probably one of the most paradoxic situations in urology is the tremendous difference in appearance of the excretory urogram and the retrograde cystogram in some cases of reflux. Not uncommonly an excretory urogram will suggest little if any ureteropyelectasis even though there seems to be reasonably good filling with contrast medium, yet a delayed cystogram or retrograde pyelogram will show an enormous degree of ureteropyelectasis. Hodson (1959) and Hodson and Edwards observed this phenomenon, in their studies of vesicoureteral reflux, as a cause of pyelonephritis and pyelonephritic atrophy (see Chapter 7). The explanation of this phenomenon is not entirely clear but appears to be damage to the wall of the ureter and renal pelvis from previous obstruction and/or infection. It has been suggested that the "tone" of these structures does not return to normal after the obstruction and infection have been eliminated. This phenomenon occurs frequently enough that the alert urologist will routinely make retrograde cystograms of all infants and children who are suffering from recurring urinary infection. *A normal excretory urogram is not sufficient evidence of a normal urinary tract in a child. In fact, the most important single urologic examination in the child is a retrograde cystogram. It takes precedence over cystoscopy.*

VISUAL DEMONSTRATION

Motzkin has suggested adding two ampules of indigo carmine to the cystographic medium to permit the visual demonstration of reflux. After cystographic films are exposed, the bladder is washed out, and cystoscopy is performed immediately. In cases of reflux, it may be possible to see the blue dye in the efflux from the ureteral orifices. There has been good correlation of the visual and urographic diagnoses of reflux. Also, it has been suggested that visual identification may indicate severe disease and retention of a large amount of refluxed material. Ekman and co-workers demonstrated that stimulation of a marked diuresis by means of the intravenous injection of mannitol can prevent the visual demonstration of vesicoureteral reflux. In their case, reflux evident while the patient had a low urinary output was no longer demonstrable 30 minutes after the initiation of the diuresis.

The Clinical Problem of Reflux

The development in recent years of improved surgical techniques of ureteroneocystostomy has provided more efficient methods of dealing with reflux.* Difficult problems remain, however, which include (1) differentiating primary from secondary reflux, (2) determining indications for medical and surgical treatment, and (3) evaluating the role of infravesical obstruction (vesical-neck obstruction, urethral stenosis, and so on) as a cause of reflux.

In children, should Y-V plasty or transurethral resection of the vesical neck be done routinely at the time of ureteroneocystostomy? Should vesical-neck surgery be tried before ureteroneocystostomy is considered? How long should medical treatment be continued before one resorts to antireflux surgery?

Obviously, answers to these questions are not obtained easily, and a pragmatic conservative approach is usually employed—for example: In the case of *iatrogenic reflux*, damage to the ureteral orifice can be detected cystoscopically in most cases without difficulty. On the other hand, obstruction of the bladder neck, especially in infants, is almost impossible to detect and be sure of (either cystoscopically or urographically). Dilated "golf hole" ureteral orifices are easily seen, but lesser degrees of dilatation are hard to evaluate. The intramural ureter compromised by a "Hutch diverticulum" usually is demonstrated easily, either cystoscopically or urographically. On the other hand, the role of infection, whether primary or secondary, is difficult to assess.

No hard and fast rules can be given, and the reader must keep abreast of the situation by watching for reports of results of management of substantial series of cases from clinical centers (Garrett and Switzer; King and associates). However, certain trends emerge from the literature which can be mentioned. If, in spite of conservative treatment (which includes continuous chemotherapy, multiple voiding technique, and overdilatation of the urethra [in little girls] to size 32 F to eliminate Lyon's "distal urethral ring"), infection persists or recurs or if there is evidence of progressive renal damage by urographic demonstration of increased pyelectasis and parenchymal atrophy, or by means of renal function tests, ureteroneocystostomy seems advisable. No firm data exist regarding the advisability of performing vesical-neck surgery at the same time. Such statements as "if it appears that vesical neck obstruction is present" are entirely meaningless in most cases, especially when the patients are infants and children. Presently many urologists prefer to perform a revision of the vesical neck at the same time, reasoning that if the vesical neck is contributing to the reflux it will be corrected; if not the patient should not be made worse because it is done.

All workers emphasize that best results are obtained when the ureters are minimally or only moderately dilated. Good results are usually not possible if the ureters are tremendously dilated.

Long-term chemotherapy may be expected to allow spontaneous correction of reflux in half the children treated. In children who have reflux but no infection and show no evidence of progressive dilatation of the upper urinary tract, operation should probably not be done (Garrett and Switzer). Gaping ureteral orifices suggest that operation should be done. Of 123 children with reflux in Garrett and Switzer's series, 58 (51%) had ureteroneocystostomy.

*See discussion of techniques of ureteroneocystostomy (page 471.)

(*Text continued on page 471.*)

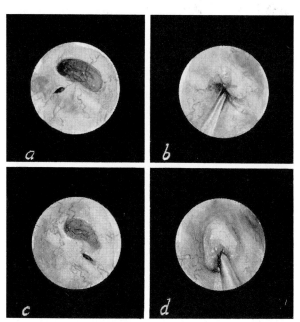

Figure 5–134. *Cystoscopic views.* **Saccules near ureteral orifices. A,** Saccule near right ureteral orifice. **B,** Catheter introduced into meatus, showing intramural ureter in floor of saccule with no muscular support. **C** and **D,** Same situation, near left ureteral orifice. (From Hutch, J. A., 1958.)

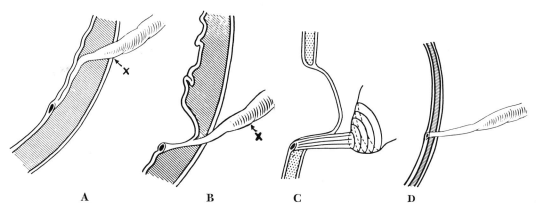

Figure 5–135. **Intramural ureters. A,** Normal ureter passes obliquely and distally through bladder wall from point "X." **B,** Much of intramural ureter (to "X") is extravesical because bladder wall is weakened by saccule adjacent to ureteral orifice. **C,** Intravesical ureter in extravesical position is obstructive even though its lumen is not occluded. Dilatation occurs only where circular muscle fibers are present. There are none in remaining intramural ureter; thus, it acts as inert tube with no peristalsis when much of it is in extravesical position. **D,** Essentially all of ureter is extravesical, result of bladder being thinned out and having no trabeculation. (From Hutch, J. A., 1958.)

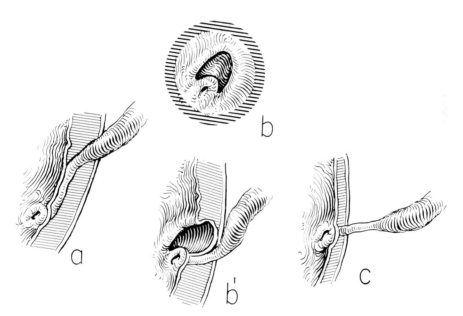

Figure 5–136.   Intramural ureter. Three dimensional illustration of principles illustrated in Figure 5–135. **a,** Normal intramural ureter. **b,** Cystoscopic appearance of ureteral orifice on edge of saccule or small diverticulum. **b′,** Bladder wall weakened by saccule adjacent to ureteral orifice. **Intramural ureter has become extravesical. c,** Same situation, which has resulted from thinned-out bladder with no trabeculation.

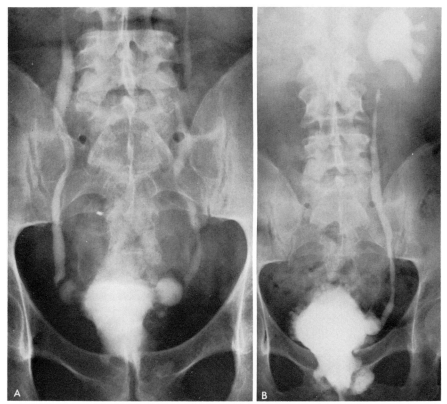

Figure 5–137.   Neurogenic bladder with bilateral "Hutch diverticula" and left ureteral reflux. (Secondary to traumatic lesion of conus medullaris and cauda equina.) **A,** *Excretory urogram.* Note wide open prostatic urethra from previous transurethral resection. **B,** *Retrograde urethrogram.* (Note filling of prostatic ducts.) **Reflux up left ureter.**

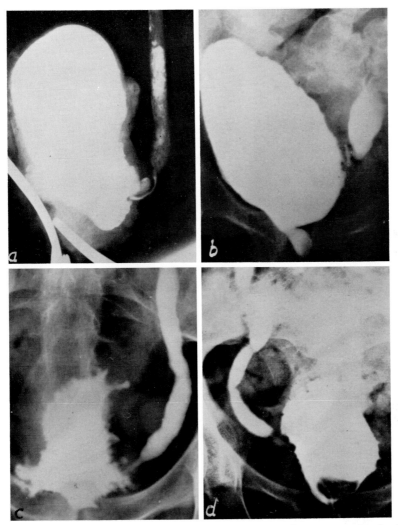

Figure 5–138. Extravesical position of normally intravesical part of ureter associated with neurologic disease. *Cystograms.* **A, Paraplegia.** Patient died of progressive renal failure. At necropsy urinary tract was removed intact, and this cystogram was made. Lateral exposure clearly shows saccule lying above intravesical ureter. Intravesical ureter can be seen passing along floor of saccule. Note that dilatation begins at juncture of intravesical and extravesical segments of ureter. **B, Meningomyelocele,** in child. In complete x-ray series, peristaltic wave was seen passing down ureter and forcing contrast medium into dilated lower portion of ureter. Note tortuous, undilated intravesical ureter in extravesical position. **C, Paraplegia and spastic bladder.** Intravesical ureter on left is clearly visible in extravesical position. **D, Paraplegia.** Intravesical ureter in extravesical position. (From Hutch, J. A., 1958.)

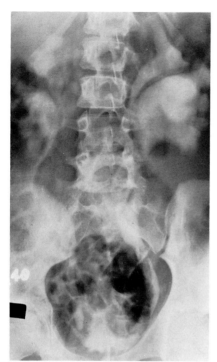

Figure 5–139. *Retrograde cystogram* of girl, 12 years of age, with myelodysplasia. Bilateral reflux, trabeculation of bladder, large bilateral saccules (or small diverticula), incomplete duplication on right, and complete duplication on left. Common right ureteral orifice was situated just inside saccule. On left, orifice serving upper pelvis was situated just on edge of saccule; that serving lower pelvis, in bottom of saccule.

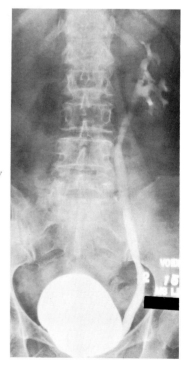

Figure 5–140. *Retrograde cystogram* of woman. Solitary kidney with reflux associated with interstitial cystitis.

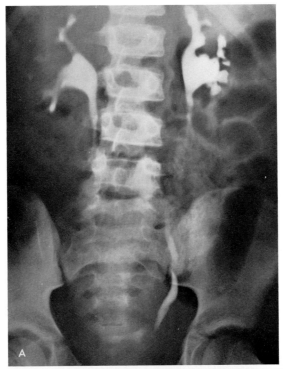

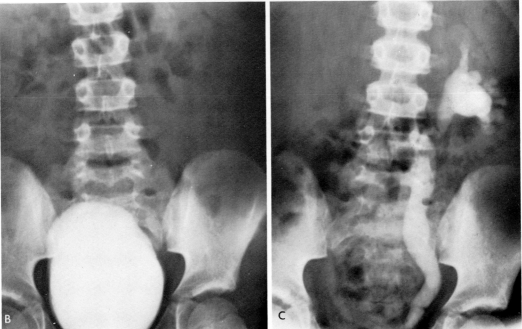

Figure 5–141. Ureteral reflux demonstrated only while patient voided. A, *Bilateral retrograde pyelogram.* Evidence of **slight pyelouretrectasis on left.** B, *Retrograde cystogram exposed while catheter was still in bladder.* No evidence of reflux up either ureter. C, *Retrograde cystogram exposed while patient was voiding.* **Reflux up left ureter,** dilated grade 3. This degree of uretrectasis would not be suspected from excretory urogram.

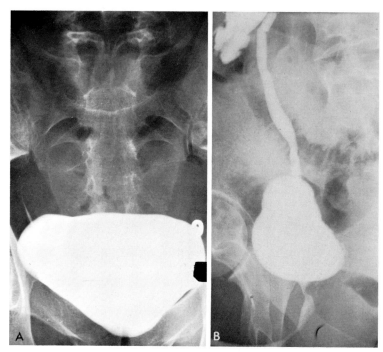

Figure 5–142.   Unilateral reflux seen principally on voiding. Transurethral removal of benign vesical tumor had been performed 8 years previously. **A,** *Retrograde cystogram.* Small amount of media has refluxed up right ureter. **B,** *Voiding cystourethrogram.* Reflux up right ureter produces complete pyeloureterogram.

SURGICAL REVISION OF THE URETEROVESICAL JUNCTION TO PREVENT REFLUX: URETERONEOCYSTOSTOMY
by
Lawrence G. Fehrenbaker

Surgical procedures to correct vesicoureteral reflux have been surprisingly successful, considering that the physiology of the ureterovesical junction remains imperfectly understood and controversial. However, standardization has not yet been possible, and several techniques of ureteroneocystostomy are currently used.

As mentioned previously, the role of the vesical neck in reflux has not been finally appraised, but currently its assigned importance seems to be on the wane. On the other hand, the role of the ureterovesical junction has received increasing attention.

Indications for Antireflux Operations

Paquin and Williams and Eckstein (1965b) have suggested the following indications for surgical correction of reflux: (1) failure of specific antimicrobial therapy to control infection and concomitant vesicoureteral reflux; (2) progressive deterioration of the kidneys and their function, even if infection is controlled; (3) persistence of vesicoureteral reflux after surgical revision of the vesical neck for "apparent" obstruction to urinary outflow; (4) association of vesicoureteral reflux with demonstrable anatomic defects of the trigone and intravesical ureter (that is, the presence of a vesical saccule or diverticulum [Hutch diverticulum] adjacent to the ureteral orifice) (see Figs. 5–134 through 5–138); (5) occurrence of vesicoureteral reflux at low intravesical pressures;[*] and (6) progressive renal damage associated with iatrogenic reflux due to

trauma of the trigone or ureteral orifice sustained during transurethral resection of the prostate or vesical neoplasm, excision of a ureterocele, ureteral meatotomy, or other surgical procedures.

Surgical Techniques

The object of all antireflux operations is to provide an intravesical ureter of adequate length and an adequate detrusor-muscle buttress to support it.

Brief descriptions of the more common antireflux operations should help the reader appraise them. As representative examples, I have chosen the following: (1) the Hutch operation, (2) the Bischoff vesicoureteroplasty, (3) the Politano-Leadbetter ureteroneocystostomy and the Kelalis modification, and (4) the Paquin operation.

The Hutch Operation (Fig. 5–143). One of the first attempts to correct reflux surgically was made by Hutch in 1952. He described a vesicoureteroplasty for paraplegics. He originally transplanted the intramural ureter intravesically, suturing the bladder mucosa under the ureter. Later Jewett, and also Ambrose and Nicolson, modified this procedure so that the bladder mucosa was sutured over the transplanted ureter. This modification is now preferred by Hutch (1966).

The Bischoff Vesicoureteroplasty. Bischoff's technique (Fig. 5–144A, B, and C) has been favored by some because it does not involve mobilization of the ureter and its orifice. Bischoff also performs a ureteroplasty on the large tortuous decompensated ureters. (The reader is referred to Bischoff's article for his description of ureteroplasty.)

The Politano-Leadbetter Ureteroneocystostomy (Fig. 5–145). This widely used operation is performed transvesically without mobilization of the bladder. For comparison, a modified Politano-Leadbetter technique described by Kelalis is also illustrated (Fig. 5–146A through P).

---

[*]There is at present considerable difference of opinion concerning the value of correlating intravesical pressure and reflux.

The Paquin Ureteroneocystostomy (Fig. 5–147A through E). The technique of Paquin, also widely used, differs from that of Politano and Leadbetter in that the ureter is mobilized extravesically. It is particularly adaptable to large tortuous ureters.

Comment. The interested reader is referred to the original articles of other investigators for variations in technique of the above four basic operations (Ambrose and Nicolson; Girgis, Veenema, and Lattimer; Jewett; Mathisen; Witherington).

Complications

Creevy (1967b) states that the most common complication of antireflux operations is *postoperative ureteral obstruction of the reimplanted ureter.* This may result from (1) inflammatory edema of the transplanted segment, (2) an inadequate submucosal tunnel, (3) excessive angulation of the ureter as it enters the bladder wall, resulting in obstruction of the extravesical segment, (4) excessive tension on the ureter, and (5) stenosis of the ureteral meatus. Although obstruction from inflammatory edema is often only temporary, not uncommonly it persists for several months after operation (Fig. 5–148A, B, and C); and it may require nephrostomy or ureteral catheterization in severe cases. Obstruction from any of the other listed causes may require secondary reimplantation (Fig. 5–149A, B, and C).

Injudicious dissection may lead to *perforation of the ureter* and *impairment of the ureteral vasculature;* these, in turn, may result in disruption of the ureterovesical anastomosis with extravasation of urine and subsequent fibrosis. *Late fibrosis,* causing fixation of the reimplanted segment and trigone, may result in persistent reflux.

Infection is not uncommon after ureteroneocystostomy. It requires continuous specific antimicrobial therapy until eradicated.

Results

Politano reported the results of 162 reimplantations on 100 patients (74 females and 26 males) during a 5-year period. The Politano-Leadbetter technique was used in all cases, a vesical-neck revision was performed simultaneously in 19%, and a previous transurethral resection of the vesical neck had been done in 21%.

Reflux was not corrected in the case of one female and five male patients. The success rate, therefore, was 99% for females and 81% for males—an overall success rate of 94%. Five males required eventual urinary diversion by means of an ileal conduit. Diversion was not required for any female patient.

In five cases, obstruction developed at the site of reimplantation. In three, this was corrected by simple dilatation with ureteral catheters. The other two patients required secondary reimplantation.

After using the Paquin technique in reimplanting 327 ureters in 226 children, McGovern and Marshall reported 90% success (average follow-up period 4.5 years). They defined *success* as absence of both reflux and obstruction at the involved ureterovesical junction. In 82% of their cases, vesical neck revision (Y-V plasty on the anterior vesical outlet) was performed at the same time. The differences in the success rates for boys (71%) and girls (96%) reflect the severity of the disease in males and may also indicate the higher incidence of vesical-neck obstruction in boys. The authors hypothesized that their failures resulted from attempting to correct vesicoureteral reflux in cases in which renal deterioration and ureteral decompensation were excessive. Infection (present in all cases preoperatively) persisted in 34% of the cases at 1 year postoperatively. However, on longer follow-up, only 17% of the patients continued to have urinary infection. The mortality rate was 1.3%.

Scott used the Politano-Leadbetter technique for 66 ureteral reimplantations and reported 100% success.

Comment. Vesicoureteral reflux can be eliminated by operation in a high percentage of cases (Fig. 5–150A and B). The surgeon's success in correcting reflux appears to depend more on his proficiency with the operation than on the specific surgical technique employed.

(*Text continued on page 480.*)

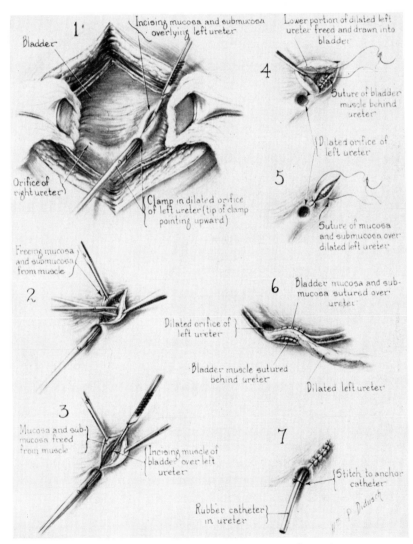

Figure 5–143. Hutch I vesicoureteroplasty as modified by Jewett. This technique is accomplished intravesically in its entirety. Note that in step 4, after freeing ureter, surgeon closes bladder muscle behind ureter, creating firm detrusor buttress. In step 5, mucosa and submucosa are sutured over new intravesical ureter. Suturing mucosa and submucosa in this manner has decreased incidence of ureteral cicatrization which was common complication in original Hutch operation. (From Jewett, H. J.)

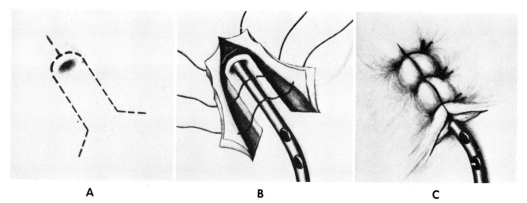

A   B   C

Figure 5–144. Bischoff's vesicoureteroplasty. **A,** Relationship of intended incision through bladder mucosa and submucosa to ureteral orifice. **B,** Splint which is not snug to ureteral orifice is positioned along proposed course of new intravesical ureter. Mucosa and submucosa are sutured over splint, enclosing original orifice. **C,** Note how new intravesical ureter and ureteral orifice have been made without mobilization of defective ureter. (From Bischoff, P.)

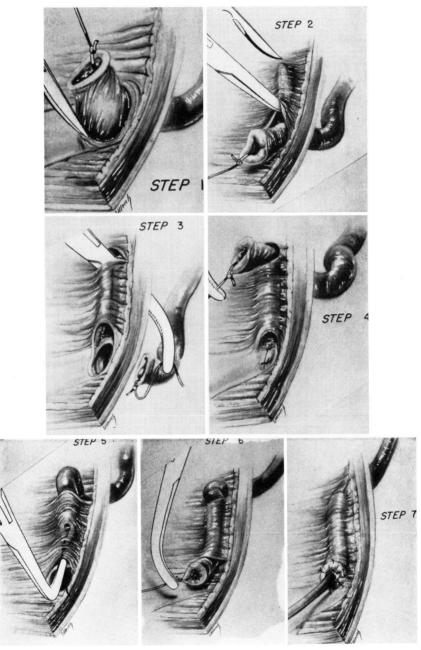

Figure 5–145. **Politano and Leadbetter's technique of ureteroneocystostomy to correct vesicoureteral reflux.** *Step 1,* Ureteral orifice is circumscribed and intramural ureter dissected free. *Step 2,* Submucosal tunnel is made by gentle spreading of clamp beneath mucosa. *Step 3,* Bladder is perforated. *Step 4,* Withdrawal of clamp pulls ureter into bladder at new site. Original muscular defect is closed with interrupted sutures. *Step 5,* Distal end of ureter is pulled through submucosal tunnel. *Step 6,* Ureter has been pulled through tunnel and is ready for mucosa-to-mucosa anastomosis. *Step 7,* Anastomosis is completed by using several interrupted fine chromic sutures. (From Politano, V. A., and Leadbetter, W. F.)

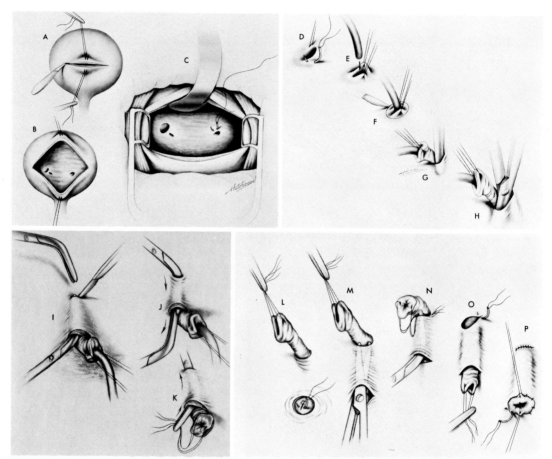

Figure 5–146. Modified Politano-Leadbetter ureteroneocystostomy, as described by Kelalis. **A,** Bladder is opened between two traction sutures. **B,** Exposure of trigone and ureteral orifices. Note "Hutch saccule" adjacent to ureteral orifice. **C,** Positioning of retractors for maximal exposure and placing of traction suture adjacent to uretral orifice. **D,** Two traction sutures are used to facilitate dissection. Note that sutures are not placed through orifice. **E,** Ureteral splint is advanced along course of ureter to aid in dissection of ureter. **F,** With aid of traction to immobilize mucosa, ureteral orifice is circumcised. **G** and **H,** By using continued traction and blunt scissor dissection, surgeon frees ureter from bladder muscle. **I,** Right angle clamp is advanced along course of ureter until it is extravesical. Incision through bladder is made over tip of clamp. **J** and **K,** By interlocking right angle clamp with another, surgeon can insert second clamp into vesical incision and subsequently draw exposed ureter extravesically. **L,** Ureter is brought back into bladder. (New entrance of ureter into bladder is at proximal end of new submucosal tunnel. This site is somewhat posterior and medial, so that good support is obtained in mobile portion of bladder.) Muscular defect in bladder is closed with interrupted sutures. **M,** Submucosal tunnel is made by means of blunt scissors dissection. (Tunnel is short, and its length is unrelated to diameter of ureter.) **N,** Ureter is placed into its new tunnel. **O,** Mucosal defect is closed. **P,** Ureteral orifice is sutured into its original site.

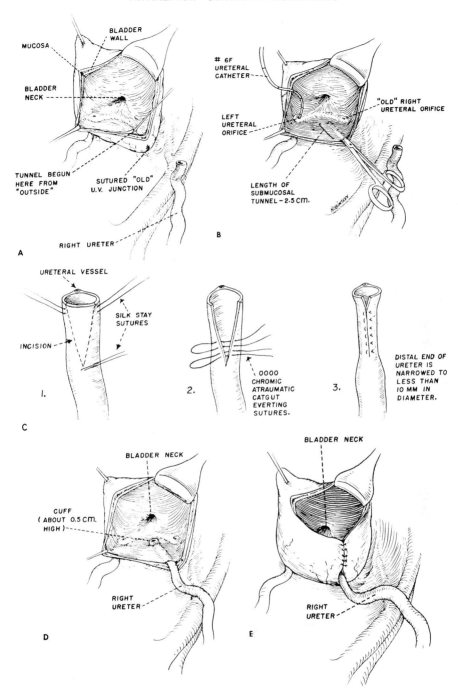

Figure 5–147.   Paquin technique of ureteroneocystostomy. A, After bladder is incised, ureter is dissected from its attachment to bladder, and creation of submucosal tunnel is begun. **B,** Submucosal tunnel is made by dissecting from incised mucosa for distance equal to five times diameter of ureteral orifice. Tunnel terminates on or near trigone. **C,** If ureter is dilated to more than 8 to 10 mm in diameter, wedge of ureter is excised proximally for about 30 to 40 mm. Paquin's original description mentioned distal ureteral cuff which he thought strengthened orifice and made it more resistant to reflux. However, on subsequent examinations ureteral cuff had disappeared, and its value has been questioned. **D,** Appearance of ureter after reimplantation. Frequently ureteral orifice is positioned on trigone. **E,** In closing bladder, no attempt is made to close bladder muscle tightly about ureter. (From Paquin, A. J.)

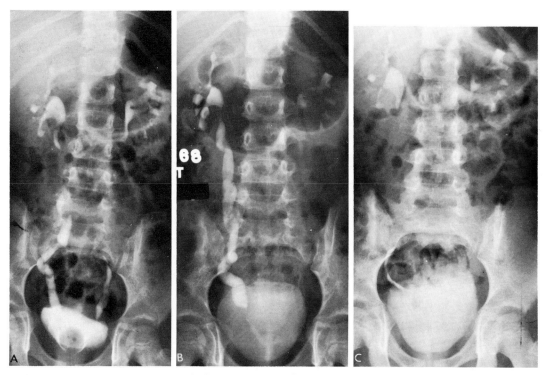

Figure 5–148.   Temporary ureteral obstruction from edema after ureteroneocystostomy to correct reflux. Patient, 6-year-old girl, had 2-year history of recurring urinary tract infections caused by bilateral vesicoureteral reflux. **A**, *Preoperative excretory urogram.* **Bilateral parenchymal thinning and ureterectasis.** Note balloon of Foley catheter in bladder. Patient had been on catheter drainage because of bilateral vesicoureteral reflux. (At cystoscopy large, thin-walled, nontrabeculated bladder was seen. Ureteral orifices were gaping, and intramural ureters were entirely absent while bladder was full.) **B**, *Excretory urogram* 9 months after bilateral ureteroneocystostomy. **Ureteropyelocaliectasis on right, secondary to residual postoperative edema.** Patient was asymptomatic and free of reflux. **C**, *Excretory urogram* 14 months after operation. Essentially normal.

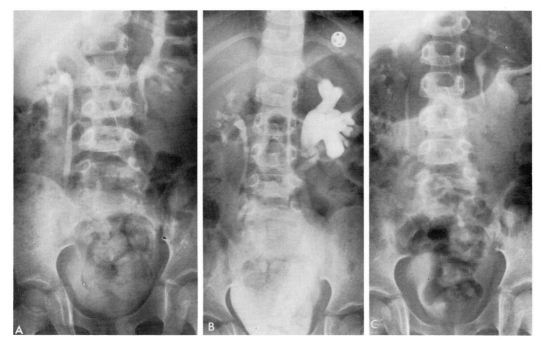

Figure 5–149. Postoperative constriction of ureter (after ureteroneocystostomy for reflux), requiring secondary operation. Patient, 3½-year-old girl, had 2-year history of pyuria and fever caused by left vesicoureteral reflux, treated initially with urethral dilatation and antibiotics. **A,** *Excretory urogram.* **Minimal left calycectasis.** (Left ureteroneocystostomy was performed, but postoperatively patient continued to have fever and pyuria.) **B,** *Postoperative excretory urogram.* **Marked ureteropyelocaliectasis.** (Patient was explored surgically and constriction of ureter at its entrance into bladder was found. Repeat left ureteroneocystostomy was done.) **C,** *Postoperative excretory urogram.* Good result.

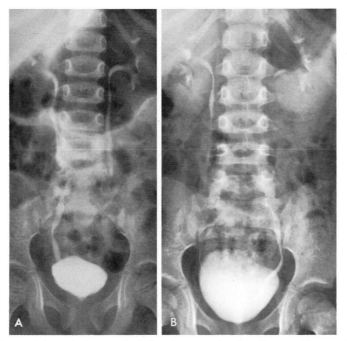

Figure 5–150. Successful surgical correction of vesicoureteral reflux. Patient, 3½-year-old girl, had 1-year history of urinary tract infections, caused by vesicoureteral reflux on right. **A,** *Excretory urogram* obtained in course of work-up. Ureterectasis of lower half of right ureter. (Cinecystourethrogram demonstrated right vesicoureteral reflux.) **B,** *Excretory urogram* 7 months after right ureteroneocystostomy. Normal.

479

STASIS INVOLVING THE LOWER PART OF THE URINARY TRACT

Neurogenic Bladder

ACQUIRED

As Ney and Duff pointed out, several abnormalities are seen in cystourethrograms of patients with neurogenic bladders; yet none of them is pathognomonic of the disease, and almost all can be simulated in the cystourethrograms of patients without neurologic disease. Furthermore, there is no common agreement on the clinical significance of these abnormal findings. The following are among the cystographic variations: trabeculated bladder of either circular or pyramidal ("pine tree") contour; hourglass bladder with pseudosphincteric formations; normal-sized or small hypertonic trabeculated bladder; large dilated hypotonic bladder without trabeculation; vesicoureteral reflux; variations in the contour of the vesical neck and prostatic urethra—such as the dilated funnel type, saccular dilatation, and contracted spastic vesical neck; and spastic or relaxed external sphincter.

The plain film should be examined carefully, especially if the patient is an infant or child with vesical and rectal dysfunction, for evidence of deformity or agenesis (partial or complete) of the sacrum. (See Figs. 3–179, 3–181, and 3–182.)

Trabeculation of the Bladder

Except for the disorders in which only the sensory pathways are compromised (such as tabes dorsalis, diabetic tabes, and vesical dysfunction from an "asymptomatic" protruded lumbar disk [the so-called silent-disk syndrome]) (Emmett and Love; Love and Emmett), almost all neurogenic bladders have some degree of trabeculation and often are associated with vesicoureteral reflux (Figs. 5–151 through 5–154; see also Fig. 5–137). Some authors

(Giertz and Lindblom; McLellan) have tried to correlate the degree of trabeculation, contour, size, and tonicity of the bladder with the level of the spinal lesion. Others (Bors, 1951; 1957) have concluded that these characteristics of the bladder relate more directly to the duration of the lesion, the degree of recovery, and the type of treatment applied to the bladder. It has been stated that trabeculation of the bladder is slight and the capacity of the bladder is large in the case of lower motor lesions (involving the conus). In my (J.L.E.) experience (Emmett, 1947; 1954; Emmett and Dunn; Emmett and Helmholz; Emmett and Simon; Emmett, Simon, and Mills), however, at least 80% of patients with congenital spina bifida and myelodysplasia (a lower motor lesion) have trabeculated bladders. In fact, the most advanced degrees of trabeculation that I have ever seen were in cases of this type or in acquired lesions of the conus and cauda equina. Giertz and Lindblom apparently have had similar experience. They stated that the trabeculated "pine tree" shaped bladder is seen almost exclusively in association with nuclear and infranuclear lesions. In the case of upper motor neuron lesions, they found that the bladder is circular and usually has less trabeculation.

The difficulty in trying to correlate the cystourethrographic or any other type of urologic findings with the level of the lesion in the spinal cord is the absence of an accurate standard method for determining whether a lesion is nuclear (involving the sacral cord which contains the reflex center for micturition), supranuclear, or infranuclear (cauda equina). Some authors, including McLellan, Langworthy, Kolb, and Lewis, and Watkins (1934), have used the cystometrogram for this purpose; Albers, Anderson, and one of us (J.L.E.) have used the sensory level plus the voiding pattern. Bors' (1951; 1957) method of determining the presence or absence of the anal and bulbocavernous reflexes seems to be more accurate and easily employed, but it has been criticized as being unreliable in some cases.

It is generally conceded that most small, spastic, trabeculated bladders are associated with upper motor neuron lesions, yet relatively efficient and balanced automatic bladders with good capacity and minimal trabeculation are encountered in association with lesions of the midthoracic cord. That almost any type or degree of trabeculated bladder, including the "pine tree" bladder, may be seen in patients with no neurologic disease who have only simple obstruction of the vesical neck should not be forgotten.

The large, smooth, thin-walled, atonic type of bladder with little or no trabeculation is seen in tabes dorsalis, diabetic tabes (Emmett and Beare, 1941; 1948; Emmett, Daut, and Sprague), and the "silent-disk syndrome" (Emmett and Love; Love and Emmett). However, it is also seen in patients without demonstrable neurologic disease who have an obstruction of the vesical neck of long standing, in which the detrusor muscle seemingly has "decompensated" rather than "risen to the challenge" by becoming hypertrophied and trabeculated. In still other cases, no obstruction can be demonstrated and the cause of the dilatation is obscure (Figs. 5-155, 5-156, and 5-157A and B).

(Text continued on page 485.)

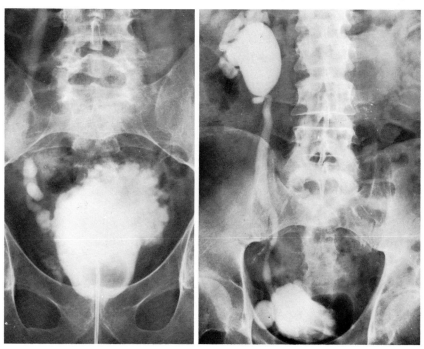

Fig. 5–151   Fig. 5–152

Figure 5–151. *Retrograde cystogram.* **Neurogenic bladder, secondary to traumatic lesion of spinal cord at C-5 in boy, 18 years of age.** Marked trabeculation of bladder with cellule formation and reflux up right ureter. Prostatic urethra wide open and filled with medium as result of previous transurethral resection of vesical neck. Negative shadow in base of bladder represents bag of catheter.

Figure 5–152. *Retrograde cystogram.* **War injury (gunshot) of spinal cord at level of T-12 and L-1.** Outline of irregular, trabeculated bladder with cellules and diverticulum on right. Reflux up right ureter, which is dilated, grade 2. Renal pelvis is dilated, grade 3.

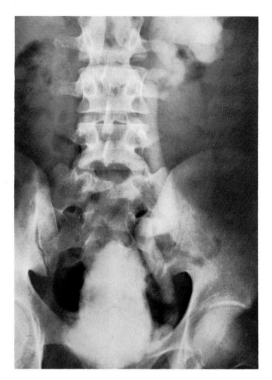

Figure 5–153. *Retrograde cystogram.* **Neurogenic bladder, resulting from transverse lesion of spinal cord secondary to surgical removal of tumor at L-1 and L-2,** in boy of 17 years; 1,200 ml of residual urine. Typical pyramid-shaped bladder with cellule formation and reflux up left ureter. **Pyeloureterectasis, grade 3.** (Urinary retention was relieved by transurethral resection of vesical neck. Patient now voids voluntarily, at regular intervals, and empties bladder completely.)

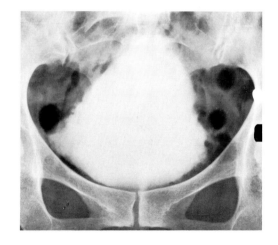

Figure 5–154. *Retrograde cystogram.* **Neurogenic bladder resulting from multiple sclerosis** in woman 46 years of age. Note trabeculation, cellule formation, and pyramidal contour.

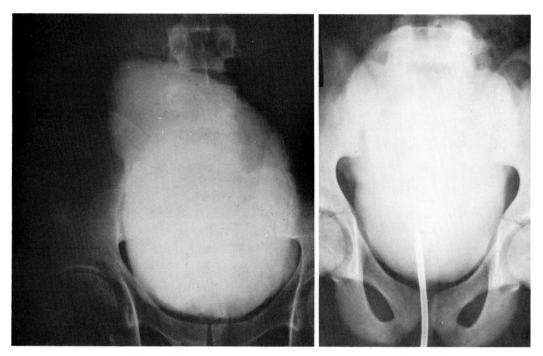

Fig. 5–155   Fig. 5–156

Figure 5–155. *Retrograde cystogram.* Huge "atonic" bladder resulting from long-standing obstruction of vesical neck. No evidence of trabeculation. Decompensation of bladder; 1,000 ml of residual urine.

Figure 5–156. *Retrograde cystogram.* Large, distended, atonic bladder of undetermined etiology. No evidence of trabeculation. Cystogram suggests long-standing congenital obstruction with decompensation of bladder.

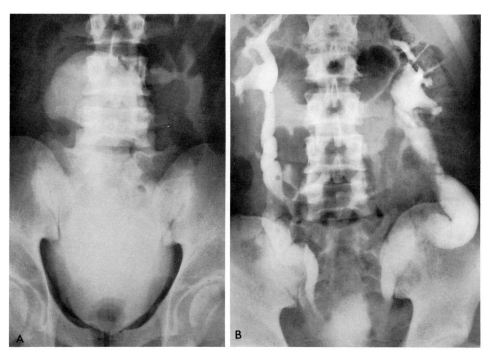

Figure 5–157.   Large atonic bladder (capacity more than 1,000 ml) of undetermined etiology. Bladder contained several hundred milliliters of residual urine, and patient (21-year-old man) had had recurrent urinary infection with fever. (Questionable obstruction of vesical neck on cystoscopy. No vesical reflux demonstrated.) **A,** *Retrograde cystogram.* Incompletely filled, huge, redundant bladder, extends to level of L3-4 interspace. **B,** *Bilateral retrograde pyelograms.* **Bilateral ureterectasis** with tortuous ureters. (Courtesy of Dr. A. A. Parrish.)

Characteristics of the Vesical Neck and External Urethral Sphincter

Attempts to correlate the various urographic contours of the vesical neck and prostatic urethra with the level of the spinal lesion, type of neurogenic vesical dysfunction, type of treatment indicated, and prognosis, generally speaking, have not been rewarding. One exception to this has been the demonstration of *spasticity of the external sphincter* by means of retrograde cystourethrography (Damanski and Kerr; Emmett, Daut, and Dunn). It has been shown (Emmett, Daut, and Dunn) that, in upper motor neuron lesions, spasticity of the striated muscle fibers of the external urethral sphincter may be the obstructive factor that prevents the bladder from emptying satisfactorily (Figs. 5-158 through 5-161). Bors (1951; 1957) has shown that some of the striated muscle fibers of the external sphincter may extend up and intertwine with smooth muscle fibers of the vesical neck,

so that the vesical neck may also become spastic. Transurethral resection of the vesical neck will eliminate the bladder-neck factor but obstruction from a spastic external sphincter may persist, allowing bladder retention to continue. Procedures to eliminate the latter factor include pudendal nerve section (Ross and Damanski), subarachnoid alcohol block (Shelden and Bors), selective spinal cordectomy (MacCarty), and resection or division of the external urethral sphincter (Ross, Damanski, and Gibbon; Ross, Gibbon, and Damanski). In a recent article on the subject, Damanski described the important role of the cystourethrogram in deciding which operative procedure (or combination of procedures) is indicated to restore acceptable bladder function for the 40% of paraplegic patients who do not respond to conservative treatment (Figs. 5-162A and B through 5-168). The rationale of the various procedures is discussed elsewhere (Emmett and Greene).

(Text continued on page 494.)

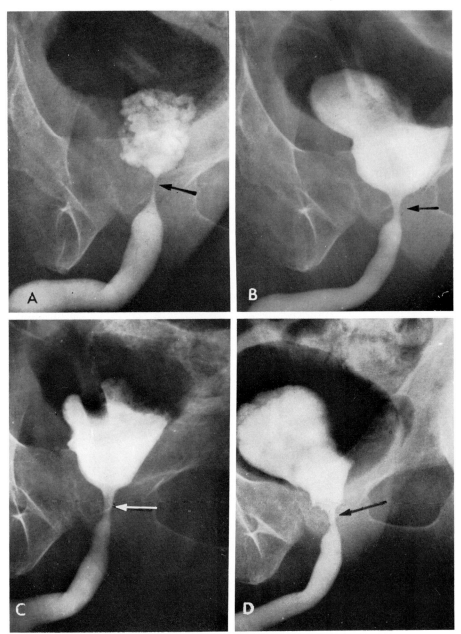

Figure 5–158. Determination of increased spasticity of external sphincter in paraplegic patient with spastic paralysis of lower extremities, associated with mass reflexes. **A,** *Retrograde cystourethrogram.* **Spastic external sphincter** (*arrow*). (Patient had undergone previous transurethral resection because of cord bladder and was unable to void.) **B,** *Cystourethrogram* during sacral block with procaine hydrochloride. Relaxation of external sphincter allowed patient to void easily. **C,** *Cystourethrogram* during bilateral pudendal block with procaine. Relaxation of external sphincter allowed patient to void easily. **D,** *Cystourethrogram* after surgical section of both anterior and posterior roots of fourth and fifth lumbar and all five sacral nerves. Relaxation of external sphincter allowed patient to void easily and empty bladder completely. (From Emmett, J. L., Daut, R. V., and Dunn, J. H.)

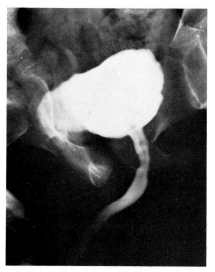

Figure 5–159. *Retrograde cystourethrogram.* Relaxation of external sphincter in paraplegic patient with flaccid paralysis of lower extremities. (From Emmett, J. L., Daut, R. V., and Dunn, J. H.)

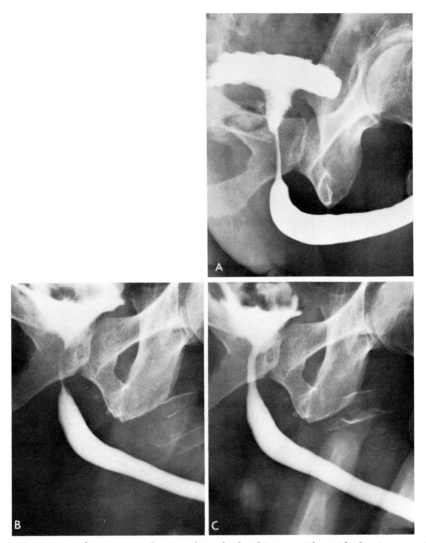

Figure 5–160. Increased spasticity of external urethral sphincter with residual urine associated with neurogenic bladder from primary lateral sclerosis of spinal cord in man, 57 years of age. (Transurethral resection of vesical neck done 3 years previously, but substantial amount of residual urine persisted.) **A,** *Retrograde urethrogram.* Note marked spasticity and elongation of external sphincter. (Exploratory cervical laminectomy done.) **B,** *Retrograde urethrogram* 1 year after laminectomy. Still spastic external sphincter, but length seems diminished. **C,** *Retrograde urethrogram* made immediately after caudal and transsacral procaine block. Note relaxation of external sphincter.

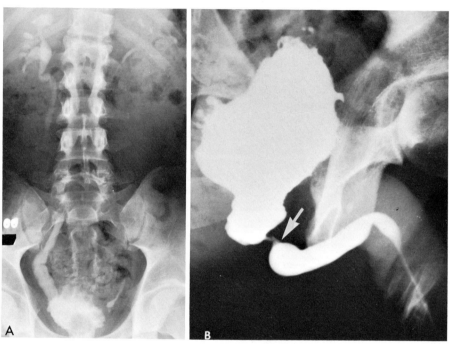

Figure 5–161.   **Neurogenic bladder with spastic external sphincter** in man, aged 21, with traumatic lesion of cauda equina. Bladder dysfunction was only residual disability from accident. Transurethral resection of vesical neck was only partially helpful. **A**, *Excretory urogram* after transurethral resection. Dilatation of lower half of right ureter, trabeculated (incompletely filled) bladder, and wide open vesical neck. **B**, *Voiding cystourethrogram*. Marked spasticity of external sphincter (*arrow*). (Transurethral excision of lower left quadrant of external sphincter resulted in substantial improvement.)

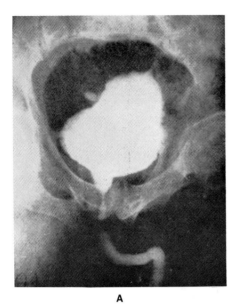
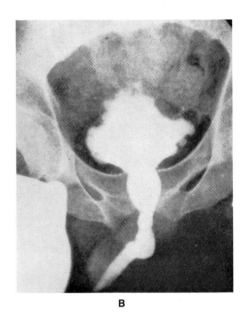

A   B

Figure 5–162.   Partial and complete relief of spastic contraction of vesical neck and external sphincter. *Retrograde urethrograms.* **A,** *After transurethral resection.* Residual urine of 300 ml persists. Vesical neck has been widened, but clinical result was not satisfactory. **B,** *After subarachnoid alcohol block.* Marked relaxation of vesical neck, entire prostatic urethra, and external sphincter. (From Damanski, M., and Kerr, A. S.)

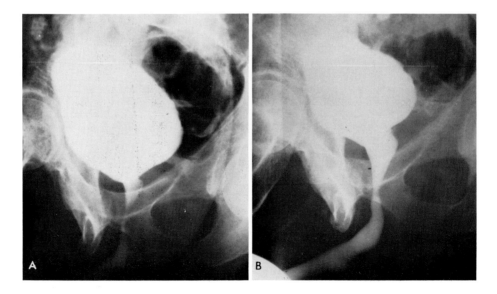

Figure 5–163.   Spastic external urethral sphincter of paraplegic patient. *Retrograde urethrograms.* **A,** *Preoperative.* Spasticity of external sphincter is evident. **B,** *After transurethral resection* of external sphincter. Note relaxation of external sphincter. (From Ross, J. C., Damanski, M., and Gibbon, N.)

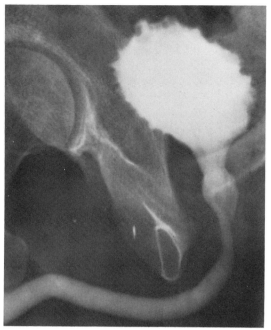

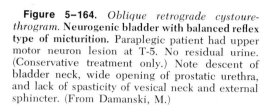

Figure 5–164. *Oblique retrograde cystoure-throgram.* **Neurogenic bladder with balanced reflex type of micturition.** Paraplegic patient had upper motor neuron lesion at T-5. No residual urine. (Conservative treatment only.) Note descent of bladder neck, wide opening of prostatic urethra, and lack of spasticity of vesical neck and external sphincter. (From Damanski, M.)

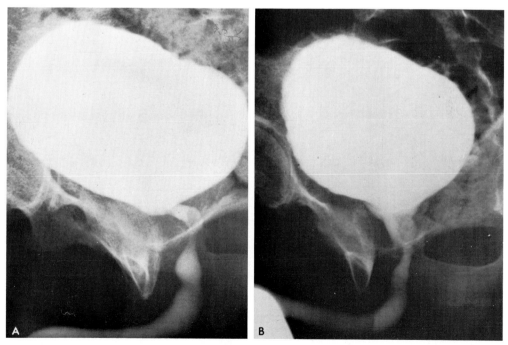

Figure 5–165. **Relief of urinary retention by transurethral resection of vesical neck** of quadriplegic patient with upper motor neuron lesion at C-7. *Retrograde cystourethrograms.* **A,** *Preoperative oblique view.* Anterior tilt and posterior ledge of vesical neck. (Complete retention with autonomic hyperreflexia.) **B,** *Postoperative oblique view.* Note wide opening of proximal part of prostatic urethra. (Residual urine was reduced to 350 ml and autonomic hyperreflexia disappeared. Patient had normal excretory urogram 4 years after spinal injury.) (From Damanski, M.)

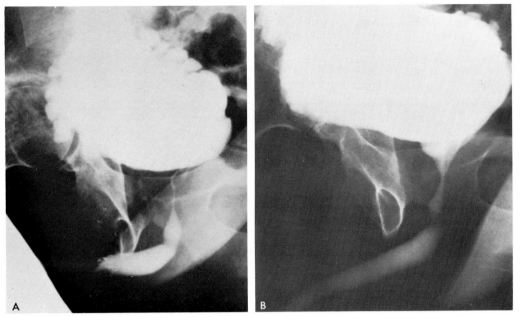

Figure 5–166. Relief of urinary retention by transurethral resection of vesical neck of paraplegic patient with upper motor neuron lesion at T-10. *Retrograde cystourethrograms.* **A,** *Preoperative oblique view.* Posterior tilt and anterior ledge. Note also **diverticulosis of bladder** resulting from urinary infection of long standing. **B,** *Postoperative oblique view.* Note funnel-shaped proximal portion of prostatic urethra. (Residual urine reduced from 480 ml to nil.) (From Damanski, M.)

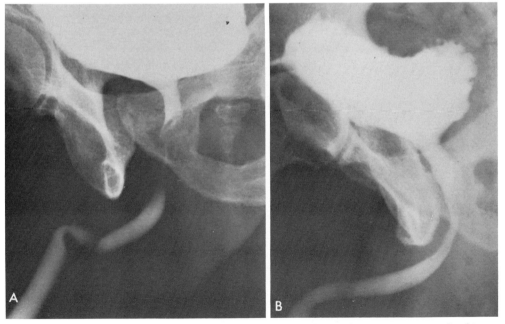

Figure 5–167. Relief, by pudendal neurectomy, of urinary retention from spastic external sphincter of paraplegic patient with upper motor neuron lesion at T-11. *Retrograde cystourethrograms.* **A,** *Preoperative oblique view.* Prostatic urethra is patent above verumontanum, and external sphincter is spastic (very narrow). (Residual urine measured 570 ml. **Hydronephrosis.** Pudendal neurectomy was performed.) **B,** *Postoperative oblique view.* Much better opening of external sphincter. (Residual urine reduced to 60 ml. Hydronephrosis improved.) (From Damanski, M.)

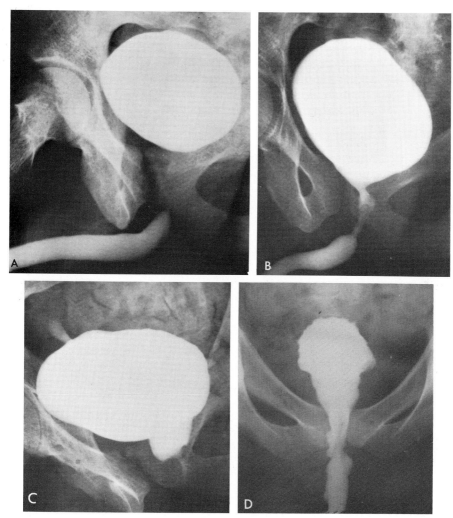

Figure 5–168. Relief of bladder retention and dilatation of upper part of urinary tract of quadriplegic patient (C-8) after (1) subarachnoid alcohol block, (2) transurethral resection of vesical neck, and (3) division of external urethral sphincter (performed in sequence). **A,** *Retrograde cystourethrogram, oblique view.* Normal anterior urethra ends abruptly at level of external urethral sphincter. (Attempt at overcoming its resistance by forceful injection might result in extravasation. Indwelling catheter was inserted to relieve complete retention.) Subarachnoid alcohol block was performed. **B,** *Retrograde cystourethrogram, oblique view, after alcohol block* (and conversion of upper motor neuron lesion into lower one). Note difference at bladder outlet. Prostatic urethra is patent, but there remains posterior ledge. Moderate relaxation of external urethral sphincter as compared to "A." Note descent of bladder base. Urinary retention persisted. (Transurethral resection of bladder neck was performed.) **C,** *Cystogram, oblique view,* after resection of bladder neck. Prostatic urethra is wide open but spasticity of external sphincter persists. (Note vesicoureteral reflux on right.) Urinary retention persisted. (By this time patient had acquired bilateral hydronephrosis. Division of external sphincter was performed.) **D,** *Micturition cystourethrogram, anteroposterior view, after division of external sphincter.* Patient reacted to introduction of contrast medium with immediate emptying of bladder, associated with wide opening of all structures at bladder outlet and external urethral sphincter. Note absence of reflux. (Residual urine eliminated. Hydronephrotic changes disappeared almost completely.) (From Damanski, M.)

CONGENITAL

Myelodysplasia; Spina Bifida Occulta; Spina Bifida Cystica; Meningocele; Meningomyelocele; Anomalies of the Sacrum; Agenesis of the Sacrum

Terminology. *Vertebral Defects and Associated Neural Abnormalities. Spina bifida* means a failure of fusion of the laminae of the vertebra. If a cystic lesion appears on the surface of the body, the combination lesion is called *spina bifida cystica*. The lesion may be designated (1) *meningocele*, if the cyst includes only the spinal membranes, (2) *meningomyelocele*, if it includes portions of the meninges and the spinal cord, and (3) *myelocele*, if the cord itself is exposed. Nerve roots also may be included.

Spina bifida occulta is the term used if there is failure of fusion of the lamina but no external swelling or "tumor" over the defect to indicate its presence. The condition may be suspected, however, from thickening or dimpling of the skin, abnormal growth of hair, abnormal pigmentation, or the presence of a lipoma or fibroma. Spina bifida may occur at any level of the spine, but it most often involves the lumbosacral levels. The laminal defect is almost always posterior and is usually filled in by a fibrofatty pad (Williams, 1958), which Campbell (1960) has described as an intramedullary lipoma. Ventral (anterior) spina bifida is rare (Fig. 5–169).

There is no correlation between the type and degree of spina bifida and the incidence or severity of the neurologic defect. For instance, it has been estimated that in routine roentgenographic examinations of the lumbar spine in "normal" adults, some defect in closure of the laminae is apparent in at least one third of cases. Karlin estimated that it is encountered in more than 50% of "normal" children. The defect varies from involvement of only the lower sacral segments ("open neural arch") to wide separation of the lamina of all the sacral and many of the lumbar vertebrae. (See Figs. 3–177 through 3–180.)

In the remainder of this discussion, the general term *myelodysplasia* will be used to include all congenital malformations of the sacral neural axis.

Sacral and Coccygeal Defects. Other types of congenital defects occur either alone or associated with spina bifida. These defects—sacral scoliosis ("twisted" sacrum) and agenesis of part or all of the sacrum—are often overlooked when one is reading urograms, especially of infants and children. (See Figs. 3–181 and 3–182.) *Agenesis of the sacrum* is the general term used when any or all segments of the sacrum are missing. To be classified as "true" sacral agenesis two or more sacral segments should be absent (Williams and Nixon). Sacral agenesis is often associated with anorectal anomalies, such as imperforate anus, anal atresia, rectourethral fisula, and so on (Williams and Nixon). In 1959, Blumel, Evans, and Eggers found approximately 50 cases in the literature and added 8 of their own. They stated that complete absence of the sacrum was found in 32 and partial absence in 18 of the 50 cases reported in the literature. Six of their eight cases had only partial absence of the sacrum. Koontz and Prout recently reported eight more cases.

There is little doubt that the condition is more common than is appreciated, because roentgenologic recognition is difficult owing to poor visualization of the sacrum—especially in children. Missing segments are often interpreted simply as "poor visualization," and even though the radiologist may suspect the lesion, exact interpretation of the x-ray films may be exceedingly difficult.

Cause of Neurologic Defects in Cases of Spina Bifida With Myelodysplasia. The reason for the neurologic disability is the arrested ascent of the spinal cord because of fixation of the cord and its coverings at the site of the laminal defect (anchored conus medullaris). This usually is seen as a confluence of the conus medullaris and intramedullary lipoma with extension into the soft tissues overlying the spina bifida* (Campbell, 1960) (Figs. 5-170 and 5-171). Because of this fixation, the cord is unable to go through the normal "shortening" process that occurs in intra-uterine growth and development. This continues after birth, and as the child grows taller, the traction on the cord may increase. As a matter of fact, this is the explanation given for cases in which symptoms and signs of myelodysplasia do not appear until several years after birth (in some cases as late as puberty, or even later). This situation and the so-called tight filum terminale or tethered-cord syndrome (Campbell, 1960) (Figs. 5-172 and 5-173) also provide the rationale for neurosurgical operations in which the bands and adhesions that are holding the cord are severed and the lipoma is removed. In addition to this mechanical problem, associated anomalous malformations of the cord—such as congenital hydromyelia and diastematomyelia—may be present.

Degree of Disability; Clinical Findings

The degree of disability associated with spina bifida depends on the extent of the defect and the degree of damage and degeneration of the sacral cord and cauda equina. Symptoms and findings in myelodysplasia vary from minimal or nonexistent to extensive and disabling. For instance, visceral innervation *only* may be affected such as that of the rectum and bladder. On the other hand, the lesion may involve the somatic (sensory and motor) nerves, producing various degrees of

anesthesia in the saddle area and over the lower extremities as well as various degrees of flaccid paralysis of the muscles of the legs. In a general way, the vesical dysfunction simulates that associated with an acquired lower motor neuron lesion, except that dribbling passive incontinence from a relaxed external urethral sphincter is much more common. Trabeculation of the bladder may be of extreme degree and there may be ureteropyelectasis and reflux. Incontinence is the most troublesome problem: Some children are totally incontinent and "leak empty," so that the upper urinary tract is protected; others have overflow incontinence and carry large amounts of residual urine which threatens death from renal insufficiency.

Vesical dysfunction associated with myelodysplasia is notoriously erratic and does not adhere to one type as does that in association with acquired lesions. For instance, although one would expect this type of case to simulate an acquired lower motor neuron lesion, often it exhibits mixed characteristics. Williams (1958) suggested three main types of vesical dysfunction as follows: (1) a flaccid thin-walled bladder with no trabeculation in a patient who has no sensation of bladder fullness, (2) a markedly trabeculated bladder with saccules and diverticula, which may be emptied by means of the manual Credé technique, and (3) a trabeculated bladder that simulates that associated with a lesion of the higher centers, such as multiple sclerosis. Patients having the last-mentioned type of bladder retain sensation of bladder fullness and do not have constant passive dribbling; rather, they have an urgency-incontinence pattern.

A study of 53 cases of myelodysplasia (Emmett and Simon) suggested that the crux of the situation was the degree of tonicity remaining in the external urethral sphincter (commonly called *urethral resistance*). If the sphincter was flaccid (see Fig. 5-159), the leakage was "passive" and constant, and the bladder tended to

---

*Normally, the conus medullaris terminates at either the inferior border of the first lumbar vertebra or the superior border of the second. The filum terminale extends on down and anchors at the back of the coccyx. The cul-de-sac of the dura (tube of the dura) ends at the level of the second sacral segment.

leak completely empty; thus, there was no residual urine, no ureteropyelectasis, and no reflux. On the other hand, if the urethral sphincter had been partially spared, residual urine, ureteropyelectasis, and reflux could be substantial. These findings are essentially in agreement with Pellman who, in discussing 61 cases of myelodysplasia, said that there was an "inverse relationship between the severity of the neuromuscular deficit and the degree of vesicoureteral reflux and residual urine." He noted reflux in 30 of his 61 cases.

Unrecognized Myelodysplasia as Cause of Vesical Dysfunction; Congenital Obstruction of the Vesical Neck. There is currently much concern that some cases of unexplained vesical dysfunction may be the result of myelodysplasia or some involvement of the cauda equina even though typical findings of myelodysplasia are absent. For instance, it is becoming more and more apparent that visceral fibers of the cauda equina (that is, those serving the bladder and rectum) may be more susceptible to impairment than are somatic fibers. This has been demonstrated in cases of vesical dysfunction secondary to "asymptomatic" midline protruded lumbar disks, the so-called silent-disk syndrome (Emmett and Love; Love and Emmett). One of us (J.L.E.) and Greene (*Campbell's Urology*, page 1,466) previously suggested the *possibility that some of the so-called congenital obstruction of the vesical neck in infants and children may result from "obscure" myelodysplasia.* At present we are not as convinced of our ability to accurately distinguish myelodysplasia from congenital obstruction as we were a few years ago (Emmett and Simon). Williams (1958) acknowledged that the problem exists by suggesting a method of differentiating the two conditions (if Credé expression will evacuate urine, myelodysplasia is likely; if not, obstruction of the vesical neck should be present). The current tendency to discount urographic and cystoscopic diagnoses of vesical-neck obstruction (Shopfner, 1967c) further supports this

thesis. Also, it is being currently pointed out (Koontz and Prout) that we have been overlooking deformities and partial or total agenesis of the sacrum in the case of many infants and children suffering from the well-known syndrome of distended bladder and extensive ureteropyelectasis, in which the diagnosis of congenital obstruction of the vesical neck has been made (Figs. 5-174, 5-175, and 5-176). This will be considered further on pages 509 through 514.

Urographic Diagnosis of Congenital Neurogenic Bladder

Roentgenographic characteristics of the bony defects in spina bifida and agenesis of the sacrum have already been described (Figs. 5-172 through 5-176).

In congenital neurogenic bladder, *from the urographic standpoint,* the bladder and upper part of the urinary tract tend to resemble those of a patient with an acquired lesion of the spinal cord, which already has been discussed. Trabeculation of the bladder and various degrees of ureteropyelectasis (often with reflux) are the most common findings (Figs. 5-177, 5-178, and 5-179), although an occasional smooth flaccid distended bladder may be seen. The similarity of urograms of children having a diagnosis of congenital obstruction of the vesical neck and of those having myelodysplasia is shown in Figures 5-180 through 5-183. Relaxation of the external urethral sphincter often can be demonstrated in the male by cysto-urethrography (see Fig. 5-159) which resembles the urethrogram of a patient with an acquired upper motor neuron lesion after subarachnoid alcohol block, pudendal neurectomy, or surgical division of the external sphincter to overcome the spasticity (see Figs. 5-162 through 5-168).

Treatment of Congenital Neurogenic Bladder

The most pressing problems from the standpoint of the urologist are (1) incontinence of bladder and bowel and (2) residual urine associated with ureteropyelectasis and ureteral reflux, both of which seriously threaten renal function. As mentioned previously the nub of the situation appears to be the degree of tonicity or flaccidity of the external urethral sphincter (so-called urethral resistance).

Nonoperative. Nonoperative treatment should be used if possible. By means of the manual Credé method of expressing urine, one may evacuate urine fairly completely unless the sphincter has good tone. If passive leakage leaves little or no residual urine, expression will not help. Penile urinals may be useful for boys, but no satisfactory urinal for girls has yet been devised. On the other hand, indwelling urethral catheters are often effective in girls, but they are not tolerated by boys.

Operative. For some boys who have substantial amounts of residual urine, a transurethral resection of the vesical neck may be helpful, although usually some

leakage continues (Emmett and Simon). Exploration or reexploration of the lower part of the cord and of the cauda equina, with release of the conus, removal of adhesions holding nerve roots, and section of the filum terminale (tight-filum, tethered-cord syndrome), results in improvement in some cases (Campbell, 1960).

Urinary diversion by means of an ileal or colonic conduit (Mogg) appears to be the most satisfactory procedure to use in moderate and severe cases. In severe cases, if rectal incontinence is also present, the colonic conduit is preferable, as a permanent colostomy may be established at the same time. Girls benefit dramatically from urinary diversion, as they are changed from pitiful wet odoriferous patients with maceration and excoriations of the vulva, perineum, and buttocks into socially acceptable young women who may marry successfully and complete normal pregnancies with uneventful deliveries.

(Text continued on page 509.)

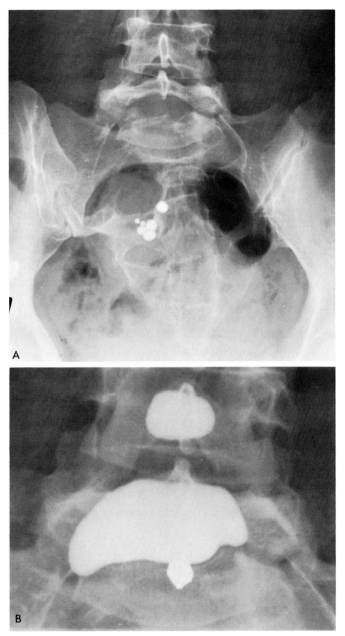

Figure 5–169. Large anterior meningocele. Woman, aged 33, had had bladder dysfunction requiring use of indwelling urethral catheter since age 20. **A,** *Plain film.* Erosion of right half of sacrum from pressure of meningocele. Residual Lipiodol from ancient myelogram. **B,** *Myelogram.* Large meningocele sac partially filled. (Patient's only disability was of bladder; she had normal bowel function and no sensory or motor impairment. Surgical exploration revealed that marked erosion had destroyed anterior wall of sacrum; posterior wall also was eroded and thin. Rectum protruded into sacral canal. Surgical repair was impossible. Note: Pressure over thin eroded portion of posterior wall of sacrum produced headache.)

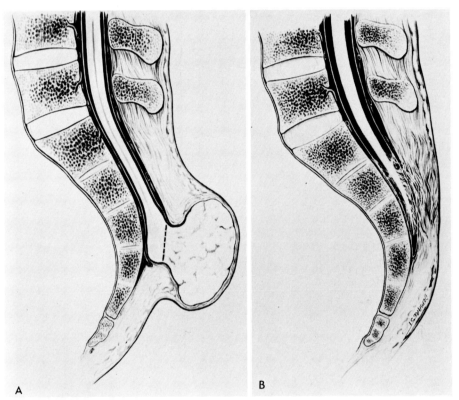

A

B

Figure 5–170.   Representation of arrested ascent of spinal cord in spina bifida. **A,** Confluence of conus medullaris and intramedullary lipoma, with extension into soft tissues overlying spina bifida. (Broken line marks site of amputation of the lipoma.) **B,** Retention of the conus medullaris at a low sacral level as the result of adhesions arising in conjunction with a **meningocele.** (From Campbell, J. B., 1960.)

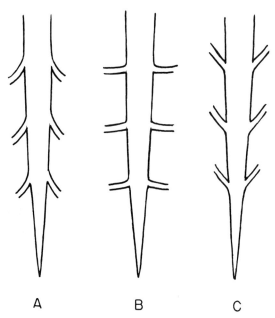

Figure 5–171. Abnormal angles that may be assumed by nerve roots in caudal portion of spinal cord when ascent of conus is prevented by fixation, by adhesions, or by intramedullary lipoma in continuity with overlying soft tissues. (From Campbell, J. B., 1960.)

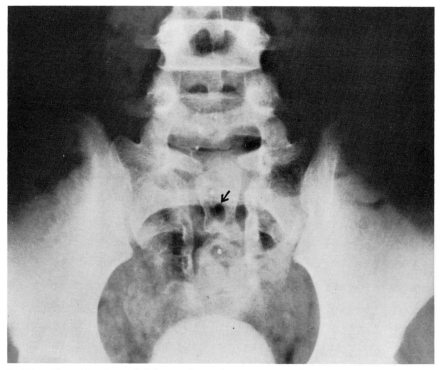

Figure 5–172. *Plain film.* **Spina bifida occulta without meningocele.** (At operation, fibrous strand containing both neural and fibrous tissue ran from conus through dura to hole [*arrow*] in bony plate which probably represents confluence of maldeveloped lamina. This probably represented "tight filum terminale" syndrome.) (From Campbell, J. B., 1960.)

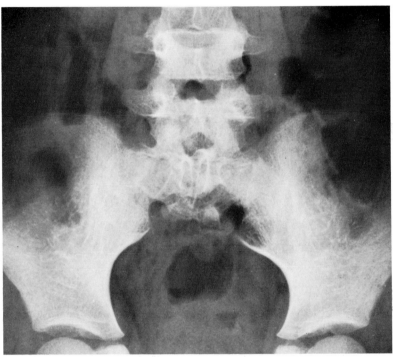

Figure 5–173. *Plain film* of little girl with dysfunction of bladder. **Absence of sacrum and coccyx, without meningocele.** Conus had ascended to level just above bony malformation and cauda equina was funneled through small bony canal. (Decompression of bony canal and removal of abnormal amount of epidural fat restored bladder function.) (From Campbell, J. B., 1960.)

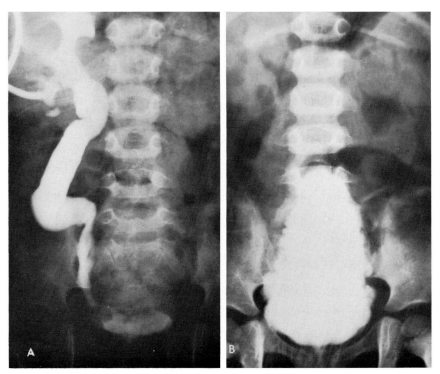

Figure 5–174. Partial absence of sacrum (S4-5 and coccyx) in girl aged 3 years. Unrecognized neurogenic vesical dysfunction. **A,** *Excretory urogram.* Absence of sacral segments 4, 5, and coccyx. Pyeloureterectasis in "solitary" right kidney. (Previous left nephrectomy for infected "hydronephrosis.") **B,** *Retrograde cystogram.* Pine tree shape trabeculated bladder typical of neurogenic dysfunction. (From Koontz, W. W., Jr., and Prout, G. R., Jr.)

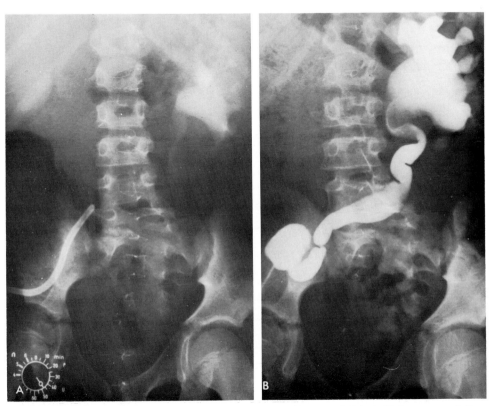

Figure 5–175. Boy aged 14 years with **right renal agenesis. Absence of right half of sacrum and distortion of left half.** Neurogenic vesical dysfunction diagnosed as congenital obstruction of vesical neck. Multiple operations on vesical neck finally culminating in urinary diversion with an ileal conduit. **A,** *Excretory urogram.* Absence of right half of sacrum with distortion of left half. Solitary left kidney. **B,** *Pyelogram* made through ileal conduit. (From Koontz, W. W., Jr., and Prout, G. R., Jr.)

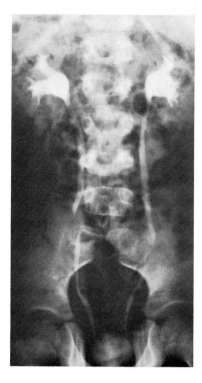

Figure 5–176. Boy aged 4 years with **complete absence of sacrum and coccyx except for hemivertebra of S1.** *Excretory urogram.* Sacral defect as noted. Normal kidneys. Note: Patient has urinary and fecal incontinence, flaccid anal sphincter, and absent ankle jerks bilaterally but no other demonstrable neurologic deficits. (From Koontz, W. W., Jr., and Prout, G. R., Jr.)

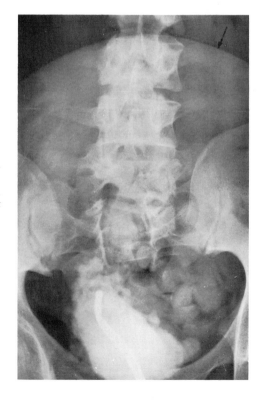

Figure 5–177. *Retrograde cystogram.* Neurogenic bladder from myelodysplasia associated with large meningomyelocele (*arrow*). Pyramid-shaped bladder with cellule formation in boy of 19 years. Note absence of most of sacrum.

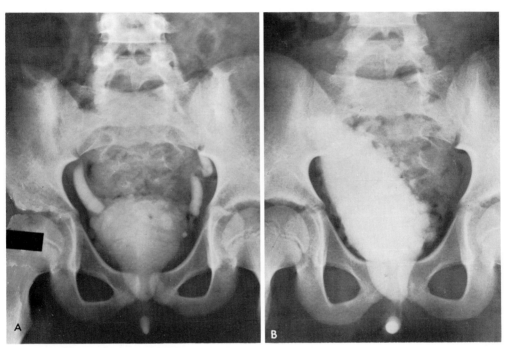

Figure 5–178. Neurogenic bladder resulting from myelodysplasia in boy, aged 9 years. **A,** *Excretory urogram.* Dilatation of lower portions of both ureters. Bladder is trabeculated and has multiple cellules. Prostatic urethra was dilated and filled with medium. Medium also was present in bulbous urethra, indicating urinary incontinence. **B,** *Retrograde cystogram.* Bladder better filled. Typical pyramidal bladder with multiple cellules. Medium is present in bulbous urethra.

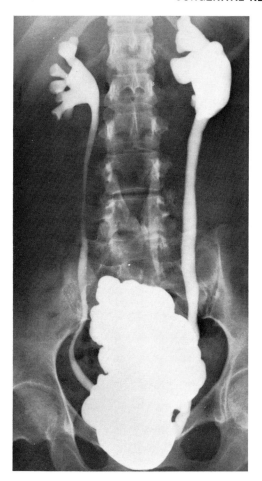

Figure 5–179. *Retrograde cystogram.* Myelodysplasia with neurogenic bladder and bilateral ureteral reflux in case of woman, aged 40. (Laminectomy, at age 12, had been performed to remove relatively asymptomatic meningomyelocele. Bladder dysfunction only since operation which also resulted in somatic sensory nerve damage with trophic ulcers, finally requiring amputation of right leg above knee.)

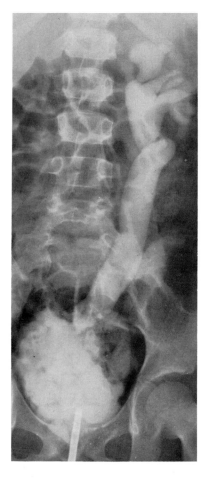

Figure 5–180. *Retrograde cystogram* of 5-year-old girl with myelodysplasia. Marked trabeculation of bladder and left pyeloureterectasis with reflux. (From Emmett, J. L., and Simon, H. B.)

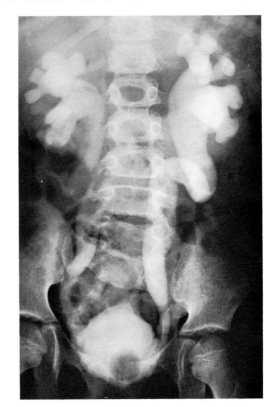

Figure 5–181. *Retrograde cystogram* of 6-year-old girl with myelodysplasia. Minimal trabeculation of bladder with bilateral pyeloureterectasis and reflux. (From Emmett, J. L., and Simon, H. B.)

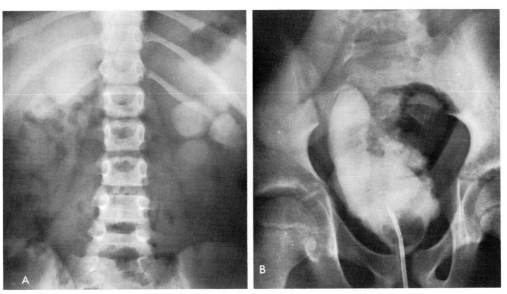

Figure 5–182. Congenital obstruction of vesical neck of boy, aged 8 years. **A,** *Excretory urogram.* Advanced bilateral hydronephrosis. Poor renal function. **B,** *Retrograde cystogram.* Trabeculated bladder with extensive right ureteral reflux. (From Emmett, J. L., and Simon, H. B.)

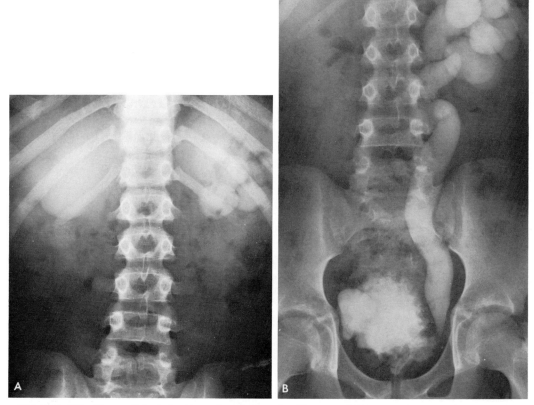

Figure 5–183.   Congenital obstruction of vesical neck of boy, aged 13 years. **A,** *Excretory urogram.* Bilateral hydronephrosis. Poor renal function. **B,** *Retrograde cystogram.* Markedly trabeculated bladder with left ureteropyelectasis and reflux. (From Emmett, J. L., and Simon, H. B.)

Congenital Obstruction of the Vesical Neck; Distal Urethral Obstruction; Stenosis of the Urethral Meatus

These lesions comprise a poorly understood clinical complex that includes a great proportion of all pediatric urologic problems and spills over into adult urology. Also, it covers a wide range of morbidity and disability—from that of the infant born with advanced renal insufficiency from extensive bilateral hydronephrosis, hydroureter, distended bladder, and vesicoureteral reflux to that of the little girl with only a mild persistent or recurring urinary infection, with little or no residual urine, with or without ureteral reflux, and with or without ureteropyelectasis.

During the last 2 or 3 decades many theories have been advanced and discarded; authorities in the field have taken positions only to abandon them later; clinical and urographic data previously considered to be important and on a firm foundation have had to be discarded; and today the problem is still far from being solved. Current opinion which we will document here may appear ridiculous 5 or 10 years from now.

CONGENITAL OBSTRUCTION OF THE VESICAL NECK

The clinical picture which first comes to mind with the diagnosis of "congenital obstruction of the vesical neck" is the newborn infant or child with urinary stasis that includes a distended bladder, greatly dilated ureters and renal pelves, and usually ureteral reflux and extensive renal damage that threaten death from renal insufficiency (Fig. 5-184). This condition may be definitely obstructive from some bona fide obstructive lesion, such as congenital posterior urethral valves in little boys. In many cases, however, no definite obstruction can be found and for want of a better term the syndrome has been called *congenital obstruction of the vesical neck* (Figs. 5-185 through 5-188). Cystoscopic and urethrographic diagnosis of this syndrome is now being seriously challenged (see pages 511 through 513). Surgical procedures to correct the "obstruction" have been of some help, but certainly not brilliant. Resort to permanent urinary diversion has only too often been the only solution.

Differential Diagnosis From Neurogenic Bladder of Myelodysplasia

For years there has been an uneasiness among urologists that this condition may be of neurogenic origin rather than obstructive. Certainly the two conditions share many similarities, and differentiation can be made only by demonstrating *somatic* neurologic deficits with their attending special disabilities. In the discussion of myelodysplasia this problem was raised. Surgical procedures on the vesical neck have been used with varying degrees of success for both disorders (Burns and Kittredge; Emmett and Helmholz; Emmett and Simon).

In 1956, one of us (J.L.E.) and Simon called attention to the similarities present in the two conditions but expressed the opinion that clinically the differentiation had not proved too difficult. To support this stand a table was prepared comparing the incidence of symptoms and findings in 105 cases diagnosed as congenital obstruction and 53 cases diagnosed as myelodysplasia. This table is reproduced here (Table 5-1).

When grossly demonstrable neurologic deficits are present, the problem is relatively easy. In the absence of such findings, however, one wonders if neurologic deficits involving the bladder *only* may be still present and not evident on routine neurologic examination. Our recent experience with vesical dysfunction and retention caused by "asymptomatic" midline protruded lumbar disks has

Table 5–1. **Comparative Incidence of Symptoms and Findings in Myelodysplasia and Congenital Obstruction of the Vesical Neck**[*]

SYMPTOMS AND FINDINGS	MYELODYSPLASIA (53 PATIENTS)	CONGENITAL OBSTRUCTION VESICAL NECK (105 PATIENTS)
Fecal incontinence	About ½	None
Urinary incontinence (day and night)	Almost all	Less than ⅓ (30)
Enuresis only	Almost none	¼
Residual urine		
Less than 30 cc	Almost none (3)	⅓ (30)
30-99 cc	⅓ (16)	⅕ (20)
100 cc or more	More than ½ (32)	Less than ½ (48)
Infected urine	85 per cent	85 per cent
"Recurring infection"	Less than ½ (21)	¾ (76)
"Obstructive" symptoms; poor stream, difficulty in voiding	⅕	⅕
Increase of blood urea	¼ (13)	⅓ (32)
Gastrointestinal symptoms only (from azotemia)	None	7
Pyelo-ureterectasis	⅗[†]	⅘[†]
Trabeculation of bladder	⅘	½

[*]From Emmett, J. L., and Simon, H. B.
[†]These represent the proportion of patients on whom satisfactory urographic studies were available.

further increased our suspicions (Emmett and Love; Love and Emmett). At the present writing we have a series of 35 such cases and wonder if the *visceral fibers* of the cauda equina which serve the bladder may be more susceptible to damage by mild degrees of pressure, stretching, and so on than are the *somatic* sensory and motor fibers.

EVALUATION OF THE VESICAL NECK

Cystoscopic

The cystoscopic diagnosis of vesical-neck obstruction in infants and children has never been an accurate procedure. The occasional marked obstruction in a boy may be easily identified, but the great majority of cases fall into the category of minor degrees of obstruction (Bodian). Thus, the cystoscopist describes such situations as a "collar" at the vesical neck with a depressed "gutter" between the vesical neck and the verumontanum. Or, he may mention that the trigone is not visible with the Foroblique lens at the

level of the verumontanum. In girls such situations as "spastic collar" or "thickening" or "hypertrophy" of the vesical neck are mentioned. All expert cystoscopists realize that these findings depend a good deal on the activity of the detrusor muscle at the time of the examination. The vesical neck is simply a part of the detrusor muscle. If the detrusor muscle contracts, the vesical neck will contract.

Most workers experienced in pediatric cystoscopy are quick to admit that only too often findings are equivocal; one cannot be sure that obstruction actually exists, and, if it does, to what degree. It is common knowledge that even experienced cystoscopists may not agree on a cystoscopic evaluation of a bladder neck. Some of the most obstructive-appearing vesical necks that I (J.L.E.) have ever seen cystoscopically in children and women have been in "normal" patients who had no vesical dysfunction. In discussing endoscopy for this condition, Kjellberg, Ericsson, and Rudhe stated, "A differential diagnosis between pure bladder neck obstruction and such caused by a urethral valve or neurogenic disturbance cannot be based on the appearance of the bladder neck."

Urographic

Because of the inaccuracy of cystoscopic appraisal of the vesical neck, various types of urographic procedures have been suggested.

Scandinavian roentgenologists were the first to advocate and employ *voiding cystourethrography* to study the vesical neck (Jorup and Kjellberg; Kjellberg, Ericsson, and Rudhe). Kjellberg, Ericsson, and Rudhe described congenital obstruction of the vesical neck as a "defective opening of the bladder neck on micturition" that may appear urographically either to *encircle the bladder neck* or to present only as an *inward bulging of the posterior aspect of the vesical neck* (like a median bar in an adult; Figs. 5–189 through 5–193). Waterhouse; Griesbach, Waterhouse, and Mellins; and Hamm and Waterhouse have questioned the validity of such urographic alterations of the vesical neck because they believe these may represent simply physiologic variations in the contractions of the trigonal region and sphincteric mechanisms during micturition, which are apparent only on instantaneous roentgenograms (see Figs. 4–192 and 4–193). Lich, Howerton, and Davis (1960), using an image intensifier and making multiple exposures during micturition of contrast medium (voiding cystourethrography), demonstrated in girls what they considered to be vesical-neck obstruction. They described this as a ring-like constriction at the vesical neck associated with a tapering dilatation or "acorn" deformity of the urethra (Fig. 5–194A, B, and C). They attributed the urethral widening to "poststenotic" dilatation as has been described in partial arterial obstruction. They also pointed out that to demonstrate this deformity the film must be exposed at the right instant, preferably at the height of voiding when a forceful stream is being ejected. Almost

simultaneously Williams and Sturdy described the same deformity. To them it resembled a "spinning top" (Fig. 5–195). They explained the urethral dilatation distal to the vesical neck as the "result of a powerful stream of urine which distends a poorly supported thin-walled urethra." Since then several investigators have demonstrated similar findings (Figs. 5–196 through 5–199).

Criticism of these concepts arose from those who wondered if the ring-like constriction might represent simply the normal contraction of the detrusor muscle, the part of detrusor around the vesical neck taking part in the contractile effort as does the fundus of the bladder (Fig. 5–200). Williams (writing with Sturdy in 1961), however, became convinced of the importance of this examination; whereas in 1959 he was critical of urologists resecting vesical necks on the seemingly inadequate indication that they "looked obstructive" cystoscopically. He and Sturdy reported favorable results with Y-V plasty procedures on the vesical necks of a substantial number of little girls with recurring urinary infection; the voiding cystourethrogram played a major role in the diagnosis of obstruction of the vesical neck, which they stated they were able to confirm visually at operation when the bladder was opened. Interpretation of the "acorn" or "spinning top" deformity was further questioned when interested workers began using it as an example of the result of distal *urethral stenosis*.

DISTAL URETHRAL STENOSIS

In 1963, Lyon and Smith and, in 1965, Lyon and Tanagho published their work on distal urethral stenosis which added another factor and concept that required a complete reevaluation of the overall problem. They demonstrated by anatomic dissections that the muscular components of the female urethra (inner longitudinal layer and outer circular layer which are continuations of the detrusor muscle at the vesical neck) end sharply at the juncture of the middle and distal thirds of the urethra by inserting into dense collagenous tissue. They also found that, in little girls with persistent urinary infection, the nonmuscular distal segment of the urethra appeared to impede urinary flow. Calibration showed it to vary from size 14 to 26 F. When this "ring" was "ruptured" by forcibly dilating it to at least size 32 F, infection was eliminated in a substantial number of cases; also, reflux was eliminated in 30% of the cases and decreased in severity in another 25%. Subsequently, other workers have used internal urethrotomy with the Otis urethrotome instead of dilatation; Richardson (1968) has used "external urethroplasty."

Although there have been criticisms of this new concept,* at the time of this writing (November 1969) many workers have confirmed the work of Lyon and his co-workers (1963; 1965) and find it applicable not only in little girls but also in adult women (Kerr, Leadbetter, and Donahue; McLean and Emmett; Richardson, 1968). Although calibration of the urethra with Otis bulbs (bougie à boule) is the procedure of choice, it was suggested that the voiding cystourethrogram might also be of help in detecting stenosis of the distal urethral segment. It was further suggested that the distal stenosis might account for the dilatation of the urethra seen in the "acorn" or "spinning top" cystourethrograms. As a matter of fact, illustrations appeared in the literature, which showed such deformities eliminated after *either* operation on the vesical neck (transurethral resection or Y-V plasty) *or* internal urethrotomy (or overdilatation) to eliminate distal urethral stenosis (so-called Lyon's ring).

In a meticulous and painstaking investigation of voiding cystourethrograms of a large number of children, Shopfner (1967a) recently has startled the profession by showing that urographic deformities which have been considered pathognomonic for either vesical-neck obstruction or distal urethral stenosis mean nothing and are of no diagnostic value in either condition.

In a communication regarding the **roentgenographic evaluation of bladder-neck obstruction**, Shopfner (1967c) pointed out that the diameter of the vesical neck and of the various parts of the urethra varies in relation to the stages of voiding. He believes it axiomatic that *to be considered contracted and obstructive a bladder neck must be smaller than any of the normally constricted points of the urethra*; that is, it must be smaller than the urethral meatus, penoscrotal junction, and membranous urethra in the male and the distal urethra and urethral meatus in the female. If urethrograms are considered in this light, the bladder neck is almost never obstructive (Fig. 5–201A through F). Furthermore, he contends that the urethral widening seen in the "spinning top" deformity is present in normal children and is a result of forceful passage of a large volume of urine which distends and widens the thin-walled urethra.

Shopfner (1967c) also thinks that segmental irregularities seen in the bladder neck should not be interpreted as anterior or posterior "obstructive ledges," "lips," or "notches" that require surgical removal as suggested by Kjellberg, Ericsson, and Rudhe. He contends that these are also present in normal persons, and he considers them variations of the trigonal plates which make up the trigonal canal. (See the new concept of physiology of micturition [Hutch, 1965; Shopfner and Hutch].) The interested reader is advised to read all of these articles carefully.

The concept of **urographic visualization of distal urethral stenosis** fares no better in Shopfner's hands (1967a). Again he points out that the variations in diameter and contour of the urethra are only ex-

---

*One of the chief objections has to do with calibration of the "normal" urethra in little girls. Immergut, Culp, and Flocks found it to be as follows: from 0 to 4 years, size 14 to 15 F; from 5 to 9 years, 16 to 17 F; from 10 to 14 years, 21 to 22 F; and from 15 to 20 years, 26 F.

pressions of the *volume* and *rate* of urinary flow during voiding (Fig. 5–202*A* through *F*). In Shopfner's opinion calibration of the urethra with diagnostic bulbs is required for accurate diagnosis. Bona fide organic stenosis of the urethral meatus should demonstrate dilatation of the urethra proximal to the narrow obstructive meatus in all films regardless of the "stage" of voiding (see Figs. 5–229 and 5–230).

RELATION OF OUTLET OBSTRUCTION AND URETERAL REFLUX; INCIDENCE OF OBSTRUCTION

The pendulum is swinging away from the concept of obstruction. Whereas a decade or two ago almost all urinary problems in children were considered to have at least some obstructive aspects, this is no longer the case. For instance, in at least half of the children diagnosed as having either myelodysplasia or congenital obstruction of the vesical neck, vesicoureteral reflux can be demonstrated, and reflux is being incriminated in such conditions as obstruction of the ureteropelvic junction, atrophic pyelonephritis, and pyelonephritis of pregnancy. More and more emphasis is being placed on methods of demonstrating reflux and methods of determining if reflux is "primary" or "secondary." Controversy still rages over such questions as, Does infection cause reflux or reflux cause infection, does reflux per se cause renal deterioration, or does the deterioration result from secondary infection?

Out of all this controversy has come the realizations that (1) reflux is much more common than appreciated and (2) elimination of reflux is an important factor in eliminating urinary infection. *The unresolved problem at the moment is the role of the vesical neck and urethra in the problem of reflux.* This is further abetted by the fact that cystoscopic and urographic evaluation of the vesical neck and urethra is now considered to be unreliable. The problem is especially critical in cases in which there is little or no residual urine to support the thesis of obstruction. It has become even more important as a result of the development, during the past decade, of efficient antireflux operations on the ureterovesical junction (ureteroneocystostomies) (see page 471). The urologist is constantly confronted with the question, "Shall I do a ureteroneocystostomy only or shall I perform a revision of the vesical neck at the same time?"

Harrow, Sloane, and Witus in a comprehensive evaluation of this subject came to the conclusion that bladder-neck obstruction in children is rare and that transurethral resection and Y-V plasty of the vesical neck are rarely indicated. They advocated that the criteria for bladder-outlet obstruction in adults should be applied to children—that is, restriction and intermittency of the urinary stream, trabeculation of the bladder, and presence of saccules and diverticula in the bladder, plus residual urine. In their excellent review of the current literature on the subject, they listed authors who still favor the concept of obstruction of the vesical neck and those who now believe it is relatively uncommon. In a review of the records of 217 children with recurring urinary infection on their pediatric hospital service, they found that only three patients proved to have bona fide congenital vesical-neck obstruction which required surgical treatment. These authors also think that determinations of vesical and urethral pressures during micturition (Gleason and Lattimer; Smith; Smith, Edwards, and Bryant) are "unreliable and capricious."

Of 26 patients with reflux treated with ureteroneocystostomy (Politano-Leadbetter technique), 24 (92%) were "cured." The vesical neck was not operated on in any case. Harrow, Sloane, and Witus think that operations on the vesical neck in children are not only ineffective and unnecessary but actually may be harmful in later life because of sterility in the male (retrograde ejaculation) and widening of the urethra in the female, which can increase susceptibility to infection.

Williams and Eckstein (1965a; 1965b) appear to be coming to similar conclusions. They now agree that bladder-neck obstruction (especially in girls) cannot be demonstrated urographically with cystourethrograms and that one must rely on such findings as residual urine, trabeculation of the bladder, and calibration of the urethra with diagnostic bulbs (to detect distal urethral stenosis). They think that in a few cases involving boys one can be certain of vesical-neck obstruction, but that in most cases doubt remains. However, they still maintain that they can be reasonably certain of the presence or absence of such obstruction by visual examination of the bladder neck when the bladder is open for ureteroneocystostomy, and they make the decision at that time to revise the vesical neck or not. In their series of 165 cases of ureteroneocystostomy done for reflux, in which follow-up studies were available, revision of the bladder neck was done also in 76 cases (52%); but they stated that "this procedure made no difference to the incidence of successful prevention of reflux." Excellent results were obtained in 86% of cases. In only 13 cases was vesical neck revision done alone, without ureteroneocystostomy. In four of these cases, reflux persisted.

Howerton and Lich who originally described the "acorn" deformity in the cystourethrogram also appear to be changing their opinion of the importance of vesical-neck obstruction. Reflux was demonstrated in 130 (23.3%) of 558 cases in which voiding cystourethrograms were made. Revision of the vesical neck *only* was done in 12 cases, and reflux was eliminated in only 4 of these. They said that this was not as effective as conservative treatment with drugs and antibiotics.

MANAGEMENT

Treatment remains highly controversial; however, a few broad statements may be appropriate. First, a trial of conservative treatment for a period of 6 to 12 months should be carried out. This should include the administration of antibiotics and other drugs to eradicate urinary infection. Double and triple voiding techniques should also be tried. Also, during this period, one should use urethral calibration and overdilatation or internal urethrotomy to detect and eliminate possible stenosis of the distal urethral segment (Lyon's ring). If these procedures are ineffective and urinary infection and ureteral reflux persist, antireflux operations on the ureterovesical junction (ureteroneocystostomy) are indicated. Unless bona fide obstruction of the vesical neck can be demonstrated, it would seem that surgical revision of the vesical neck at the same time is not indicated. However, I suspect that, at least until more information is available, most operators will choose to include a revision of the vesical neck as part of the operative procedure— assuming that if any vesical-neck obstruction is present, it will be taken care of; if not, no great harm is likely to be done.

(*Text continued on page 526.*)

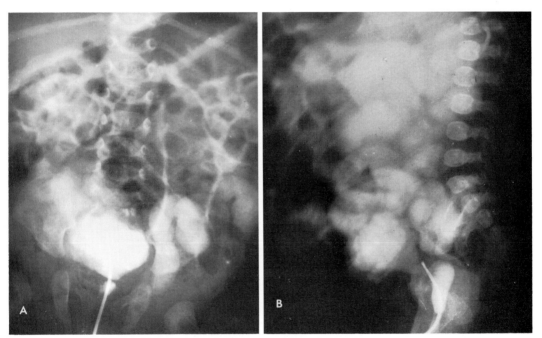

Figure 5–184.   Advanced hydronephrosis and hydroureter with renal insufficiency. Etiology considered to be either congenital obstruction of vesical neck or congenital urethral stricture. *Retrograde cystograms of baby boy, aged 7 weeks.* **A,** *Anteroposterior view.* **B,** *Lateral view.*

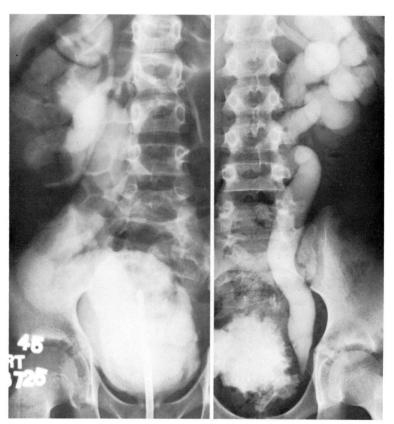

Fig. 5–185   Fig. 5–186

Figure 5–185. *Retrograde cystogram.* Advanced unilateral ureterectasis with reflux associated with congenital obstruction of vesical neck of boy, 8 years of age.

Figure 5–186. *Retrograde cystogram.* Unilateral ureterectasis with reflux associated with congenital obstruction of vesical neck of boy, 10 years of age.

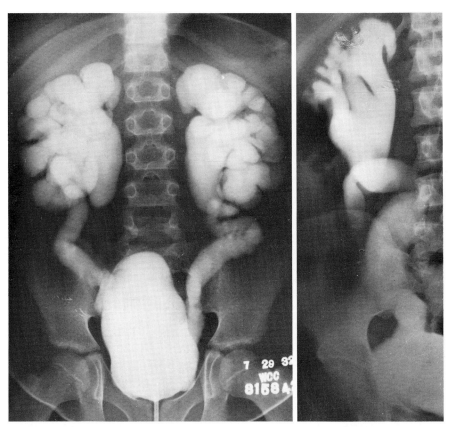

Fig. 5–187   Fig. 5–188

Figure 5–187. *Retrograde cystogram.* Advanced bilateral ureteropyelectasis with reflux associated with congenital obstruction of vesical neck of boy, 12 years of age. Upper and lower parts of urinary tract constitute almost one common continuous reservoir for urine.

Figure 5–188. *Retrograde cystogram.* Marked reflux up right ureter, outlining hugely dilated ureter. Atrophic type of kidney, with pyelocaliectasis of moderate degree.

Fig. 5–189   Fig. 5–190

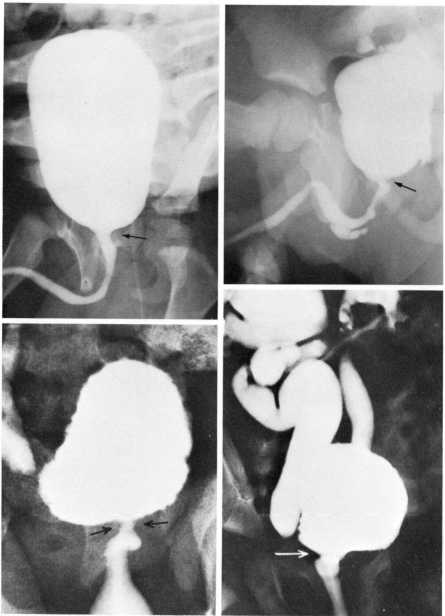

Fig. 5–191   Fig. 5–192

Figure 5–189. *Expression cystourethrogram* of boy, 1 year of age, with palpable bladder and 200 ml of residual urine. **Posterior commissural indentation at vesical neck** (*arrow*), thought clinically to be obstructing. Confirmed by cystoscopy. (Obstruction relieved by Y-V plasty on vesical neck.)

Figure 5–190. *Expression cystourethrogram* (made under general anesthesia) of boy, 4 years of age. **Congenital obstruction of vesical neck with definite median-bar type of obstruction** (*arrow*) which was proved cystoscopically. False passage in bulbous urethra resulted from recent instrumentation. Large vesical diverticulum is obscured by vesical outline.

Figure 5–191. *Voiding cystourethrogram* of girl, 18 months of age. **"Circular bladder-neck obstruction"** (*arrows*) **with right ureteral reflux.** (From Kjellberg, S. A., Ericsson, N. D., and Rudhe, U.)

Figure 5–192. *Voiding cystourethrogram* of male infant, 3 weeks of age. **"Circular bladder-neck obstruction"** (*arrow*) **with bilateral ureteropyelectasis and reflux.** (From Kjellberg, S. A., Ericsson, N. D., and Rudhe, U.)

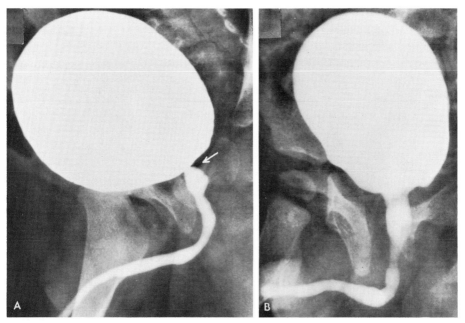

Figure 5–193. Operative relief of obstruction of vesical neck. *Voiding cystourethrograms* of boy, 7 months of age. **A,** *Preoperative.* Note inward bulging of posterior vesical lip (*arrow*). **B,** *After transurethral resection.* (From Kjellberg, S. A., Ericsson, N. D., and Rudhe, U.)

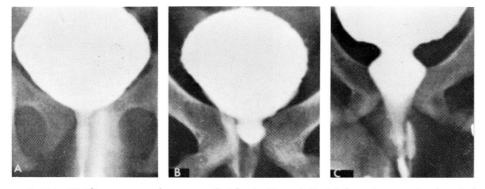

Figure 5–194. *Voiding cystourethrograms* of girls. **A, Normal. B, Moderately constricted vesical neck due to hyperplasia of bladder outlet.** Mild trabeculation. Dilatation of urethra distal to vesical neck ("**acorn deformity**") interpreted as "**poststenotic**" **dilatation. C, More advanced obstruction of vesical neck,** with acorn deformity from poststenotic dilatation. (From Lich, R., Jr., Howerton, L. W., and Davis, L. A.)

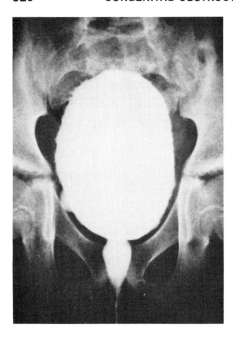

Figure 5–195. *Voiding cystourethrogram* of girl, 7 years of age. Trabeculation of bladder, saccule on right side of bladder, and "spinning top" deformity of vesical neck and urethra, considered to represent congenital obstruction of vesical neck. (From Williams, D. I., and Sturdy, D. E.)

Figure 5–196. *Voiding cystourethrogram* of girl, aged 6½. "Acorn" or "spinning top" contour of bladder neck and urethra interpreted as representing contracture of bladder neck and poststenotic dilatation of urethra. (From Gould, H. R., and Peterson, C. G., Jr.)

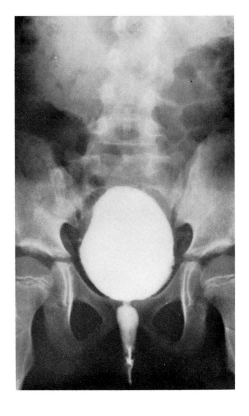

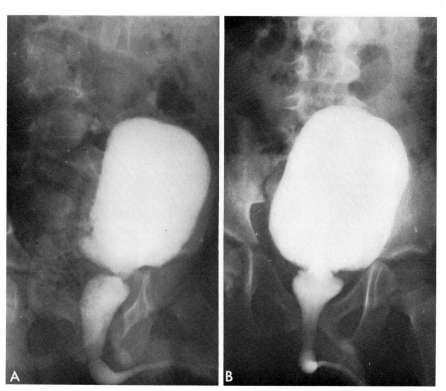

Figure 5–197. Narrowing at bladder neck interpreted as representing marked contracture of bladder neck (mainly posterior). *Voiding cystourethrograms* of boy, aged 8. **A,** *Preoperative.* **B,** *After transurethral resection.* Lumen at vesical neck has increased in diameter. (From Gould, H. R., and Peterson, C. G., Jr.)

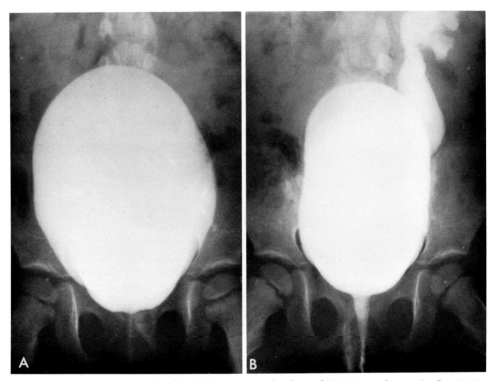

Figure 5–198. Demonstration of reflux. **A**, *Cystogram* of girl, aged 3½. No evidence of reflux. **B**, *Voiding cystourethrogram.* **Marked reflux up dilated left ureter.** Bladder neck and urethra appear as normal. (From Gould, H. R., and Peterson, C. G., Jr.)

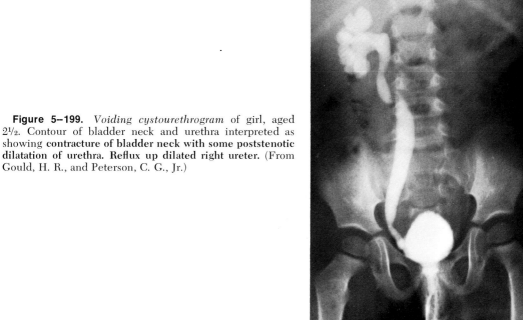

Figure 5–199. *Voiding cystourethrogram* of girl, aged 2½. Contour of bladder neck and urethra interpreted as showing **contracture of bladder neck with some poststenotic dilatation of urethra. Reflux up dilated right ureter.** (From Gould, H. R., and Peterson, C. G., Jr.)

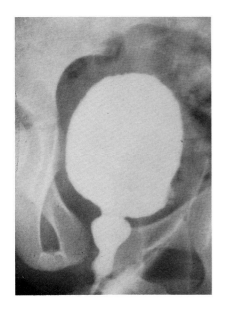

Figure 5–200. *Voiding cystourethrogram.* "Acorn" or "spinning top" deformity of vesical neck and urethra of girl, 14 years of age. No residual urine. Negative cystoscopic examination.

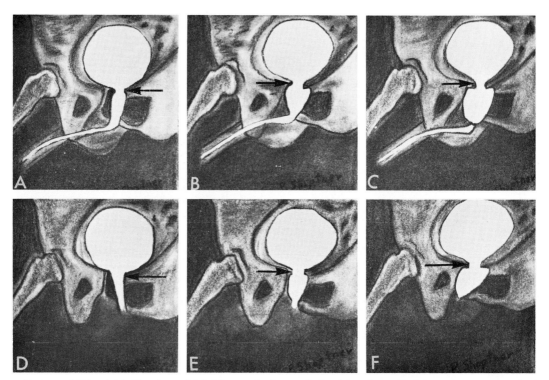

Figure 5–201. A-F, Sketches of bladder neck show relationship of so-called contracture to urethral caliber. **A-C**, Male urethra. **D-F**, Female urethra. Diameter of bladder neck is actually same in all; degree of apparent "contracture" appears to increase as urethra is distended and becomes wider. (*Arrows* indicate bladder neck.) (From Shopfner, C. E., 1967c.)

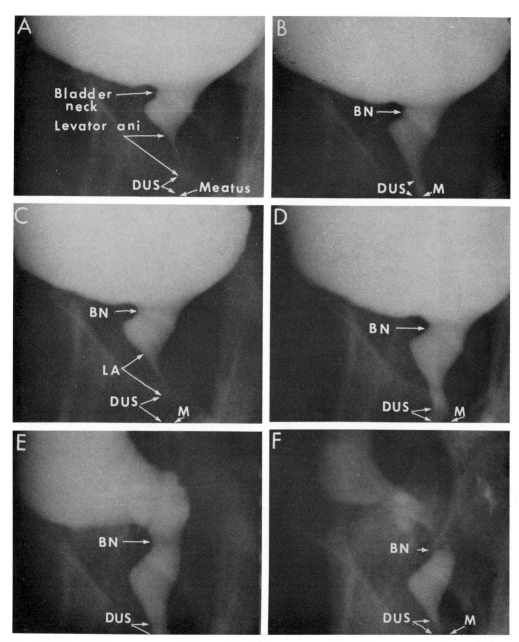

Figure 5–202. Voiding sequence of 10-year-old girl **demonstrates effect of constrictor urethrae contraction and volume and velocity of flow on width of distal urethral segment (DUS). A,** Voiding has just started, and urethral flow is not fully established. **B,** Urethral flow has been fully established, and DUS is wide. **C,** Voluntary contraction of constrictor urethrae muscle has caused interruption of urethral flow and produced same appearance as in A. Tapering of urethra above DUS is due to simultaneous contraction of levator ani muscle (external sphincter). **D** and **E,** Voiding is again fully established with DUS maximally distended. **F,** Volume and velocity of urethral flow have decreased during late phase of voiding and have resulted in narrowing of DUS. Tapering of urethra in **A, C,** and **F** could be erroneously interpreted as stenosis without proper identification of meatus and sequential filming. (From Shopfner, C. E., 1967a.)

Congenital Urethral Valves

CONGENITAL VALVES IN THE MALE URETHRA

Posterior Urethral Valves

Congenital urethral valves occur almost exclusively in the male. They have been the most poorly diagnosed lesions in pediatric urology. Urographic diagnosis has been inaccurate because in most cases only *retrograde* cystourethrograms have been used, and the valves are not obstructive to the retrograde flow of fluid. For the same reason, endoscopic diagnosis is also inaccurate. One type of endoscopic error has been "overdiagnosis," urethral valves being diagnosed when they were not present because small folds of urethral mucosa (greatly magnified by small-lens cystoscopes) have been misinterpreted. Small mucosal folds in the floor of the urethra, running from the verumontanum or crista urethralis proximally to the vesical neck and distally to the membranous urethra (plica colliculi), are normal findings. A second error, of course, has been "underdiagnosis," urethral valves not being recognized. Even the experienced pediatric endoscopist has difficulty identifying true valves. The retrograde flow of water from the cystoscope collapses the valves against the walls of the urethra so that they cannot be seen. Also, small instruments with lens magnification provide inadequate and distorted views which are difficult to evaluate.

In the classic paper on the subject of urethral valves by Young, Frontz, and Baldwin in 1919, three types of valves were described (Fig. 5–203). A most lucid anatomic description of these three types of posterior urethral valves by Ellis, Fonkalsrud, and Smith follows (italics and boldface added):

Posterior urethral valves are thin, membranous structures in the male posterior urethra. Although numerous variations have been described, the anatomical classification of Young is generally accepted. **Type 1**, the most common, usually consists of two *thin, cusp-like membranes that are attached to the verumontanum proximally, sometimes being fused at this point and, coursing distally, diverge from one another to be attached to the respective lateral urethral wall proximal to the external sphincter.* Laterally the entire leaflet is attached to the urethral wall, whereas medially a free edge remains. The urethral lumen between the valve leaflets is dorsally located. **Type 2** is similar but originates from the proximal end of the verumontanum and courses toward the bladder neck. This is the least common type mentioned by Young, who only described 1 case. Stephens states that Young's description may have been made from endoscopic findings and not confirmed radiographically. One case of this type was encountered early in our series. *Some surgeons who have had considerable experience with posterior urethral valves have never encountered type 2.* **Type 3** consists of diaphragms, usually with central openings which occur at, above or below the verumontanum. The aperture in the diaphragm may be centrally or eccentrally placed, or the diaphragm may be incomplete peripherally. Except for one early case, all valves encountered in our series were type 1. The basic pathology of all valves is obstruction that causes proximal urinary tract dilation and damage. *In general the damage has been most severe in type 1.*

From the standpoint of etiology, Williams and Eckstein (1965a) said the lesions "are clearly an exaggeration [sic] of the normal ridges of mucous membrane which extend from the verumontanum or from the midline dorsal ridge of the urethra,* downwards and laterally almost to surround the urethra a little above the membranous region."

The Clinical Problem. Congenital posterior urethral valves may be the cause of some of the most obstructive uropathies of infants and children. They are commonly encountered at birth, the kidneys being almost destroyed from advanced hydronephrosis and hydroureter. Paradoxically, at birth the infant may appear to be in good general condition and may have a relatively normal level of blood urea, because during fetal life the waste products

---

*Crista urethralis.

of metabolism were eliminated by the placental circulation. His condition then rapidly deteriorates and the level of urea rises.

Of Williams and Eckstein's 104 patients, the majority presented in the first year of life—one half within the first 3 months. Of Ellis, Fonkalsrud, and Smith's 29 patients (from Children's Hospital, Columbus, Ohio), 8 were seen on the first day of life, 17 were seen within the first 4 weeks of life, and 12 were seen between the ages of 1 and 8 years. On the other hand, of Nesbit and Labardini's 51 patients (Ann Arbor, Michigan) only 5 were less than 1 year of age; 7 were 10 years old or older. Our experience with this condition at the Mayo Clinic has likewise been limited, and many of our cases have been in older children. The differences in experience are not difficult to explain. Most patients present at birth, when they already have serious disease. They die rapidly unless prompt diagnosis is made and unless adequate treatment exists and is available. Patients with serious trouble do not live long enough to be taken long distances to large clinical centers for diagnosis and treatment. Large population centers are necessary to provide pediatric urologic services with clinical material of such relatively rare conditions. Affected patients who reach early or late childhood before treatment becomes imperative have relatively mild obstruction.

As is the case in all types of urinary obstruction in infants and children, presenting symptoms may be urinary or systemic (that is, vomiting from azotemia, failure to thrive, and so on), and the physical findings may include palpation of the bladder or kidneys. The presenting signs and symptoms vary according to the age of the patient as indicated in Table 5-2 which shows the modes of presentation in Williams and Eckstein's series of 104 cases from the Hospital for Sick Children in London, England.

An infant with extensive renal damage and azotemia usually requires immediate

Table 5-2. **Presenting Symptoms and Signs in 104 Infants and Children With Congenital Posterior Urethral Valves Correlated With Age of Child**[*]

	< 3-MOS.-OLD	> 3-MOS.-OLD	TOTAL
Failure to thrive	15	4	19
Vomiting	8	5	13
Palpable kidney or bladder	14	1	15
Recurrent infections	2	19	21
Retention of urine	6	6	12
"Enuresis"	–	3	3
Incontinence	–	9	9
Abdominal pain	–	4	4
Hematuria	–	2	2
Incidental (palp. bladder)	–	1	1
Ascites	1	–	1
Abdominal distension	1	–	1
Frequency	–	1	1
Difficulty (micturition)	–	1	1
Pain in legs (rickets)	–	1	1

[*]From Williams, D. I., and Eckstein, H. B., 1965a.

life-saving urinary diversion either by ureterostomy or nephrostomy (Ellis, Fonkalsrud, and Smith; Williams and Eckstein). Definitive surgical attack on the valves can be delayed until the patient's general condition has improved. Williams and Eckstein think preliminary suprapubic cystostomy may be sufficient for the child but not for the infant. In the case of a child without extensive damage of the upper urinary tract and with adequate renal function, primary surgical removal of the valve (usually done transurethrally) may be considered.

Urographic Diagnosis; Voiding Cystourethrograms. Interest in voiding or expression cystourethrography to demonstrate urethral valves began with the study of Jorup and Kjellberg in 1948. Since that time many reports of urethral valves demonstrated by this method have appeared (Fisher and Forsythe; Griesbach, Waterhouse, and Mellins; Hamm and Waterhouse; Raper; Williams and Sturdy). The urographic deformity consists of a bulging dilatation of the prostatic urethra which is sharply demarcated from the narrow distal urethra; the prostatic urethra also appears to bulge forward over the bulbous urethra. The deformity is quite characteristic and is not difficult to recognize after several have been seen (Figs. 5-204 through 5-214). In addition to the characteristic "bulge," negative defects from the valves themselves may be recognized. Kjellberg, Ericsson, and Rudhe have emphasized this aspect of the urethrogram (Figs. 5-215 through 5-219), but generally it is not considered to be especially important. Another fairly commonly associated finding is the apparent "ring-like" constriction of the vesical neck which is now thought to be of no clinical significance. It probably represents a thickened detrusor muscle which has become hypertrophied by repeated forceful contraction to force urine past the valvular obstruction. Experience has shown that if the valves are adequately removed, urinary obstruction is relieved and revision of the vesical neck is unnecessary.

The valves that seem to be the most obstructive are those that arise from the lower (distal) border of the verumontanum.

Kjellberg, Ericsson, and Rudhe emphasized the importance of anterior fusion of the urethral valves. They found that valves situated principally in the ventral half (roof) of the urethra are far more obstructive than are those situated only in the dorsal half (floor). As a matter of fact, they suggested that small folds or "fins" in the floor of the urethra, extending proximally and distally and simulating Young and associates' valves of types I and II, can be entirely innocent, normal findings. They concluded that obstruction to flow of urine results only when a *ventral* transverse fold joins these "fins." Griesbach, Waterhouse, and Mellins were not able to substantiate this finding. They stated that the most obstructive valves are predominantly in the floor of the urethra.

Kjellberg, Ericsson, and Rudhe encountered the type I valve in 13 of their 52 cases and the circular diaphragm type III in 39 cases; there were no instances of the type II valve. This experience contrasts with that of Williams and Eckstein, who had 104 cases of the Young type I valve and no cases of type II or III.

Anterior Urethral Valves

Anterior urethral valves are extremely rare. About 10 cases have been reported in the literature (Chang; Daniel, Stewart, and Blair). Symptoms are similar to those associated with posterior valves, but the degree of obstruction—as evidenced by the condition of the upper urinary tract—appears to be much less. Diagnosis is made by means of the voiding cystourethrogram (Figs. 5-220, 5-221, and 5-222). Surgical excision of such a valve is carried out through an external urethrotomy incision.

CONGENITAL VALVES IN THE FEMALE URETHRA

Structures resembling valves have also been encountered in girls and women (Lowsley and Kerwin; Mitchell, Makhuli, and Frittelli; Nesbit, McDonald, and Busby; Stevens, 1936). In the cases reported, the valves have caused obstruction during voiding, and voiding cystourethrograms have demonstrated dilated ballooned urethras proximal to the valve and narrowing distally (Figs. 5-223 through 5-226). The valves also can be demonstrated with a blunt probe, the end of which has been bent into the shape of a buttonhook. The probe is passed first through the urethra to the region of the vesical neck and then is withdrawn slowly. If a valve is present, it will be caught by the hook; and, usually, it can be pulled out beyond the meatus and incised with the scalpel.

Valves have been encountered both in the floor and roof of the urethra; all have been close to the urethral meatus. In one of Nesbit, McDonald, and Busby's cases (Fig. 5-224), the obstructing lesion proved to be a tough fibrous transverse band that "cut like cartilage."

In all cases reported, the obstructive symptoms have been relieved, and the cystourethrogram has returned to normal.

(Text continued on page 543.)

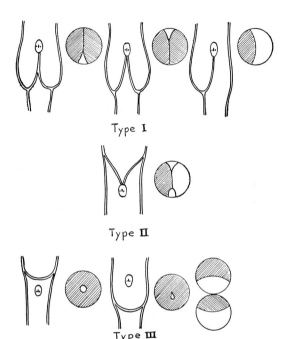

Figure 5-203. Types of congenital valves of posterior urethra with indications of cystoscopic appearances. (Modified from Young, H. H., Frontz, W. A., and Baldwin, J. C.)

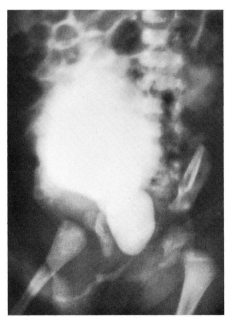

Figure 5-204. *Voiding cystourethrogram* of newborn infant boy. Huge dilatation of prostatic urethra apparently result of **congenital urethral valves.** (From Griesbach, W. A., Waterhouse, R. K., and Mellins, H. Z.)

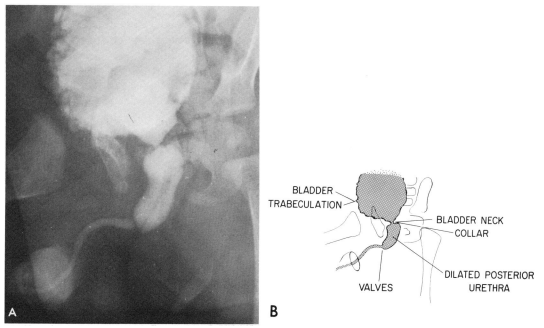

Figure 5–205.   Congenital posterior urethral valves in male infant. **A,** *Voiding cystourethrogram.* **B,** Drawing, illustrating findings on cystourethrogram. (From Ellis, D. G., Fonkalsrud, E. W., and Smith, J. P.)

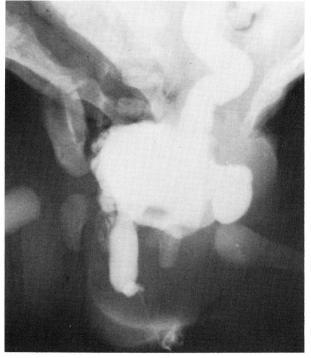

Figure 5–206.   *Voiding cystourethrogram* of male infant, aged 2 days. **Congenital posterior urethral valves.** Note bilateral vesicoureteral reflux and ureterectasis. (From Ellis, D. G., Fonkalsrud, E. W., and Smith, J. P.)

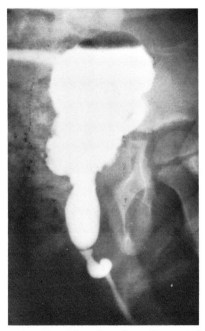

Figure 5–207. *Voiding cystourethrogram* of male infant. **Congenital posterior urethral valves.** (From Lapides, J., Anderson, E. C., and Petrone, A. F.)

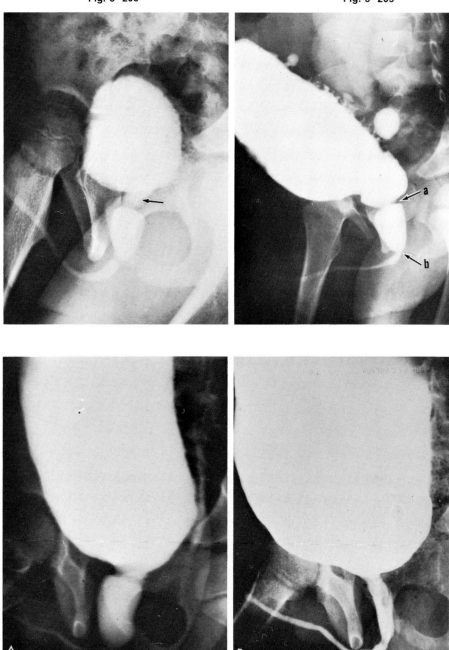

Fig. 5–210

Figure 5–208. *Voiding cystourethrogram* of boy, 7 years of age. **Congenital posterior urethral valves,** producing characteristic dilatation of prostatic urethra below grossly hypertrophied bladder neck (*arrow*). (From Griesbach, W. A., Waterhouse, R. K., and Mellins, H. Z.)

Figure 5–209. *Voiding cystourethrogram* of boy, 22 months of age. **Congenital valve** (*b*) **of posterior urethra** with typical dilatation of prostatic urethra. Note narrowing in region of vesical neck (*a*). This is apparently due to hypertrophy of vesical neck, which is part of general hypertrophy of detrusor muscle. (From Griesbach, W. A., Waterhouse, R. K., and Mellins, H. Z.)

Figure 5–210. **Congenital urethral valves.** *Voiding urethrograms.* **A,** *Preoperative.* Obstructive dilatation of prostatic urethra. Moderate secondary hypertrophy of vesical neck was considered to be part of generalized hypertrophy of detrusor muscle. **B,** *Seven days after transurethral removal of valve.* Prostatic urethra has returned almost to normal caliber. (From Hamm, F. C., and Waterhouse, K.)

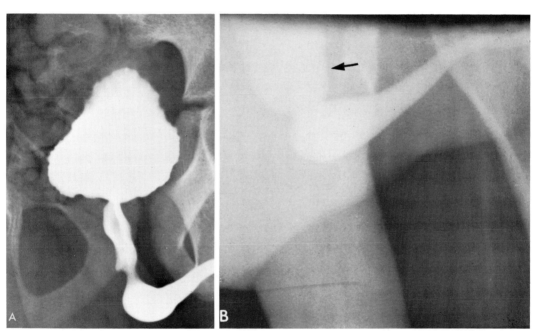

Figure 5–211.   Congenital urethral valves in boy, 10 years of age. **A,** *Retrograde urethrogram.* Rather peculiar elongated prostatic urethra with spreading. **B,** *Voiding cystourethrogram.* Greatly dilated prostatic urethra secondary to obstructive valves (*arrow*).

Fig. 5–212

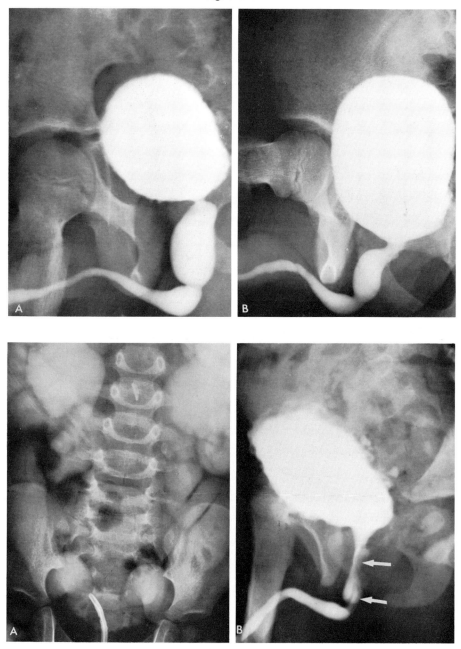

Fig. 5–213

Figure 5–212. Congenital urethral valves in boy, 7 years of age. *Voiding cystourethrograms.* A, *Before operation.* B, *Five days after transurethral fulguration of valves.*

Figure 5–213. Congenital urethral valves in boy, 21 months of age. A, *Excretory urogram, 4-hour film.* Bilateral advanced pyeloureterectasis. B, *Voiding cystourethrogram.* Verumontanum and valves visible (*arrows*).

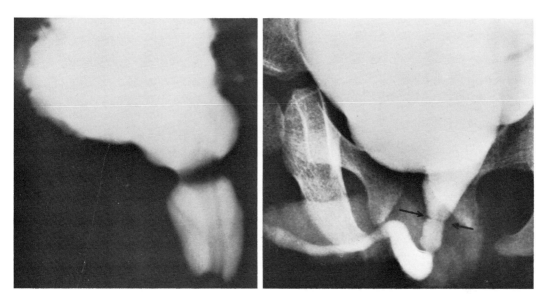

Fig. 5–214   Fig. 5–215

Figure 5–214. *Cystourethrogram* made with catheter in urethra of boy with **congenital urethral valves.** Radiolucent lines are considered to be valves causing great dilatation of prostatic urethra. Indentation in region of vesical neck is considered to indicate obstruction. (From Lich, R., Jr., Howerton, L. W., and Davis, L. A.)

Figure 5–215. *Voiding urethrogram.* **Semicircular valves** (*arrows*) at level of verumontanum in boy, 3 years of age. (From Kjellberg, S. A., Ericsson, N. D., and Rudhe, U.)

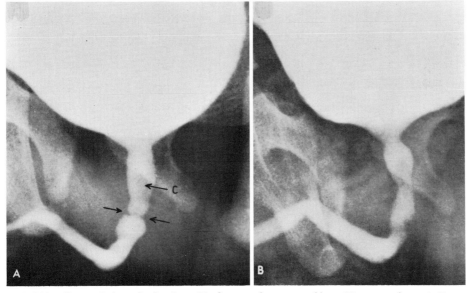

Figure 5–216. **Congenital urethral valves.** *Voiding urethrograms* of boy, 1½ years of age. **A,** *Preoperative film.* Negative shadows of semicircular valves (*arrows*) slightly below level of verumontanum (*c*). **B,** *Postoperative film.* (From Kjellberg, S. A., Ericsson, N. D., and Rudhe, U.)

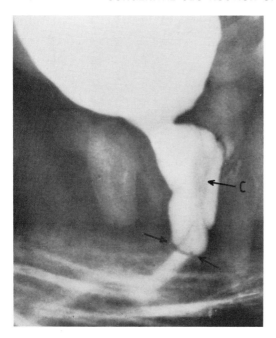

Figure 5–217. *Voiding cystourethrogram* of male infant, 6 days old. **Bicuspid type of urethral valves** (*arrows*), well below verumontanum (*c*), at level of urogenital diaphragm. (From Kjellberg, S. A., Ericsson, N. D., and Rudhe, U.)

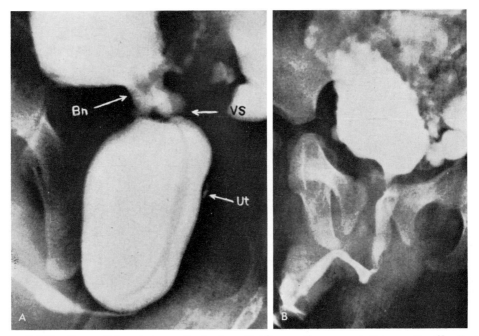

Figure 5–218. Congenital posterior urethral valves. *Voiding urethrograms.* **A,** *Preoperative film.* Posterior urethral valves at level of urogenital diaphragm, producing enormous dilatation of prostatic urethra. Utricle (*Ut*) and seminal vesicles (*VS*) also are filled with contrast medium. *Bn* = bladder neck. **B,** *Postoperative film.* Prostatic urethra is smaller. Note vesicoureteral reflux. (From Kjellberg, S. A., Ericsson, N. D., and Rudhe, U.)

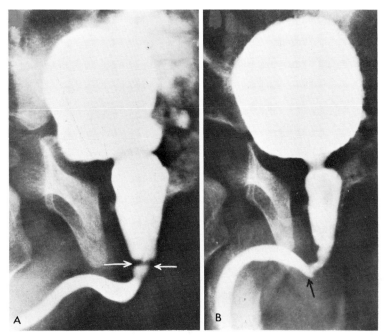

Figure 5–219. Congenital posterior urethral valves in boy, 10 months of age. *Voiding cystourethrograms.* **A,** *Preoperative film.* Valves (*arrows*) at level of urogenital diaphragm, with considerable dilatation of prostatic lumen above. **B,** *Postoperative film.* Valves are gone. Dilatation of prostatic urethra is greatly diminished. Arrow points to depression where external urethral incision was made. (From Kjellberg, S. A., Ericsson, N. D., and Rudhe, U.)

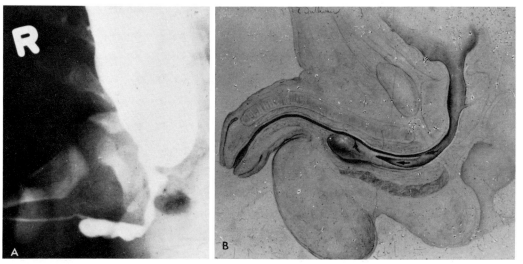

Figure 5–220. Anterior urethral valve in male infant aged 3½ months. **A,** *Cystourethrogram.* Note dilatation proximal to valve. Negative linear shadow represents valve. **B,** Position of valve and mechanism of obstruction during micturition. (From Chang, C.-Y.)

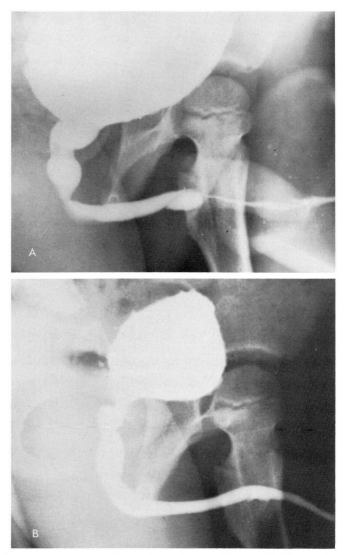

Figure 5–221.   Congenital anterior urethral valve in boy aged 6 years. *Voiding cystourethrograms.* **A,** *Preoperative film.* Note trabeculation of bladder. (At operation, thin circumferential "sail-like" valve was found and excised.) **B,** *Postoperative film.* (From Daniel, J., Stewart, A. M., and Blair, D. W.)

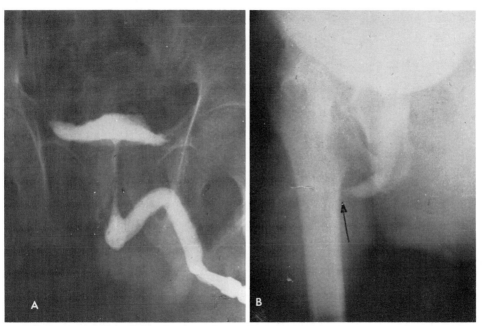

Figure 5–222. Anterior urethral valve in male, aged 25. **A,** *Retrograde urethrogram.* Valve not demonstrated. **B,** *Voiding cystourethrogram.* Abrupt narrowing of anterior part of urethra distal to bulb (*arrow*). Surgical exposure of urethra revealed valves which were removed. (Upper urinary tract was normal.) (From Colabawalla, B. N.)

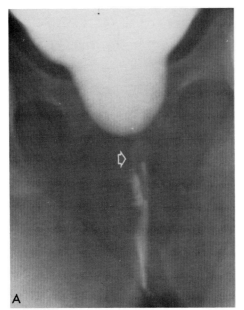

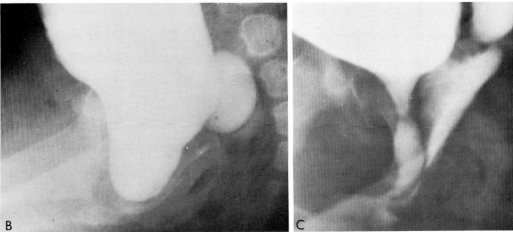

Figure 5–223. Congenital urethral valve in female. *Voiding cystourethrograms.* **A,** *Preoperative film, frontal view.* Urethra dilated proximal to valve. Tiny stream of contrast medium (*arrow*) seen in distal part of urethra. **B,** *Preoperative film, lateral view.* Note small vesical diverticulum. **C,** *Postoperative film, oblique view.* Proximal part of urethra is now of normal size and distal part is of good caliber. (From Mitchell, G. F., Makhuli, Z., and Frittelli, G.)

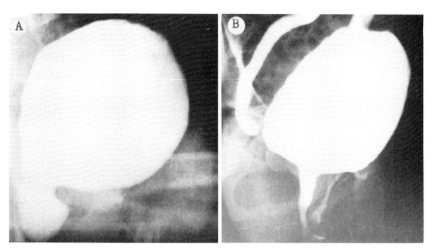

Figure 5–224. Congenital urethral valve or fibrotic band in young girl. *Voiding cystourethrograms.* **A,** *Preoperative film.* Dilatation of urethra; obstructive point appears to be near urethral meatus. (Obstructive band near meatus was demonstrated by pulling partially inflated Foley balloon catheter through urethra. Stricture was incised—"cut like cartilage.") **B,** *Postoperative film.* Urethra now appears normal. (From Nesbit, R. M., McDonald, H. P., Jr., and Busby, S.)

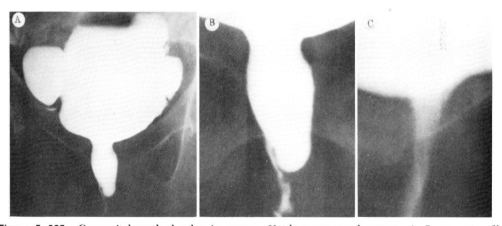

Figure 5–225. Congenital urethral valve in woman. *Voiding cystourethrograms.* **A,** *Preoperative film.* Ballooned proximal part of urethra and very narrow distal part. Note diverticula of bladder. **B,** *Close-up view of urethra.* Shadow between dilated and narrow portions of urethra has appearance of valve. (Valve was hooked with silver probe with end bent like buttonhook, pulled down through urethra, and incised.) **C,** *Postoperative film.* Obstruction relieved. (From Nesbit, R. M., McDonald, H. P., Jr., and Busby, S.)

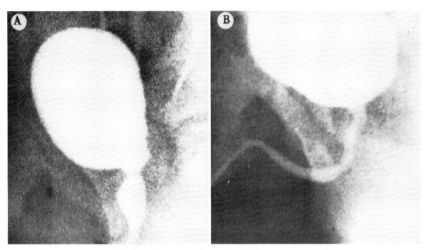

Figure 5–226. Congenital urethral valve in little girl. *Voiding cystourethrograms.* **A,** *Preoperative film.* Ballooning of urethra. (Buttonhook-shaped probe was passed into and pulled back through urethra. It hooked valve on floor of urethra near meatus. Valve was incised.) **B,** *Postoperative film.* Urethra appears normal. (From Nesbit, R. M., McDonald, H. P., Jr., and Busby, S.)

Urethral Polyps in Boys

A true pedunculated polyp is composed of a stalk of loose connective tissue containing blood vessels and covered with transitional epithelium. They occur exclusively in boys and are located in the prostatic urethra. In most cases, they are attached to the dorsal half (floor) of the prostatic urethra near the verumontanum. They are not common; Meadows and Quattlebaum were able to find reports in the literature of only eight cases, since the first was reported by Scott, Collins, and Singer in 1938. At rest, the polyp usually lies near the bladder neck; during micturition, it may prolapse into the membranous urethra. The degree of obstruction depends on the size and location, and the symptoms are similar to those of any infravesical obstruction. In Meadows and Quattlebaum's four cases, the patients were boys from 5 to 9 years of age; the excretory urogram showed no evidence of obstruction of the upper urinary tract in any case, but one boy had 150 ml of residual urine. On the other hand, ureteropyelectasis was present in three of Williams and Abbassian's four cases. The ages of their patients were 8 years, 3 years, 3 years, and 7 months, respectively. In the *cystourethrogram,* the polyp appears as a negative shadow which may be round, ovoid, or teardrop in shape. Because of its mobility, the shadow may assume different shapes and occupy different locations in sequential films (Figs. 5–227 and 5–228).

Congenital Stenosis of the Urethral Meatus

Campbell (1951) stated that approximately 20% of children with urologic disease have congenital stricture of the urethra, chiefly stenosis of the urethral meatus. Certainly the condition is so common that it should be given first consideration in the urologic investigation of every child. It is the first thing to consider in enuresis.

Many physicians are familiar with this problem in little boys but are not aware that it occurs with almost equal frequency in girls. This subject has been considered previously under the subject of distal urethral stenosis (pages 511 through 513) which also includes data concerning the caliber of the normal urethra in girls of various ages.

It is more difficult to try to set up a table of standards for the caliber of the urethra for male infants and little boys than to do so for little girls. The pediatrician and urologist soon learn to recognize degrees of meatal narrowing in little boys and, by watching them void, can decide whether urethral narrowing exists. Calibration of the meatus with small Otis diagnostic bulbs (bougie à boule) will settle the problem if there is any uncertainty. The occasional inflammatory granulomatous eczematoid-appearing lesion involving the meatus and glans penis in cases of meatal stenosis has been described repeatedly. Confronted by such a case, the pediatrician and urologist should instantly suspect meatal stenosis as the underlying cause. Generally speaking, little boys who are normal have a much larger stream than most physicians realize.

It is important to remember that the narrowest portion of the urethra in boys and girls is the urethral meatus. In boys, there is also a second site of narrowing, namely the penoscrotal juncture. The voiding cystourethrogram is not so important in cases of meatal stenosis as it is in those of congenital obstruction of the vesical neck and congenital urethral valve. Nevertheless, it may be helpful and corroborative and is easily made. Kjellberg, Ericsson, and Rudhe pointed out that the actual site of the meatal narrowing may be difficult or impossible to demonstrate urographically. Dilatation of the urethra proximal to the meatus during all stages of micturition (polyview filming while patient voids) is pathognomonic of meatal narrowing (Figs. 5–229 and 5–230).

Congenital, Iatrogenic, and Traumatic Strictures of the Urethra in Infants and Children

Bona fide congenital stricture of the urethra (excluding meatal stenosis) is rare. Kjellberg, Ericsson, and Rudhe encountered it in one case in their study—the case of a male infant who had been operated on at the age of 1 day for anal atresia with scrotal fistula (Fig. 5-231). In our experience most so-called congenital strictures are iatrogenic and have resulted from ill-advised urethral instrumentation. Many so-called congenital strictures would disappear if a cystourethrogram were made on each child needing urologic investigation before any rigid or semirigid instruments were introduced through the urethra. If, after a cystourethrogram and excretory urogram have been made, cystoscopy is considered necessary, it should be done under general anesthesia, and the urethra should be carefully calibrated with small Otis diagnostic bulbs before the cystoscope is introduced. Only in this way can the caliber of the meatus and penoscrotal junction be accurately determined. Also, if areas of narrowing do exist in the urethra, their exact size and location can be charted. It is impossible to obtain this information accurately by calibration with sounds (Emmett, Kirchheim, and Greene).

Almost all **congenital strictures** occur in boys and are usually located at the junction of the bulbous urethra (of ectodermal origin—from the genital fold) with the prostatic and membranous urethra (of entodermal origin—from the cloaca). These are usually "soft" strictures that dilate quite easily, although Cobb, Wolf, and Ansell have shown that they may persist in spite of dilation and be the cause of irritative symptoms in young men when they are usually diagnosed as "prostatitis" (Figs. 5-232 and 5-233). They found two peak ages for congenital stricture, (1) infancy and young childhood and (2) young adulthood—the early twenties.

The caliber of congenital strictures can vary in degree from complete atresia (Campbell, 1951; Engle and Schlumberger) to almost normal urethral caliber. In a series of 26 male patients less than 14 years of age (average age, 5½, range, newborn to 13 years), Cobb, Wolf, and Ansell found the average caliber of the strictures to be 10 F. They defined a stricture as a narrowing of smaller caliber than the urethral meatus (based on calibration with Otis bulbs). The largest caliber, in a 12-year-old boy, was 16 F and the smallest, in an 8-year-old boy, was 6 F. Treatment consisted of urethral dilatation with infant sounds or pediatric Kollman dilators; if this was ineffective, internal urethrotomy was performed with an infant Otis urethrotome.

In an article on urethral strictures in boys, Leadbetter and Leadbetter reported a series of cases in which dilatation was ineffective, so that open operation (urethroplasty) was required (Figs. 5-234 and 5-235). In two of these cases, the stricture was located in the penile urethra just proximal to the fossa navicularis; in the other four, it was located in the "proximal bulb." In only two of these cases were the strictures regarded as congenital; in four, they resulted from trauma (straddle injury or kicks), while in two, they were iatrogenic (one from instrumentation and one from repair of a hypospadias). Most **traumatic strictures** in little boys result from straddle injuries and are located in the "proximal bulb" of the urethra (Fig. 5-236).

Iatrogenic strictures occur most commonly at the penoscrotal junction and the meatus, the two narrowest points of the male urethra, although almost any part of the pendulous urethra may be involved. Urologists should appreciate the caliber of the normal urethra in the infant and child, since attempts to "dilate" a normal urethra usually result in traumatic avulsion which is followed too often by disabling stricture. If instruments too large to be easily accommodated by the urethra are required, it is preferable to introduce them through an external urethrotomy incision into the bulbous urethra which is normally the largest part of the male urethra. If the bulbous urethra is too small, a suprapubic approach is usually the procedure of choice (Figs. 5–237 through 5–240).

Diagnosis

In the diagnosis of urethral stricture, as in that of any "obstructive" problem of an infant or child, it is good judgment always to begin the investigation urographically with (1) an excretory urogram and (2) a cystourethrogram. A voiding or expression cystourethrogram may be made in conjunction with the excretory urogram if there has been adequate excretion of concentrated contrast medium. If not, a small urethral catheter should be passed, the bladder filled with contrast medium, the catheter withdrawn, and a voiding or expression cystourethrogram obtained. If it is impossible to introduce a catheter, a retrograde cystourethrogram may be made to demonstrate the stricture. If it proves necessary, instrumentation can be done later, when it should be done with the child under general anesthesia to preclude his making sudden movements that might result in trauma or perforation of the urethra.

(Text continued on page 553.)

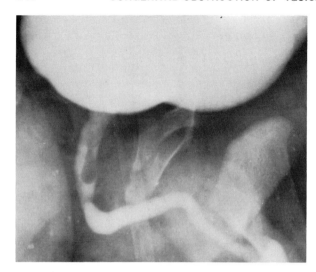

Figure 5–227. *Voiding cystourethrogram* of boy. **Polyp of prostatic urethra.** Note teardrop shape of negative shadow from polyp. (From Williams, D. I., and Abbassian, A.)

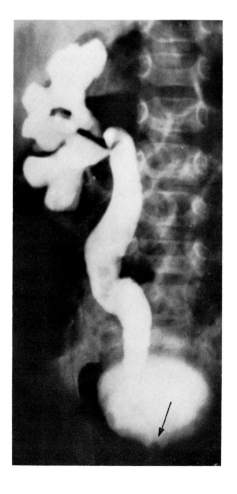

Figure 5–228. *Cystogram* of boy. Reflux up dilated ureter showing marked pyeloureterectasis caused by obstruction from **polyp of prostatic urethra,** which can be seen as small, circular negative filling defect in midline at vesical neck (*arrow*). (From Williams, D. I., and Abbassian, A.)

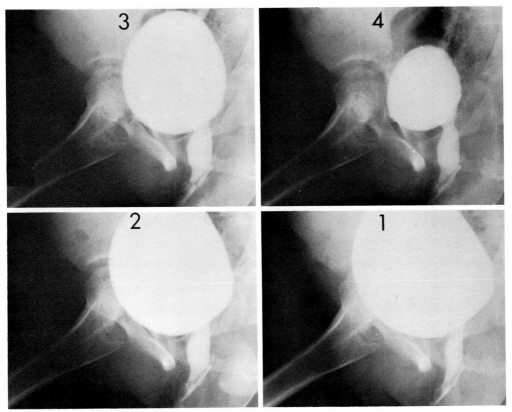

Figure 5–229. *Polyview voiding cystourethrogram* of 8-year-old girl. **Meatal stenosis.** (Films taken during several stages of voiding.) (From Thornbury, J. R., and Immergut, M. A.)

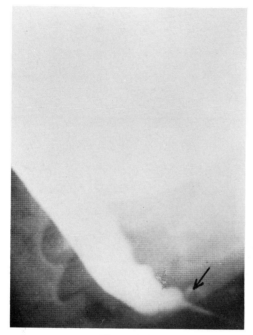 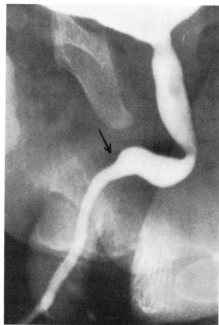

Fig. 5–230   **Fig. 5–231**

Figure 5–230. *Voiding urethrogram* of girl, 9 years of age. **Stenosis of urethral meatus** (*arrow*), with proximal dilatation of urethra. (From Kjellberg, S. A., Ericsson, N. D., and Rudhe, U.)

Figure 5–231. *Voiding cystourethrogram* of male infant, 10 months of age. **Constriction of entire cavernous portion of urethra** (*distal to arrow*). Considered to be congenital anomaly. (From Kjellberg, S. A., Ericsson, N. D., and Rudhe, U.)

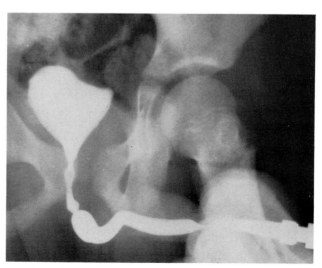

Figure 5–232. *Retrograde urethrogram* of infant. **Congenital stricture of proximal part of bulbous urethra.** (From Cobb, B. G., Wolf, J. A., and Ansell, J. S.)

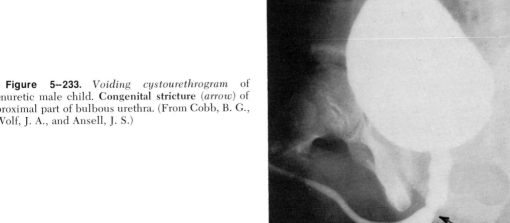

Figure 5–233. *Voiding cystourethrogram* of enuretic male child. **Congenital stricture** (*arrow*) of proximal part of bulbous urethra. (From Cobb, B. G., Wolf, J. A., and Ansell, J. S.)

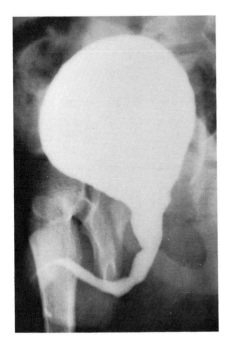

Figure 5–234. *Voiding cystourethrogram* of boy. **Stricture of distal part of pendulous urethra,** causing dilatation of proximal part of urethra and of vesical neck. (From Leadbetter, G. W., and Leadbetter, W. F.)

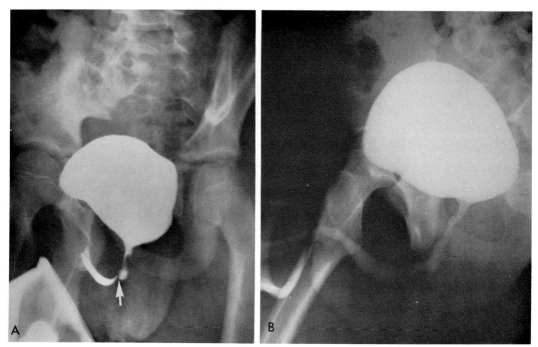

Figure 5–235. Stricture of bulbous portion of urethra of boy, age 8 years. *Voiding cystourethrograms.* **A,** *Preoperative film.* (Stricture was excised and pedicle-flap procedure performed.) **B,** *Postoperative film.* (From Leadbetter, G. W., and Leadbetter, W. F.)

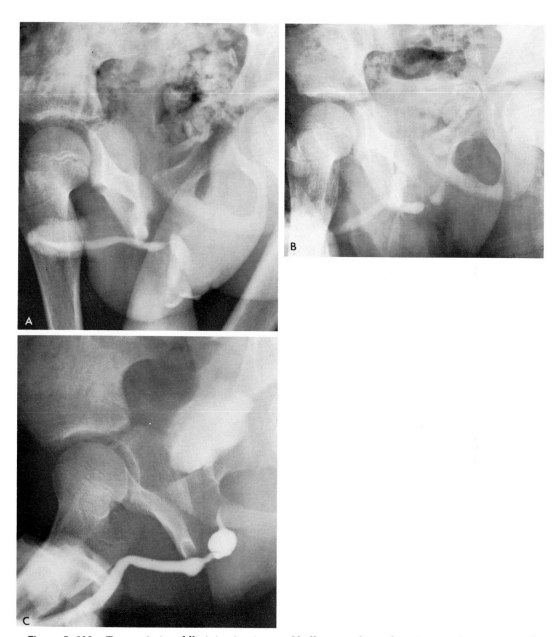

Figure 5–236.   Traumatic (straddle injury) stricture of bulbous urethra in boy, 9 years of age. *Retrograde urethrograms.* **A,** *Two months after injury and rupture of urethra.* Contrast medium is running out through perineum at site of urethral defect. **B,** *One month after* **A.** Short filiform stricture in bulb. (Perineal operation with excision of stricture and end-to-end anastomosis was performed.) **C,** *Eight months postoperatively.* Recurring stricture with some dilatation of bulbous urethra proximal to stricture. (Patient responded well to periodic dilatations.)

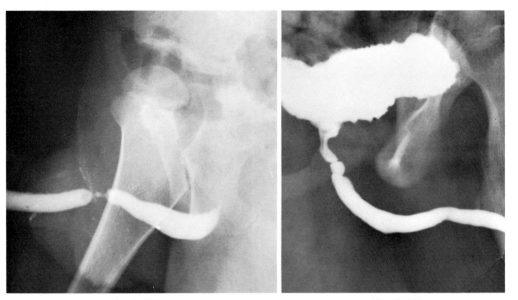

Fig. 5–237   Fig. 5–238

Figure 5–237. *Retrograde urethrogram* of boy, 3 years of age. Iatrogenic (postcystoscopic) stricture of urethra at penoscrotal juncture.

Figure 5–238. *Retrograde urethrogram* of boy, 11 years of age, with myelodysplasia. Iatrogenic stricture of membranous urethra from perineal transurethral resection of vesical neck at age 2 years.

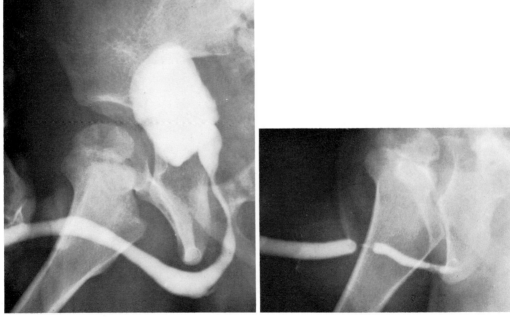

Fig. 5–239   Fig. 5–240

Figure 5–239. *Retrograde urethrogram* of boy, 2½ years of age. Congenital obstruction of vesical neck with large-caliber stricture in proximal part of bulbous urethra. Note small false passage in floor of urethra. Stricture was either congenital or result of previous cystoscopy. Instruments larger than size 14 F could not be passed. (Heineke-Mikulicz operation on vesical neck was performed with good result.)

Figure 5–240. *Retrograde urethrogram* of boy, 3 years of age. Postoperative stricture at penoscrotal juncture caused by previous transurethral resection of vesical neck.

Vesical Diverticula

Diverticula of the bladder may be single or multiple, large or small. Small diverticula that empty are similar to large cellules and as a general rule are of no surgical importance. Larger diverticula may assume bizarre shapes and positions and at times may reach such huge proportions that the diverticulum may be larger than the bladder (Figs. 5–241 through 5–248). Although a diverticulum usually is diagnosed by cystoscopic examination, it may be easily missed if its neck is small, unless a cystogram is made. Not only will the cystogram reveal diverticula overlooked on cystoscopy, but it will determine their capacity and the degree of retention and stasis. Diverticula that are capable of emptying themselves are of little or no clinical significance in the absence of infection. Inability to empty results in stagnation of retained urine in the diverticulum and predisposes to infection and formation of stone. The size of the orifice of the diverticulum may be no indication of its capacity or of its ability to empty.

In many cases the orifice of the diverticulum is *adjacent to a ureteral meatus.* Not uncommonly the ureteral orifice is situated on the edge of the neck of the diverticulum and in an occasional case it may open into the diverticulum itself. Ureterectasis may result from pressure of the diverticulum on the terminal portion of the ureter as it courses around the diverticulum (Fig. 5–249), or as it passes between the diverticulum and the wall of the bladder. It also may result from the disturbance of the normal ureterovesical junction as described by Hutch (1958), allowing the intramural ureter to become extravesical, producing both obstructive ureterectasis and reflux.

Although in most cases diverticula are easily identified in the cystogram, one may encounter a large diverticulum with a small neck which may not fill with urographic medium. In such a case the diverticulum may be confused with a filling defect from a tumor or nonopaque stone, or from an extravesical mass which is displacing the bladder. In some cases error in interpretation may be avoided by observing a characteristic displacement of the ureter as it curves around the diverticulum to enter the bladder (Figs. 5–250 through 5–255).

It is important to know the degree of retention associated with diverticula. To obtain this information a cystogram is made after the patient voids the urographic medium. Another cystogram is then made after the bladder has been drained with a catheter. From these two cystograms one can estimate the degree of urinary stasis in the bladder and in the diverticulum (Fig. 5–256).

It must not be forgotten that vesical diverticula may be the sites of **tumors** and **calculi.** Calculi usually are quite easily visualized in plain films and cystograms. Tumors, on the other hand, may be more difficult to recognize and often require cystoscopy for accurate diagnosis. (These conditions will be discussed in the chapters devoted to stone [Chapter 6] and tumor [Chapter 10].)

(Text continued on page 562.)

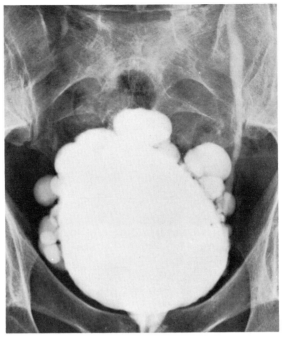

Figure 5–241. *Retrograde cystogram.* Multiple small vesical diverticula and large cellules associated with benign prostatic hyperplasia.

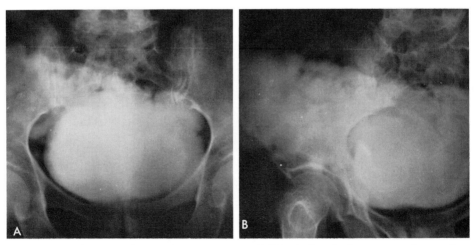

Figure 5–242. Huge vesical diverticulum in woman with 700 ml of residual urine secondary to **obstruction of vesical neck.** *Retrograde cystograms.* **A,** *Anteroposterior film.* Large vesical diverticulum extending to right side. **B,** *Oblique film.* Better filling of huge vesical diverticulum which extends beyond right ilium. (Transurethral resection of vesical neck relieved obstruction.) (Courtesy of Dr. David Cristol.)

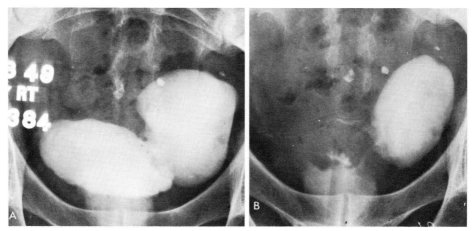

Figure 5–243. Large vesical diverticulum. *Retrograde cystograms* soon after transurethral resection of prostate gland and neck of diverticulum. **A,** *With bladder full.* Diverticulum arises from left posterior wall of bladder. Note prostatic urethra is wide open and filled with medium. **B,** *Immediately after voiding.* Bladder is empty, but there is some medium still trickling through into prostatic urethra from diverticulum.

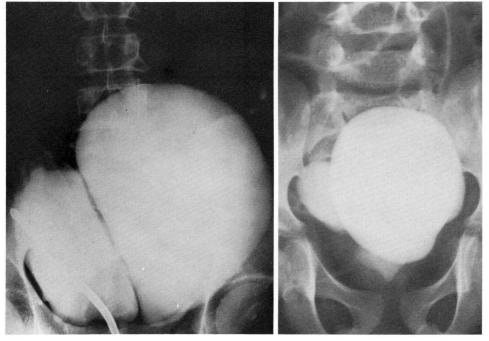

| Fig. 5–244 | Fig. 5–245 |

Figure 5–244. *Retrograde cystogram.* **Huge vesical diverticulum,** much larger than bladder, arises from left wall of bladder and displaces bladder to right of midline. Urethral catheter is in bladder.

Figure 5–245. *Cystogram made through cystostomy tube.* **Large diverticulum** arises from left side of bladder; smaller one from right. Necks of both diverticula were situated near ureteral orifices. Bladder is posterior. (Diverticulectomy and transurethral resection of vesical neck were done.)

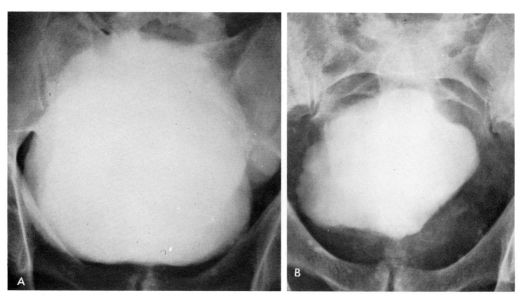

Figure 5–246. Vesical diverticulum obscured by over-filling of bladder with contrast medium. *Retrograde cystograms.* **A,** *Bladder overdistended with contrast medium.* Suggestion of superimposed shadows. **B,** *After bladder emptied with catheter.* Medium remains in large diverticulum arising from midposterior wall of bladder.

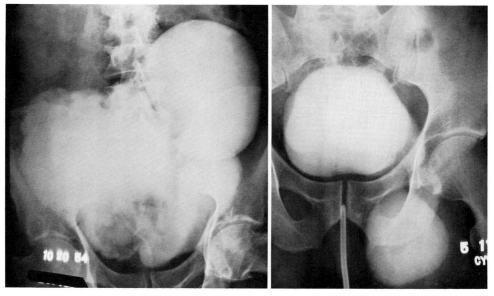

Fig. 5–247   **Fig. 5–248**

Figure 5–247. *Retrograde cystogram.* Multiple huge vesical diverticula in patient with hypertrophy of prostate. (Diverticulectomy and suprapubic prostatectomy were performed.)

Figure 5–248. *Retrograde cystogram.* Two moderate-sized vesical diverticula with incorporation of bladder in recurring inguinal (scrotal) hernia.

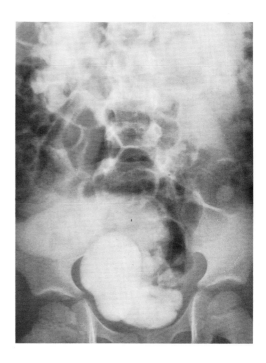

Figure 5–249. *Excretory urogram, 75-minute film* of boy, 4 years of age. **Large vesical diverticulum on right** associated with congenital obstruction of vesical neck and **marked bilateral ureterectasis** (without reflux). Right kidney functioned better than left. Note hugely dilated right ureter curving around diverticulum to reach right ureteral orifice (which was normal in appearance and situated 1 cm medial to neck of diverticulum).

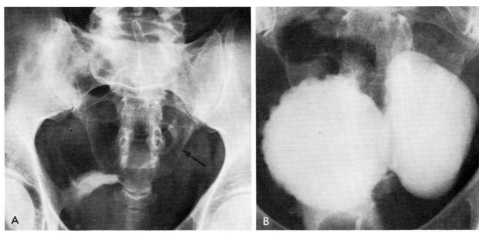

Figure 5–250. Large vesical diverticulum. **A,** *Excretory cystogram.* **Diverticulum arising from left half of bladder** does not fill with contrast medium. Small amount of medium in right side of bladder could be mistaken for deformity from large carcinoma of bladder. Pathognomonic finding here is displacement of lower portion of left ureter upward and to midline (*arrow*), denoting presence of large vesical diverticulum which does not fill with medium. **B,** *Retrograde cystogram* made after transurethral prostatic resection and excision of neck of diverticulum. Diverticulum now fills with medium. Note bag catheter in prostatic urethra, which is open wide as result of prostatic resection.

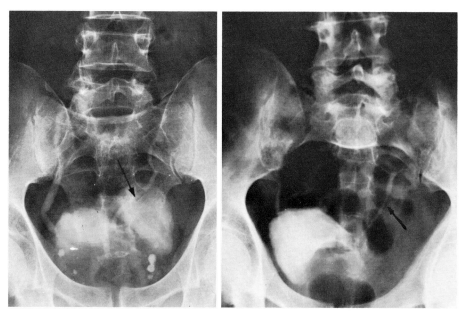

Fig. 5–251 **Fig. 5–252**

Figure 5–251. *Excretory cystogram.* **Large vesical diverticulum** arising from left wall of bladder. Note displacement of lower third of left ureter (*arrow*) as it encircles diverticulum.

Figure 5–252. *Excretory cystogram.* **Apparent filling defect of left half of bladder,** from **large unfilled vesical diverticulum,** might be mistaken for carcinoma of bladder. Displacement of lower third of left ureter (*arrow*), however, suggests correct diagnosis.

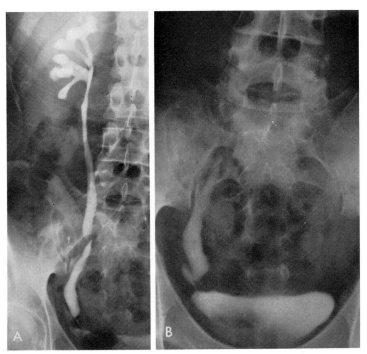

Figure 5–253. Ureteral obstruction from small vesical diverticulum. **A,** *Right retrograde pyelogram.* Dilatation of entire ureter, especially terminal portion, with calycectasis but no pyelectasis. Note abrupt termination of ureter, suggesting stricture or obstruction. **B,** *Fifteen-minute delayed pyelogram.* Medium retained in lower third of dilated ureter. There is small vesical diverticulum adjacent to ureter at point where outline of ureter is abruptly terminated. (Cystoscopy showed small diverticulum in right base adjacent to ureteral orifice. Surgical exploration revealed ureter to lie between wall of diverticulum and wall of bladder, where it was compressed and obstructed. Reimplantation of ureter into bladder was done.)

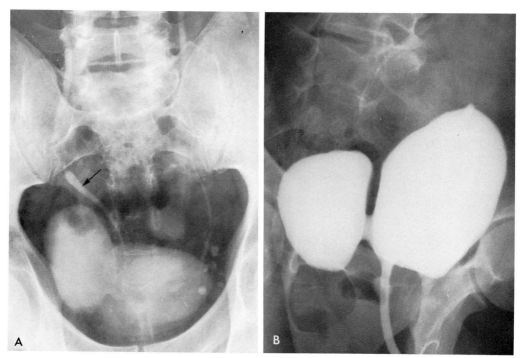

Figure 5–254. Vesical diverticulum displacing lower portion of ureter medially. **A,** *Excretory urogram.* Note displacement of right ureter to left (*arrow*). **B,** *Retrograde cystogram, oblique view.* Neck of diverticulum communicates with bladder.

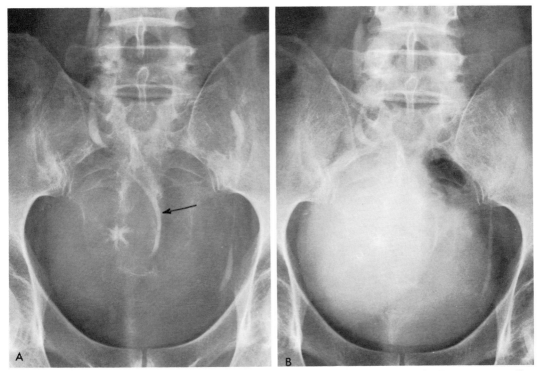

Figure 5–255. **Vesical diverticulum containing jackstone.** Excretory urograms. **A,** *Twenty-minute film.* Medial displacement of right ureter (*arrow*) around partially filled diverticulum. **B,** *One-hour film.* More complete filling of diverticulum.

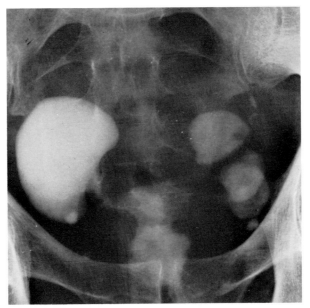

Figure 5–256. *Retrograde cystogram.* **Multiple vesical diverticula.** Cystogram had been made and bladder emptied with urethral catheter. Medium, seen running into base of bladder and prostatic urethra, was retained in large diverticulum on right and two small ones on left.

Obstruction of the Bladder Outlet in Adult Men

BENIGN PROSTATIC HYPERPLASIA

The commonest cause of obstruction of the vesical neck in adult men is benign prostatic hyperplasia. Diagnosis is usually made on the basis of symptoms, digital rectal examination, the finding of residual urine in the bladder, and (when necessary) cystoscopic examination. Urography is usually only a confirmatory test, but at times it can be important in diagnosis. It is impossible to determine the size of the prostate gland accurately by radiographic means (Vermooten and Schweinsberg).

Long-standing obstruction of the vesical neck with residual urine may result in dilatation of the ureters and renal pelves (Figs. 5–257A and B and 5–258). Even though the bladder may not be outlined with contrast medium in the excretory urogram, vesical distention may be suspected by the abnormally wide separation of the terminal portions of the ureters (Figs. 5–259, 5–260, and 5–261). Trabeculation of the bladder is common (Figs. 5–262 and 5–263). The cystogram (either excretory or retrograde) may reveal a characteristic smooth negative filling defect in the base of the bladder caused by the projection of the enlarged prostate gland up into the bladder. Intravesical projections of lateral or median lobes yield typical filling defects, which may be confused at times with the negative shadows of pedunculated bladder tumors. Diagnostic errors may be made because of overlying gas in the rectum, nonopaque vesical calculi, or the inflated bag of a Foley catheter, all of which may simulate prostatic filling defects in the cystogram (Figs. 5–264 through 5–274). Enormous enlargements of the prostate gland may displace the bladder upward almost out of the pelvis (Figs. 5–275 and 5–276). When large glands elevate the trigone and base of the bladder, the terminal ureters may have a "fishhook" appearance that is pathognomonic (Figs. 5–277 and 5–278).

Cystourethrography. Some urologists are enthusiastic about urethrography in the diagnosis of prostatic hyperplasia. We have never employed it extensively, because we thought that the information obtained is either unnecessary or can be obtained more easily and directly by cystoscopic examination. Flocks and Kerr and Gillies have combined air cystograms with retrograde urethrograms with interesting results (see Chapter 1). Belker, Flocks, Culp, and Immergut have also used cystourethrography as a teaching aid in prostatic surgery to determine if the adenomatous tissue has been adequately removed.

The urethrographic deformity depends on the type and position of the prostatic enlargement. *Enlargement of the lateral lobes* produces pressure on the urethra so that it becomes flattened in its lateral diameter but widened in its anteroposterior diameter. This urographic phenomenon is spoken of as *spreading*. The prostatic urethra also becomes *longer*. If the *posterior commissure* or *median lobe* is enlarged, a sharp anterior displacement of the urethra occurs in its proximal part where it lies against this hypertrophied lobe. This results in an angulation of the prostatic urethra with its apex directed posteriorly in the region of the verumontanum. This deformity is called *anterior tilting*. Inasmuch as most cases of adenofibromatous hyperplasia involve all three lobes to various degrees, many combinations of the foregoing urographic deformities are encountered (Figs. 5–279 through 5–283).

CARCINOMA OF THE PROSTATE

What has been said about the need for cystourethrography in the diagnosis of benign prostatic hyperplasia applies also to carcinoma of the prostate. The plain film (KUB) is important in the detection of metastasis to bone (see Chapter 3). Trabeculation of the bladder and ureterectasis may be demonstrated by excretory urography. Negative filling defects in the bladder from intravesical projection of the gland are not as commonly seen as in benign hyperplasia. When present, however, they tend to be more irregular (Fig. 5–284) and may be difficult to distinguish from those of infiltrating bladder tumors.

The retrograde cystourethrogram is not as pathognomonic as it is in benign hyperplasia. There is narrowing in both the anteroposterior and lateral diameters of the prostatic urethra, so that instead of manifesting the "spreading" phenomenon, it appears as a narrow tube. It may lose its normal curve and become straight and elongated (Fig. 5–285).

(Text continued on page 576.)

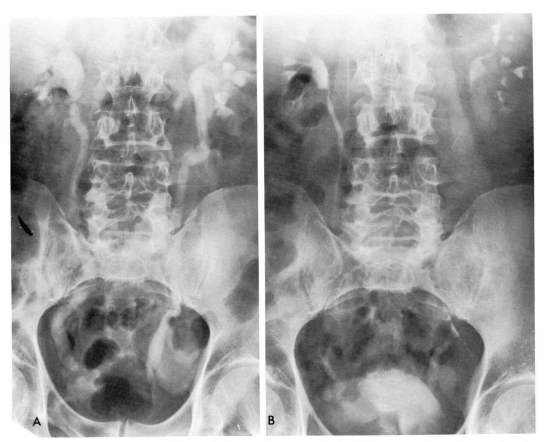

Figure 5–257. Moderate-sized vesical diverticulum associated with ureteropyelectasis secondary to urinary obstruction from benign prostatic hyperplasia. *Excretory urograms.* **A,** *Preoperative film.* **B,** *Film made 5 months after transurethral resection.* Ureteropyelectasis has almost disappeared.

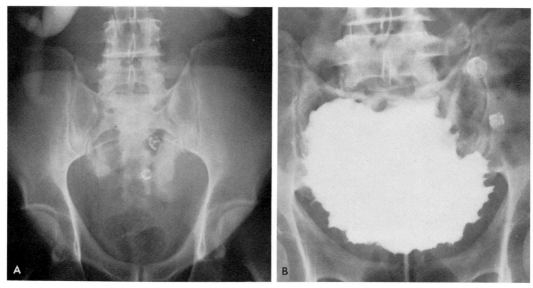

Figure 5–258. Bilateral hydronephrosis and hydroureter from long-standing distention of bladder secondary to prostatic obstruction. A, *Excretory urogram.* B, *Retrograde cystogram.*

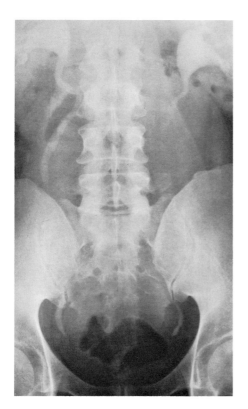

Figure 5–259. *Excretory urogram.* **Huge distended bladder** (2,000 ml of residual urine) **secondary to congenital obstruction of vesical neck** of man, aged 49. There is wide separation of terminal portions of ureters and of ureteral orifices.

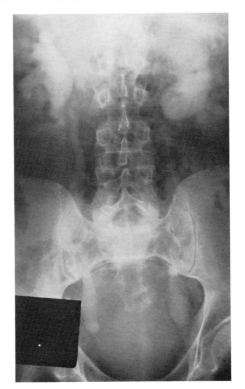

Figure 5–260. *Excretory urogram.* Huge distended bladder secondary to prostatic obstruction. Distance between terminal portions of ureters is increased.

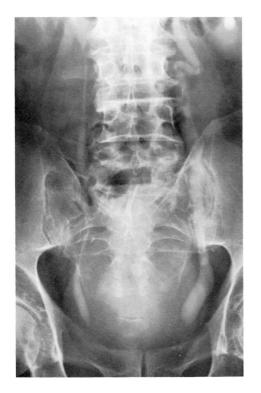

Figure 5–261. Widely separated terminal ureters from greatly distended bladder secondary to prostatic obstruction. Terminal portions of ureters are widely separated.

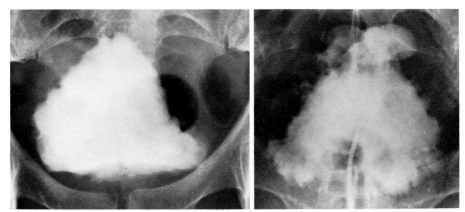

Fig. 5–262   Fig. 5–263

Figure 5–262. Moderate trabeculation of bladder associated with moderate obstruction secondary to benign prostatic hyperplasia. Pear-shaped outline of bladder commonly seen in cases of obstruction of vesical neck.

Figure 5–263. *Retrograde cystogram.* Moderate trabeculation of bladder and cellule formation caused by urinary obstruction from benign prostatic hyperplasia. Note pyramidal shape of bladder.

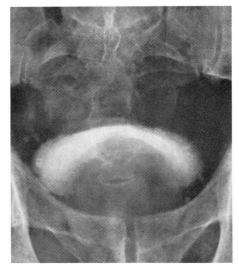

Figure 5–264. *Retrograde cystogram.* Filling defect in base of bladder with typical smooth outline, from benign prostatic hyperplasia.

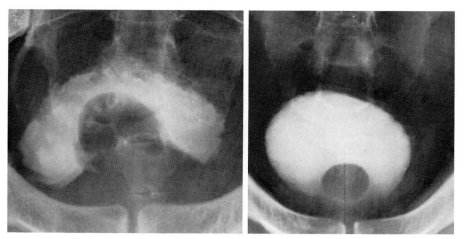

Fig. 5–265   Fig. 5–266

Figure 5–265. *Excretory cystogram.* Filling defect in base of bladder from intravesical enlargement of median lobe of prostate gland. Note trabeculation of bladder and small cellules.

Figure 5–266. *Excretory cystogram.* Unusually well-defined filling defect from small subcervical benign prostatic enlargement. Could be confused with filling defect from bag catheter.

Fig. 5–267   Fig. 5–268

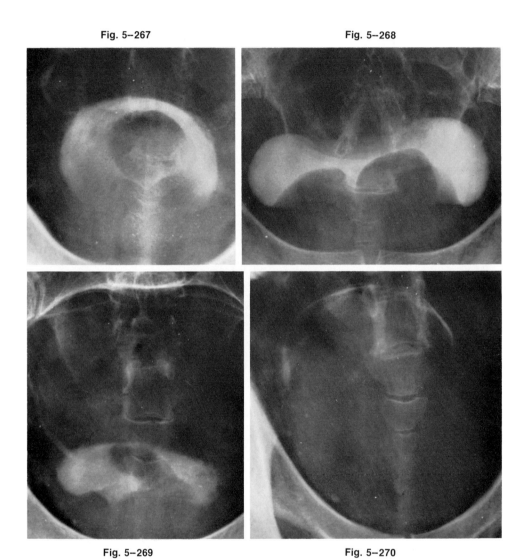

Fig. 5–269   Fig. 5–270

Figure 5–267. *Excretory cystogram.* Filling defect in bladder from intravesical trilobar benign prostatic hyperplasia. Could be confused with filling defect from tumor.

Figure 5–268. *Excretory cystogram.* Filling defect in base of bladder from intravesical benign hyperplasia of lateral lobes of prostate.

Figure 5–269. *Excretory cystogram.* Irregular filling defect in bladder from intravesical projection of benign prostatic hyperplasia. Could be mistaken for filling defect from tumor of bladder.

Figure 5–270. *Excretory cystogram.* Marked intravesical projection of huge benign prostatic hyperplasia, which seems to fill bladder completely except for medium seen in periphery anteriorly.

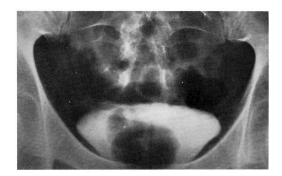

Figure 5–271. *Excretory cystogram.* Gas in rectum, which might be mistaken for filling defect from benign prostatic hyperplasia.

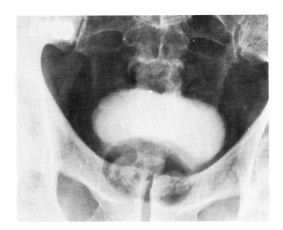

Figure 5–272. *Excretory cystogram.* Filling defect from benign prostatic hyperplasia and superimposed gas in rectum.

Figure 5–273. *Excretory cystogram.* Filling defect in bladder from huge intravesical hyperplasia of prostate gland.

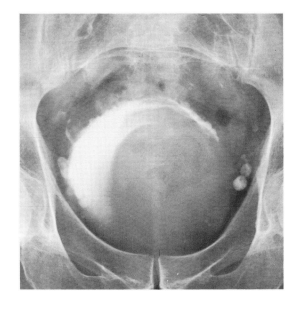

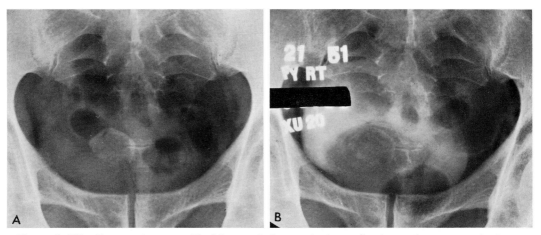

Figure 5–274. Encrustation on residual intravesical prostatic tissue after incomplete transurethral resection. Lesion simulates encrusted bladder tumor. **A,** *Plain film.* **B,** *Excretory cystogram.*

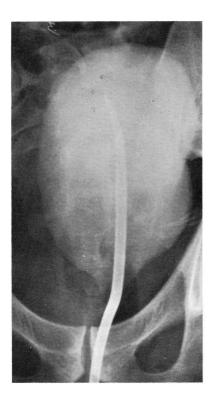

Figure 5–275. *Retrograde cystogram.* Marked displacement of bladder upward and to left due to enormous benign prostatic hyperplasia. (Suprapubic prostatectomy was done; prostate gland weighed 787 gm.)

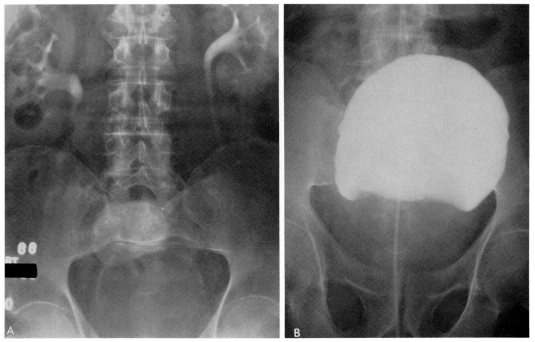

Figure 5–276. Upward displacement of bladder by large hyperplastic prostate gland (384 gm). **A,** *Excretory urogram, 10-minute film.* Normal kidneys and ureters. **Large vesical calculus** overlying upper part of sacrum. Thin rim of contrast medium surrounds intravesical protrusion of prostate. **B,** *Retrograde cystogram.* Bladder pushed upward almost out of pelvis.

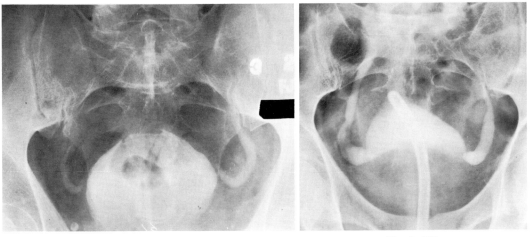

Fig. 5–277   Fig. 5–278

Figure 5–277. *Excretory urogram.* Characteristic "fish hook" contour of terminal portions of ureters caused by upward displacement of trigone and base of bladder from enlarged prostate gland.

Figure 5–278. *Excretory urogram.* "Fish hook" contour of terminal portions of ureters from hypertrophied prostate gland.

A

B

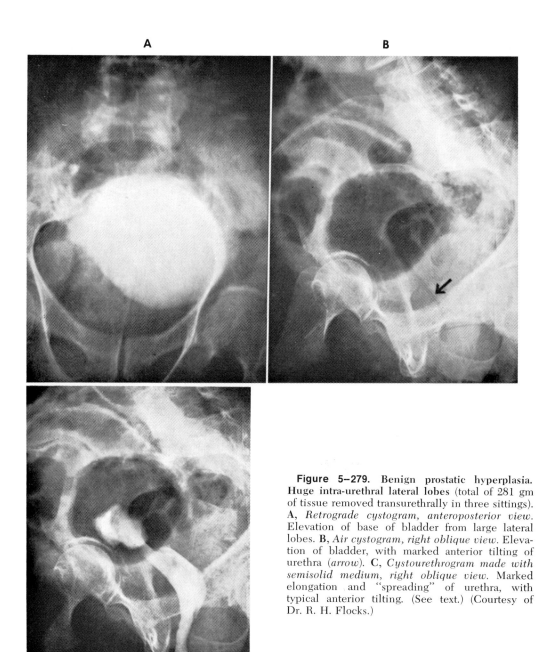

C

Figure 5–279. Benign prostatic hyperplasia. Huge intra-urethral lateral lobes (total of 281 gm of tissue removed transurethrally in three sittings). **A,** *Retrograde cystogram, anteroposterior view.* Elevation of base of bladder from large lateral lobes. **B,** *Air cystogram, right oblique view.* Elevation of bladder, with marked anterior tilting of urethra (*arrow*). **C,** *Cystourethrogram made with semisolid medium, right oblique view.* Marked elongation and "spreading" of urethra, with typical anterior tilting. (See text.) (Courtesy of Dr. R. H. Flocks.)

A

B

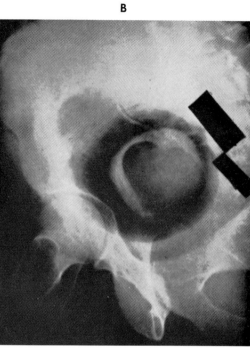

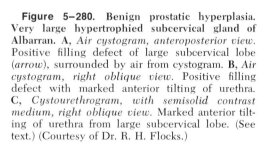

C

Figure 5–280. Benign prostatic hyperplasia. Very large hypertrophied subcervical gland of Albarran. **A,** *Air cystogram, anteroposterior view.* Positive filling defect of large subcervical lobe (*arrow*), surrounded by air from cystogram. **B,** *Air cystogram, right oblique view.* Positive filling defect with marked anterior tilting of urethra. **C,** *Cystourethrogram, with semisolid contrast medium, right oblique view.* Marked anterior tilting of urethra from large subcervical lobe. (See text.) (Courtesy of Dr. R. H. Flocks.)

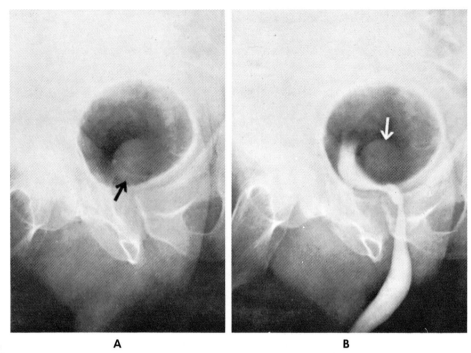

A   **B**

Figure 5–281. **Benign prostatic hyperplasia. Large intravesical median lobe. A,** *Air cystogram, right oblique view.* Positive filling defect from median lobe *(arrow).* **B,** *Cystourethrogram made with semisolid medium, right oblique view.* Marked anterior tilting of urethra from enlarged median lobe, which also casts shadow of positive filling defect in air cystogram *(arrow).* (Courtesy of Dr. R. H. Flocks.)

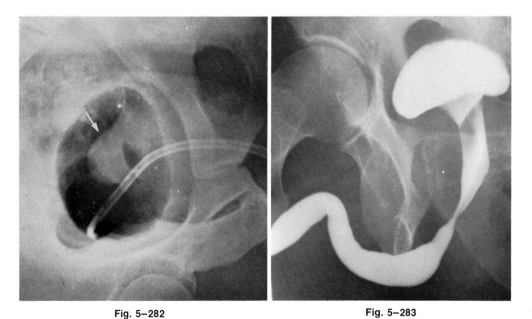

Fig. 5–282   **Fig. 5–283**

Figure 5–282. *Air cystogram, right oblique view.* **Filling defect from intravesical median lobe** *(arrow).* Marked anterior tilting of urethra.

Figure 5–283. *Retrograde urethrogram* of patient with **benign hyperplasia of prostate.** Spreading and elongation of prostatic urethra are pathognomonic of marked intra-urethral enlargement of lateral lobes.

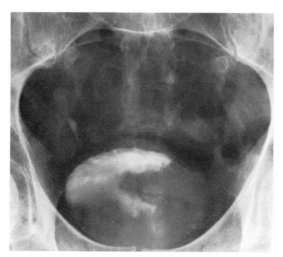

Figure 5–284. *Excretory cystogram.* **Recurrent carcinoma of prostate gland,** with irregular intravesical projection of tissue, which simulates carcinoma of bladder.

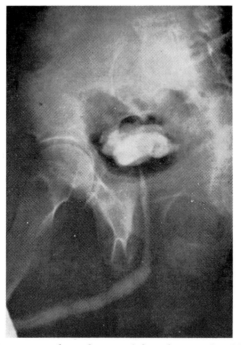

Figure 5–285. *Cystourethrogram made with semisolid medium, right oblique position.* **Carcinoma of prostate gland.** Straight narrow prostatic urethra is typical of this disease. (Three preliminary films gave negative findings, showing no deformity of the vesical outline.) (Courtesy of Dr. R. H. Flocks.)

POSTOPERATIVE CONTRACTURE OF THE VESICAL NECK

by

Laurence F. Greene

This condition, consisting of the formation of scar tissue at the vesical neck, may follow a suprapubic, perineal, or transurethral prostatectomy. In its mildest form, it produces an elevation of the posterior lip of the vesical neck or a slight circumferential narrowing and rigidity; in its severest form, complete or nearly complete occlusion of the vesical neck occurs. On the basis of experimental and clinical studies, Greene, Robinson, and Campbell suggested that the formation of a contracture after transurethral prostatic resection results from excessive electroexcision and electrocoagulation of the vesical neck.

A diagnosis of postoperative contracture of the vesical neck should be considered if a patient's urinary symptoms are relieved by adequate prostatic resection but return shortly thereafter. An impediment or obstruction blocking the passage of instruments in the region of the vesical neck suggests the diagnosis. Retrograde urethrography usually fails to show distinctive changes which will permit the diagnosis of a mild or moderate contracture. Severe or diaphragmatic contractures, on the other hand, may be diagnosed readily by retrograde urethrography; such contractures offer resistance to the free flow of contrast medium into the bladder and the resulting increased intraurethral pressure causes dilation of the distensible unscarred segments of the prostatic, bulbous, and pendulous portions of the urethra (Figs. 5–286, 5–287, and 5–288). The contracted vesical neck is visualized, and from this point the medium spreads, in a fan shape, into the bladder. If the urethrographic contrast medium is more viscid than usual, it will retain its shape as it passes through the small opening in the diaphragm and will form coils or layers in the bladder. Greene and Robinson (1965; 1966) called this appearance of the medium in the roentgenogram the *toothpaste sign of diaphragmatic contracture* (Figs. 5–289, 5–290, and 5–291). Ureteral obstruction from inclusion of the ureteral orifices in the scar tissue is a not uncommon complication (Fig. 5–292).

Finally, the diagnosis may be established by using urethroscopy to visualize the contracture. For this purpose, the panendoscope with a Foroblique lens is the instrument of choice. The instrument is passed under vision to the contracture and the various degrees of circumferential narrowing of the vesical neck are appreciated. When the ureteral orifices are "caught" in the scar tissue and pulled down into the region of the vesical neck they may be very difficult to see.

Prophylaxis against postoperative contractures consists in recognizing the prostatic configuration in which trauma to the vesical neck is likely to occur during resection and modifying the operation accordingly. In such cases, the resection should be limited to the adenoma, thereby preventing trauma to the vesical neck and adjacent structures.

Conservative treatment is advisable not only for patients with mild or moderate postoperative contractures but also for selected patients with severe or even diaphragmatic contractures; occasionally, the latter will disappear, not to reappear, after one dilatation with sounds. Unfortunately, in most instances, dilatation affords only temporary relief and the contracture and associated symptoms soon recur. Nevertheless, patients whose symptoms can be controlled by the infrequent passage of sounds should follow such a regimen. If this type of therapy is unsuccessful, resection of the contracture, repeated if necessary, can be undertaken. However, a decision to treat a contracture by transurethral incision or excision should not be arrived at lightly, because in an appreciable number of cases, the severity of the contracture and of the associated symptoms will be increased by such procedures. Finally, if these measures fail, an open, surgical revision of the vesical neck may be necessary. In the case of marked stenosis of one or both ureteral orifices, transvesical meatotomy or ureteroneocystostomy may be necessary.

(Text continued on page 581.)

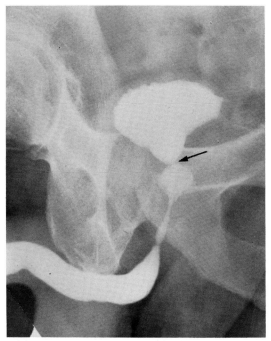

Figure 5–286. *Retrograde urethrogram.* **Severe postoperative contracture (diaphragm) of vesical neck** (*arrow*), which occurred after transurethral prostatic resection.

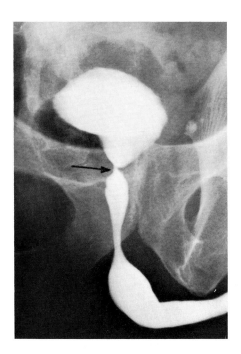

Figure 5–287. *Retrograde urethrogram.* **Severe contracture (diaphragm) of vesical neck** (*arrow*) after transurethral resection.

Figure 5–288. *Retrograde urethrogram.* **Severe contracture (diaphragm) of vesical neck** (*arrow*) after transurethral resection.

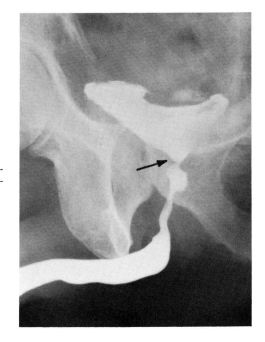

Fig. 5–289

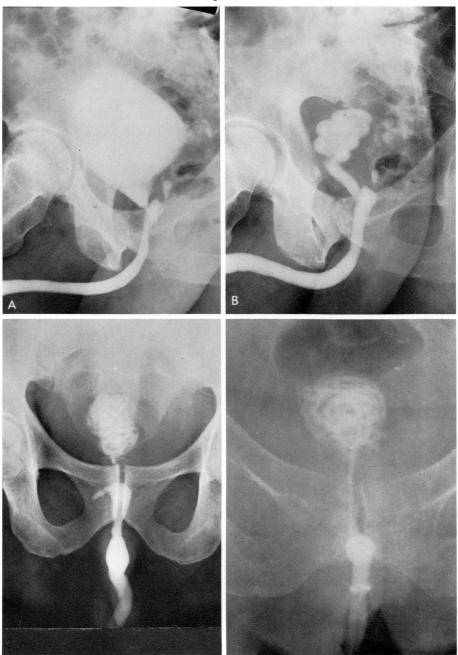

Fig. 5–290   Fig. 5–291

Figure 5–289. A, Severe contracture of vesical neck after transurethral prostatic resection. *Retrograde urethrograms.* **A,** *Made with usual medium.* Ventral position of small aperture of vesical neck (as seen cystoscopically in roof of prostatic urethra) is clearly shown. **B,** *Made with more viscid medium.* Medium being squeezed through contracted vesical neck layers in bladder ("toothpaste" sign).

Figure 5–290. *Retrograde urethrogram made with viscid contrast medium.* **Severe contracture of vesical neck** after transurethral prostatic resection. Note "toothpaste" sign due to medium being forced through small aperture at vesical neck and layering out in bladder.

Figure 5–291. *Retrograde urethrogram made with viscid contrast medium.* **Severe contracture of vesical neck of woman,** which occurred after repeated resections of vesical neck. Note "toothpaste" sign.

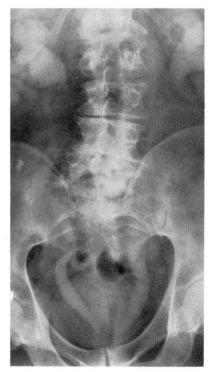

Figure 5–292. Bilateral ureteropyelectasis from ureteral obstruction from postoperative contracture of vesical neck.

Urethral Diverticula in the Male*

Congenital (primary) urethral diverticulum in the male is a relatively rare condition. Acquired (secondary) diverticulum is more common and usually results from trauma and infection of the urethra secondary to transurethral resection. In a review of the literature in 1955 Warren found 236 cases of which 96 were considered to be congenital. Primary or congenital diverticula are lined by normal urethral epithelium, whereas acquired diverticula are not. Lesions of either type may be located in the pendulous or bulbous portions of the urethra.

CONGENITAL (PRIMARY) DIVERTICULA

Mandler and Pool found three cases of congenital diverticulum that had been treated at the Mayo Clinic during 21 years, 1945 through 1965. One patient was a boy, age 3½ years; the other two were men, age 31 and 44.

Abeshouse stated that congenital diverticula become symptomatic during the first 20 years of the patient's life. In Mandler and Pool's cases, one presented in childhood; the other two adult patients had not developed symptoms until adolescence or adulthood.

---

*Diverticula in the female is considered in Chapter 18, pages 1954–1957. See also discussion in Chapter 12, page 1548.

Symptoms consist primarily of "incontinence" characterized by prolonged terminal dribbling of urine after voiding, as the diverticulum gradually empties itself. If the diverticulum is fairly large with considerable stasis from poor emptying, urinary infection may be superimposed. All three of Mandler and Pool's patients apparently had adequate drainage, and there was no urinary infection.

Diagnosis is made by means of retrograde urethrography (Figs. 5–293, 5–294, and 5–295) and confirmed by urethroscopic examination with the panendoscope.

Treatment consists of surgical excision and urethral reconstruction. Usually temporary urinary diversion is not necessary. Because of the high incidence of fistula formation after reconstruction of the pendulous urethra the two-stage urethroplasty (Culp, 1959) may be necessary.

ACQUIRED (SECONDARY) DIVERTICULA

Acquired diverticula are usually the result of trauma and periurethritis or periurethral abscess. The penoscrotal junction is the most common location for those which follow transurethral resection or prolonged drainage with indwelling urethral catheters, as in cases of paraplegia (Figs. 5–296, 5–297, and 5–298).

(Text continued on page 585.)

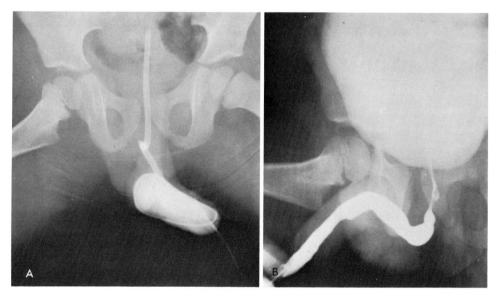

Figure 5–293.   Congenital diverticulum of pendulous urethra in 3½-year-old boy. **A,** *Retrograde diverticulogram.* Urethral catheter in bladder. Ureteral catheter was passed alongside and into diverticulum and injected with contrast medium, filling diverticulum. (Surgical excision was done.) **B,** *Postoperative retrograde urethrogram.* (From Mandler, J. I., and Pool, T. L.)

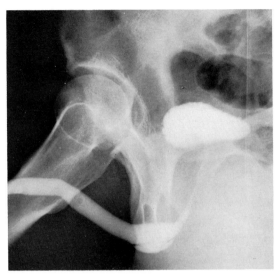

Figure 5–294. *Retrograde urethrogram.* **Congenital (?) diverticulum of bulbous urethra** in man, aged 31 (patient had had postmicturition dribbling since age 16). (With panendoscope, 3-mm opening into diverticulum could be seen in floor of urethra. Surgical excision was performed.) (From Mandler, J. I., and Pool, T. L.)

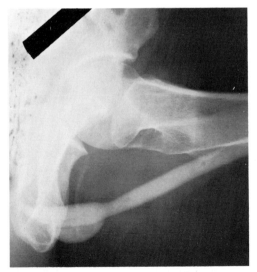

Figure 5–295. *Retrograde urethrogram.* **Diverticulum of bulbous urethra** of man, aged 44. (Etiology unknown.) (Patient had had postmicturition dribbling for 1 year.) (Cystoscopy [panendoscope] showed 1.5-mm opening into diverticulum in floor of urethra. Surgical excision was performed.) (From Mandler, J. I., and Pool, T. L.)

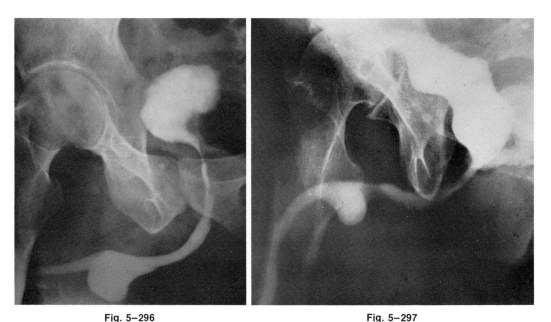

Fig. 5–296   Fig. 5–297

Figure 5–296. *Retrograde cystourethrogram.* Acquired diverticulum (result of periurethral abscess) in anterior urethra of male patient.

Figure 5–297. *Micturition cystourethrogram* of man, 72 years of age. Urethral diverticulum, probably secondary to periurethral abscess. Note wide prostatic fossa. (Patient had had retropubic prostatectomy 1 year previously.) (Courtesy of Dr. H. W. ten Cate.)

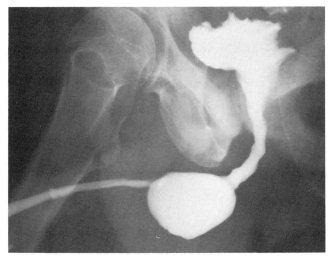

Figure 5–298. *Retrograde cystourethrogram.* Acquired (post-transurethral resection) urethral diverticulum. (Diverticulum resulted from postoperative periureteritis and periurethral abscess.)

Urethral Stricture in Adult Males*

Cystourethrography is of distinct value in the diagnosis of urethral stricture. It is of especial value in accurately localizing the site of the stricture and outlining irregularities, old false passages (from previous instrumentation), abscess pockets, and fistulas. The smaller the caliber of the stricture the easier it is to demonstrate. Lapides and Stone's study indicates that strictures of 20-F caliber and smaller are easily identified with the urethrogram; those of larger caliber, they consider more difficult to identify.

INFLAMMATORY STRICTURES

Inflammatory strictures (chiefly from previous Neisserian urethritis) are becoming less common. The majority of these old gonorrheal strictures are located in the bulbous urethra, although the anterior urethra may be involved. A characteristic finding in inflammatory strictures is that, although the main stricture appears to be confined to one relatively short segment, the entire urethra is narrowed (Figs. 5-299 through 5-303). The urethrogram can illustrate **false passages** made by sounds during dilatation of strictures. Often **communication of these false passages with the venous circulation** may be seen, providing a graphic explanation of the frequency of chills and fever following urethral instrumentation (Figs. 5-304 through 5-311). Perineal fistula resulting from Neisserian stricture (so-called watering-pot perineum) was common before the introduction of sulfonamides and penicillin. Today they are relatively infrequent (Fig. 5-312; see Chapter 15).

---

*Urethral stricture in children has been discussed previously (page 544).

TRAUMATIC AND IATROGENIC STRICTURES

Traumatic strictures result from either accidents (fracture of the pelvis, saddle injuries, and others) or urethral instrumentation. Because of the large numbers of transurethral prostatic resections and transurethral resections of bladder tumors being done, iatrogenic instrumental strictures (caused by the resectoscope) are now encountered much more commonly. They are caused by the use of instruments of too large caliber for the urethra.

Traumatic strictures differ from inflammatory strictures in that they usually are shorter and more localized, and the caliber of the remainder of the urethra may be normal or relatively normal. In the case of *fracture of the pelvis* the urethra may be sheared off near the apex of the prostate and the stricture occurs at that point (in the membranous urethra). *Straddle injuries*, blows, and other injuries may cause stricture near the penoscrotal junction where the urethra impinges on the symphysis pubis (Fig. 5-313). Stricture at the site of vesicourethral nastomosis, after radical perineal prostatectomy, is occasionally encountered (Fig. 5-314).

Iatrogenic (instrumental) strictures are most commonly located in the anterior urethra at its two normally narrow points: (1) the penoscrotal junction and (2) the urethral meatus and fossa navicularis. As in traumatic strictures, they may remain localized and short, with the remainder of the urethra of more or less normal caliber (Figs. 5-315 through 5-318). On the other hand, the entire anterior urethra may have been damaged so that it may be completely strictured (Figs. 5-319 through 5-322). Also, iatrogenic (post-transurethral resection) strictures of the bulbomembranous urethra do occur (Fig. 5-323). They usually follow use of the "hot loop" resectoscope; in contrast, lesions of the penoscrotal junction are more common after use of the "cold punch" instrument.

Instrumental strictures may be prevented by preliminary careful calibration of the urethra with Otis diagnostic bulbs. If the anterior urethra does not admit a size 30-F bulb easily, three procedures are available: (1) use of a size 24-F resectoscope, (2) introduction of the resectoscope through an external urethrotomy boutonniere in the large bulbous urethra, or (3) enlargement of the urethra by means of internal urethrotomy. At this clinic, we employ the last procedure (Emmett, Kirchheim, and Greene).

POSTOPERATIVE INCONTINENCE IN THE MALE

Urinary incontinence occurring after various types of prostatectomy usually results from damage to the external urethral sphincter. In some cases this can be demonstrated by a retrograde urethrogram which will show reduction or absence of the normal tonicity of the external sphincter (Figs. 5–324 and 5–325). See discussion of the external urethral sphincter under the heading of neurogenic bladder (page 485).

(References begin on page 600.)

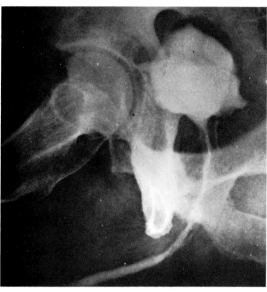
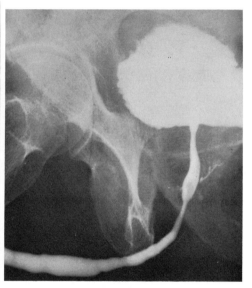

Fig. 5–299   **Fig. 5–300**

Figure 5–299. *Retrograde cystourethrogram, right oblique view.* **Inflammatory stricture of urethra.** Although main portion of stricture is in bulbomembranous segment, entire urethra seems to be considerably narrowed, as is typical of these cases. (Courtesy of Dr. J. J. Alvarez-Ierena.)

Figure 5–300. *Retrograde urethrogram.* **Long-standing stricture involving primarily bulbous urethra.** Stricture is long and diffuse, and there is also some reduction in caliber of anterior urethra. Ejaculatory ducts and some prostatic ducts are outlined with contrast medium.

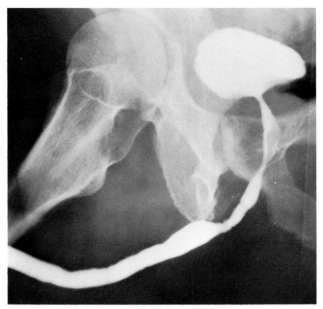

Figure 5–301. *Retrograde urethrogram.* **Old Neisserian stricture of bulbous urethra.** Note minimal narrowing of entire urethra (compare with retrograde urethrogram of normal urethra [Figs. 4–182, 4–183, and 4–184]).

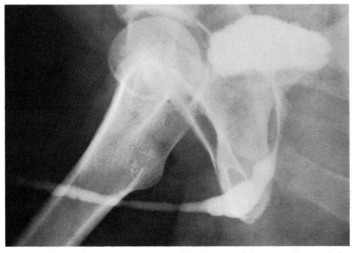

Figure 5–302. *Retrograde urethrogram.* **Stricture of entire pendulous urethra and distal half of bulbous urethra.** Etiology not known.

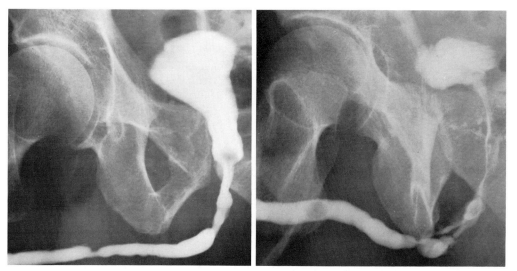

Fig. 5–303   Fig. 5–304

Figure 5–303. *Retrograde urethrogram.* Inflammatory stricture primarily of penoscrotal juncture but, to lesser degree, involving both pendulous and bulbous portions of urethra.

Figure 5–304. *Retrograde urethrogram.* Stricture of bulbomembranous urethra with false passage from recent dilatation.

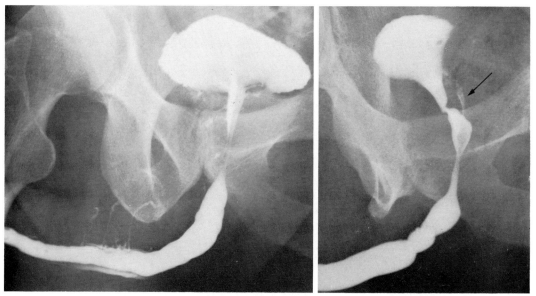

Fig. 5–305   Fig. 5–306

Figure 5–305. *Retrograde urethrogram.* Recently dilated stricture in region of penoscrotal juncture. Note some extravasation of contrast medium filling veins which apparently communicate with dorsal vein of penis.

Figure 5–306. *Retrograde urethrogram.* Stricture of bulbomembranous urethra recently dilated. Note false passage (*arrow*) between floor of prostatic urethra and trigone of bladder (under posterior vesical lip).

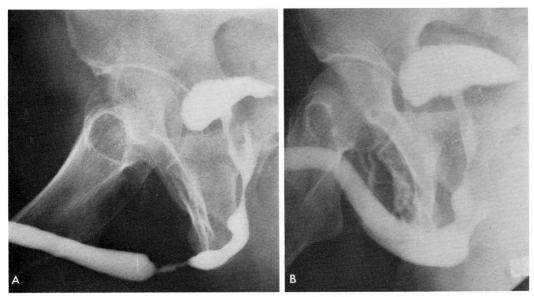

Figure 5–307. Stricture of perineal urethra just proximal to penoscrotal juncture. *Retrograde urethro-grams.* **A,** *Before dilatation.* **B,** *Immediately after dilatation.* "False passage" and extravasation of contrast medium. Note contrast medium filling periurethral veins anteriorly.

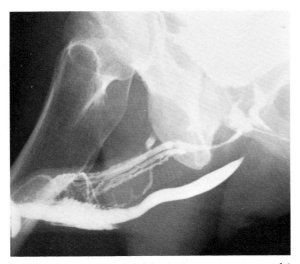

Figure 5–308. *Retrograde urethrogram.* **Large-caliber stricture at penoscrotal junction** in man, 30 years of age. Periurethral extravasation of medium fills dorsal vein of penis and communicating veins. Urethrogram made prior to dilatation of stricture.

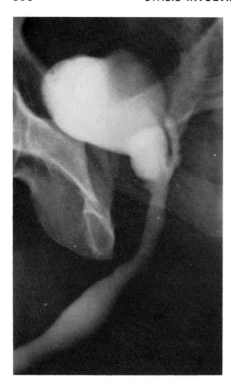

Figure 5–309. *Cystourethrogram.* Fistula between bladder and bulbous urethra after dilatation of urethral stricture with sounds, during which false passage was made. Patient was incontinent as result of this fistula.

Figure 5–310. Stricture of bulbous urethra with false passage made on attempted dilatation. *Retrograde urethrograms.* **A,** *Initial film.* False passage is evident. **B,** *Second film,* after injection of more contrast medium. Extravasation of contrast medium which outlines dorsal vein of penis.

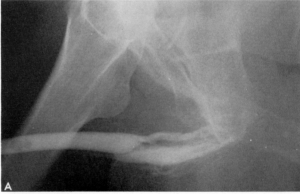

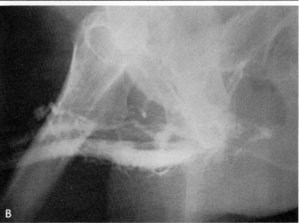

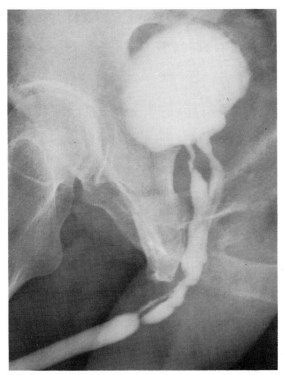

Figure 5–311. *Retrograde urethrogram.* Urethral stricture of bulbous urethra with false passage extending into bladder.

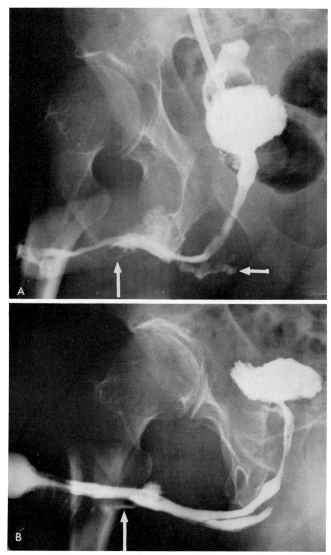

Figure 5–312. Multiple small-caliber strictures of pendulous portion of urethra with urethrocutaneous fistula at penoscrotal junction and false passage in perineal portion of urethra. **A,** *Voiding cystourethrogram* (contrast medium introduced through suprapubic cystostomy tube). Fistula at penoscrotal junction (*vertical arrow*) and false passage proximally (*horizontal arrow*). **B,** *Retrograde urethrogram,* made after internal urethrotomy and drainage with indwelling catheter (suprapubic tube had been removed). Small amount of medium is escaping from fistula (*arrow*). Well-filled false passage appears to begin in region of penoscrotal junction and to extend into bulbous urethra.

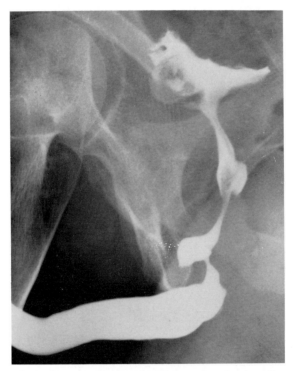

Figure 5–313. *Retrograde urethrogram.* Traumatic stricture of perineal portion of urethra from previous fracture of pelvis. Urethra had been repaired through perineum, resulting in deformity and reforming of stricture.

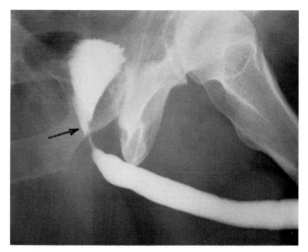

Figure 5–314. *Retrograde urethrogram.* Postoperative stricture at site of vesicourethral anastomosis (*arrow*) which followed radical perineal prostatectomy.

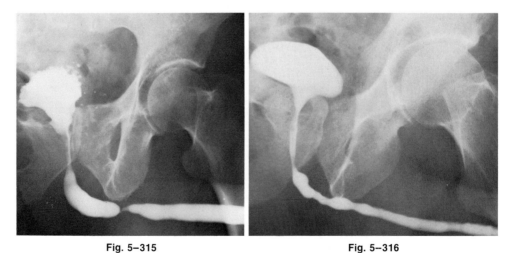

Fig. 5–315   Fig. 5–316

Figure 5–315. *Retrograde urethrogram.* Iatrogenic stricture at penoscrotal junction from previous transurethral resection.

Figure 5–316. *Retrograde urethrogram.* Iatrogenic (instrumental) stricture of entire urethra.

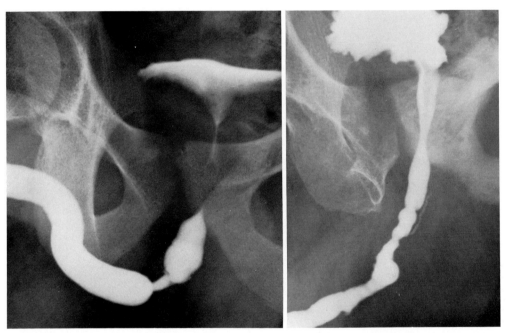

Fig. 5–317   Fig. 5–318

Figure 5–317. *Retrograde urethrogram.* **Iatrogenic stricture of bulbous urethra** in boy, 17 years of age, caused by prolonged use of indwelling catheter after automobile accident. (Patient had severe brain injury.)

Figure 5–318. *Retrograde urethrogram.* **Iatrogenic stricture of urethra in region of penoscrotal juncture and extending proximally.** Stricture had persisted in spite of Johannsen's operation. Note contrast medium outlining vein parallel to bulbous urethra.

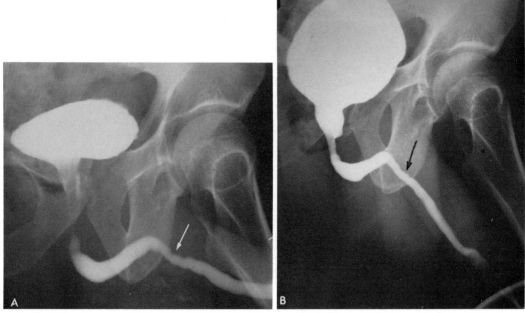

Figure 5-319. Iatrogenic (post-transurethral resection) stricture mainly at penoscrotal junction (*arrows*), but it also involves pendulous portion of urethra. **A,** *Retrograde urethrogram.* **B,** *Voiding cystourethrogram.*

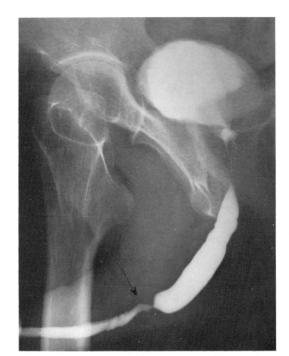

Figure 5–320. *Retrograde urethrogram.* Iatrogenic (post-transurethral resection) stricture at penoscrotal junction (*arrow*) and pendulous urethra. Postoperative contracture of vesical neck also is present.

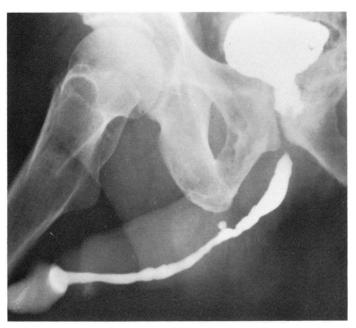

Figure 5–321. Iatrogenic (post-transurethral resection) stricture involving penoscrotal junction, entire pendulous portion of urethra, and distal half of bulbous portion.

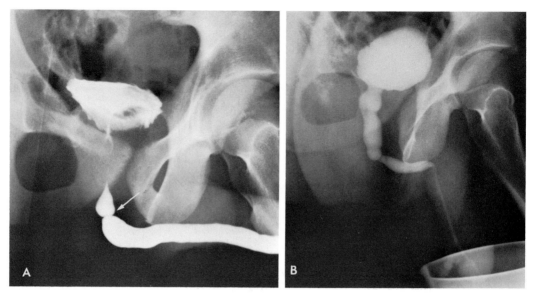

Figure 5–322. Iatrogenic stricture of bulbous urethra of boy, aged 18, after transurethral removal of bladder polyps. **A,** *Retrograde urethrogram.* Stricture (*arrow*) is short. **B,** *Voiding cystourethrogram.* Note dilatation of urethra proximal to stricture.

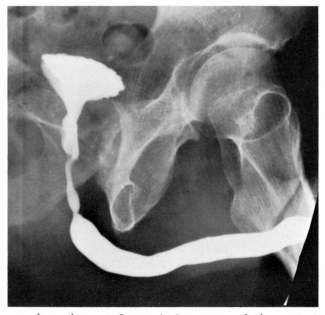

Figure 5–323. *Retrograde urethrogram.* Iatrogenic (post-transurethral resection) stricture of bulbous portion of urethra. Remainder of urethra is normal.

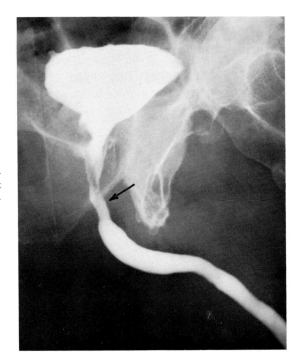

Figure 5–324. *Retrograde urethrogram.* **Post-transurethral-resection incontinence.** Note lack of tonicity of external urethral sphincter (*arrow*).

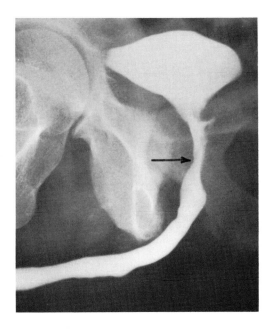

Figure 5–325. *Retrograde urethrogram.* **Post-transurethral-resection incontinence.** Note relaxation (lack of tonicity) of external urethral sphincter (*arrow*). Also, some residual adenomatous prostatic tissue remains near apex of prostatic urethra.

REFERENCES

Abeshouse, B. S.: Diverticula of the Anterior Urethra in the Male: A Report of Four Cases and a Review of the Literature. Urol. & Cutan. Rev. 55:690-707, 1951.

Ambrose, S. S., and Nicolson, W. P., III: Vesicoureteral Reflux Secondary to Anomalies of the Ureterovesical Junction: Management and Results. J. Urol. 87:695-700 (May) 1962.

Anderson, K. N., and Ansell, J. S.: Congenital Valves of the Posterior Urethra. J. Urol. 95:783-784 (June) 1966.

Ansell, J. S.: The Bischoff Submucosal Ureteroplasty: A Clinical Evaluation. J. Urol. 95:768-770 (June) 1966.

Ansell, J. S., and Paterson, J. R. S.: Intermittent Hydronephrosis. New England J. Med. 267:447-448 (Aug. 30) 1962.

Beard, D. E., Goodyear, W. E., and Weens, H. S.: Radiologic Diagnosis of the Lower Urinary Tract. Springfield, Illinois, Charles C Thomas, 1952, 143 pp.

Becker, J. A., and Pollack, H.: Cinefluorographic Studies of the Normal Upper Urinary Tract. Radiology 84:886-893 (May) 1965.

Belker, A. M., Flocks, R. H., Culp, D. A., and Immergut, M. A.: Cystourethrography as a Teaching Aid in Prostatic Surgery. J. Urol. 95:818-826 (June) 1966.

Benham, A. M., Halikiopoulos, H. J., and Hodges, C. V.: Urinary Tract Infection in Girls: A Ten Year Followup Report. J. Urol. 86:669-672 (Nov.) 1961.

Bettex, M., Genton, N., and Schärli, A.: Results of Uretero-cysto-neostomy in Vesico-ureteric Reflux in Infants and Children. Arch. Dis. Childhood 41:160-164 (Apr.) 1966.

Bischoff, P.: Megaureter. Brit. J. Urol. 29:416-423, 1957.

Bischoff, P. F.: Operative Treatment of Megaureter. J. Urol. 85:268-274 (Mar.) 1961.

Bischoff, P. F., and Bresch, H. G.: Origin, Clinical Experiences and Treatment of Urinary Obstructions of the Lower Ureter in Childhood. J. Urol. 85:739-748 (May) 1961.

Blumel, Johanna, Evans, E. B., and Eggers, G. W. N.: Partial and Complete Agenesis or Malformation of the Sacrum with Associated Anomalies: Etiologic and Clinical Study With Special Reference to Heredity; a Preliminary Report. J. Bone & Joint Surg. 41A:497-518 (Apr.) 1959.

Bodian, M.: Some Observations on the Pathology of Congenital "Idiopathic Bladder-Neck Obstruction" (Marion's Disease). Brit. J. Urol. 29:393-398, 1957.

Bors, E.: Neurogenic Bladder. In Piersol, G. M.: The Cyclopedia of Medicine, Surgery Specialties. Philadelphia, F. A. Davis Company, Ed. 3, vol. 9, 1951, pp. 603-614.

Bors, E.: Neurogenic Bladder. Urol. Survey 7:177-250 (June) 1957.

Bourne, R. B.: Intermittent Hydronephrosis as a Cause of Abdominal Pain. J.A.M.A. 198:1218-1219 (Dec. 12) 1966.

Bumpus, H. C., Jr., Nourse, M. H., and Thompson,

G. J.: Urologic Complications in Injury of the Spinal Cord. J.A.M.A. 133:366-368 (Feb. 8) 1947.

Bunge, R. G.: Further Observations With Delayed Cystograms. J. Urol. 71:427-434 (Apr.) 1954.

Burns, E., and Kittredge, W. E.: Surgical Procedures on the Vesical Neck. Tr. Am. A. Genito-Urin. Surgeons 49:204-207, 1957.

Bustos, F., Lichtwardt, J. R., and Lichtwardt, H. E.: Benign Non-epithelial Tumors of the Ureter. J. Urol. (In press.)

Campbell, J. B.: Neurosurgical Treatment of Bladder and Bowel Dysfunction Resulting From Anomalous Development of the Sacral Neural Axis. Clin. Neurosurg. 8:133-156 (Oct.) 1960.

Campbell, M. F.: Clinical Pediatric Urology. Philadelphia, W. B. Saunders Company, 1951, 1,113 pp.

Campbell, M. F.: Urology. Ed. 2, Philadelphia, W. B. Saunders Company, 1963.

Chang, C.-Y.: Anterior Urethral Valves: A Case Report. J. Urol. 100:29-31 (July) 1968.

Cobb, B. G., Wolf, J. A., Jr., and Ansell, J. S.: Congenital Stricture of the Proximal Urethral Bulb. J. Urol. 99:629-631 (May) 1968.

Colabawalla, B. N.: Anterior Urethral Valve: A Case Report. J. Urol. 94:58-59 (July) 1965.

Creevy, C. D.: The Atonic Distal Ureteral Segment (Ureteral Achalasia). J. Urol. 97:457-463 (Mar.) 1967a.

Creevy, C. D.: Vesicoureteral Reflux in Children: A Review. Urol. Survey 17:279-306 (Oct.) 1967b.

Culp, O. S.: Treatment of Ureteropelvic Obstruction. Am. Urol. A., North Central Sect., Postgrad. Seminar 278-288, 1955.

Culp, O. S.: Experiences With 200 Hypospadiacs: Evolution of a Therapeutic Plan. S. Clin. North America 39:1007-1023 (Aug.) 1959.

Culp, O. S.: Choice of Operations for Ureteropelvic Obstruction: Review of 385 Cases. Canad. J. Surg. 4:157-165 (Jan.) 1961.

Culp, O. S., and DeWeerd, J. H.: A Pelvic Flap Operation for Certain Types of Ureteropelvic Obstruction: Observations After Two Years' Experience. J. Urol. 71:523-529 (May) 1954.

Damanski, M.: Cystourethrography in Paraplegia as a Guide to Catheter-Free Life: 17 Years' Experience of a Paraplegic Center. J. Urol. 93:466-471 (Apr.) 1965.

Damanski, M., and Kerr, A. S.: The Value of Cystourethrography in Paraplegia. Brit. J. Urol. 44:398-407, 1956-1957.

Daniel, J., Stewart, A. M., and Blair, D. W.: Congenital Anterior Urethral Valve – Diagnosis and Treatment. Brit. J. Urol. 40:589-591 (Oct.) 1968.

Daut, R. V., Emmett, J. L., and Kennedy, R. L. J.: Congenital Absence of Abdominal Muscles With Urologic Complications: Report on a Patient Successfully Treated. Proc. Staff Meet., Mayo Clin. 22:8-13 (Jan. 8) 1947.

Edwards, D.: The Lower Urinary Tract. Proc. Roy. Soc. Med. 59:417-419 (May) 1966.

Ekman, H., Jacobsson, B., Kock, N. G., and Sundin, T.: High Diuresis, a Factor in Preventing Vesicoureteral Reflux. J. Urol. 95:511-515 (Apr.) 1966.

Eliason, O. D., and Smith, J. P.: Ureteral Advancement for Correction of Vesicoureteral Reflux: Experience With 50 Patients in a 3-Year Period. J. Urol. 98:331-334 (Sept.) 1967.

Ellis, D. G., Fonkalsrud, E. W., and Smith, J. P.: Congenital Posterior Urethral Valves. J. Urol. 95:549-554 (Apr.) 1966.

Emmett, J. L.: Further Observations in the Management of Cord Bladder by Transurethral Resection. J. Urol. 57:29-41 (Jan.) 1947.

Emmett, J. L.: Neuromuscular Disease of the Urinary Tract. 1. Physiology of the Normal Bladder: Neurophysiology of Micturition. 2. Neurogenic Vesical Dysfunction (Cord Bladder) and Neuromuscular Ureteral Dysfunction. In Campbell, M. F.: Urology, Philadelphia, W. B. Saunders Company, vol. 2, 1954, pp. 1255-1383.

Emmett, J. L., Albers, D. D., and Anderson, R. E.: Statistical and Analytic Review of the Final Results of Transurethral Resection for Cord Bladder. J. Urol. 65:36-59 (Jan.) 1951.

Emmett, J. L., and Beare, J. B.: Bladder Difficulties of Tabetic Patients: With Special Reference to Treatment by Transurethral Resection. J.A.M.A. 117:1930-1934 (Dec. 6) 1941.

Emmett, J. L., and Beare, J. B.: Transurethral Resection for Vesical Dysfunction in Cases of Tabes Dorsalis. J.A.M.A. 136:1093-1096 (Apr. 24) 1948.

Emmett, J. L., Daut, R. V., and Dunn, J. H.: Role of the External Urethral Sphincter in the Normal Bladder and Cord Bladder. J. Urol. 59:439-454 (Mar.) 1948.

Emmett, J. L., Daut, R. V., and Sprague, R. G.: Transurethral Resection for Neurogenic Vesical Dysfunction in Cases of Diabetic Neuropathy. J. Urol. 61:244-257 (Feb.) 1949.

Emmett, J. L., and Dunn, J. H.: Transurethral Resection in the Surgical Management of Cord Bladder. Surg., Gynec. & Obst. 83:597-612 (Nov.) 1946.

Emmett, J. L., and Greene, L. F.: Neurogenic Vesical Dysfunction (Cord Bladder) and Neuromuscular Ureteral Dysfunction. In Campbell, M. F.: Urology. Ed. 2, Philadelphia, W. B. Saunders Company, 1963, vol. 2, pp. 1406-1504.

Emmett, J. L., and Helmholz, H. F.: Transurethral Resection of the Vesical Neck in Infants and Children. J. Urol. 60:463-478 (Sept.) 1948.

Emmett, J. L., Kirchheim, D., and Greene, L. F.: Prevention of Postoperative Stricture From Transurethral Resection by Preliminary Internal Urethrotomy: Report of Experience With 447 Cases. J. Urol. 78:456-465 (Oct.) 1957.

Emmett, J. L., and Love, J. G.: Urinary Retention in Women Caused by Asymptomatic Protruded Lumbar Disk: Report of 5 Cases. Tr. Am. A. Genito-Urin. Surgeons 59:130-139, 1967.

Emmett, J. L., and Simon, H. B.: Transurethral Resection in Infants and Children for Congenital Obstruction of the Vesical Neck and Myelodysplasia. J. Urol. 76:595-608 (Nov.) 1956.

Emmett, J. L., Simon, H. B., and Mills, S. D.: Neuromuscular Disease of the Urinary Tract in Infants and Children. Pediat. Clin. North America 803-818 (Aug.) 1955.

Engle, W. J., and Schlumberger, F. C.: Urinary Extravasation in New-Born Infant Associated With Congenital Stenosis of Urethra: Report of Case. Cleveland Clin. Quart. 5:278-283, 1938.

Falk, D.: Intermittent Obstruction at the Ureteropelvic Juncture. J. Urol. 79:16-20 (Jan.) 1958.

Fisher, O. D., and Forsythe, W. I.: Micturating Cystourethrography in the Investigation of Enuresis. Arch. Dis. Child. 29:460-471 (Oct.) 1954.

Flocks, R. H.: The Roentgen Visualization of the Posterior Urethra. J. Urol. 30:711-736 (Dec.) 1933.

Frates, R., and DeLuca, F. G.: Urethral Polyps in Male Children. Radiology 89:289-291 (Aug.) 1967.

Freedman, B.: Congenital Absence of the Sacrum and Coccyx: Report of a Case and Review of the Literature. Brit. J. Surg. 37:299-303 (Jan.) 1950.

Fuqua, F., Alexander, J. C., King, K. B., and Ware, E. W., Jr.: The Operative Correction of Vesicoureteral Reflux in the Nonparaplegic Child: Indications, Technique and Results. J. Urol. 80:443-447 (Dec.) 1958.

Garrett, R. A., and Switzer, R. W.: Antireflux Surgery in Children. J.A.M.A. 195:636-638 (Feb. 21) 1966.

Gatewood Baghdassarian, Olga M., Calhoun, R. C., and Levin, S.: Pedunculated Polyp of the Posterior Urethra. J. Urol. 97:1052-1055 (June) 1967.

Giertz, G., and Lindblom, K.: Urethrocystographic Studies of Nervous Disturbances of the Urinary Bladder and the Urethra: A Preliminary Report. Acta Radiol. 36:205-216 (Sept.) 1951.

Girgis, A. S., Veenema, R. J., and Lattimer, J. K.: Triangular Flap Ureterovesical Anastomosis: A New Technique for Correction or Prevention of Ureteral Reflux. J. Urol. 95:19-26 (Jan.) 1966.

Gleason, D. M., and Lattimer, J. K.: The Pressure-Flow Study: A Method for Measuring Bladder Neck Resistance. J. Urol. 87:844-852 (June) 1962.

Glenn, J. F., and Anderson, E. E.: Distal Tunnel Ureteral Reimplantation. J. Urol. 97:623-626 (Apr.) 1967.

Gould, H. R., and Peterson, C. G., Jr.; Voiding Cystourethrography in Children. Am. J. Roentgenol. 98:192-199 (Sept.) 1966.

Graves, R. C., and Davidoff, L. M.: Studies on the Ureter and Bladder With Especial Reference to Regurgitation of the Vesical Contents. J. Urol. 10:185-231 (Sept.) 1923.

Graves, R. C., and Davidoff, L. M.: II. Studies on the Ureter and Bladder With Especial Reference to Regurgitation of the Vesical Contents. J. Urol. 12:93-103 (Aug.) 1924.

Graves, R. C., and Davidoff, L. M.: III. Studies on the Bladder and Ureters With Especial Reference to Regurgitation of the Vesical Contents: Regurgitation as Observed in Cats and Dogs. J. Urol. 14:1-17 (July) 1925.

Greene, L. F., Emmett, J. L., Culp, O. S., and Kennedy, R. L. J.: Urologic Abnormalities Associated With Congenital Absence or Deficiency of Abdominal Musculature. J. Urol. 68:217-229 (July) 1952

Greene, L. F., and Leary, F. J.: Contractures of the Vesical Neck Following Transurethral Prostatic Resection. Surg., Gynec. & Obst. 124:1277-1282 (June) 1967.

Greene, L. F., Priestley, J. T., Simon, H. B., and Hempstead, R. H.: Obstruction of the Lower Third of the Ureter by Anomalous Blood Vessels. J. Urol. 71:544-548 (May) 1954.

Greene, L. F., and Robinson, H. P.: Postoperative Contracture of the Vesical Neck. V. Clinical Findings, Symptoms and Diagnosis. J. Urol. 94:141-147 (Aug.) 1965.

Greene, L. F., and Robinson, H. P.: Postoperative Contracture of the Vesical Neck. VI. Prophylaxis and Treatment. J. Urol. 95:520-525 (Apr.) 1966.

Greene, L. F., Robinson, H. P.., and Campbell, J. C.: Postoperative Contracture of the Neck of the Bladder. Abstr. Am. Acad. Gen. Pract. 431-432, 1961.

Griesbach, W. A., Waterhouse, R. K., and Mellins, H. Z.: Voiding Cysto-urethrography in the Diagnosis of Congenital Posterior Urethral Valves. Am. J. Roentgenol. 82:521-529 (Sept.) 1959.

Grieve, J.: Bladder Neck Stenosis in Children—Is It Important? Brit. J. Urol. 39:13-16 (Feb.) 1967.

Gross, R. E., Randolph, J., and Wise, H. M., Jr.: Surgical Correction of Bladder-Neck Obstruction in Children. New England J. Med. 268:5-14 (Jan. 3) 1963.

Gruber, C. M.: III. The Function of the Urethrovesical Valve and the Experimental Production of Hydroureters Without Obstruction. J. Urol. 23:161-179 (Feb.) 1930.

Hamm, F. C., and Waterhouse, K.: Changing Concepts in Lower Urinary-Tract Obstruction in Children. J.A.M.A. 175:854-857 (Mar. 11) 1961.

Hanley, H. G.: The Pelvi-ureteric Junction: A Cine-pyelographic Study. Brit. J. Urol. 31:377-384, 1959.

Hanley, H. G.: Hydronephrosis. Lancet 2:664-667 (Sept. 24) 1960.

Harrow, B. R.: The Myth of the Megacystis Syndrome. J. Urol. 98:205 (Aug.) 1967a.

Harrow, B. R.: How Not to Re-implant Double Ureters Into the Bladder. J. Urol. 98:345-346 (Sept.) 1967b.

Harrow, B. R., Sloane, J. A., and Witus, W. S.: A Critical Examination of Bladder Neck Obstruction in Children. J. Urol. 98:613-617 (Nov.) 1967.

Hinman, F.: The Principles and Practice of Urology. Philadelphia, W. B. Saunders Company, 1935, 1,111 pp.

Hodson, C. J.: The Radiological Diagnosis of Pyelonephritis. Proc. Roy. Soc. Med. 52:669-672 (Aug.) 1959.

Hodson, C. J.: Analysis of Hydronephrosis: Back Pressure Atrophy. Postgrad. Seminar, unit 7, pp. 1-6 (Mar.) 1967.

Hodson, C. J., and Craven, J. D.: The Radiology of Obstructive Atrophy of the Kidney. Clin. Radiol. 17:305-320 (Oct.) 1966.

Hodson, C. J., and Edwards, D.: Chronic Pyelonephritis and Vesico-ureteric Reflux. Clin. Radiol. 11:219-231 (Oct.) 1960.

Holm, H.: On Pyelogenic Renal Cysts. Acta radiol. 29:87-94, 1948.

Hope, J. W.: Personal communication to the author.

Hope, J. W., Jameson, P. J., and Michie, A. J.: Diagnosis of Anterior Urethral Valve by Voiding Urethrography: Report of Two Cases. Radiology 74:798-801 (May) 1960.

Howerton, L. W., and Lich, R., Jr.: The Cause and Correction of Ureteral Reflux. J. Urol. 89:672-675 (May) 1963.

Huffman, G. C., and Keitzer, W. A.: Urodynamics of the Lower Urinary Tract. Invest. Urol. 3:1-9 (July) 1965.

Hutch, J. A.: Vesico-ureteral Reflux in the Paraplegic: Cause and Correction. J. Urol. 68:457-467 (Aug.) 1952.

Hutch, J. A.: The Treatment of Hydronephrosis by Sacral Rhizotomy in Paraplegics. J. Urol. 77:123-134 (Feb.) 1957.

Hutch, J. A.: The Ureterovesical Junction. Berkeley and Los Angeles, Univ. of California Press, 1958, 178 pp.

Hutch, J. A.: Saccule Formation at the Ureterovesical Junction in Smooth Walled Bladders. J. Urol. 86:390-399 (Oct.) 1961a.

Hutch, J. A.: Theory of Maturation of the Intravesical Ureter. J. Urol. 86:534-538 (Nov.) 1961b.

Hutch, J. A.: Ureteric Advancement Operation: Anatomy, Technique and Early Results. J. Urol. 89:180-184 (Feb.) 1963.

Hutch, J. A.: A New Theory of the Anatomy of the Internal Urinary Sphincter and the Physiology of Micturition. Invest. Urol. 3:36-58 (July) 1965.

Hutch, J. A.: Personal communication to the authors, 1966.

Hutch, J. A., Ayres, R. D., and Loquvam, G. S.: The Bladder Musculature With Special Reference to the Ureterovesical Junction. J. Urol. 85:531-539 (Apr.) 1961.

Hutch, J. A., and Bunts, R. C.: The Present Urologic Status of the Wartime Paraplegic. J. Urol. 66:218-228 (Aug.) 1951.

Hutch, J. A., and Tanagho, E. A.: Etiology of Nonocclusive Ureteral Dilatation. J. Urol. 93:177-184 (Feb.) 1965.

Immergut, M., Culp, D., and Flocks, R. H.: The Urethral Caliber in Normal Female Children. J. Urol. 97:693-695 (Apr.) 1967.

Jewett, H. J.: Upper Urinary Tract Obstructions in Infants and Children: Diagnosis and Treatment. Pediat. Clin. North America 737-754 (Aug.) 1955.

Johnston, J. H.: Vesico-ureteric Reflux: Its Anatomical Mechanism, Causation, Effects and Treatment in the Child. Ann. Roy. Coll. Surgeons England 30:324-341 (May) 1962.

Jorup, S., and Kjellberg, S. R.: Congenital Valvular Formations in the Urethra. Acta Radiol. 30:197-208, 1948.

Karlin, I. W.: Incidence of Spina Bifida Occulta in Children With and Without Enuresis. Am. J. Dis. Child. 49:125-134 (Jan.) 1935.

Kaufman, J. J.: Unusual Causes of Extrinsic Ureteral Obstruction. J. Urol. 87:319-337 (Mar.) 1962.

Keitzer, W., and Allen, J.: Transurethral Incisions for Recurring Chronic Cystitis. (Unpublished data.)

Keitzer, W. A., and Benavent, C.: Bladder Neck Obstruction in Children. J. Urol. 89:384-388 (Mar.) 1963.

Keitzer, W. A., Cervantes, L., Demaculongan, A., and Cruz, B.: Transurethral Incision of Bladder Neck for Contracture. J. Urol. 86:242-246 (Aug.) 1961.

Keitzer, W. A., and Huffman, G. C.: The Voiding

Audiograph: A New Voiding Test. J. Urol. 96:404-410 (Sept.) 1966.

Kelalis, P. P.: Personal communication to the authors, 1969.

Kendall, A. R., and Karafin, L.: Intermittent Hydronephrosis: Hydration Pyelography. J. Urol. 98:653-656 (Dec.) 1967.

Kerr, H. D., and Gillies, C. L.: The Urinary Tract: A Handbook of Roentgen Diagnosis. Chicago, Year Book Publishers, Inc. 1944, 320 pp.

Kerr, W. S., Jr., Leadbetter, G. W., Jr., and Donahue, J.: An Evaluation of Internal Urethrotomy in Female Patients With Urethral or Bladder Neck Obstruction. J. Urol. 95:218-221 (Feb.) 1966.

King, L. R., Surian, M. A., Wendel, R. M., and Burden, J. J.: Vesicoureteral Reflux: A Classification Based on Cause and the Results of Treatment. J.A.M.A. 203:169-174 (Jan. 15) 1968.

Kjellberg, S. R., Ericsson, N. D., and Rudhe, U.: The Lower Urinary Tract in Childhood: Some Correlated Clinical and Roentgenologic Observations. [Tr. by Erica Odelberg.] Almqvist, Year Book Publishers, Inc., 1957, 298 pp.

Koontz, W. W., Jr., and Prout, G. R., Jr.: Agenesis of the Sacrum and the Neurogenic Bladder. J.A.M.A. 203:481-486 (Feb. 12) 1968.

Langworthy, O. R., Kolb, L. C., and Lewis, L. G.: Physiology of Micturition: Experimental and Clinical Studies With Suggestions as to Diagnosis and Treatment. Baltimore, The Williams & Wilkins Co., 1940, 232 pp.

Lapides, J., Anderson, E. C., and Petrone, A. F.: Urinary-Tract Infection in Children. J.A.M.A. 195:248-253 (Jan. 24) 1966.

Lapides, J., and Stone, T. E.: Usefulness of Retrograde Urethrography in Diagnosing Strictures of the Anterior Urethra. J. Urol. 100:747-750 (Dec.) 1968.

Lattimer, J. K.: Conservative Management of Neurogenic Bladder, Including Re-exploration of the Spinal Cord. Tr. Am. A. Genito-Urin. Surgeons 49:203, 1957.

Lattimer, J. K., Dean, A. L., Jr., and Furey, C. A.: The Triple Voiding Technique in Children With Dilated Urinary Tracts. J. Urol. 76:656-660 (Nov.) 1956.

Leadbetter, G. W., Jr., and Leadbetter, W. F.: Urethral Strictures in Male Children. J. Urol. 87:409-415 (Mar.) 1962.

Leuzinger, D. E., Lattimer, J. K., and McCoy, C. B.: Reflux Is Dangerous but Not Always Disastrous: Conservative Treatment Often Effective. J. Urol. 82:294-303 (Sept.) 1959.

LeVine, M., Allen, A., Stein, J. L., and Schwartz, S.: The Crescent Sign. Radiology 81:971-973 (Dec.) 1963.

Lich, R., Jr., Howerton, L. W., and Davis, L. A.: Vesicourethrography. Tr. Am. A. Genito-Urin. Surgeons 52:43-44, 1960.

Lich, R., Jr., Howerton, L. W., and Davis, L. A.: Vesicourethrography. J. Urol. 85:396-397 (Mar.) 1961a.

Lich, R., Jr., Howerton, L. W., and Davis, L. A.: Recurrent Urosepsis in Children. J. Urol. 86:554-558 (Nov.) 1961b.

Love, J. G., and Emmett, J. L.: "Asymptomatic" Protruded Lumbar Disk as a Cause of Urinary Retention: Preliminary Report. Mayo Clin. Proc. 42:249-257 (May) 1967.

Lowsley, O. S., and Kerwin, T. J.: Clinical Urology. Ed. 3, Baltimore, Williams & Wilkins Company, 1956, vol. 1.

Lyon, R. P., and Smith, D. R.: Distal Urethral Stenosis. J. Urol. 89:414-421 (Mar.) 1963.

Lyon, R. P., and Tanagho, E. A.: Distal Urethral Stenosis in Little Girls. J. Urol. 93:379-388 (Mar.) 1965.

MacCarty, C. S.: The Treatment of Spastic Paraplegia by Selective Spinal Cordectomy. J. Neurosurg. 11:539-545 (Nov.) 1954.

Mandler, J. I., and Pool, T. L.: Primary Diverticulum of the Male Urethra. J. Urol. 96:336-338 (Sept.) 1966.

Markland, C., Koos, G., and Creevy, C. D.: Evaluation and Treatment of Recurrent Urinary Infection in Girls. Univ. Minnesota M. Bull. 36:373-375 (June) 1965.

Mathisen, W.: Vesicoureteral Reflux and Its Surgical Correction. Surg., Gynec. & Obst. 118:965-971 (May) 1964.

McGovern, J. H., and Marshall, V. F.: Reimplantation of Ureters Into the Bladders of Children. Tr. Am. A. Genito-Urin. Surgeons 59:116-118, 1967.

McGovern, J. H., Marshall, V. F., and Paquin, A. J., Jr.: Vesicoureteral Regurgitation in Children. J. Urol. 83:122-149 (Feb.) 1960.

McLean, P., and Emmett, J. L.: Internal Urethrotomy in Women for Recurrent Infection and Chronic Urethritis. J. Urol. 101:724-728 (May) 1969.

McLellan, F. C.: The Neurogenic Bladder. Springfield, Illinois, Charles C Thomas, 1939, 206 pp.

Meadows, J. A., Jr., and Quattlebaum, R. B.: Polyps of the Posterior Urethra in Children. J. Urol. 100:317-320 (Sept.) 1968.

Mitchell, G. F., Makhuli, Z., and Frittelli, G.: Congenital Urethral Valve in a Female. Radiology 89:690-693 (Oct.) 1967.

Mogg, R. A.: The Treatment of Urinary Incontinence Using the Colonic Conduit. J. Urol. 97:684-692 (Apr.) 1967.

Moore, T.: Hydrocalicosis. Brit. J. Urol. 22:304-317, 1950.

Moore, T., and Hira, N. R.: The Role of the Female Urethra in Infections of the Urinary Tract. Brit. J. Urol. 37:25-33 (Feb.) 1965.

Motzkin, D.: The Clinical Significance of Visually Determined Vesicoureteral Reflux. J. Urol. 95:711-712 (May) 1966.

Murnaghan, G. F.: The Dynamics of the Renal Pelvis and Ureter With Reference to Congenital Hydronephrosis. Brit. J. Urol. 30:321-329, 1958.

Nesbit, R. M.: Diagnosis of Intermittent Hydronephrosis: Importance of Pyelography During Episodes of Pain. J. Urol. 75:767-771 (May) 1956.

Nesbit, R. M.: The Genesis of Benign Polyps in the Prostatic Urethra. J. Urol. 87:416-418 (Mar.) 1962.

Nesbit, R. M., and Labardini, M. M.: Urethral Valves in the Male Child. J. Urol. 96:218-228 (Aug.) 1966.

Nesbit, R. M., McDonald, H. P., Jr., and Busby, S.:

Obstructing Valves in the Female Urethra. J. Urol. 91:79-83 (Jan.) 1964.

Ney, C., and Duff, J.: Cysto-urethrography: Its Role in Diagnosis of Neurogenic Bladder. J. Urol. 63:640-652 (Apr.) 1950.

Paquin, A. J., Jr.: Ureterovesical Anastomosis: The Description and Evaluation of a Technique. J. Urol. 82:573-583 (Nov.) 1959.

Paquin, A. J., Jr., Marshall, V. F., and McGovern, J. H.: The Megacystis Syndrome. J. Urol. 83:634-646 (May) 1960.

Pasquier, C. M., Jr., St. Martin, E. C., and Campbell, J. H.: The Problem of Vesicoureteral Reflux in Children. Tr. Southeast. Sect., Am. Urol. A., 1957, pp. 77-87.

Pellman, C.: The Neurogenic Bladder in Children With Congenital Malformations of the Spine: A Study of 61 Patients. J. Urol. 93:472-475 (Apr.) 1965.

Peters, P. C., Johnson, D. E., and Jackson, J. H., Jr.: The Incidence of Vesicoureteral Reflux in the Premature Child. J. Urol. 97:259-260 (Feb.) 1967.

Politano, V. A.: One Hundred Reimplantations and Five Years. J. Urol. 90:696-699 (Dec.) 1963.

Politano, V. A., and Leadbetter, W. F.: An Operative Technique for the Correction of Vesicoureteral Reflux. J. Urol. 79:932-941 (June) 1958.

Prather, G. C.: Calyceal Diverticulum. J. Urol. 45:55-64 (Jan.) 1941.

Raper, F. P.: The Recognition and Treatment of Congenital Urethral Valves. Brit. J. Urol. 25:136-141, 1953.

Richardson, F. H.: Lysis or Excision of the Urethrovaginal Septum. (Unpublished data.)

Richardson, F. H.: External Urethroplasty in Women: Technique and Clinical Evaluation. J. Urol. 101:719-723 (May) 1969.

Robinson, H. P., and Greene, L. F.: Postoperative Contracture of the Vesical Neck. I. Review of Cases and Proposed Theory of Etiology. J. Urol. 87:601-609 (Apr.) 1962a.

Robinson, H. P., and Greene, L. F.: Postoperative Contracture of the Vesical Neck. II. Experimental Production of Contractures in Dogs: Transurethral Series. J. Urol. 87:610-616 (Apr.) 1962b.

Ross, J. C., and Damanski, M.: Pudendal Neurectomy in the Treatment of the Bladder in Spinal Injury. Brit. J. Urol. 25:45-50, 1953.

Ross, J. C., Damanski, M., and Gibbon, N.: Resection of the External Ureteral Sphincter in the Paraplegic—Preliminary Report. J. Urol. 79:742-746 (Apr.) 1958.

Ross, J. C., Gibbon, N. O. K., and Damanski, M.: Division of the External Urethral Sphincter in the Treatment of the Neurogenic Bladder: A Preliminary Report on a New Procedure. Brit. J. Urol. 30:204-212, 1958.

Russell, H. E., and Aitken, G. T.: Congenital Absence of the Sacrum and Lumbar Vertebrae With Prostatic Management: A Survey of the Literature and Presentation of Five Cases. J. Bone & Joint Surg. 45A:501-508 (Apr.) 1963.

Sampson, J. A.: Ascending Renal Infection: With Special Reference to the Reflux of Urine From the Bladder Into the Ureters as an Etiological Factor in Its Causation and Maintenance. Bull. Johns Hopkins Hosp. 14:334-350 (Dec.) 1903.

Schoenberg, H. W., Tristan, T. A., and Murphy, J. J.: The Effect of Urethral Meatotomy in Girls With Bladder Neck Dysfunction. J. Urol. 96:921-923 (Dec.) 1966.

Scott, J. E. S.: Results of Operations for Ureteric Reflux. Arch. Dis. Childhood 41:165-167 (Apr.) 1966.

Scott, W. F., Collins, T. A., and Singer, P. L.: Papilloma of Urethra in Infant. J.M.A. Alabama 7:370-371 (Apr.) 1938.

Shelden, C. H., and Bors, E.: Subarachnoid Alcohol Block in Paraplegia: Its Beneficial Effect on Mass Reflexes and Bladder Dysfunction. J. Neurosurg. 5:385-391 (July) 1948.

Shopfner, C. E.: Changing Concepts of Pediatric Uroradiology. Journal-Lancet 85:525-531 (Nov.) 1965.

Shopfner, C. E.: Ureteropelvic Junction Obstruction. Am. J. Roentgenol. 98:148-159 (Sept.) 1966a.

Shopfner, C. E.: Nonobstructive Hydronephrosis and Hydroureter. Am. J. Roentgenol. 98:172-180 (Sept.) 1966b.

Shopfner, C. E.: Roentgen Evaluation of Distal Urethral Obstruction. Radiology 88:222-231 (Feb.) 1967a.

Shopfner, C. E.: Analysis of Hydronephrosis. Postgrad. Seminar, unit 6, pp. 1-6 (Mar.) 1967b.

Shopfner, C. E.: Roentgenological Evaluation of Bladder Neck Obstruction. Am. J. Roentgenol. 100:162-176 (May) 1967c.

Shopfner, C. E., and Hutch, J. A.: The Trigonal Canal. Radiology 88:209-221 (Feb.) 1967.

Siegelman, S. S., and Bosniak, M. A.: Renal Arteriography in Hydronephrosis. Radiology 85:609-616 (Oct.) 1965.

Smith, J. C.: Some Theoretical Aspects of Urethral Resistance. Invest. Urol. 1:477-481 (Mar.) 1964.

Smith, J. C., Edwards, D., and Bryant, G. H.: A Practical Method of Measuring Urethral Resistance to Micturition. Brit. J. Urol. 38:542-546 (Oct.) 1966.

Spence, H. M., Steward, C. M., Marshall, V. F., Leadbetter, W. F., and Hutch, J. A.: Panel on Ureteral Reflux in Children. J. Urol. 85:119-144 (Feb.) 1961.

Stephens, F. D.: Urethral Obstruction in Childhood: The Use of Urethrography in Diagnosis. Australian & New Zealand J. Surg. 25:89-109 (Nov.) 1955.

Stevens, W. E.: Urology in Women. J.A.M.A. 81:1917-1924 (Dec. 8) 1923.

Stevens, W. E.: Congenital Obstructions of the Female Urethra. J.A.M.A. 106:89-92 (Jan. 11) 1936.

Stewart, C. M.: Delayed Cystograms. J. Urol. 70:588-593 (Oct.) 1953.

Stewart, C. M.: Cystography and Voiding Cystoureterography. J. Urol. 74:749-759 (Dec.) 1955.

Stewart, C. M.: Congenital Bladder Neck Obstruction: Diagnosis by Delayed and Voiding Cystography and Surgical Removal by Use of a New Cold, Crush-Cutting Punch. J. Urol. 83:679-681 (May) 1960.

Swenson, O., MacMahon, H. E., Jaques, W. E., and Campbell, J. S.: A New Concpet of Etiology of Megaloureters. New England J. Med. 246:41-46 (Jan. 10) 1952.

Tanagho, E. A., and Hutch, J. A.: Primary Reflux. J. Urol. 93:158-164 (Feb.) 1965.

Tanagho, E. A., Hutch, J. A., Meyers, F. H., and Rambo, O. N., Jr.: Primary Vesicoureteral Reflux: Experimental Studies of Its Etiology. J. Urol. 93:165-176 (Feb.) 1965.

Tanagho, E. A., and Pugh, R. C. B.: The Anatomy and Function of the Ureterovesical Junction. Brit. J. Urol. 35:151-165, 1963.

Thompson, G. J.: Cord Bladder: Restoration of Function by Transurethral Operation. U.S. Nav. M. Bull. 45:207-214 (Aug.) 1945.

Thornbury, J. R., and Immergut, M. A.: Polyview Voiding Cystourethrography in Children. Am. J. Roentgenol. 95:475-478 (Oct.) 1965.

Vermooten, V.: Congenital Cystic Dilatation of the Renal Collecting Tubules. Yale J. Biol. & Med. 23:450-453 (June) 1951.

Vermooten, V., and Schweinsberg, M.: Radiographic Estimation of the Size of the Prostate. Radiology 182:1010-1015 (June) 1964.

Warren, J. W., Jr.: Congenital Diverticulum of the Urethra. Am. Surgeon 21:385-387, 1955.

Waterhouse, K.: Voiding Cystourethrography: A Simple Technique. J. Urol. 85:103-104 (Jan.) 1961.

Waterhouse, K., and Scordamaglia, L. J.: Anterior Urethral Valve: A Rare Cause of Bilateral Hydronephrosis. J. Urol. 87:556-559 (Apr.) 1962.

Watkins, K. H.: The Clinical Value of Bladder Pressure Estimations. Brit. J. Urol. 6:104-118, 1934.

Watkins, K. H.: Cysts of the Kidney Due to Hydrocalycosis. Brit. J. Urol. 11:207-215, 1939.

Wesson, M. B., and Fulmer, C. C.: Influence of Ureteral Stones on Intravenous Urograms. Am. J. Roentgenol. 28:27-33 (July) 1932.

Widén, T.: Renal Angiography During and After Unilateral Ureteric Occlusion: A Long-Term Experimental Study in Dogs. Acta radiol., suppl. 162, 1958, pp. 1-103.

Williams, D. I.: The Chronically Dilated Ureter: Hunterian Lecture. Ann. Roy. Coll. Surgeons England 14:107-123 (Feb.) 1954a.

Williams, D. I.: The Radiological Diagnosis of Lower Urinary Obstruction in the Early Years. Brit. J. Radiol. 27:473-481 (Sept.) 1954b.

Williams, D. I.: Urology in Childhood. In Encyclopedia of Urology. XV. Berlin, Springer-Verlag, 1958, pp. 127-137.

Williams, D. I.: Megacystis and Mega-ureter in Children. Bull. New York Acad. Med. 35:317-327 (May) 1959.

Williams, D. I.: Rhabdomyosarcoma of the Genitourinary Tract. Proc. Roy. Soc. Med. 59:413-414 (May) 1966.

Williams, D. I., and Abbassian, A.: Solitary Pedunculated Polyp of the Posterior Urethra in Children. J. Urol. 96:483-486 (Oct.) 1966.

Williams, D. I., and Eckstein, H. B.: Obstructive Valves in the Posterior Urethra. J. Urol. 93:236-246 (Feb.) 1965a.

Williams, D. I., and Eckstein, H. B.: Surgical Treatment of Reflux in Children. Brit. J. Urol. 37:13-24 (Feb.) 1965b.

Williams, D. I., and Mininberg, D. T.: Hydrocalycosis: Report of Three Cases in Children. Brit. J. Urol. 40:541-545 (Oct.) 1968.

Williams, D. I., and Nixon, H. H.: Agenesis of the Sacrum. Surg., Gynec. & Obst. 105:84-88 (July) 1957.

Williams, D. I., Scott, J., and Turner-Warwick, R. T.: Reflux and Recurrent Infection. Brit. J. Urol. 33:435-441 (Dec.) 1961.

Williams, D. I., and Sturdy, D. E.: Recurrent Urinary Infection in Girls. Arch. Dis. Child. 36:130-136 (Apr.) 1961.

Witherington, R.: Experimental Study on Role of Intravesical Ureter in Vesicoureteral Regurgitation. J. Urol. 89:176-179 (Feb.) 1963.

Young, H. H., Frontz, W. A., and Baldwin, J. C.: Congenital Obstruction of the Posterior Urethra. J. Urol. 3:289-354, 1919.

Vascular Obstruction of Superior Infundibulum of the Upper Calyx

Baum, S., and Gillenwater, J. Y.: Renal Artery Impressions on the Renal Pelvis. J. Urol. 95:139-145 (Feb.) 1966.

Doppman, J. L., and Fraley, E. E.: Arteriography in the Syndrome of Superior Infundibular Obstruction: A Simplified Technic for Identifying the Obstructing Vessel. Radiology 99:1039-1041 (Nov.) 1968.

Fraley, E. E.: Vascular Obstruction of Superior Infundibulum Causing Nephralgia: A New Syndrome. New England J. Med. 275:1403-1409 (Dec. 22) 1966.

Fraley, E. E.: Surgical Correction of Intrarenal Disease. I. Obstructions of the Superior Infundibulum. J. Urol. 98:54-64 (July) 1967.

Kreel, L., and Pyle, R.: Arterial Impressions on the Renal Pelvis. Brit. J. Radiol. 35:609-613 (Sept.) 1962.

Nebesar, R. A., Pollard, J. J., and Fraley, E. E.: Renal Vascular Impressions: Incidence and Clinical Significance. Am. J. Roentgenol. 101:719-727 (Nov.) 1967.

Tille, D.: Nicht pathologische Füllungsdefekte des Nierenbeckens und der Nierenkelche. Deutsche med. Wchnschr. 85:1414-1415 (Aug.) 1960.

INDEX

Boldface numbers indicate pages on which illustrations appear.
Italic numbers indicate pages on which tables appear.

Cyst(s) (*Continued*)
  renal, 931–1042. See also *Cystic disease* and *Polycystic disease.*
    calcification in, **204**
    classification of, 931
    congenital, 981–1021. See also *Cystic disease, renal, congenital.*
    echinococcus, 1022–1024, **1024–1032**
    in duplex kidney, **1441**
    in renal duplication, 1453, **1467, 1468**
    management of, 970
    multilocular, 1007, **1009**
    multiple, 934, **949–953**
    nephrogenic polycythemia and, 933
    pyelogenic, stones in, 648
    renal angiography in, 133, **134**
    renal tuberculosis and, 896, **900**
    renovascular hypertension and, 1632–1633
    simple, 931–976
      histopathogenesis of, 932
      tumor incidence with, 932, **935**
      urographic diagnosis of, 933–935, **936–956**
      vs. renal tumor, 934, **954–956,** 1087, **1090–1114**
        arteriography in, 957, **967–969**
        nephrotomography in, 957, **958–966**
        percutaneous renal cystography in, 970, **971–976**
    retroperitoneal, 1190, **1200–1203**
    sebaceous, of scrotum, **1938**
    splenic, vs. retroperitoneal tumor, **1209**
    urachal, 1330, **1335,** 1532, **1537**
Cystadenocarcinoma, papillary mucous, confusing shadows from, 189, **193, 194**
Cystadenoma
  of renal cortex, 1049–1050, **1053, 1056**
  ovarian, ureteral obstruction from, 1974, **1978**
  pancreatic, **1204**
  retroperitoneal, **1200**
Cystic adenoma, 820–821, **823, 824**
Cystic disease. See also *Polycystic disease.*
  of renal pyramids, 1013–1014, **1015–1021**
  renal, congenital, 981–1021
    classification and pathogenesis of, 981–982
    with lower urinary tract obstruction, 989
Cystic dysplasia, familial bilateral, 983, **986, 987**
Cystic lymphangioma, **1203**
Cystic necrotic adenoma of adrenal gland, 1235, **1246**
Cystine calculi, 608, **611**
Cystitis, 818–821, **822–824**
  amicrobic, 818, **822**
  eosinophilic, 819, **823**
  interstitial, 818–819
  panmural, 818–819
  tuberculous, 818
Cystitis cystica, 819–820
Cystitis emphysematosa, 787, 788, **795–797**
Cystitis glandularis, 820–821, **823, 824**
Cystitis granuloma, 820–821, **823, 824**
Cystocele, 1962, **1962–1964**
  stress incontinence with, **1970**
Cystogram, 58–63
  definition of, 7
  distortion of, by uterus, 350, **352, 353**
  errors in interpretation of, 351, **356, 357**

Cystography, 58–63
  air, 60
  delayed, 61
    for demonstration of urinary retention in children, 62
  excretory, 350–357
    definition of, 58
    in papillary vesical tumors, 1258, **1260–1262**
    in ureteral reflux, 461, **468–470**
  percutaneous renal, in renal cyst vs. renal tumor, 970, **971–976**
  retrograde, 350–357
    definition of, 58
    in vesical and ureteral hernias, 1860, **1861–1863**
    technique of, 59–60
  superimposition, 60
  triple-voiding, 62
Cystorectostomy, 1786, **1790**
Cystoscopy
  excretory urography prior to, 40
  in diagnosis of congenital vesical neck obstruction, 510
  in ectopic ureteral orifice, 1485
  urethroscopy and, in urethral diverticulum in female, 1955
Cystostomy, suprapubic, 1785–1786, **1788**
Cystourethrography, 63–71, 358–366
  chain, in stress incontinence, 1966, **1969–1971**
  evacuation, 63
    contrast media for, 65
    techniques of, 68–70
  expression, 63
    technique of Williams, 69, **70**
  in adult male, 358, **360–363**
  in female, 360, **366**
  in male infants and children, 359, **363–365**
  in urethral stricture, 585
  micturition, 63
    definition of, 59
  retrograde, contrast media for, 64–65
    definition of, 59
    technique of, 65–68
      Flock's, 63, 67
      in female, 66, **67**
      in male, 65, **69**
  voiding, 63, 70–71
    in congenital anterior urethral valves, 528, **537–539**
    in congenital posterior urethral valves, 527, **529–537**
    in congenital urethral valves in females, 528, **540–542**
    in congenital vesical neck obstruction, 511, **518–523**
    in urethral diverticulum in female, 1955, **1960, 1961**
    technique of, 68, **69**

Davis, intubated ureterotomy technique of, Y-plasty and, for long constriction of ureter, 429
Delayed cystography, 61
  for demonstration of urinary retention in children, 62